UNDERSTANDING
SURGICAL DISEASE

The Miami Manual of Surgery

UNDERSTANDING SURGICAL DISEASE

The Miami Manual of Surgery

Edited by

Mark G. McKenney, M.D.
Associate Professor of Surgery
Division of Trauma Services
Department of Surgery
University of Miami School of Medicine
Miami, Florida

Patrick C. Mangonon, M.D.
Resident in General Surgery
Department of Surgery
University of Miami School of Medicine
Miami, Florida

Joseph A. Moylan, M.D.
Professor and Chairman
Department of Surgery
University of Miami School of Medicine
Miami, Florida

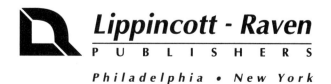

Lippincott - Raven

PUBLISHERS

Philadelphia • New York

Acquisitions Editor: Lisa McAllister
Developmental Editor: Emilie Linkins
Manufacturing Manager: Dennis Teston
Production Manager: Jodi Borgenicht
Production Editor: Christina Zingone
Cover Designer: Jeanette Jacobs
Indexer: Lynne E. Mahan
Compositor: Lippincott–Raven Electronic Production
Printer: Courier Kendallville

Printed in the United States of America

9 8 7 6 5 4 3 2 1

Library of Congress Cataloging-in-Publication Data

Understanding surgical disease : the Miami manual of surgery / edited by Mark G. McKenney, Patrick
C. Mangonon, Joseph A. Moylan.
     p.   cm.
     Includes bibliographical references and index.
     ISBN 0-316-56001-4
     1. Surgery, Operative—Handbooks, manuals, etc. 2. Surgical diseases—Pathophysiology—
Handbooks, manuals, etc.   I. McKenney, Mark G.   II. Mangonon, Patrick C.   III. Moylan, Joseph A.
IV. University of Miami. School of Medicine.
     [DNLM: 1. Surgery, Operative—methods. 2. Surgery, Operative—examination questions.   WO
500 U55 1998]
RD37.U53   1998
671—DC21
DNLM/DLC
for Library of Congress

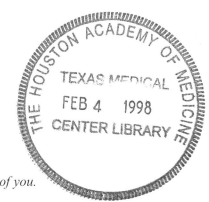
To my wife, Kimberley and our son, Kyle, each day is a joy because of you.

Also, to my parents, Betty and Al, I still look up to you for who you are and what you have done.

Finally, to Joyce, thanks for all the help.

—M.G.McK.

*To my parents, Pat and Aurora—thanks for the lifetime of love that you have given me. I live my life
as you have taught me—with humility, honor, and integrity.*

To my brother, Michael–Godspeed, young man!

To Dr. Joseph Civetta—thanks for guiding me and helping me realize my true potential in surgery.

*To my dear wife, Imelda—thanks for your unconditional love and support that makes me whole
and gives me motivation to succeed. I love you!*

—P.C.M.

*To Nicholas and Madeline and future grandchildren. Tomorrow's medical progress in education
and care is secure because of your potential.*

—J.A.M.

Contents

III. Surgical Specialties

IV. Examination

Contributing Authors

University of Miami School of Medicine
P.O. Box 016960 (D-40)
Miami, Florida 33101

Jose I. Almeida, M.D.
Resident in General Surgery

John H. Armstrong, M.D.
Fellow in Critical Care

Jodeen E. Boggs, M.D.
Assistant Professor of Surgery

Mark Brown, M.D.
Professor and Chairman
Department of Orthopedics

Donald M. Buckner, M.D.
Professor of Pediatric Surgery

Patricia M. Byers, M.D.
Associate Professor of Surgery
Section Chief, Nutritional and Metabolic
  Support Services

Francisco J. Civantos, M.D.
Assistant Professor of Otolaryngology

Joseph M. Civetta, M.D.
Professor of Surgery, Medicine,
  and Anesthesia Pathology
Medical Director, Intensive Care Unit

Stephen M. Cohn, M.D.
Professor of Surgery
Chief, Division of Trauma and Surgical
  Critical Care

Marc Davison, M.D.
Resident in General Surgery

Nestor de la Cruz-Munoz, M.D.
Resident in General Surgery

Jorge de la Pedraja, M.D.
Resident in General Surgery

Utpal S. Desai, M.D.
Resident in General Surgery

James Dygert, M.D.
Resident in General Surgery

Ricardo Estape, M.D.
Fellow in Gynecologic Oncology

Ara J. Feinstein, B.A.
Research Fellow

Enrique Ginzburg, M.D.
Assistant Professor of Surgery

Anthony M. Gonzalez, M.D.
Resident in General Surgery

Barth A. Green, M.D.
Professor and Chairman
Department of Neurological Surgery

Rene Hartmann, M.D.
Associate Professor of Surgery
Chief, Division of Colorectal Surgery

Duane G. Hutson, M.D.
Professor of Surgery
Director, Surgical Residency Program

James J. Jacque, M.D.
Associate Professor of Anesthesia

Orlando C. Kirton, M.D.
Associate Professor of Surgery
Director, Trauma Intensive Care Unit

Tammy Kopelman, M.D.
Fellow in Trauma Surgery

David M. Levi, M.D.
Resident in General Surgery

Joe U. Levi, M.D.
Professor of Surgery

Alan S. Livingstone, M.D.
Professor and Vice-Chairman
Department of Surgery

Cristina Lopez, M.D.
Resident in General Surgery

Marilu Madrigal, M.D.
Fellow in Gynecologic Oncology

Patrick C. Mangonon, M.D.
Resident in General Surgery
Department of Surgery

Larry C. Martin, M.D.
Associate Professor of Surgery

Rodolfo Martinez, M.D.
Resident in General Surgery

Mark G. McKenney, M.D.
Associate Professor of Surgery
Division of Trauma Services
Department of Surgery

Joshua Miller, M.D.
Professor of Surgery
Chief, Division of Transplant Surgery

L. Stacy Mitchell, M.D.
Resident in Orthopedic Surgery

Frederick L. Moffat, Jr., M.D.
Associate Professor of Surgery

Orlando Morejon, M.D.
Resident in General Surgery

Joseph A. Moylan, M.D.
Professor and Chairman
Department of Surgery

Nicholas Namias, M.D.
Fellow in Trauma Surgery

Itzhak Nir, M.D.
Resident in General Surgery

Anselmo Nunez, M.D.
Professor of Surgery
Chief, Division of Vascular Surgery

Claudio Oiticica, M.D.
Associate Professor of Surgery

Eduardo Parra-Davila, M.D.
Resident in General Surgery

Manuel A. Penalver, M.D.
Professor of Obstetrics and Gynecology

Richard A. Perryman, M.D.
Professor and Chief
Division of Cardiac Surgery

Henri T. Pham, M.D.
Resident in Urology

Hector Pombo, M.D.
Resident in General Surgery

David S. Robinson, M.D.
Associate Professor of Surgery

Carl Schulman, M.D.
Resident in General Surgery

David V. Shatz, M.D.
Associate Professor of Surgery

Shishir Sheth, M.D.
Resident in Otolaryngology

Danny Sleeman, M.D.
Associate Professor of Surgery
Director, Surgical Intensive Care Unit

Mark S. Soloway, M.D.
Professor and Chairman
Department of Urology

Magesh Sundaram, M.D.
Fellow in Surgical Oncology

Richard J. Thurer, M.D.
Professor of Surgery
Chief, Division of Thoracic Surgery

Sydney J. Vail, M.D.
Fellow in Critical Care

Willem Van der Werf, M.D.
Resident in General Surgery

Albert J. Varon, M.D.
Professor of Anesthesia
Director, Anesthesia Critical Care

C. Gillon Ward, M.D.
Professor of Surgery
Chief, Division of Burn Surgery

Brian Weider, M.D.
Resident in Neurosurgery

Marla Weissler, M.D.
Resident in General Surgery

Jimmy Windsor, M.D.
Resident in General Surgery

Dyann Yarish, M.D.
Resident in General Surgery

Gregory A. Zych, D.O.
Associate Professor of Surgery
Chief, Orthopediatric Trauma Surgery

Preface

Medical student education is undergoing major changes to assure that current curriculum and content meet the changing needs of the practice of medicine. The multiple factors include managed care, emphasis on a personal physician, and balance of specialists versus generalists. Within the medical school, the need to train more primary care physicians has altered the time allotted to surgical education. The third-year clerkship has been reduced from 12 or 16 weeks to 8 weeks in many institutions.

The goal of this book is to assure an adequate and broad basis of understanding of surgical diagnosis and treatment for medical students whose careers may be in primary care or other nonsurgical specialties, while providing additional information for those students who will pursue training in traditional surgical careers. The emphasis is on practical and frequently treated surgical diseases, which will allow future physicians the understanding of surgery's role in a team approach to diagnosis and therapy. Finally, this textbook provides the student with topical information to assure sufficient knowledge to perform well on standardized tests such as UMSLE II + III, which are increasingly required for graduation or residency selection.

The editorship of this text combines three levels of surgical experience: a surgical faculty member who has completed his medical school experience and surgical training within the last decade, a chief resident in the surgical training program, and a senior faculty member with multiple years of experience to allow focus on current important topics, involvement in national examinations, and a longitudinal experience that brings all aspects into a solid balance. The contributors of the chapters join the experience of faculty members with surgeons-in-training to reinforce this focus.

Each chapter presents the history of one disease, including its pathophysiology and the tools used for diagnosis to understand the role of surgery and the team approach. The current therapy including surgical alternatives are outlined without overemphasis on the technical aspect of the surgery. Important complications are detailed so that all members of the future health team can appreciate and participate in the management of these issues. Alternatives other than surgical interventions are included since today's multiple approaches to treatment are possible.

This textbook also incorporates chapters of specialty areas of surgery such as neurosurgery, orthopaedics, and urology to familiarize the students with these areas so that during their medical school experience, a broad exposure is provided particularly for those going into a primary care practice.

SECTION I

Basic Science

CHAPTER 1

Neurohumoral Response to Injury

Jimmy Windsor and Orlando C. Kirton

Surgery and trauma can result in substantial tissue damage with significant intravascular, interstitial, and intracellular fluid and electrolyte imbalance that leads to cellular and systemic derangements. To preserve physiologic balance, homeostasis, and maintain adequate oxygen and glucose delivery, a complex yet integrated cascade of neural, immunologic, hematologic, endocrine, paracrine, and autocrine events occurs. The surgical incision or trauma initiates a complex inflammatory response that alters the microcirculation of the traumatized tissue by increasing blood flow to the injury site and promoting increased vascular permeability.

SYSTEMIC METABOLIC RESPONSE

The immediate and long-term temporal events of the physiologic response to injury and stress were described by Sir David Cuthbertson >50 years ago. The systemic response to injury is triggered by stimuli propagated along neuronal pathways that are integrated at the level of the central nervous system. The strongest stimuli for these neuronal pathways are local and systemic hypoxia, acidosis, low systemic perfusion pressure, and direct injury to tissues. The response to injury and surgery is mediated by hormones from the pituitary gland and neurotransmitters from the sympathetic nervous system. The paramount goal of these responses is to optimize the organism's chances for survival by providing the substrates necessary for healing.

"Ebb" Phase

The initiating phase of the response has been termed the "Ebb" phase because of a decrease in the metabolic rate observed for the first 24 to 48 hr following significant trauma and complicated major surgery. This decreased metabolic energy cost is due to a decrease in

blood flow to the splanchnic, renal, and peripheral circulation. Oxygenation and glucose delivery to the vital organs (e.g., brain, heart, lungs, liver) is maintained at the expense of an oxygen debt accumulating from anaerobic metabolism in the remaining tissues until such time that splanchnic circulation is restored.

The first attempt to restore normal circulatory volume is the use of the reserve fluid volumes found in the interstitial and cellular fluid compartments. When peripheral perfusion pressure falls, interstitial fluid is recruited into the circulation. At the same time, systemic perfusion pressure to vital organs is augmented by vasoconstriction induced by release of catecholamines, e.g., norepinephrine. Additionally, increased sympathetic neuronal discharge accelerates the rate of sinus node discharge and conduction rate through all cardiac tissues as well as augmenting atrial and ventricular muscular contractions, resulting in improved cardiac performance, which further increases central blood flow. Sympathetic outflow is further increased by hypoxia and acidosis.

A decrease in circulating blood volume is sensed by baroreceptors (Fig. 1) distributed in the walls of large arteries, e.g., aortic arch and internal carotid arteries, as well as low-pressure areas, e.g., atria and pulmonary arteries. Chemoreceptors located in specialized tissues such as the carotid and aortic bodies are stimulated by systemic hypercarbia, acidosis, and hypoxia. When these receptors are stimulated, the respiratory center and medullary vasomotor centers are triggered resulting in tachypnea and tachycardia, respectively.

The sympathetic nervous system also stimulates secondary target glands, the products of which contribute to systemic perfusion pressure and increase plasma levels of glucose. Increased sympathetic tone upon the adrenal medulla stimulates release of norepinephrine and epinephrine, causing splanchnic and peripheral circulatory vasoconstriction. These substances also increase glycogenolysis and gluconeogenesis in the liver to increase the

3

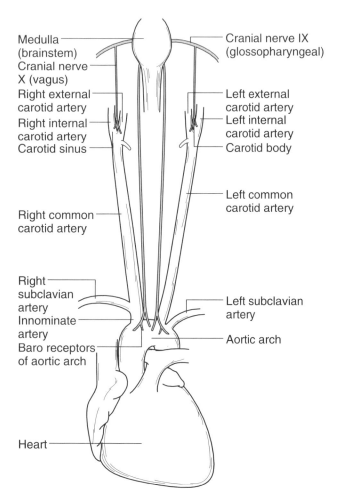

FIG. 1. Baroreceptors of aortic arch and carotid bifurcation (carotid sinus) involved in the ebb phase of neurohumoral response to stress.

levels of circulating glucose. Glucagon stimulates gluco-neogenesis directly and causes the breakdown of glycogen by raising levels of intracellular cAMP, increasing serum glucose levels. This store of glucose, in branched chains of glycogen, though, is exhausted within 24 hr. In order to promote the hyperglycemic state, circulating catecholamine, alpha adrenergic activity, and somatostatin decrease the release of insulin from the beta cells of the pancreas. Glucagon and epinephrine also stimulate lipolysis through the peripheral activation of hormone sensitive lipase, liberating free fatty acids to be transported to the liver by albumin. Direct hepatic stimulation and the increase transport of free fatty acids lead to increased ketone body production (acetoacetone, beta-hydroxy-buterate, and acetone).

The sympathetic nervous system also directly innervates the juxtaglomerular apparatus of the kidney to stimulate renin release. Renin is also released in the presence of decreased renal blood flow to the juxtaglomerular cells

or when there is decreased plasma chloride levels sensed by the macula densa of the distal nephron. Plasma renin converts angiotensinogen to angiotensin I. Angiotensin converting enzyme present in the pulmonary vasculature then catalyzes the conversion of angiotensin I into angiotensin II. Angiotensin II is the most potent circulating vasoconstrictor. It stimulates the release of antidiuretic hormone (ADH) and adrenocorticotrophic hormone (ACTH) from the pituitary, and catecholamine and aldosterone from the adrenal glands. ADH, also known as vasopressin, increases renal tubular fluid reabsorption and is a potent vasoconstrictor of splanchnic and peripheral arterioles. ADH is also stimulated by increases in serum electrolyte concentration and diminished intravascular volume. Aldosterone increases the resorption of sodium by renal nephron distal tubules in exchange for hydrogen ions and potassium.

The endocrinologic response to injury is initiated by the afferent neuronal signals, which are interpreted and integrated at the level of the hypothalamus. In turn, the hypothalamus secretes a range of stimulatory products that mediate the endocrinologic efferent response (Fig. 2). Corticotropin-releasing factor is secreted by the hypothalamus, which stimulates the release of ACTH. The adrenal cortex synthesizes and releases cortisol and corticosterone, as well as aldosterone, when stimulated by ACTH.

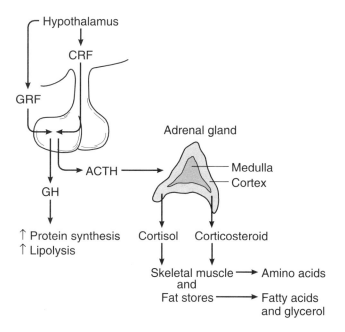

CRF = Corticoptropic releasing factor
GRH = Growth releasing hormone
GH = Growth hormone
ACTH = Adreno corticotropic hormone

FIG. 2. The hypothalamus secretes stimulatory products that mediate the endocrinologic efferent response.

Cortisol initiates the breakdown of skeletal muscle (amino acids) and peripheral fat stores (fatty acids and glycerol) to provide the elements for gluconeogenesis (also stimulated by cortisol). Growth hormone is under the control of the hypothalamus. During stress, growth hormone promotes protein synthesis and inhibits protein catabolism. It enhances the use of fat deposits as a more efficient energy source by stimulating lipolysis. Growth hormone will also increase insulin secretion from the pancreas by promoting a state of glucose intolerance peripherally through postreceptor impairment of insulin action.

"Flow" Phase

If the patient survives the 24- to 48-hr period after the initial stress of injury or extensive surgery and is adequately resuscitated to provide the proper volume that maintains perfusion pressure, a period termed the "flow" phase is entered in which wound healing becomes the prime goal. In the early period of this phase, healing is characterized by weight loss (as much as 80 g/day). The major mediators of this phase are increased levels of insulin and glucagon. Fatty acids liberated by lipolysis from adipose tissue and gluconeogenesis are the principal fuel source during this time period. This is due in part to the fact that glycogen stores are depleted in 24 hr; therefore, the body turns to fat and protein stores as

potential sources of glucose needed to meet the body's anabolic requirements. This release from peripheral fat stores is stimulated by cortisol, glucagon, and catecholamine. The liver metabolizes fatty acids to ketones, acetoacetate, and beta-hydroxybutyrate, which can be readily oxidized by the brain and all other tissues. During states of starvation, these ketone bodies cross the blood-brain barrier and can supply ~50% of the brain's metabolic energy needs.

Recruitment of amino acids as substrates for gluconeogenesis by the liver is also stimulated during the flow phase by catecholamine. Protein catabolism is reflected by the increased excretion of electrolytes, such as potassium, magnesium, and phosphorus in urine, as well as by the increases of urinary creatinine and nitrogen. If the patient is in a state of starvation, though, protein catabolism decreases due to a shutdown of gluconeogenesis. The catabolism of peripheral proteins continues in the face of sepsis or following injury. Therefore, nutritional supplementation becomes a lifesaving maneuver in these patients. The hyperglycemia that is maintained for wound healing during the flow phase is also due to an attenuation of insulin sensitivity by the liver and peripheral muscles. Muscle cells decrease their glucose extraction from the circulation, and hepatocytes increase their output of glucose. The lactate and pyruvate produced is recycled by the process of gluconeogenesis by the liver, known as the Cori cycle (Fig. 3). The flow phase is fol-

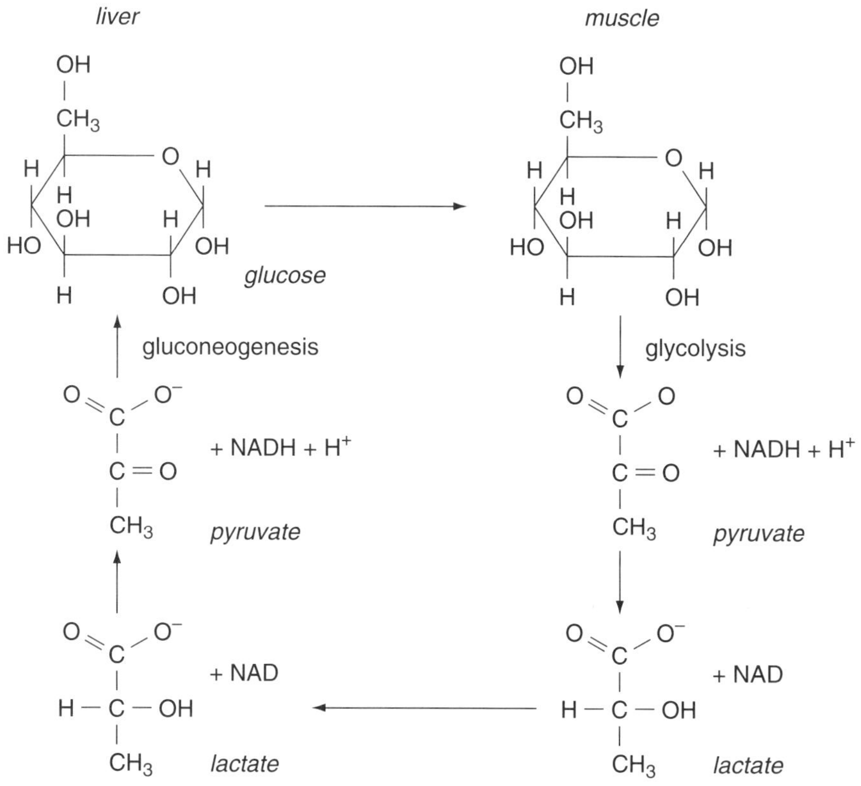

FIG. 3. CORI cycle.

lowed by the phases of anabolism and recovery, which are characterized by nitrogen retention as evidenced by decreased urinary nitrogen loss, positive nitrogen balance, and absence of the systemic inflammatory response syndrome (SIRS).

SYSTEMIC INFLAMMATORY RESPONSE

The interleukins, particularly IL-1, IL-6, and TNF, are primarily secretory products of monocytes and macrophages, and play a vital role in the mobilization of resources to respond to surgical stress. These cytokines are also synthesized by a whole host of cell populations, such as fibroblasts, neutrophils, B cells, skin keratinocytes, mesangial cells, endothelial cells, and glial cells. Excessive action of these immunologic mediators contributes to protein wasting from skeletal muscle and exhaustion of body nitrogen stores, and has been linked in increased metabolism. This is because the endogenous levels of these cytokines are directly proportional to the degree of systemic illlnesses, such as severe gram-negative sepsis. The interplay of these three immunologic mediators can cause decreased food consumption, increased gluconeogenesis, glucose oxidation, and synthesis of free fatty acids by hepatocytes. This increased rate leads to increases of the basal (resting) energy expenditure and oxygen consumption.

IL-1 production is stimulated predominantly by endotoxin, but other stimuli include exotoxin production by staphylococcus and streptococcus, viruses, complement components, bile salts, thrombin, and androgens. The increased levels of IL-1 cause hepatic synthesis of specific proteins, such as fibrinogen, complement components, and clotting factors. Fatty acid synthesis is also stimulated, as previously mentioned. Messenger RNA coding by hepatocytes for albumin, and transferrin and liproprotein lipase is decreased in the face of increased IL-1 levels. Insulin production is affected by IL-1 in a dose-dependent manner, with low concentrations stimulating mRNA production of pre-proinsulin and high concentrations suppressing insulin production. IL-1 works synergistically with IL-6 to induce steroid synthesis by induction of ACTH release during stress. An important metabolic effect shared by both IL-1 and TNF is the induction of fever by their direct ability to stimulate hypothalamic PGE_2 synthesis. Systemic IL-1 also increases pituitary secretion of CRF, ACTH, vasopressin, and somatostatin. Tumor necrosis factor (alpha), also known as cachectin, is released in considerable amounts in response to a wide variety of stimuli and is a mediator of protein depletion by increasing the rate of skeletal muscle and hepatic proteolysis. Tumor necrosis factor directly mediates catabolism of lipid stores found in adipocytes and stimulates hepatic lipogenesis. This combined effect on fatty acid metabolism of increased hepatic

production and decreased peripheral fat clearance from blood by adipocytes is responsible for the increased levels of triglycerides in plasma during stress.

IL-6 production appears to be under the control of IL-1 and TNF. Like IL-1 and TNF, IL-6 is also an endogenous pyrogen and contributes to the acute phase response. It has been speculated that, since IL-6 production can be induced by IL-1 and TNF, it may serve as a mediator of IL-1 and TNF, impinging in the hypothalamic-pituitary axis, increasing the levels of cortisol through an increase of ACTH levels.

IMMUNOLOGIC REACTION

The immunologic reaction describes activation of the complement pathway of functionally linked proteins that participate in humoral immunity and inflammation. Products of the cascade stimulate a cellular response and enhance the activity of the cells that are recruited to the injured site. Activators of the complement system impart specificity to the complement cascade, allowing only damage to foreign antigens. The binding of C1 to at least two of the Fc portions of the immunoglobulin classes IgM and IgG causes the activation of the classical pathway (Fig. 4). Activation of the alternative pathway (Fig. 5) is initiated directly on the surface of foreign antigens. The activated complement system produces proteolytic products that are chemotactic, attracting inflammatory cells to the site of complement activation. Other proteolytic products, called anaphylatoxins (C3a, C4a, C5a), stimulate leukocytes, such as granulocytes and mast cells, to release chemical mediators that cause local venous constriction, increased permeability of capillaries (C3a), and recruitment of effector cells (neutrophils and monocytes, C5a).

The complement pathways serve to opsonize foreign particles and destroy bacteria by lysis through the creation of pores in the cell membranes. The binding of complement products also serves to limit the tissue damage caused by circulating immune complexes. The anaphylatoxin, when bound to mast cells and basophils, causes degranulation with the concomitant release of histamine, which increases vascular permeability and stimulates visceral smooth muscle contraction. The anaphylatoxins, especially C5a, also directly bind and stimulate smooth muscle contraction, causing increased vascular permeability by affecting endothelial cells. C5a also has chemoattractant effects on neutrophils and can increase oxidative metabolism and degranulation. C5a is an essential chemical recruiter to the area of inflammation.

The last phase of the acute inflammatory response is mediated by recruited circulating effector cells. The binding of C5a to neutrophils is an important first step to cellular activation. The binding of this anaphylatoxin causes increased nondirected movement, increased adherence

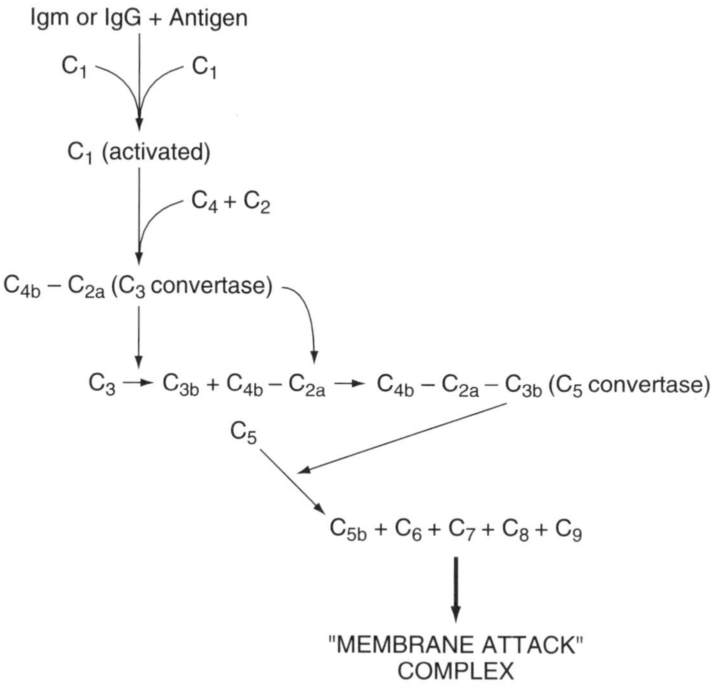

Igm or IgG + Antigen

C_1 ⟍ ⟋ C_1

C_1 (activated)

⟋ $C_4 + C_2$

$C_{4b} - C_{2a}$ (C_3 convertase) ⟍

$C_3 \rightarrow C_{3b} + C_{4b} - C_{2a} \rightarrow C_{4b} - C_{2a} - C_{3b}$ (C_5 convertase)

C_5

$C_{5b} + C_6 + C_7 + C_8 + C_9$

"MEMBRANE ATTACK"
COMPLEX

FIG. 4. Classic pathway of complement activation.

and aggregation of neutrophils, and exocytosis of neutrophils granules (which includes expression of the aforementioned receptors). Microorganisms must first be coated by particles, such as C3b or immunoglobulin, that will be recognized by neutrophils. The exocytosis of receptors for these coating agents begins the process of

phagocytosis, which is initialized by the binding of enough receptors to the opsonizing particles (IgG and C3b). The neutrophil is able to surround the antigen with a plasma membrane and then combine the internalized particle with a primary granule. Prior exposure to C5a causes an increase in the number and clustering of recep-

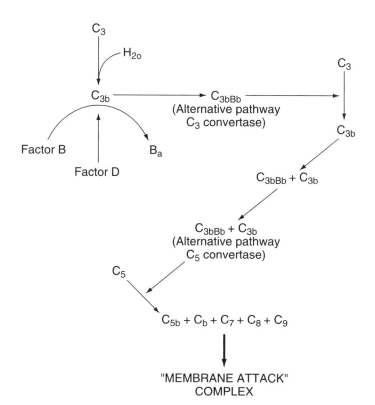

C_3

⟍ H_{2o}

C_3

C_{3b} → C_{3bBb} (Alternative pathway C_3 convertase) →

C_{3b}

Factor B B_a

Factor D

$C_{3bBb} + C_{3b}$

$C_{3bBb} + C_{3b}$ (Alternative pathway C_5 convertase)

C_5

$C_{5b} + C_b + C_7 + C_8 + C_9$

"MEMBRANE ATTACK"
COMPLEX

FIG. 5. Alternative pathway of complement activation.

tors on the neutrophil surface and thereby enhances the rate of phagocytosis. The N-formylated peptides are also potent chemoattractant agents and cause important changes in cellular metabolism, such as changes in cellular pH, cAMP, and concentrations of calcium. The previously released protein mediators that caused the activation of the coagulation pathway produce a fibrin matrix for the cellular effectors of inflammation.

Coagulation System

The local inflammatory response is at first chemically mediated by direct contact of plasma elements with the negatively charged basement membrane of the subendothelium of blood vessels and collagen exposed by damage to the endothelium. This leads to the initiation of the coagulation, fibrinolysis, kinin, and complement pathways, through the interaction of four plasma elements: Hageman factor, prekallikrein, high molecular weight kininogen, and factor XI (HMWK). Normally HMWK is complexed with prekallikrein and factor XI in the circulation. Upon exposure to these activating, negatively charged surfaces, these complexes of HMWK/prekallikrein and HMWK/factor XI bind to the exposed surfaces. Exposure to these sufaces also causes the activation of Hageman factor, whose active form is an activator of prekallikrein and factor XI. Activated Hageman factor is also an activator of the complement pathway through its activation of C1 and participates in the activation of coagulation through the activation of factor VII. Furthermore, activated kallikrein causes in turn the cleaving of HMWK to bradykinin (which can cause increased capillary permeability, vasodilation, and pain). Other substrates of kallikrein include plasminogen to form plasmin, which causes fibrinolysis, and prorenin, which is cleaved to become renin (cleaves angiotensinogen to become angiotensin I). The activation of these protein mediators of inflammation, therefore, alters the local circulatory surroundings by increasing permeability.

SUMMARY

The neurohumoral response to surgery or trauma is a complex interplay of cellular and humoral elements design to maintain homeostasis, combat infection, and enhance the chance of survival of the human organism. Uncontrolled activation and propagation of these pathways have been implicated in the development of the multiple organ system failure syndrome.

STUDY QUESTIONS

1. Describe the "ebb" phase.
2. Describe the "flow" phase.
3. Describe the physiologic compensatory mechanisms for decreased intravascular volume.
4. What are some other attendant physiologic effects of the mechanisms in the previous question?
5. What objective data implys that the patient is in a catabolic state—an anabolic state?

SUGGESTED READING

Abbas AK, Lichtman AH, Pober JS. The complement system. In: *Cellular and molecular immunology.* Philadelphia: Saunders, 1991:259.
Gann DS, Foster AH. Endocrine and metabolic response to injury. In: Schwartz SI, Shires TG, Spencer FC, eds. *Principles of surgery.* 6th ed. New York: McGraw-Hill, 1994:3.
Goldfien A. Adrenal medulla. In: Greenspan FS, ed. *Basic and clinical endocrinology.* Norwalk, CT: Appleton and Lange, 1991:380.
Hunt TK, Mueller RV. Wound healing. In: Way LW, ed. *Current surgical diagnosis and treatment.* East Norwalk, CT: Appleton and Lange, 1994: 80.
Scher AM. Cardiovascular control. In: Patton HD, Fuchs AF, Hille B, Scher AM, Steiner R, eds. *Textbook of physiology.* Philadelphia: Saunders, 1989:972.

CHAPTER 2

Hemostasis and Transfusion Therapy

James Dygert and David V. Shatz

In patients without preexisting bleeding tendencies, intra- or postoperative bleeding usually results from a surgically correctable cause. A working knowledge of the mechanisms of hemostasis, the pathophysiology of hemostatic disorders, the pharmacology of their treatment, and basic concepts behind clinical methods of blood replacement and evaluating hemostasis is a necessity for those managing surgical patients.

MECHANISMS OF HEMOSTASIS

Vascular Endothelium

Vascular endothelium is a dynamic surface. Under normal conditions, it assists in maintaining a clot-free vasculature. Once the endothelial surface is damaged, it both promotes clot formation and helps prevent an inappropriate, uncontrolled, and dangerous disseminated clotting response. It accomplishes this through vasomotor activity and the release of protein products.

Vasoconstriction is mediated by the nervous system and paracrine acting platelet products, such as thromboxane A2 (TXA2) and serotonin. The vasoconstricting and platelet aggregating actions of TXA2 are balanced by the vasodilating and platelet disaggregating actions of prostacyclin (PGI2), also produced and secreted by platelets. Arachidonic acid is the precursor for both TXA2 and PGI2; the balance between the amounts of each produced is governed by many factors. A similar hemostatic balancing act is performed by the vascular endothelium in the production of both anti- and proclotting factors. Anticlotting endothelial products include thrombomodulin, when complexed with thrombin on the activated platelet surface, thrombomodulin accelerates the activation of protein C, a coagulation inhibitor, nearly 20,000 times; endothelial ADPase, which destroys ADP, a platelet activator; heparan sulfate, which is similar to heparin and potentiates thrombin inactivation by antithrombin III

(ATIII); and tissue plasminogen activator (tPA), which triggers the fibrinolytic system which lyses already formed clot. Proclotting endothelial products are coagulation factors V and VIII, von Willebrand's factor (vWF), alpha 2 antiplasmin, and tPA inhibitor.

Arteries, because of thicker muscular coats, display a greater vasoconstrictive response than veins. Even capillaries have contractile properties, mediated not by muscle but through contractile proteins. In partially transected vessels, vasoconstriction may widen defects or keep them open, and perpetuate bleeding. In contrast, completely transected vessels tend to vasoconstrict and retract, and thereby cease further bleeding.

Platelets

When the vessel wall is damaged, the exposure of subendothelial collagen triggers the platelet/vessel wall interaction. The adhesion of platelets to subendothelial collagen is mediated by platelet binding of vWF. The platelet surface receptor for vWF is glycoprotein (gp) Ib.

The externalization of platelet factor three (PF3, a phospholipid) during platelet activation allows the assembly of the prothrombinase and Xase coagulation complexes (see "Coagulation" below) on the platelet membrane surface. These two assemblies greatly accelerate the events of coagulation. Platelet activation initiates the platelet release of arachidonic acid, the precursor to TXA2 and PGI2. Activated platelets degranulate and release their contents in a reaction stimulated by ADP (released from damaged cells), platelet factor 4 (PF4), calcium, magnesium, thrombin, and fibrinogen, and inhibited by cyclic AMP. Platelet ADP, PF4, and calcium are themselves released, forming a positive feedback loop for further platelet activation. Also released are serotonin (which along with ADP mediates platelet adhesion and aggregation) and platelet-derived growth factor.

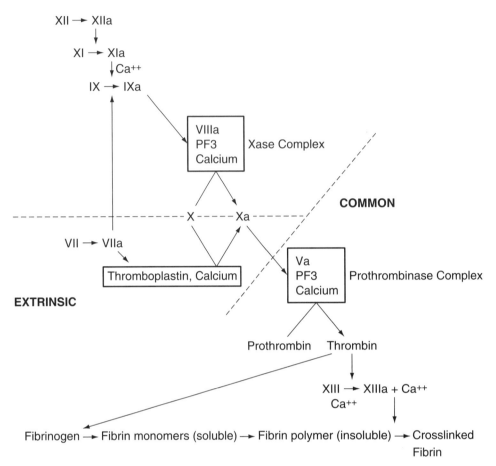

INTRINSIC

XII → XIIa

XI → XIa

↓ Ca++

IX → IXa

VIIIa
PF3
Calcium   Xase Complex

COMMON

X ---- Xa

VII → VIIa

Thromboplastin, Calcium

EXTRINSIC

Va
PF3
Calcium   Prothrombinase Complex

Prothrombin   Thrombin

XIII → XIIIa + Ca++
Ca++

Fibrinogen → Fibrin monomers (soluble) → Fibrin polymer (insoluble) → Crosslinked Fibrin

FIG. 1. Coagulation cascade. Ca++, calcium; PF3, platelet factor 3.

GpIIb:IIIa is the platelet receptor for fibrinogen, vWF, fibronectin, and thrombin. It is hidden on inactive platelets but is present in high density on the surface of activated platelets. Exposure of the gpIIb:IIIa receptor by activated platelets allows platelet aggregation. When bound to gpIIb:IIIa, fibrinogen allows for platelet/platelet interactions and aggregation because of its dimeric nature.

Coagulation

The coagulation cascade (Fig. 1) is a complex set of events that leads to both local and systemic coagulation. Initiated and propagated by coagulation factors (Table 1), both the intrinsic and extrinsic coagulation pathways lead to the common pathway. Here, factor X is activated by joining the Xase complex (a grouping of factor IXa, with "a" following a factor signifying the activated form of that factor; factor VIIIa; ionized calcium; and PF3) on the surface of activated platelets. Subsequently, thrombin is formed from prothrombin in a reaction catalyzed by the

prothrombinase complex (a grouping of the newly activated factor Xa, factor Va, ionized calcium and PF3) on the activated platelet's surface. The prothrombinase complex accomplishes the formation of thrombin 300,000 times faster than by Xa alone. The newly formed thrombin catalyzes the transformation of fibrinogen into fibrin

TABLE 1. *Coagulation factors*

Number	Factor
I	Fibrinogen
II	Prothrombin
III	Thromboplastin (tissue factor)
IV	Calcium
V	Proaccelerin
VI	Same as factor V
VII	Proconvertin
VIII	Antihemophilic factor
IX	Christmas factor
X	Stuart-Prower factor
XI	Plasma thromboplastin antecedent
XII	Hageman factor
XIII	Fibrin stabilizing factor

monomers (soluble), which quickly polymerize (insoluble). These polymers are subsequently cross-linked by the action of factor XIIIa (activated by thrombin and calcium). Thrombin additionally activates factors V and VIII, platelets, and protein C.

The intrinsic pathway is a cascade of enzymatic reactions that leads to the formation of the Xase complex. Factor XII is activated by binding to exposed subendothelial collagen. Factor XIIa in turn activates factor XI, which, when complexed with calcium, activates factor IX. Factor IXa is then able to participate in the Xase complex of the common pathway.

The extrinsic pathway begins with the activation of factor VII by tissue factor, also known as thromboplastin, a phospholipid released from injured cells. The tissue factor/factor IIa complex, along with ionized calcium, activates factor X, thereby beginning the common pathway.

The extrinsic and intrinsic pathways are linked by activated factors crossing over from one pathway to activate a factor of the other pathway. For example, factor VIIa of the extrinsic pathway may activate factor IX of the intrinsic pathway, initiating the steps of the intrinsic pathway and circumventing the classical steps leading to factor IX activation. The coagulation cascade is also associated with inflammatory cytokines. For example, factor XIIa can activate prekallikrein to kallikrein, thereby initiating subsequent steps of the inflammatory process.

There are several proteins that inhibit coagulation. Protein C, protein S, and ATIII are prominent coagulation inhibitors. Also, activated factor IX and kallikrein are inhibited by C1 protease inhibitor, and alpha 1 antitrypsin inhibits activated factor XI.

Fibrinolysis

Coagulation of an injured vessel usually remains a localized process. Reactants in the coagulation process that disperse into the systemic circulation are quickly diluted, leading to a tremendous decrease in activity. Passage through the liver leads to degradation by the reticuloendothelial system, further preventing distant, disseminated coagulation.

To prevent unchecked coagulation, mechanisms must be present to dissolve established clot. This is known as fibrinolysis (Fig. 2). Plasmin, a serine protease, is the main fibrinolytic enzyme in the body and catalyzes the breakdown of fibrin into one fibrin E and two fibrin D fragments (when linked, these form the D dimer). Plasmin has its greatest efficacy against fibrin in newly formed clot, but can also degrade fibrinogen and factors II, V, VIII, IX, and XI. It can also activate factor XII. Fibrin-bound plasminogen, the precursor of plasmin, is more susceptible to activation than free-circulating plasminogen, thus limiting fibrinolysis to the clot site. Plasminogen deficiency leads to thrombotic states.

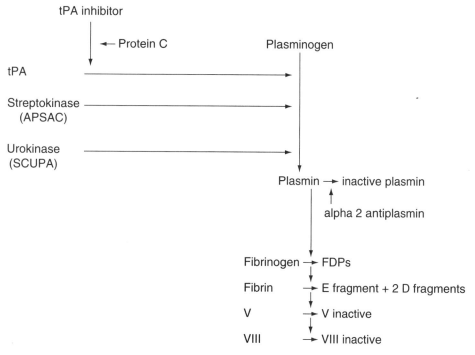

FIG. 2. Fibrinolysis. tPA, tissue plasminogen activator; APSAC, acylated plasminogen/streptokinase activator complex; SCUPA, single chain urokinase-type plasminogen activator; FDP, fibrinogen degradation products.

tPA catalyzes the transformation of plasminogen into plasmin. Its release from endothelial cells is promoted by thrombin. tPA has a catalytic site and a fibrin binding site that are widely separated from one another. This allows tPA, bound to fibrin, to convert plasminogen to plasmin. This molecular property of tPA helps limit its activity away from the clot surface in the systemic vasculature, where it can be harmful.

Fibrinolysis itself is influenced by a number of circulating inhibitors. The secretion of tPA inhibitor by endothelial cells is increased by thrombin, interleukin-1, and endotoxin. Protein C inactivates TPA inhibitor and promotes fibrinolysis. Circulating tumor necrosis factor (TNF) decreases protein C activity and thereby decreases fibrinolysis. These reactions link fibrinolysis and the inflammatory process through tPA inhibitor.

Alpha 2 antiplasmin, secreted by endothelial cells, is a natural inhibitor of plasmin. Alpha 2 antiplasmin, plasminogen, and tPA are all absorbed to the surface of the freshly formed clot. Alpha 2 antiplasmin has its greatest efficacy away from the clot surface in the systemic vasculature where it inhibits plasmin that has dispersed systemically. Deficiency of alpha 2 antiplasmin leads to hemorrhagic states and can be treated by epsilon aminocaproic acid, a competitive inhibitor of tPA.

HEMOSTATIC DISORDERS

Platelets

Thrombocytopenia is defined as a circulating platelet count of <100,000. Bleeding complicating surgical procedures typically occurs with counts of <50,000. Spontaneous bleeding, usually from the gastrointestinal mucosa, does not typically occur until platelet counts are <20,000. Platelet transfusions are rarely necessary when platelet counts are >50,000.

Increased destruction, increased utilization, and decreased production of platelets can cause thrombocytopenia. Increased platelet destruction can be due to a variety of etiologies, including sepsis, drugs (e.g., heparin), acute alcohol intoxication, viruses, and immunologic mechanisms. In idiopathic thrombocytopenic purpura (ITP), destructive autoantibodies are directed at platelets; corticosteroids, plasmapheresis, or splenectomy may improve platelet counts. Very low platelet counts (<10,000) can be tolerated preoperatively in patients with ITP since circulating platelets are all newly formed and have not yet lost functional ability like senescent platelets. Thrombotic thrombocytopenic purpura (TTP) and hemolytic uremic syndrome (HUS) are different expressions of the same disease process. This is a syndrome of diverse etiologies (idiopathic, pregnancy, bacterial toxin, cancer, and drugs) causing diffuse endothelial damage and disseminated platelet thrombi.

The classic pentad of findings includes fever, thrombocytopenia, microangiopathic hemolytic anemia, neurologic abnormalities, and renal dysfunction. Normal coagulation studies differentiate TTP-HUS from disseminated intravascular coagulation (DIC). The cornerstone of treatment is plasma exchange, replacing the patient's plasma with fresh frozen plasma (FFP).

Pooling of platelets in an enlarged spleen causes thrombocytopenia. Normally, the spleen sequesters ~30% of circulating platelets, but up to 90% of platelets may be sequestered in an enlarged spleen. Splenic enlargement and hypersplenism may be due to a variety of etiologies, including portal hypertension, leukemia, lymphoma, sarcoidosis, and Gaucher's disease.

Thrombocytopenia may be caused by decreased platelet production due to bone marrow suppression from cytotoxic chemotherapy or radiation. Bone marrow infiltration in leukemic states and hypoplastic marrow conditions are associated with deficiencies in megakaryocyte function as well as number, leading to decreased functional platelet production. Folate and vitamin B_{12} deficiencies cause pancytopenia and thus thrombocytopenia due to ineffective platelet production.

Dysfunctional platelets may cause bleeding problems even though platelet numbers are normal. Hypothermia produces relative thrombocytopenia by liver and splenic sequestration at <25°C. The use of cardiopulmonary bypass pumps during open cardiac procedures can also cause a bleeding diathesis, not by a quantitative defect in platelets, but by a qualitative defect. Fibrinogen and IgG bind to the bypass circuit, activate platelets, and lead to a hemostatic defect. Synthetic vascular grafts invoke similar changes, but systemic abnormalities are rare.

Uremia causes abnormal hemostasis through defective platelet adhesion and aggregation. The exact mechanism is unknown and is probably multifactorial, but a likely component is a deficiency of circulating high molecular weight forms of vWF. Dialysis, the administration of 1-deamino-8-D-arginine vasopressin (DDAVP), conjugated estrogens, and cryoprecipitate have been found to improve the bleeding time in uremic patients. In uremic patients, anemia secondary to decreased erythropoietin production can potentiate a bleeding diathesis. With hematocrits of <25%, the location of platelets in the flowing bloodstream is altered. Platelets become scattered throughout the stream of blood instead of normally flowing in a peripheral, circumferential layer next to the vascular endothelium. Therefore, platelets are rendered even less functional by redistribution away from the vascular endothelium, the site where clotting events begin.

Thrombocytosis is an elevation of the platelet count above the normal upper limit of 400,000/dl. It is associated with myeloproliferative, malignant, and inflammatory diseases, as well as postsplenectomy states. Thrombocytosis can cause hemostatic defects due to disordered presentation of platelets to the vessel wall, a mechanism similar to that found in anemia, though thrombosis is the more commonly associated complication.

Deficiency of vWF may be inherited in an autosomal dominant or autosomal recessive manner and is as common as hemophilia A. A prolonged bleeding time and decreased factor VIII activity are characteristic laboratory findings. The only significant source of vWF is cryoprecipitate, with 10 to 40 IU/kg given every 12 hr for correction, beginning 1 day before a surgical procedure.

Coagulation Factors

Factor VIII and factor IX deficiencies are the most common congenital coagulation disorders (Table 1). A lack of either of these factors affects the intrinsic pathway and is thus characterized by prolonged partial thromboplastin time (PTT) values. Hemophilia A (classic hemophilia) is a deficiency of factor VIII and accounts for 80% of inherited factor deficiencies. It is a sex-linked condition occurring in one of 10,000 live births with variable manifestations. Historically, males are affected, although, rarely, a female carrier and affected male will give rise to a homozygous female child. Two-thirds of patients have family members with the disease. Standard treatment is transfusion of factor VIII concentrate, which is derived from pooled donor collections and has a half-life of 12 hr. A measured factor VIII level of 30% to 40% is necessary to treat minor bleeding or before minor surgical procedures, and a level of 80% to 100% is necessary to treat major bleeding and bleeding in critical locations (such as the central nervous system), and before major surgery. One unit of a factor concentrate is defined as that normally present in 1 ml of plasma. One unit per kilogram of body weight is required to raise plasma factor VIII activity by 2%. Cryoprecipitate has 9.6 U/ml of factor VIII activity. Antibodies to factor VIII may occur with chronic therapy and may necessitate increased dosing for a given clinical effect.

Hemophilia B (Christmas disease or factor IX deficiency) is clinically indistinguishable from hemophilia A and occurs in one of 100,000 live births with sex-linked transmittance. In contrast to hemophilia A, lesser factor levels (30% to 40%) are required to treat major bleeding. Factor IX is more stable than factor VIII, with a half-life of 24 hr. Unlike hemophilia A, antifactor antibody formation is rare.

The remaining inherited deficiencies of the intrinsic, extrinsic, and common pathways are rarely encountered in clinical surgery (Table 2). In general, they are inherited in an autosomal recessive manner and can be treated with FFP, with one-half of the initial dose being administered after an interval equal to the half-life of the individual factor (Table 2). Factor XII deficiency requires no specific treatment. Factor XI deficiency is usually detected after finding a prolonged PTT and excluding the more common hemophilias A and B.

Extrinsic pathway factor VII deficiency produces a bleeding diathesis of variable severity. It is associated with prolonged prothrombin times (PTs). Patients with levels of <1% of normal may experience severe bleeding.

Deficiencies of common pathway factors II, V, and X are associated with PT and PTT values. Factor X deficiency is an extremely rare disorder associated with familial carotid body tumors. Factor V deficiency occurs in one of 500,000 births and is associated with a serious hemorrhagic diathesis. Factor II is the rarest of all congenital deficiencies.

Vitamin K Deficiency

Vitamin K is a necessary cofactor in the synthesis of factors II, VII, IX, and X. It is derived from dietary plant sources or is synthesized by intestinal bacteria. Fat-soluble, dietary vitamin K is absorbed in the terminal ileum; vitamin K produced by bacteria is passively absorbed in the colon. Therefore, dietary insufficiency, inanition with

TABLE 2. *Coagulation factor replacement*

Factor	Production site	$T_{1/2}$	Stability in banked blood	Replacement agent	Necessary level for surgery
I	Liver	72–100 hr	Stable	FFP cryoprecipitate	>100 mg/dl
II	Liver[a]	72 hr	Stable	FFP or stored platelets	15%–20%
V	Liver, endothelium	15–36 hr	Labile	FFP	25%
VII	Liver[a]	5 hr	Stable	FFP or stored platelets	10%
VIII	Endothelium	8–12 hr	Labile	Cryoprecipitate	80–100%
IX	Liver[a]	12–24 hr	Stable	Factor concentrate	50%–70%
X	Liver[a]	40–50 hr	Stable	FFP or stored plasma	15%–20%
XI	Liver	40–80 hr	Stable	FFP	10%
XII	?	60 hr	Stable	Not required	—
XIII	Liver	4–7 days	Stable	FFP, cryoprecipitate, or factor concentrate	<10%
vWF	Endothelium	10–12 hr	Labile	Cryoprecipitate	50%–70%

[a]Vitamin K–dependent factor.

inadequately supplied parenteral vitamin K, antibiotic administration, ileal resection, steatorrhea, and biliary obstruction lead to inadequate body stores. Newborn infants have insufficient hepatic synthetic capacities for factors II, VII, IX, and X and have a temporary deficit of vitamin K secondary to a lack of intestinal flora. Coagulopathy due to biliary obstruction, not liver failure, will correct 24 hr after parenteral vitamin K administration.

Hepatic Failure

Derangements in hepatic function will lead to defects in coagulation. Of the clotting factors, only factors IV and VIII are not produced in the liver. The liver is the sole production site for factors II, VII, IX, and X as well as proteins C and S. The reticuloendothelial system of the liver clears fibrin degradation products (FDP), activated factor X, and plasmin. Liver fibrinogen synthetic capacity is only lost in the late stages of liver failure.

Renal Disease

The nephrotic syndrome can lead to coagulopathy secondary to depletion of coagulation factors by urinary protein loss. The absolute amounts of factors are decreased below levels compatible with normal coagulation, and production of new factors cannot compensate for the quantity lost.

As previously stated, end-stage renal disease can cause qualitative platelet dysfunction. Uremic coagulopathy can usually be controlled with hemodialysis, correction of anemia, cryoprecipitate, DDAVP, conjugated estrogens, or platelet transfusion as needed.

Disseminated Intravascular Coagulation

DIC, or consumptive coagulopathy, is characterized by simultaneously triggered coagulation and fibrinolysis, leading to the depletion of coagulation factors and a hypocoagulable state. Heparin may be given in an attempt to slow the depletion of coagulation factors, but the most important therapeutic goal is reversal of the inciting event. The causes of DIC are numerous; however, a common element is the release of tissue factor (tissue thromboplastin) into the circulation, with the consequent triggering of diffuse coagulation through extrinsic pathway factor VII activation. A compounding factor usually involved is decreased hepatic perfusion during shock. This leads to decreased hepatic clearance of FDP, which decrease the polymerization of fibrin and decrease platelet aggregation; decreased hepatic clearance of plasmin, which is free to further attack factors II, V, VII, and fibrinogen; and decreased liver synthetic capacity for the already low coagulation factors, specifically II and V. Causes of DIC include retained necrotic tissue, obstetric

catastrophes, transfusion reactions with intravascular hemolysis, trauma, crush injury, burns, thromboplastin-rich tumors (lung, prostate and pancreas), tissue embolism (brain, amniotic fluid, fat and bone marrow), ischemia/reperfusion injury, sepsis, and hypoperfusion with liver ischemia. Already low plasma levels of factors V and VIII may be diluted by transfusion of stored blood containing low levels of these factors. Clinically, factors V and VIII, fibrinogen, and platelets are found to be more deficient than factors II, VII, IX, X, and XIII. Laboratory abnormalities include elevated PT and PTT, decreased platelet count, decreased fibrinogen level, and increased FDP levels. On peripheral smear, a microangiopathic picture is usually seen with fragmented, damaged red blood cells (RBCs). The most common cause of intraoperative DIC is a transfusion reaction.

Hypercoagulable States

Protein C inactivates factor Va, factor VIIIa, and tPA inhibitor, thereby decreasing coagulation and increasing fibrinolysis. Its activation by thrombin is accomplished 20,000 times faster in the presence of the thrombin/thrombomodulin complex on the surface of activated platelets. Protein S is a cofactor for protein C, enhancing the formation of the protein C/factor Va complex. Deficiency of one of these two proteins leads to a hypercoagulable state. Treatment is with lifelong warfarin anticoagulation following the initial thrombotic episode.

ATIII deficiency is associated with 2% of thrombotic events and must be considered when thrombosis occurs in patients receiving heparin. Treatment consists of administration of FFP to replace ATIII and warfarin anticoagulation. (The administration of warfarin is associated with an increase in ATIII levels.)

A hypercoagulable state is also associated with the lupus anticoagulant, an antiphospholipid antibody found in 5% to 37% of patients with systemic lupus erythematosus, and occasionally in the settings of cancer, infection, and some drugs (e.g., procainamide). Elevated PT and PTT are present, as well as a falsely positive syphilis test secondary to the antibody's reaction with cardiolipin. One-third of patients will have thrombotic complications (70% in the venous system). Proposed mechanisms include direct activation of platelets by the antibody, decreases in prostacyclin release from endothelial cells, or a decrease in protein C activation.

PHARMACOLOGIC INTERVENTIONS IN HEMOSTASIS

Antiplatelet Agents

Aspirin permanently inhibits cyclooxygenase, the enzyme responsible for the production of TXA_2, a platelet aggregator and vasoconstrictor. The life span of normal platelets is 7 to 10 days; the antiplatelet effect of aspirin is seen until new platelets can be generated

The nonsteroidal antiinflammatory drugs (NSAIDs), such as ibuprofen, also inhibit cyclooxygenase, producing similar defects in platelet aggregation. However, in contrast to aspirin, this inhibition in NSAIDs is reversible, resulting in an aggregation defect lasting only as long as the drug is present.

Several agents inhibit platelet aggregation by inhibiting the exposure of gpIIb:IIIa. Methylxanthines (e.g., dipyridamole) inhibit phosphodiesterase, an enzyme that degrades cAMP in platelets. This leads to a higher intraplatelet cAMP level, which inhibits gpIIb:IIIa exposure and thereby decreases platelet aggregation. Nitric acid, nitroprusside, and nitroglycerin inhibit platelet aggregation by increasing intracellular cyclic GMP levels, which, similar to increased cAMP levels, inhibit gpIIb:IIIa exposure. Prostacyclin and prostaglandin E1 increase the intraplatelet level of adenylate cyclase, used in the production of cAMP, increasing levels of cAMP and once again inhibiting exposure of gpIIb:IIIa and thus platelet aggregation.

Anticoagulation

Warfarin is an oral anticoagulant that induces the production of inactive forms of the vitamin K–dependent clotting factors II, VII, IX, and X, protein C, and protein S. Warfarin prevents reduction of oxidized vitamin K, which is necessary for the conversion of glutamic acid residues of newly formed proteins to gamma carboxy glutamic acid residues. The converted amino acid allows these proteins to bind to phospholipid membranes, an important activity in the formation of the prothrombinase and Xase complexes on activated platelets.

Clinical administration is guided by monitoring the PT. Anticoagulation that maintains PT levels from 1.3 to 1.4 times that of control values is effective and associated with one-fifth of the bleeding complications associated with higher PT values. There is a 1- to 3-day delay between warfarin administration and anticoagulation as reflected by the PT. Acute anticoagulation is maintained with heparin until warfarin-induced anticoagulation is established.

A complication of warfarin therapy seen in patients with protein C deficiency is skin necrosis over fatty areas such as the breast and buttocks. This is due to inhibition of protein C, producing a hypercoagulable state before the inhibition of factors with long half-lives (5 to 7 days). These include factors II, VII, IX, and X. Heparin must be administered before starting warfarin therapy to prevent this rare complication.

Heparin is a mixture of sulfated polysaccharides, with molecular weights ranging from 2,000 to 40,000. Heparin

binds to ATIII, inducing a conformational change and thereby increasing ATIII activity. ATIII inhibits thrombin, factors IX, X, XI, and XII, and plasmin. The effect of heparin may vary depending on circulating ATIII levels, which are decreased in the postoperative period, in trauma, and in DIC. Administration of heparin, which has a half-life of 1 hr, is guided by monitoring the PTT, with a goal of 1.5 times the control. Only trace amounts of heparin are needed for its inhibition of activated factor X. Mini-dose heparin administration (5,000 U s.c. twice daily) has been shown to be effective in the prophylaxis of deep venous thrombosis (DVT) and pulmonary embolism (PE). Use in less than high-risk postoperative patients, however, is not indicated due to an associated increased incidence of bleeding complications.

Protamine is used to reverse the action of heparin, at a dose of 1 U/100 U of residual heparin. Hemodynamic and hematologic complications, such as hypotension and shock, can occur and are most frequently seen in patients with previous protamine exposure (e.g., diabetic patients taking NPH insulin).

In heparin-induced thrombocytopenia (HIT), antiheparin antibodies induce platelet aggregation. These multiple aggregates may then lead to arterial and venous thrombosis, stroke, PE, and myocardial infarction. Treatment consists of removal of all heparin sources and protamine reversal if needed. Platelet counts of <100,000 are seen in <10% of heparinized patients. It is suggested that platelet counts be monitored every other day after day 4 of therapy, since HIT frequently occurs between days 5 and 15.

Fibrinolytic Agents

Streptokinase, isolated from group C beta hemolytic, triggers fibrinolysis through a plasmin/streptokinase complex (Fig. 2). Urokinase and tPA act directly on plasmin. TPA, acylated plasminogen/streptokinase activator complex (APSAC), and single-chain urokinase-type plasminogen activator (SCUPA), are fibrin-selective agents, acting more on fibrin bound to plasminogen than on circulating plasminogen. Acylation of the catalytic site of streptokinase to form APSAC makes the complex inert to circulating plasminogen. However, after binding to fibrin, the acetyl group leaves the complex, thereby reactivating the catalytic site. This results in a fibrin-specific fibrinolytic effect.

Urokinase, produced by urinary tract epithelial cells, is a two-chain polypeptide formed from cleavage of single-chain urokinase by plasmin. Fibrin-specific SCUPA activates plasminogen 10 times more rapidly at the fibrin surface than in the circulation.

Bleeding complications can be seen with these agents, with an increased risk of bleeding associated with fibrinogen levels of <100 mg/dl. Hemostatic defects are secondary to hypofibrinogenemia, circulating FDPs, and decreases in factors V and VIII secondary to the actions of plasmin. In the early phases following thrombolysis, platelet activation may contribute to recurrent thrombosis; however, subsequent impaired platelet adhesion and aggregation are found.

Indications for fibrinolytic agents include DVT (with or without heparin), PE with cardiogenic shock, peripheral arterial thrombosis (infused through a catheter placed into the thrombus), and peripheral arterial embolization, with critical ischemia following incomplete balloon embolectomy. Probably the most frequent use of fibrinolytic agents is in the setting of acute myocardial infarction (streptokinase reduces in-hospital mortality by 25%).

Primary contraindications include active internal bleeding, cerebrovascular accident (CVA) within the previous 2 months, surgery or trauma within 10 days, documented left heart thrombus, active gastrointestinal bleeding, or uncontrolled hypertension. Alternative means of anticoagulation or thrombus removal must be used.

Dextran

Dextran is a high molecular weight polysaccharide, one form having a molecular weight of 40,000 and the other 70,000. Dextran causes hemodilution due to an osmotic effect. Simultaneously, blood viscosity, platelet adhesiveness, and factor VIII activity decrease.

EVALUATION OF HEMOSTASIS

The most important step in the preoperative detection of an underlying defect in hemostasis is obtaining a thorough patient history. One should inquire about a history of prolonged bleeding with previous surgery, minor cuts, dental extractions, menstrual periods, or circumcisions. A history of easy bruising, gingival bleeding, epistaxis, hemarthroses, and a family history of a bleeding tendency should all be investigated. Physical examination may reveal the petechiae, purpura, ecchymosis, hematoma, hematuria, or oozing from phlebotomy sites.

Numerous laboratory investigations are available to evaluate the hemostatic mechanism. Examination of the peripheral smear, platelet count, fibrinogen, and FDP levels are self-explanatory. The bleeding time assesses the platelet/vessel wall interaction and platelet function. In the modified Ivy method, a standardized cut is made on a relatively avascular area of the forearm. The appearance of clot after 10 min is abnormal and reflects a qualitative or quantitative platelet dysfunction.

The PT measures the speed of the extrinsic pathway and is altered by exogenous heparin. Deficiencies in factors II, V, VII, X, or fibrinogen will abnormally prolong the PT. The PTT measures the time required to

form clot via the intrinsic pathway and therefore detects deficiencies of factors VIII, IX, XI, and XII. It can also detect deficiencies of all factors detected by the PT, except VII.

The thrombin time is measured when thrombin is added to a patient's plasma. It is prolonged in the presence of FDPs, heparin, and deficiencies of fibrinogen and is used clinically to detect the presence of fibrinogen deficiency in DIC. Hereditary fibrinogen disorders—afibrinogenemia, hypofibrinogenemia, and qualitative fibrinogen defects—are rare and are detected by abnormal thrombin test values and assays for fibrinogen.

The activated clotting time (ACT) measures the ability of whole blood to clot. It is useful for monitoring heparin levels intraoperatively and responds in a linear fashion to increasing heparin dosages. Acceptable values during extracorporeal circulation are 300 to 600 sec.

A thromboelastogram (TEG) is a graphic representation of clotting. It can give information about clotting time, speed of fibrin polymerization, and clot strength and solubility.

TRANSFUSION

The fractionation of whole blood into its components allows preservation of those components that would be lost in storage and allows a more efficient distribution of this precious resource. Whole blood (1 U = 450 ml blood + 63 ml citrate anticoagulant) is rarely used now, except in cases of massive transfusion (>2,500 or 5,000 ml/24 hr). Stored at 4°C, it has a shelf life of 40 ± 5 days with newer preservatives. Seventy percent of transfused RBCs are viable 24 hr after transfusion. It is a poor source of platelets because platelets rarely survive 24 hr of storage.

Generally, transfusion of RBCs (unit volume, ~300 ml in CPDA-1 anticoagulant; average unit hematocrit, 75%) is performed when the need exists to improve the oxygen-carrying capacity. Intravascular volume expansion can be carried out using crystalloid or colloid solutions, but these solutions lack the ability to transport oxygen. The transfusion threshold should be individualized for each patient, as defined by varied physiologic needs. A rise in hemoglobin and hematocrit levels with each unit of RBC transfusion of 1 g/dl and 3%, respectively, can be expected. For patients with a demonstrated hypersensitivity to leukocytes or platelets, leukocyte-poor, washed red cells are available.

Prior to RBC or whole blood transfusion, serologic compatibility is established for the ABO and Rh groups of donor and recipient blood, and a cross-match is performed between the donor cells and the recipient's serum. Type O negative or type-specific blood is acceptable for emergency transfusion.

Platelet concentrates (unit volume, ~50 ml) have an average concentration of 5.5×10^{10} platelets/U. An increase in the platelet count of 10,000 for each unit of platelets transfused can be expected.

FFP (unit volume, ~225 ml) provides factors V and VIII, which deteriorate in stored blood. It is often given to correct coagulopathies associated with liver disease, to rapidly reverse warfarin effects or vitamin K deficiency, in DIC, and in massive transfusion to prevent coagulopathy from factor dilution.

Cryoprecipitate (unit volume, ~15 ml) is a single-donor product and is a source of factors V and VIII, vWF, and fibrinogen. It is composed of the cold precipitable proteins of plasma, formed by fractionating blood for component therapy. It can be used to treat von Willebrand's disease and severe DIC.

ABO compatibility is a requirement for platelet, FFP, and cryoprecipitate transfusions. Platelets should also be Rh compatible.

Complications of Transfusion

Fatal hemolytic reaction (one in 100,000 U infused) due to blood group incompatibility is most commonly the result of human administration error. Intravascular hemolysis occurs, and acute tubular necrosis of the kidney may result from the toxic effects of free hemoglobin on the nephron and precipitation of hemoglobin in the renal tubules. DIC may be triggered by the red cell stromal lipid released and antigen/antibody complex formation. Clinical signs and symptoms include chills, fever, respiratory distress, tachycardia, hypotension, pain along the vein used for infusion, lumbar pain, constrictive chest pain, or flushing. Treatment consists of stopping the transfusion immediately, diuresis with mannitol, and alkalinization of the urine to prevent hemoglobin precipitation within the renal tubules.

Allergic reactions occur during 1% of transfusions. Reactions ranging from fever to anaphylactic shock can occur. Sepsis resulting from transfusion of blood contaminated with bacteria can also complicate transfusion.

Massive transfusion may be accompanied by circulatory overload, hypothermia (from nonwarmed blood), citrate toxicity (binds calcium, more so in young children and those with liver disease), presence of functionally abnormal hemoglobin (intracellular 2,3-diphosphoglycerate deficiency developed during storage impairs oxygen delivery by increasing hemoglobin's oxygen affinity), dilutional thrombocytopenia, and coagulation factor dilution. Transmission of blood-borne pathogens (hepatitis, human immunodeficiency virus) is a known risk and

must be considered before blood transfusions are ordered.

SUMMARY

Hemostasis is a complex set of events requiring coordination among the vascular endothelium, platelets, coagulation factors, and the fibrinolytic system. Disorders of any one or combination of these components may result in alterations of hemostasis. Blood component therapy, antiplatelet agents, anticoagulants, or fibrinolytic agents may be required for correction of defective hemostasis. Abnormalities are detectable by a variety of laboratory investigations.

Blood component therapy in the practice of surgery requires knowledge of the indications and complications associated with its use. Directed use of components allows for efficient utilization of this limited resource and correction of specific deficits.

STUDY QUESTIONS

1. Draw an outline of the reactions of the intrinsic, extrinsic, and common pathways of coagulation.
2. Draw an outline of the reactions of fibrinolysis, including the sites of action of pharmacologic fibrinolytic agents and the fibrinolytic inhibitors.
3. List the differences between the anticoagulants heparin and warfarin. Include routes of administration, T_{fi}, mechanisms of action, chemical class, and coagulation pathway affected.
4. Describe the pathophysiology, causes, laboratory abnormalities, and treatment of DIC.
5. List the causes of quantitative and qualitative platelet defects.

SUGGESTED READING

Beutler E, Lichtman M, Coller B, Kipps T, eds. *Williams hematology.* 5th ed. New York: McGraw-Hill, 1995.

Collins JA. Blood transfusion and disorders of surgical bleeding. In: Sabiston DC, ed. *Textbook of surgery.* 14th ed. Philadelphia: Saunders, 1991: 85–102.

Colman RW, Hirsh J, Marder VJ, Salzman EW, eds. *Hemostasis and thrombosis: basic principles and clinical practice.* 2nd ed. Philadelphia: Lippincott, 1987.

Schwartz SI. Hemostasis, surgical bleeding and transfusion. In: Schwartz SI, Shires GT, Spencer FC, eds. *Principles of surgery.* 6th ed. New York: McGraw-Hill, 1994:95–118.

Wakefield TW. Hemostasis. In: Greenfield LJ, Mulholland MW, Oldham KT, Zelenock GB, eds. *Surgery: scientific principles and practice.* Philadelphia: Lippincott, 1993:102–124.

CHAPTER 3

Wounds and Wound Healing

Itzhak Nir and Larry C. Martin

Surgery may be described as the art of creating a controlled wound. Wound healing involves a very specific set of cellular events that serve to bring about the normal realignment of the injured tissues. These events are continuous and overlapping. Here, we describe the normal events involved in wound healing and the important aspects of surgery as they apply to the wound healing process.

CLASSIFICATION OF WOUNDS

Wounds can be classified into four general categories: (a) clean, (b) clean-contaminated, (c) contaminated, and (d) dirty. Wound classification is important because the operative, as well as postoperative, management of the wound types may significantly differ.

Clean Wounds

Clean wounds are wounds that are relatively new (<6 hr) and do not involve the violation of a viscus. These wounds have a low infection rate (<2%), and if infection occurs, it is most likely the result of a break in the aseptic technique during surgery. The most likely infecting organisms in these types of wounds are *Staphylococcus aureus* and *Staphylococcus epidermidis* as well as other endogenous skin flora. Usually no antibiotic prophylaxis is required for these types of wounds, but, if given, should include coverage for skin flora (e.g., first-generation cephalosporin). Examples of clean wounds are inguinal hernia repairs, cutaneous surgery, or a highly selective vagotomy.

Clean-Contaminated Wounds

Clean-contaminated wounds are wounds in which a viscus is purposely or accidentally penetrated with minimal or no spillage. The infection rate in these procedures is usually <10%. The most likely pathogenic organisms in this type of wound are Enterobacteriaceae, Enterococci, and Anaerobes (*Streptococcus faecalis*, Bacteroides). Antibiotic prophylaxis is necessary and usually consists of a second-generation cephalosporin, with the addition of anaerobic coverage (metronidazole, clindamycin) if contamination is thought to have occurred. Esophageal, stomach/duodenum, hepatobiliary, small intestinal, and adequately prepared large bowel surgeries are all classified as clean-contaminated (e.g., cholecystectomy, small bowel resection, gastrectomy).

Contaminated Wounds

Contaminated wounds are wounds in which there is excessive spillage or inflammation, or in which the local bacterial count is excessive. All unprepared large bowel and anorectal surgeries are considered contaminated. The bacteria are similar in nature to those found in clean-contaminated surgeries but are present in much larger numbers. The infection rate can be as high as 20% in these cases. Antibiotic prophylaxis, as well as a postoperative regimen of antibiotics, is required. Examples of procedures with contaminated wounds are appendectomy with inflammation, colectomy with spillage, and hemorrhoidectomy.

Dirty Wounds

Dirty wounds are wounds that are grossly contaminated. The bacterial count is excessive, and debridement of tissue with copious irrigation is required to lower the number of bacteria present. The infection rate is >60%, and a prolonged antibiotic course is required. Causes of dirty wounds are colonic perforations, abscesses, and wounds that are a result of trauma (skin avulsions, open fractures, etc.).

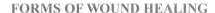

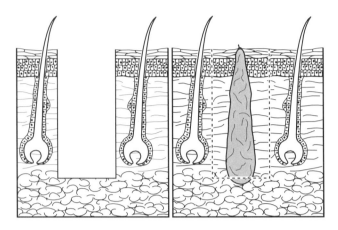

FIG. 1. In primary wound healing, the wound is closed by direct approximation of the tissues.

FIG. 3. In tertiary wound healing, or delayed primary closure, a wound is initially left open for a few days and is then surgically reapproximated.

FORMS OF WOUND HEALING

Wound healing can be divided into three distinct forms: (a) primary, (b) secondary, and (c) tertiary or delayed primary closure. In primary wound healing (primary intention), a wound is closed by the direct reapproximation of the tissues (Fig. 1). Skin grafts, or flaps, which are often used to cover a large area, are also forms of primary healing. Most surgical incisions are repaired by primary intention. In secondary wound healing (secondary intention), a wound is left open and is allowed to granulate in (Fig. 2). This process usually takes several weeks to achieve complete wound epithelialization. This is often done when the wound is contaminated or dirty, or when there is not enough tissue to properly reapproximate the wound. In tertiary wound healing, also known as delayed primary closure, a wound is initially left open for several days (usually 3 to 5 days), followed by surgical reapproximation of the wound edges (Fig. 3). This form

of healing reduces the incidence of infection in a wound that is considered too risky to close by primary intention.

STAGES OF WOUND HEALING

An injury disrupts the normal chemical and architectural environment of the involved tissue. This sets off a series of cellular and biochemical events designed to make the system whole once again. Regardless of the size of the wound, the basic steps remain the same. Wound healing can be divided into three essential and overlapping stages (Fig. 4), including (a) an inflammatory or exudative stage, (b) a fibroblastic or proliferative stage, and (c) a remodeling or maturation stage. In the inflammatory stage, the wound is erythematous and edematous, and may be difficult to distinguish from early infection. As the wound enters the proliferative stage, the wound becomes less inflamed, and the scar, which appears at this time, is raised and hard. During the maturation phase, the scar gradually flattens, fades, and becomes less noticeable.

Inflammatory or Exudative Stage

When a tissue is injured, the damaged endothelial cells release cytokines that serve to attract platelets and leukocytes into the area (Fig. 5 and Table 1). Histamine, serotonin, and kinins cause vasoconstriction initially as an aid in hemostasis followed shortly by vasodilation. Additionally, these inflammatory components cause the vessel endothelium to become more porous allowing the further influx of inflammatory cells into the area. Activated platelets release platelet-derived growth factor (PDGF), insulin-like growth factor (IGF-1), and transforming growth factor β (TGF-β), which prepare the local inflammatory cells to multiply and serve to attract other inflammatory cells (monocytes and polymorphonuclear cells

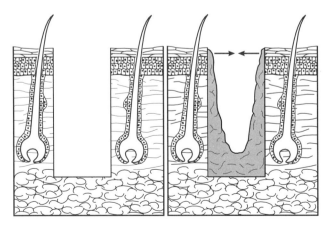

FIG. 2. In secondary wound healing, a wound is left open to granulate in over a number of weeks.

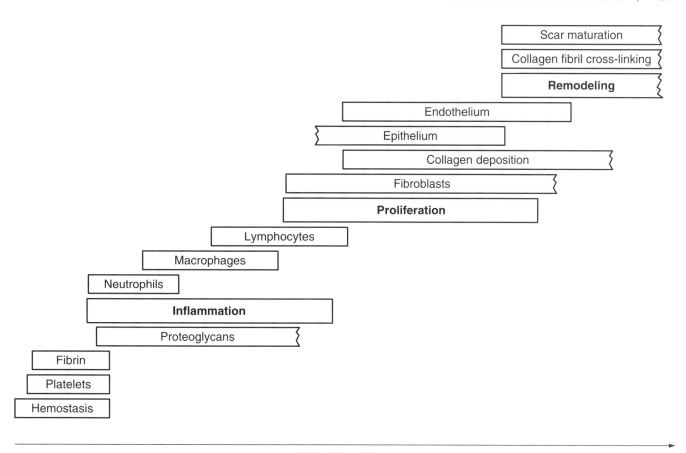

FIG. 4. Stages of wound healing.

Time from injury

[PMNs]). The neutrophils become the dominant cells within the first 24 hr (Fig. 6), but after 48 hr their numbers decline, giving way to macrophages and fibroblasts (Fig. 7). Neutrophils serve to phagocytize debris and remove contaminating bacteria but are nonessential to proper wound healing. In the absence of infection, neutrophil-

deprived wounds heal normally. The macrophage, on the other hand, is essential for proper wound healing. These specialized monocytes serve to remove debris and kill pathogenic bacteria. Additionally, the macrophage secretes a variety of products that serve to recruit fibroblasts and promote angiogenesis. Interleukin 1 (IL-1), secreted by the macrophage, has been demonstrated to enhance fibroblast activity and collagen deposition. Wounds experimentally deprived of macrophages exhibit a marked inhibition of fibroblast migration and proliferation, as well as diminished collagen synthesis. Macrophages will remain present in the wound for several weeks (Fig. 8).

Epithelialization begins within hours of injury. A cleanly incised wound will reepithelialize within 6 to 48 hr. Cellular movement is initiated by a loss of contact with neighboring ectodermal cells (skin or mucosa) and, barring debris, will continue until the wound edges are reapproximated. When this occurs, the epithelial movement is stopped automatically by a process called "contact inhibition." The proliferative and maturation stages of wound healing can begin only after epithelialization has occurred.

In a wound healing by primary intention, the inflammatory phase lasts for ~4 days. In wounds that are

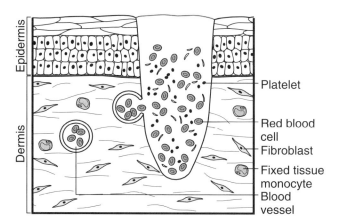

FIG. 5. In the inflammatory, or exudative phase, platelets release factors that attract inflammatory cells and fibroblasts to the wound site.

TABLE 1. *Cytokines involved in wound healing*

Factor	Abbreviation	Source	Functions regulated
Platelet-derived growth factor	PDGF	Platelets and macrophages	Fibroblast proliferation, chemotaxis, and collagenase production
Transforming growth factor β	TGF-β	Platelets, polymorphonuclear neutrophil leukocytes, T lymphocytes, and macrophages	Fibroblast proliferation, chemotaxis, collagen metabolism, and action of other growth factors
Transforming growth factor α	TGF-α	Activated macrophages and many tissues	Similar to EGF functions
Interleukin-1	IL-1	Macrophages	Fibroblast proliferation
Tumor necrosis factor	TNF	Macrophages, mast cells, and T lymphocytes	Fibroblast proliferation
Fibroblast growth factor	FGF	Brain, pituitary, macrophages, and many other tissues and cells	Fibroblast proliferation, stimulates collagen deposition and angiogenesis
Epidermal growth factor	EGF	Saliva, urine, milk, and plasma	Stimulates epithelial cell proliferation and granulation tissue formation
Insulin-like growth factor	IGF	Liver, plasma, and fibroblasts	Stimulates synthesis of sulfated proteoglycans, collagen, and cell proliferation
Human growth factor	HGF	Pituitary and thus plasma	Anabolism

Adapted from Greenfield LJ, Mulholland MW, Oldham KT, Zelenock GB, eds. Wound healing. In: Greenfield LJ, Mulholland MW, Oldham KT, Zelenock GB, eds. *Surgery: scientific principles and practice.* Philadelphia: Lippincott, 1993.

allowed to heal by secondary intention, the inflammatory phase continues until epithelialization is complete.

Proliferative or Fibroblastic Stage

Once the ectodermal elements of the wound are approximated, the second stage (proliferative stage) of wound healing can begin. The depth of the wound is healed by the fibroblasts. PDGF is a potent chemoattractant for fibroblasts. The activated fibroblasts move into the wound as quickly as the clot and debris are removed by the phagocytic cells. They migrate across strands of fibrin and fibronectin to begin the reparative process. On approximately days 4 or 5 of wound healing, collagen synthesis begins. Collagen production is stimulated by IGF-1, tumor growth factor–β, and lactate. Collagen is

secreted initially by the fibroblasts as procollagen, a left-handed triple-helix. The procollagen is then cleaved by procollagen peptidase to produce tropocollagen. The tropocollagen molecules then aggregate and cross-link to produce collagen fibrils. A specialized fibroblast, the myelofibroblast, has the properties of both a smooth muscle and a fibroblast. This cell is thought to be responsible for the wound contracture that begins in this stage.

Collagen production increases rapidly for the first 3 weeks and plateaus at ~6 weeks. After this time, there is no net gain of collagen. The wound's tensile strength rises in proportion to the initial collagen production but continues to increase through collagen remodeling, even though there is no net gain in the amount of collagen (Fig. 9).

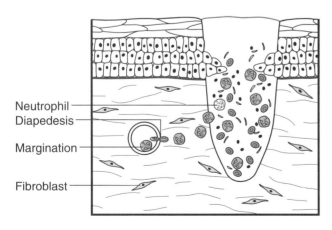

FIG. 6. Wound site at 24 hr; the neutrophil is the dominant cell in the wound site.

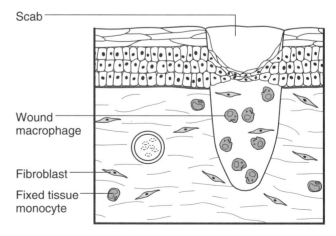

FIG. 7. Wound site at 48 hr; the macrophage is the dominant cell in the wound site, and fibroblasts appear in the wound.

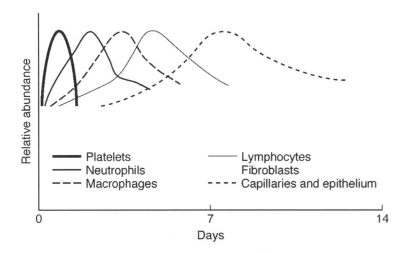

FIG. 8. Diagram of cellular appearance at the wound site.

Angiogenesis begins at ~2 days by the proliferation of endothelial cells of the cut venules. By the fourth day, a new microvascular system is in place to continue bringing nutrients into the injured area. Angiogenesis continues into the proliferative and remodeling stages.

Remodeling or Maturation Stage

This stage is marked by the intermolecular cross-linking of collagen. After ~6 weeks, collagen is produced and degraded at an equal rate, with no net gain in the amount of collagen. The scar is continuously remodeled, causing a steady increase in its tensile strength. The remodeling phase overlaps the proliferative stage and continues in the adult for up to 2 years.

FACTORS AFFECTING WOUND HEALING

The primary goal of every surgeon is to achieve maximal wound healing. A complete understanding of the many factors involved in wound healing may allow the surgeon to avoid the complications of wound breakdown. Many factors contribute to proper wound healing, including oxygenation, nutrition, immunosuppression, infection, radiation, diabetes, and mechanical influences.

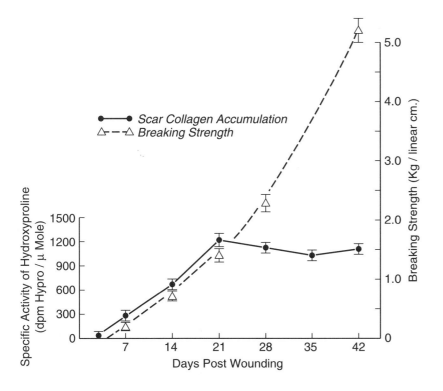

FIG. 9. The breaking strength of rat skin compared with net scar collagen accumulation. Collagen production and wound tensile strength increase rapidly for the first 3 weeks, followed by no net gain in collagen but a continued increase in wound tensile strength. (Adapted from Madden JW, Peacock EE Jr. Studies on the biology of collagen during wound healing. III. Dynamic metabolism of scar collagen and remodeling of dermal wounds. *Ann Surg* 1971;174:511.)

Oxygenation

When a tissue is injured, the major influx of inflammatory cells into the area causes an increased metabolic demand and, therefore, decreases the local oxygen tension to 30 to 40 mm Hg. This is a normal response to injury, and, in fact, the diminished oxygen tension serves to stimulate angiogenesis and collagen formation. Problems arise when the oxygen tension falls too low. Oxygen is essential for the release of collagen from the fibroblasts and is important in the formation of the toxic superoxide radicals that are used to kill the bacteria phagocytized by the macrophages and neutrophils. A low oxygen tension, as a result of hypoxia, vasoconstriction, hypovolemia, or cold, makes a wound more susceptible to infection and more prone to breakdown. Supplemental systemic oxygenation, as well as hyperbaric (local and systemic) oxygen, elevates the local oxygen tension and promotes proper wound healing. If the oxygen tension is excessively elevated (>200 mm Hg), angiogenesis is inhibited and wound healing is actually depressed.

Nutrition

Proper nutrition is essential for wound healing. Patients who had lost >10% of their body weight prior to surgery were found to have an impaired physiological response. Protein deficiency will extend the inflammatory phase, decrease fibroblast collagen synthesis, and increase the incidence of wound dehiscence. Carbohydrate (glucose) is essential for oxidative metabolism, and its deficiency will lead to diminished cell proliferation and phagocytic activity. Fat is important in the formation of cell membranes. Vitamin A deprivation diminishes the rate of wound epithelialization and wound closure. Vitamin B deficiency is thought to alter the immune system and increase the risk of infection. Vitamin K deficiency creates a propensity to bleed and may lead to hematoma formation. Vitamin C deficiency leads to impaired collagen synthesis, and a diet completely devoid of vitamin C may lead to the reopening of previously healed wounds, such as occur in the disease called "scurvy." Iron deficiency may increase the risk of tissue ischemia and may decrease the wound's tensile strength. A zinc deficiency will impair DNA and RNA synthesis, and can lead to altered collagen synthesis.

Nutritional support may be requires for malnourished patients. If a patient is malnourished prior to elective surgery, the surgery should be delayed until proper nutrition is achieved. This may be accomplished by either a well-balanced diet, enteral nutrition, or parenteral nutrition.

Immunosuppression

A properly functioning immune system is essential for adequate wound healing. Immune system suppression is associated with AIDS, sepsis, multiple trauma, malnutrition, diabetes, advanced age, chemotherapy, radiation therapy, and medications (e.g., corticosteroids). These conditions will lead to diminished cellular migration, proliferation, and function, and have the potential of turning a minor wound into a major complication.

Infection

Bacteria are found in low numbers throughout the body and, in low numbers (<10^2 organisms/g of tissue), have even been found to enhance wound healing and promote chemotaxis and bactericidal activity. When the bacterial count reaches a critical number (10^5 organisms/gram of tissue), wound healing is impaired. This is thought to occur due to the bacterial release of proteases, hemolysins, and inhibitors of leukocyte chemotaxis. The infected wound also forms a thickened connective tissue and excessive angiogenesis, leading to excessive scar formation.

Wounds with $\geq 10^5$ organisms/g of tissue are well debrided and are usually left open to heal by secondary intention. Supplemental topical or systemic antibiotics may be of value to promote wound healing.

Radiation

Irradiated tissues heal poorly as a result of both obliterative endarteritis with a decreased blood flow and poor fibroblast function and proliferation. Irradiated wounds heal slowly and have a tendency to break down frequently. These wounds have a low tensile strength and a decreased collagen deposition. Changes in irradiated wounds are often unnoticeable for several months, after which breakdown may occur. Management of irradiated wounds entails meticulous wound care. Oftentimes, the wound has to be debrided to viable tissue, and a graft may be needed for coverage.

Diabetes

Diabetes mellitus and its resulting hyperglycemia are associated with diminished leukocyte function and impaired chemotaxis and phagocytosis. The concomitant microvascular disease of diabetic patients leads to the decreased delivery of oxygen and nutrients to the healing wound. These factors lead to the increased incidence of wound infections and poor wound healing seen in the diabetic population. Stringent control of blood sugar and

TABLE 2. *Classification of tetanus-prone and non–tetanus-prone wounds*

Clinical features	Tetanus-prone wounds	Non–tetanus-prone wounds
Age of wound	>6 hr	≤6 hr
Configuration	Stellate wound, avulsion	Linear wound, abrasion
Depth	>1 cm	≤1 cm
Mechanism of injury	Missile, crush, burn, frostbite	Sharp surface (e.g., knife, glass)
Signs of infection	Present	Absent
Devitalized tissue	Present	Absent
Contaminants (dirt, feces, grass, saliva, and so on)	Present	Absent
Denervated and/or ischemic tissue	Present	Absent

Adapted from Ross SE. Prophylaxis against tetanus in wound management. *Bull Am Coll Surg* 1996;81:42–43.

meticulous wound care are essential to promote adequate wound healing.

Mechanical Influences

Mechanical factors that influence wound healing are wound site tension, edema, hematoma, and the presence of a foreign body.

Excessive wound tension can lead to tissue necrosis by jeopardizing the local blood supply. Additionally, excessive wound tension may delay the rate of repair, diminish the tensile strength, and increase the final width of a scar. It is extremely important to plan the repair carefully in order to avoid these complications.

Edema at the wound site, for any reason, may delay wound healing by altering the hydrostatic capillary pressure and may lead to diminished angiogenesis. This will suppress the proliferation of granulation tissue and lead to a prolonged inflammatory stage. Compressive dressings and elevation may be used to decrease the amount of wound edema and to promote wound healing.

A hematoma creates a space-occupying lesion that leads to diminished fibroblast migration and wound contracture, which can lead to the formation of a weaker wound with a larger scar. The hematoma also serves as a perfect culture medium for bacteria and, if infected, will lead to wound breakdown. Careful hemostasis at the time of repair is essential to avoid this complication.

Foreign bodies in a wound act as a mechanical barrier to epithelialization and fibroblast migration. They can also serve as a nidus of infection by harboring pathogenic bacteria. Devitalized tissue, as well as all foreign substances (dirt, gravel, suture, etc.), must be completely removed prior to wound closure. This is usually accomplished by copious irrigation and debridement.

TETANUS PROPHYLAXIS

Tetanus, or lockjaw, is a condition caused by the organism *Clodtridium tetani*. After an incubation period ranging from 2 days to several weeks, the exotoxin produced by this organism leads to symptoms, including restlessness, headache, jaw stiffness, and muscular contractions at the wound site. If untreated, violent muscular spasms occur within 24 hr, culminating in respiratory arrest. All traumatic wounds should receive thorough debridement of devitalized tissues and removal of foreign bodies, using meticulous aseptic technique. Active immunization against tetanus with tetanus toxoid should be administered to (a) any tetanus-prone wound (Table 2) in a patient who was last vaccinated >5 years ago, (b) any non–tetanus-prone wound in a person last vaccinated >10

TABLE 3. *Recommended tetanus immunization and prophylaxis according to wound classification and prior tetanus prophylaxis history*

History of adsorbed tetanus toxoid (doses)	Tetanus-prone wounds		Non–tetanus-prone wounds	
	Tt[a]	TIG	Tt[a]	TIG
Unknown or <3	Yes	Yes	Yes	No
≥3[b]	No[c]	No	No[d]	No

[a]For children younger than 7 years old, DPT may be considered.
[b]If only three doses of fluid toxoid have been received previously, a fourth dose, preferably an adsorbed toxoid, should be given.
[c]Yes, if >5 years since last dose.
[d]Yes, if >10 years since last dose (more frequent boosters are not needed and can accentuate side effects).
Tt, tetanus toxoid adsorbed (for adult use); TIG, tetanus immune globulin (human).
Adapted from Ross SE. Prophylaxis against tetanus in wound management. *Bull Am Coll Surg* 1996;81:42–43.

years ago, or (c) any person with an incomplete history of vaccination. Human tetanus immunoglobulin should be added to the regimen in a tetanus-prone wound in a person with an incomplete history of vaccination (Table 3).

SURGICAL MANAGEMENT OF LACERATIONS

Cleaning the Wound

Prior to repairing a laceration, the surgeon must make sure that all devitalized tissue and foreign bodies are removed. The wound has to be irrigated copiously with sterile normal saline or sterile water. These are occasionally mixed with some betadine (povidone iodine) solution or some other antiseptic solution. On occasion, the wound may be deeply contaminated, and the foreign bodies cannot be removed by irrigation alone. When this occurs, surgical debridement and irrigation is often indicated. Any material left in the wound has the potential for complications, such as infection and wound breakdown.

Draping and Anesthesia

Once the laceration has been carefully irrigated, it should be draped with either a prefabricated sterile drape or sterile towels. This process is extremely important since a break in the draping process could lead to wound contamination. Once this is accomplished, adequate anesthesia should be applied. Small wounds and lacerations usually do well with local anesthetics. The patient should be asked about adverse reactions or drug allergies prior to administering the anesthetic. An adequate amount of anesthesia should be administered, being careful not to approach the toxic dosages. The toxic dose for plain lidocaine is 3 to 5 mg/kg, and the toxic dose for lidocaine with epinephrine is 5 to 7 mg/kg. Remember, a 1% solution of lidocaine has 10 mg of lidocaine per cc and a 0.5% solution has 5 mg of lidocaine per cc. The addition of epinephrine to the anesthetic serves to cause a local vasoconstriction and thereby reduce the amount of bleeding from the wound site. Epinephrine should not be in tissues with a limited or an end blood supply, such as fingers, toes, nose, or ears.

Debridement

Once the anesthetic is administered and is effective, local debridement can be performed. The devitalized tissues are removed until healthy tissue is attained. Once debridement is completed, the wound should be irrigated once again. Only now can the actual wound closure begin.

Wound Closure

The purpose of wound closure is to reapproximate the tissues so that wound healing can occur at the optimal rate. Wounds are usually closed in two layers, deep and superficial. The purpose of deep layer closure is to eliminate any potential dead space. A dead space results from the separation of wound edges that have been improperly approximated or from air being trapped within the wound. Usually, this occurs in tissues that lack a sufficient blood supply, such as the subcutaneous fatty tissue. Serum or blood may collect within the dead space and provide an excellent medium for bacterial colonization. This may lead to a wound infection and a potential wound breakdown.

The superficial layer of the wound can be reapproximated in a variety of techniques. Usually, suture material or skin staples are used, but if the wound is small enough, steri-strips are all that may be necessary to approximate the edges. There are several key points to remember whenever closing skin:

1. Carefully approximate the wound edges. This is accomplished by taking bites of equal length and depth on both sides of the wound. Failure to do so may lead to impaired healing and an aesthetically unpleasing scar.
2. Avoid excessive tension on the wound. If the edges do not come together easily and excessive tension is applied, the wound is predisposed to dehiscence. Usually, other maneuvers, such as skin undermining, may be used to try and minimize the wound tension, but when these fail, alternative means of coverage (grafts) may be necessary.
3. Avoid excessive tightening of the sutures. Doing so may lead to wound edge strangulation and necrosis.

Types of Suture Material

In order to achieve proper wound closure, the surgeon must first decide on what type of suture material to use. Over the years, a variety of materials has been used. Each one has specific properties that make it preferable over another for a specific closure. Sutures can be divided into three broad categories: natural/synthetic, absorbable/nonabsorbable, and monofilament/braided (polyfilament). The ideal suture material would be one that is strong, easy to tie, minimally reactive, and not predisposed to infection.

Stainless steel wire is strong and inert, and does not harbor bacteria. It is difficult to manipulate and tie.

Catgut is a naturally absorbable braided suture made from sheep and bovine intestinal submucosa. It has a variable rate of absorption and causes a large inflammatory response. It loses its strength rapidly and unevenly.

Silk suture is a braided, nonabsorbable natural fiber that is relatively inert in human tissue. It is easy to tie and maintains its strength in the short term. Due to the braided polyfilament nature of the fiber, it can serve as a nidus of infection and on occasion has produced abscesses that penetrate through the skin and do not heal until the suture is removed.

Synthetic nonabsorbable sutures are strong and inert. They can be further divided into monofilament sutures (nylon, proline) and polyfilament sutures (mersilene). They are used frequently in vascular anastamoses and prosthetic grafts. These sutures do not handle as well as silk and have to be knotted at least four times to prevent knot slippage. The polyfilament sutures are just as likely as silk to harbor bacteria and form abscesses.

Synthetic absorbable sutures are strong and minimally reactive, and have a standard rate of dissolution/absorption. They can be either monofilament (monocryl, PDS) or polyfilament (vicryl). They are used for a variety of gastrointestinal, urologic, and gynecologic anastamoses, as well as frequently in skin closures.

Surgical staples are composed of a steel-tantalum alloy, incite minimal reaction, and can be used either internally or externally. There is little difference in the wound healing that follows either suture or staple placement. Staples simplify the placement process but usually cannot accommodate special situations as well as sutures. Staples do not penetrate the skin and therefore do not serve as a conduit for contaminating bacteria.

Skin tapes are ideal for closing small superficial wounds. They do not penetrate the skin and therefore do not introduce foreign organisms into the wound. They may not be used on actively bleeding wounds or wounds with complex surfaces, such as the perineum.

Postoperative Wound Care

Postoperative wound care involves the maintenance of wound cleanliness, protection of the wound from trauma, and maximal support of the patient to prevent wound breakdown.

Postoperative wound care begins with the application of the surgical dressing. Three types of surgical dressings are commonly used: dry, wet to dry, and occlusive. A dry dressing simply involves the placement of a dry sterile material (gauze, telfa) over the wound to keep it protected and to absorb any drainage. This type of dressing is usually changed daily or when the bandage is excessively saturated. A wet to dry dressing is frequently used on open granulating or infected wounds. This type of dressing involves the placement of a moistened gauze over the open surface of the wound, which is then covered by a dry dressing. As the moisture evaporates, the dressing sticks to the surface of the wound. When the dressing is removed, the superficial layer of the wound is debrided, allowing further granulation of the tissue. This type of dressing is usually changed three times daily. An occlusive dressing, as the name implies, involves the placement of an occlusive material over the wound. The mate-

rial may be either air permeable or impermeable, but all occlusive materials are fluid impermeable. This type of dressing serves to keep the wound environment humid and moist. Recent studies have shown that this type of environment serves to accelerate wound healing by allowing the epithelial cells to migrate more easily. The bacterial count in these wounds is slightly elevated, but this serves to promote the wound healing rather than inhibit it. When the bacterial count becomes excessive ($>10^5$ organisms/g of tissue), then the wound is more likely to break down. These types of dressings are usually left in place for 3 to 4 days prior to being removed.

Wound care continues with the daily inspection of the wound. Early wound healing can be confused with early infection since the process of inflammation is common to both. It is at this time that the clinical judgment of the surgeon comes into play. Excessive inflammation and erythema, excessive serous drainage, purulent drainage, or persistent fevers are suspicious for a wound infection. A closed surgical wound that is suspicious for infection must be dealt with promptly and effectively. The skin over the inflamed area must be opened to allow drainage, and antibiotics must be started. Oftentimes, drainage of the infected collection is sufficient to promote healing and the antibiotics may be stopped. The wound is then left open to heal by secondary intention. When the wound infection is more severe and involves the fascia, the patient must be taken back to the operating room, where the fascia and wound edges must be debrided down to healthy tissue.

If the surgeon adheres to good surgical technique, insures adequate blood volume, oxygenation, and nutrition, and provides effective wound care, most wounds will heal without complications.

Suture Removal

Suture removal is variable and depends on the location of the wound, on the patient's medical condition, and on the experience of the surgeon.

In a healthy patient, sutures from the skin of the face and neck may be removed in 2 to 5 days. Other skin sutures may be removed within 5 to 8 days. Retention sutures (wide sutures placed for additional wound support) are usually removed anywhere from 2 to 6 weeks after placement.

In patients with poor medical conditions or on medication that prevent wound healing, the time of suture placement is extended. There is no fixed time period, and this usually depends on the experience of the surgeon with the particular type of problem involved.

SUMMARY

Wound healing involves a very specific set of cellular events that occur in a continuous and overlapping manner. A surgeon should have a thorough understanding of these biological processes. The combination of the science of wound healing and the art of surgery will lead to optimal results. New advances in wound care and management are ever forthcoming. Careful study and utilization of these advances are essential for the progression of surgery.

STUDY QUESTIONS

1. Describe the various stages of wound healing and the major events that occur in each stage.
2. Describe the type of tetanus prophylaxis that is to be given to a 26-year-old migrant farmer with an incomplete vaccination history and a tetanus-prone wound.
3. What is the maximal dose of lidocaine (with and without epinephrine) that may given to a 70-kg man with a forehead laceration?
4. Describe how a wet to dry dressing serves to promote wound healing.
5. Briefly describe the factors affecting wound healing and how they may be optimized.

SUGGESTED READING

Albina JE. Nutrition and wound healing. *JPEN J Parenter Enteral Nutr* 1994;18:367–376.

Ehrlickman RJ, Seckel BR, Bryan DJ, Moschella CJ. Common complications of wound healing. Prevention and management. *Surg Clin North Am* 1991;71:1323–1351.

Evans RB. An update on wound management. *Hand Clin* 1991;7:402–432.

Gerstein AD, Phillips TJ, Rogers GS, et al. Wound healing and aging. *Dermatol Clin* 1993;11:749–757.

Hulten L. Dressings for surgical wounds. *Am J Surg* 1994;167:42s–44s.

Kerstein MD. Introduction: moist wound healing. *Am J Surg* 1994;167:1s–6s.

Lawrence JC. Dressings and wound infection. *Am J Surg* 1994;167:21s–24s.

Leaper DJ. Prophylactic and therapeutic role of antibiotics in wound care. *Am J Surg* 1994;167:15s–19s.

Mertz PM, Ovington LG. Wound healing microbiology. *Dermatol Clin* 1993;11:739–747.

Moy LS. Management of acute wounds. *Dermatol Clin* 1993;11:759–766.

Pierce GF, Mustoe TA. Pharmacological enhancement of wound healing. *Ann Rev Med* 1995;46:467–481.

Robinson CJ. Growth factors: therapeutic andvances in wound healing. *Ann Med* 1993;25:535–538.

Ross SE. Prophylaxis against tetanus in wound management. *Bull Am Coll Surg* 1996;81:42–43.

Telfer NR, Moy RL. Drug and nutrient aspects of wound healing. *Dermatol Clin* 1993;11:729–737.

Thomas DW, O'Neill ID, Harding KG, et al. Cutaneous wound healing: a current prospective. *J Oral Maxillofac Surg* 1995;53:442–447.

Thomson PD, Smith DJ Jr. What is infection? *Am J Surg* 1994;167:7s–11s.

Wijetunge DB. Management of acute and traumatic wounds: main aspects of care in adults and children. *Am J Surg* 1994;167:56s–60s.

CHAPTER 4

Principles of Surgical Nutrition

Patricia M. Byers and Marla Weissler

The importance of perioperative nutrition has been appreciated by surgeons since the 1930s, when Studley documented an increase in postoperative mortality in malnourished gastrectomy patients. However, the birth of surgical nutrition awaited the 1950s with Francis Moore's description of the ratio of fuel to nitrogen that was necessary for anabolism. Shortly thereafter, Jonathan Rhoads and Stanley Dudrick demonstrated the feasibility of intravenous nutrition. The debilitating gastrointestinal (GI) illnesses and complications that surgeons continually face have fueled the development of sophisticated techniques to aliment those with intestinal failure.

Here, we describe normal, fasting, and starvation metabolism. The changes that occur during periods of metabolic stress are then outlined. The clinical need for nutritional assessment and for calculation of requirements is delineated. Finally, the technique and superiority of enteral nutrition are summarized, along with a description of the solutions utilized for parenteral nutrition. Finally, the complications of therapy that may potentially harm the patient are described.

METABOLIC RESPONSES IN THE FED AND FASTING STATES

Intermediary metabolism refers to the patterns of protein, carbohydrate, and fat use that allow for energy generation and synthetic function. A typical diet that reflects normal patterns of substrate use consists of carbohydrate and fat, with 30% to 35% of caloric support in the form of lipid. Carbohydrate, primarily in the form of glucose, is the required source of energy for leukocytes, erythrocytes, the renal medulla, and the nervous system. Meanwhile, cardiac and skeletal muscle and visceral organs are able to use the byproducts of fat metabolism for their energy needs. The following section discusses substrate metabolism in the fed and the fasted but nonstressed states.

Normal Metabolism

Normal metabolism can be subdivided into states of synthesis, where energy and substrate availability is high, and deficit, where energy and substrate availability is low. Following a meal, synthesis is favored. As serum insulin levels rise in response to available glucose, glycogen synthetase is activated, thus increasing production of glycogen. In addition, glucose that enters the glycolytic pathway is used to form pyruvate. Because energy stores are abundant, pyruvate is converted to acetyl-CoA, which is then used for lipid synthesis. The high levels of citrate, ATP, and NADH act as inhibitory influences on the tricarboxylic acid (TCA) cycle, glycolysis, and the beta-oxidation pathway of lipids (Fig. 1).

Fasting Metabolism

During nonstressed periods of short-term fasting (<3 days), there is a different hormonal and metabolic environment. Glucose and insulin levels fall, and glucagon levels rise. Under these circumstances, the levels of citrate, ATP, and NADH will fall, indicating depressed energy and substrate stores. This leads to the inhibition of synthesis and favors the breakdown of glycogen and fatty acids to provide energy. Carbohydrate metabolism during the fasting state consists of both glycogen breakdown and glycolysis, as well as gluconeogenesis. Glycogen breakdown is mediated by the enzyme glycogen phosphorylase, which is activated by rising levels of glucagon. Glycolysis is the nonreversible breakdown of glucose to pyruvate. Under anaerobic conditions where the TCA cycle is not functional, pyruvate will be converted to lactate, with resulting lactic acidosis.

Gluconeogenesis is the process of forming new glucose from amino acids and other substances. It is necessary when glycogen stores have been depleted and there is no carbohydrate intake. Gluconeogenic pathways may

CYTOSOL

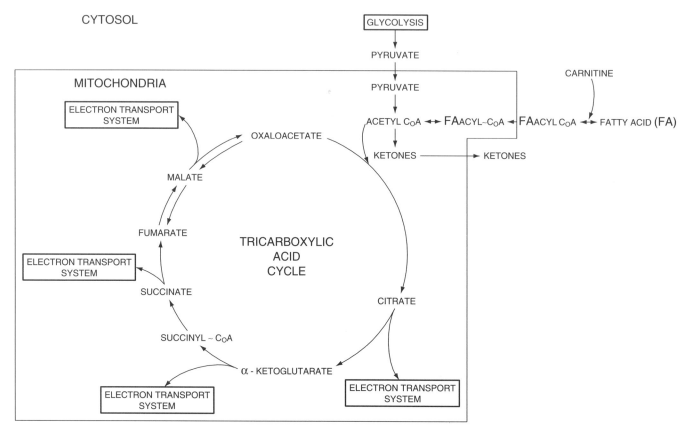

FIG. 1. Oxidation of carbohydrate and fat. (From Byers P. Trauma and nutritional support. In: Kreis DJ Jr, Gomez GA. *Trauma management.* Boston: Little, Brown, 1989:491–522.)

utilize pyruvate and lactate as substrate. Pyruvate is converted into oxalacetate and then to phosphoenolpyruvate prior to its final transformation into glucose. If this process continues, oxalacetate levels are depleted and thus unavailable for acetyl-CoA to enter the TCA cycle (Fig. 1). Lactate is reutilized via the Cori cycle. By recycling lactate and pyruvate, glucose stores are maintained at the expense of fatty acid oxidation in the liver.

In the fasting state, protein breakdown is favored, which acts to provide substrate for the formation of new glucose by gluconeogenesis (Fig. 2). In order for amino acids to be used in the synthesis of glucose, their amino groups must first be removed, which is accomplished by transamination with an alpha-keto acid. For example, alanine is deaminated in the liver to pyruvate, which can then be used in gluconeogenesis. The amino group is eliminated in the urine via the urea cycle.

Fatty acids are released by adipocytes during the fasting state and converted into acetyl units in the liver by beta-oxidation. The acetyl units are then converted into ketone bodies. Two molecules of acetyl-CoA combine to form acetoacetyl-CoA and then to acetoacetate or beta-hydroxybutyrate. Ketone body synthesis is favored during the fasting state due to the depletion of oxaloacetate during gluconeogenesis (Fig. 1). In the liver, ketone bodies are then exported for use by other tissues. Ketone bodies are broken down to acetyl-CoA, which can be used for energy generation by entry into the TCA cycle in the peripheral tissues. It has been found that cardiac muscle and the renal cortex use ketone bodies in preference to glucose. In starvation, 75% of the fuel needs of the brain are met by acetoacetate. This adaptation decreases the needs of the body for glucose, gluconeogenesis, and protein catabolism.

Starvation Metabolism

Starvation is defined as >3 days of fasting. It is perhaps the most common situation leading to compensatory changes in intermediary metabolism because of the obligate daily requirement for glucose. Hepatic glycogen stores are depleted after 24 to 72 hr, causing a decrease in serum glucose concentrations with a resultant drop in insulin secretion and an increase in glucagon secretion by the pancreas. This stimulates the breakdown of lipids into free fatty acids, which provides an ample energy source for the majority of peripheral tissues (Fig. 3).

Protein breakdown is the major source for the needed glucose. Lipid is a poor source of glucose, since only the

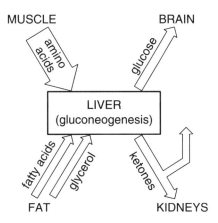

FIG. 2. Fasting metabolism. In early starvation, glycogenolysis, gluconeogenesis, and proteolysis are brisk. In fasting, protein breakdown for increased amino acids is favored. (From Wolfe BM, Ruderman RI, Pollard A. Principles of surgical nutrition: metabolic response to starvation, trauma, and sepsis. In: Dietel M, ed. *Nutrition in clinical surgery.* 2nd ed. Baltimore: Williams and Wilkins, 1985:13–18.)

glycerol portion of the triglyceride molecule can be utilized in the gluconeogenesis pathway. The breakdown of amino acids to their alpha-keto acid analogues allows them to be used for gluconeogenesis. Early in starvation, ~75 g/day of protein is catabolized. After a period of several days, the brain, which has the largest obligate requirement for glucose, is able to shift to the use of ketone bodies, thus decreasing the need for protein breakdown. Thus, protein breakdown drops to only 20 g/day. Ketone body transport across the blood-brain barrier is enhanced, allowing adaptation to occur (Fig. 3).

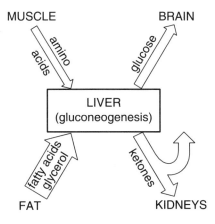

FIG. 3. Starvation metabolism. In late starvation, breakdown of protein and triglyceride must make up for the loss of glycogen reserves. Ketone body formation is prominent. The main energy source for liver and muscle shifts from glucose to fatty acids. (From Wolfe BM, Ruderman RI, Pollard A. Principles of surgical nutrition: metabolic response to starvation, trauma, and sepsis. In: Dietel M, ed. *Nutrition in clinical surgery.* 2nd ed. Baltimore: Williams and Wilkins, 1985:13–18.)

Sepsis and injury are characterized by a change in the hormonal environment that is responsible for the progressive alteration in the metabolism of substrates used for energy production. Energy requirements may increase dramatically, depending on the extent of injury or infection. The adaptations of protein, lipid, and carbohydrate metabolism are discussed in the following section.

Protein Metabolism

Skeletal muscle proteolysis and urinary nitrogen excretion are increased compared with the fasting state. Following trauma or sepsis, protein catabolism proceeds at a rate far exceeding synthesis at a time when nutritional intake is absent and metabolic demands are great. Markers of muscle proteolysis, urinary nitrogen and 3-methylhistidine, are markedly increased as a result of breakdown of muscle protein, leading to muscle wasting. The amino acids released are utilized for new protein synthesis, as oxidative fuels, or as substrate for gluconeogenesis. During stress, there is a great need for new protein synthesis by the liver, the bone marrow, and the wound. In the liver, acute-phase proteins are synthesized, which include the third component of complement, fibrinogen, C-reactive protein, and the antiproteases alpha-2-macroglobulin and alpha-1-antitrypsin. There is a reprioritization in the liver that allows for the synthesis of these crucial proteins from amino acids provided by skeletal muscle, while synthesis of less essential proteins such as albumin are put on hold. The amino acids are also used to produce glucose, the primary fuel of the cells infiltrating the wound. If new glucose could not be synthesized from protein, leukocyte dysfunction and overwhelming infection would occur. The high branch chain amino acids are utilized in their keto acid form as fuel in the periphery. Glutamine becomes the major oxidative fuel of the enterocyte and is felt to be conditionally essential during stress. In this way, protein catabolism is essential for survival in the initial phase of host stress (Fig. 4).

As sepsis worsens and organ failure develops, liver function often deteriorates. Amino acid clearance of the aromatic amino acids is impaired, and the plasma concentration of these amino acids rises. The aromatic amino acids may be metabolized to false neurotransmitters, which may compete with catecholamines for binding sites on sympathetic nerve terminals. This may lead to vasodilation, hypotension, and septic encephalopathy. Nitric oxide, a product of L-arginine, may also play a role in the hypotension of sepsis. As hepatic function worsens, acute-phase protein synthesis and synthesis of coagulation proteins are depressed.

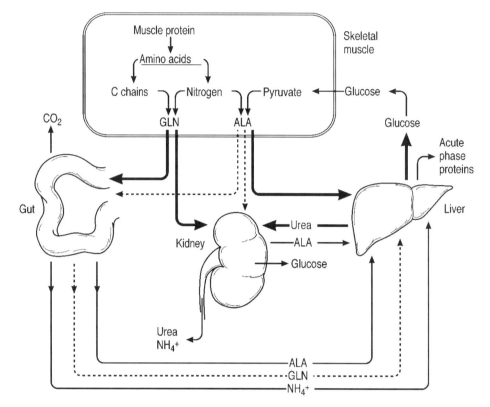

FIG. 4. Major catabolic pathways during stress metabolism. Protein catabolism supports energy requirements for peripheral muscle and intestinal mucosa, gluconeogenesis, and acute-phase protein synthesis. (Adapted from Souba WW Jr, Wilmore DW. Diet and nutrition in the care of the patient with surgery, trauma and sepsis. In: Shils ME, Olson JA, Shike M, eds. *Modern nutrition in health and disease*. 8th ed. Philadelphia: Lea and Febiger, 1994:1220.)

Lipid Metabolism

Lipid is increasingly used as a fuel source during stress to decrease the need for glucose utilization.

Lipid metabolism is altered in stress and sepsis. Endogenous lipids appear to act as a major fuel source in the septic traumatized patient. Marked elevation in triglycerides and increases in turnover rates of free fatty acids are noted. The elevated free fatty acid and glycerol production is thought to result from increased lipolysis due to elevated levels of catecholamine and cortisol and a marked elevation in the glucagon/insulin ratio. The free fatty acids are utilized for oxidation, ketone formation, or resynthesis of triglycerides.

Carbohydrate Metabolism

Glucose production by the liver increases, and peripheral glucose utilization is impaired.

Hyperglycemia is characteristically observed in the early and late periods after stress. Early hyperglycemia is related to an inhibition in pancreatic insulin release caused by elevated levels of epinephrine, as well as decreased pancreatic blood flow. This early hyperglycemia increases blood osmolarity and favors restoration of circulating blood volume.

Late hyperglycemia is characterized by elevated plasma catecholamines that favor gluconeogenesis. A marked increase in glucagon and insulin secretion and a rise in cortisol inhibit peripheral glucose use. The activity of the rate-limiting enzyme, pyruvate dehydrogenase, declines in sepsis. The rate at which pyruvate can be converted to acetyl-CoA and enter the TCA cycle in the peripheral tissues is diminished. This results in an increase of substrates, which are subsequently shuttled to the liver for gluconeogenesis. In both sepsis and stress, there is ongoing fatty acid oxidation despite the presence of high glucose concentrations.

Role of Cytokines in Intermediary Metabolism

Macrophage and monocyte cell products may be responsible for a number of the sequelae of infection and the development of septic syndromes. It is hypothesized that the translocation of bacteria and endotoxin from the intestinal lumen into the portal venous system, due to the loss of mucosal integrity during stress states, is one of the major stimuli for cytokine release. The monokines that seem to have the greatest metabolic effects are interleukin-1 (IL-1), tumor necrosis factor (TNF), and interleukin-6 (IL-6), all of which are primarily macrophage products. IL-1, or one of its breakdown products known as proteolysis inducing factor, stimulates skeletal muscle proteolysis with amino acid release in vitro as is seen in sepsis. IL-1 also produces an increase in the production of some hepatic acute-phase proteins including complement 3, with a subsequent decrease in albumin production. TNF is also involved in inhibiting albumin production while augmenting the production of the third component of the complement cascade. TNF has a significant effect on lipid metabolism through the inhibition of lipoprotein lipase, contributing to the hypertriglyceridemia of infection. IL-6 has been noted to play a significant role in hepatic acute-phase protein synthesis.

NUTRITIONAL ASSESSMENT

Adequate nutrition is essential for function, growth, and healing. Many patients cannot maintain optimal nutrient intake because of anorexia, depression, GI tract dysfunction, or endotracheal intubation. Additionally, catabolic stress and metabolic disorders alter nutritional requirements and utilization. The following section details the nutritional assessment for surgical patients as well as the basic components of therapy.

Nutritional Assessment

Although most patients do not require nutritional intervention, one must be aware of the factors that contribute to malnutrition in the hospitalized patient. In general, nutritional support should be considered in patients who have been without nutrition for 3 to 5 days. In a well-nourished individual, body stores are generally adequate to provide nutrients during shorter periods of stress without compromising physiologic functions, altering resistance to infection, or impairing wound healing. However, individuals with severe peritonitis, pancreatitis, major injury, or extensive burns are examples of patients that require immediate nutritional support. In addition, patients with poor nutritional reserves, characterized by a 10% weight loss at the time of admission, are at risk and should receive nutritional support. As weight loss approaches 30% of usual body weight, morbidity and mortality rapidly increase and approach 95%. Patients who initially do not meet one of these general indications should be reassessed every 3 to 5 days to determine whether nutritional intervention is needed.

The purpose of nutritional assessment is to determine the patient's nutritional reserves as well as predict nutritional requirements during hospitalization. The first step in assessing nutritional adequacy is the history and physical examination. One should document diet habits, weight loss, and whether or not there are any symptoms of early satiety. The physical examination should be done with special attention to signs of fat and muscle

TABLE 1. *Vitamins in human nutrition*

Vitamin	Coenzyme or active form	Deficiency	Daily requirements	
			RDA	Parenteral
Vitamin A	Retinol (in rhodopsin)	Xerophthalmia, keratomalacia, impaired epithelial integrity, hypogonadism	4,000–5,000 IU	3,300 IU
Vitamin D	1,25-dihydroxy-cholecalciferol	Rickets, osteomalacia	400 IU	200 IU
Vitamin E	α-Tocopherol	Hemolytic anemia, ataxia, nystagmus, loss of deep tendon reflexes, myopathy, edema	12–15 IU	10 IU
Vitamin K	Menaquinones	Coagulopathy	0.5–1.0 mg/kg	0.7–1 mg
Thiamine	Thiamin pyrophosphate	Wernicke's encephalopathy, peripheral neuropathy, beriberi, heart failure	1.0–1.5 mg	3.0 mg
Riboflavin	Flavin mononucleotide, flavin adenine dinucleotide	Dermatitis, glossitis, anemia, neuropathy, photophobia, lipid abnormalities	1.1–1.8 mg	3.6 mg
Niacin	Nicotinamide adenine	Pellagra (dermatitis, diarrhea, dementia, death)	12–20 mg	40 mg
Pantothenic acid	Coenzyme A	Erythromelalgia, altered mental status, GI complaints	5–10 mg	15 mg
Vitamin B_6	Pyridoxal phosphate	Sideroblastic anemia, pellagra, mucositis, peripheral neuropathy	1.6–2.0 mg	4.0 mg
Folate	Tetrahydrofolate	Megaloblastic anemia	200 µg	400 µg
Vitamin B_{12}	Cobalamine	Megaloblastic anemia, mental changes, periphal neuropathy	3.0 µg	5.0 µg
Vitamin C	Ascorbic acid	Scurvy, Sjögren's syndrome	45 mg	100 mg
Biotin	Biotinyl-lys-enzyme	Dermatitis, mucositis, GI complaints, altered mental status, paresthesias	0.50–300 µg	60 µg

TABLE 2. *Biochemical functions and manifestations of deficiency of essential trace elements*

Element	Key biochemical functions	Signs of deficiency
Zinc	Metabolism of lipids, protein, carbohydrates, and nucleic acids	Acrodermatitis enteropathica, hypogonadism
Chromium	Mediates insulin, effects membranes	Impaired glucose clearance
Cobalt	Methionine synthesis	Pernicious anemia, methylmalonicaciduria
Copper	Mitochondrial function, collagen metabolism, melanin formation	Menkes syndrome, anemia, leukopenia, neutropenia
Iodine	Cellular oxidation process	Thyroid diseases
Manganese	Oxidative phosphorylation; fatty acid metabolism; synthesis of proteins, mucopolysaccharides, and cholesterol	Defective growth, bony anomalies, reproductive dysfunction, central nervous system abnormalities
Molybdenum	Xanthine, hypoxanthine metabolism, cysteine metabolism as component of sulfite oxidase	Impaired urate clearance, mental disturbances
Selenium	Degradation of intracellular peroxides, oxidation of glutathione	Muscle pain, cardiomyopathy
Silicon	Connective tissue structure	Impaired bone function and composition

wasting and manifestations of vitamin, mineral, and essential fatty acid deficiency. These include skin rash, pallor, cheilosis, glossitis, gingival lesions, hepatomegaly, edema, Trousseau's sign, neuropathy, and dementia (Tables 1 and 2). The history and physical examination are effective tools in determining nutritional status. Anthropometric measurements, height, and weight are useful in monitoring patients requiring long-term nutritional support. Body weight is the most commonly used of these measures. Actual body weight should be interpreted relative to ideal weight and in view of current body fluid status. Anthropometric measures of limb size include mid-arm muscle circumference, which correlates with skeletal muscle mass, and triceps skin-fold thickness, which estimates subcutaneous fat stores. The 24-hr urinary creatinine is proportional to skeletal muscle mass and can also be used to monitor anabolism or catabolic loss of muscle stores. Visceral protein status is assessed by measuring the serum concentrations of selected hepatically synthesized transport proteins that have been shown to correlate with nutritional status (Table 3). These include albumin, transferrin, prealbumin, and retinol-binding protein. Depletion can be categorized as mild, moderate, or severe. Delayed hypersensitivity to skin testing is an additional sign that correlates with the adequacy of the visceral protein compartment.

Malnourished patients may be grouped into three categories. Patients with marasmus are malnourished due to a prolonged period of semistarvation; weight loss is

prominent, and anthropometric measurements are depressed. Typically, serum protein levels remain at normal levels, and skin tests are reactive. In contrast, hypoalbuminemic malnutrition or kwashiorkor-like syndrome develops rapidly in victims of trauma or sepsis as a consequence of severe metabolic stress. The serum albumin is typically <2.5 g/dl, and skin tests demonstrate anergy. Patients with mixed malnutrition usually are marasmic patients who are subjected to stress. The serum albumin of the marasmic patient falls dramatically in response to increased metabolic demands, and anergy becomes evident. These patients suffer the highest nutrition-related morbidity and mortality.

Energy Requirements

The simplest technique for estimating energy expenditure uses a kcal/kg approach. This method is limited in the edematous, obese, and elderly patient population.

Another, more accurate technique calculates the patient's basal energy expenditure (BEE) from the Harris-Benedict equations:

$$\text{BEE (women)} = 665 + (9.6\ W) + (1.7\ H) - (4.7\ A);$$

$$\text{BEE (men)} = 66 + (13.7\ W) + (5\ H) - (6.8\ A)$$

where W = weight in kg, H = height in cm, and A = age in years.

These equations better account for the decreasing metabolic rate seen with advancing age. However, as this

TABLE 3. *Protein markers*

Protein	Normal value	Mild deficiency	Moderate deficiency	Severe deficiency	$T^{1/2}$ (days)
Albumin g/dl	3.5–5.0	2.8–3.5	2.1–2.7	<2.1	20
Transferrin mg/dl	200–400	150–200	100–150	<100	8.5
Prealbumin mg/dl	21–40	15–20	11–15	<11	1.3

is a resting, basal calculation, stress factors must be used to adjust for stress states or anabolism.

Finally, one may calculate energy expenditure from measured oxygen consumption and CO_2 production, a technique known as indirect calorimetry. Oxygen consumption and CO_2 production are measured as the patient breathes into a spirometer where immediate gas analysis is performed. Energy expenditure is calculated according to the following equation:

$$\text{Metabolic rate} = [(3.9) \times VO_2 \text{ (L/min)}] + 1.1 \times VCO_2 \text{ (L/min)}] \times 60(\text{min/hr}) \; // \; \text{Body area (M}^2)$$

where VO_2 = oxygen consumption; VCO_2 = CO_2 consumption; L = liters; m^2 = meters squared. This technique allows for the calculation of the metabolic rate in $kcal/m^2/hr$ and also defines the substrate utilization patterns through the respiratory quotient (RQ). The RQ is the ratio of CO_2 production to oxygen consumption. The RQ of glucose oxidation is 1.0, that of fat is 0.7, and that of protein is 0.8. Decreasing the RQ may aid in ventilatory weaning because of decreased CO_2. Although indirect calorimetry is an accurate technique, it is labor intensive and expensive.

Estimating energy requirements for the patient who is starving mandates the development of a plan that slowly increases the level of support to avoid the occurrence of the refeeding syndrome. Rapid refeeding can result in fluid overload, hypokalemia, and hypophosphatemia. Initially, in starvation, only 80% of the kilocalories predicted by the BEE, or usually 20 kcal/kg/day, should be administered. After the patient has converted from a catabolic to an anabolic state, energy requirements can slowly be increased to anabolic levels. When anabolism is the goal, the nonprotein calories administered should approximate 1.75 times the BEE.

Nonprotein calories may be supplied as carbohydrate or fat. When carbohydrate is ingested orally, it supplies 4 kcal of energy per gram of substrate. However, when it is given intravenously, only 3.4 kcal/g are available. Limited carbohydrate reserves consist of 300 g of glycogen stored in both skeletal muscle and liver. These stores are depleted in 24 to 72 hr during fasting and may be depleted in as little as 6 hr during periods of stress due to increased energy needs. Stressed patients exhibit a maximum glucose oxidation rate of 3 to 5 mg/kg/min, regardless of the quantity infused. Their needs may be approximated by multiplying a stress factor of 1.3 to 1.5 by the calculated BEE. Seventy to 80% of the nonprotein calories should be supplied as carbohydrate. A conservative estimate of energy needs should be used, as excessive exogenous glucose may contribute to fatty liver and abnormal liver function tests. Hepatic failure may occur in patients dependent on long-term parenteral feedings.

Another source of nonprotein calories is lipid. Fat is a high-density energy source that supplies 9 kcal/g of substrate. Fatty acids are a major fuel of the heart, liver, and skeletal muscle. During stress or anabolism, 20% to 30% of calories should be supplied as lipid.

Protein Requirements

Although there are ~14 kg of protein in a 70-kg adult, only 7 kg are in a state of dynamic flux and contribute to the amino acid pool. It must be remembered that the use of endogenous protein as fuel compromises structure and function, as there are no available reserves. Protein supplies 4 kcal/g of energy, and 6.25 g of protein are needed to supply 1 g of nitrogen. Twenty common amino acids comprise most dietary proteins. There are eight essential amino acids (isoleucine, leucine, valine, lysine, methionine, phenylalanine, threonine, and tryptophan), which must be supplied from exogenous sources. The daily oral protein requirement of unstressed adults is ~0.8 g/kg/day. Children and critically ill patients require up to 2.5 g/kg/day.

Recognizing that proteins and amino acids are in dynamic equilibrium, global nitrogen balance can be calculated from total input and output and used for adjusting protein support in patients with metabolic stress:

$$\text{Nitrogen balance} = \frac{\text{Dietary protein(g)} -}{6.25} \\ [(\text{UUN(g)} + \text{GI losses(g)} + \text{cutaneous losses(g)}]$$

where UUN is urinary urea nitrogen measured in grams in a 24-hr collection. Two to 4 g of nitrogen are added to the urinary nitrogen to account for GI losses and 0 to 4 g for cutaneous losses. In stressed states, a correction factor must be added, as the UUN only accounts for 80% of the total urinary nitrogen. Measurements should be performed weekly in complicated patients.

Nitrogen balance depends not only upon the quantity of nitrogen intake, but also upon potassium, magnesium, phosphate, and vitamin intake. Of greatest importance is the intake of adequate nonprotein calories. A desirable kilocalorie/nitrogen ratio in unstressed states approximates 150:1. During stress, more nitrogen is required as protein is utilized for fuel, and the kilocalorie/nitrogen ratio is reduced to 100:1.

Vitamins, minerals, and trace elements are essential to many metabolic processes (Tables 1 and 2). Most vitamins are enzyme cofactors. During deprivation or stress, most water-soluble vitamins are prone to depletion because body stores are small. Calcium is the most abundant cation in the body and plays a vital role in muscular and cardiac contractility, neuromuscular excitability, coagulation, and membrane permeability. The Recommended Daily Allowance (RDA) for calcium is 800 mg/day, but increases to 1.2 to 1.5 g/day in adolescents and postmenopausal women because of bone growth and poor calcium balance. Normal adults absorb 30% to 50% of dietary calcium.

Magnesium is the second most abundant intracellular cation and serves as a cofactor for innumerable enzymes and as a regulator of membrane permeability and neuromuscular excitability. Normal serum levels are 1.5 to 2.5 meq/L. The RDA for magnesium is 300 to 350 mg/day, of which 40% of an oral dose is absorbed.

Iron is an abundant metal, which is vital for aerobic metabolism. It has a role in the functional groups of the Krebs cycle enzymes, is an electron carrier in cytochromes, and transports O_2 and CO_2 in hemoglobin. The average daily intake of iron in North America and Europe is between 10 and 30 mg. Its absorption is dependent on gastric acid, with the most efficient absorption occurring in the duodenum.

Essential trace elements include the minerals zinc, manganese, cobalt, chromium, copper, molybdenum, selenium, and iodine. Alcoholics and patients with malabsorption are at risk for zinc deficiency. Selenium deficiency may result in muscle pains and cardiomyopathy. Other deficiency states of trace elements may present as multiple organ dysfunction or with a variety of skin lesions (Table 2).

ENTERAL NUTRITION

Safe Use of the Gastrointestinal Tract for Feeding

Enteral nutrition is the provision of nutrient diets by mouth or tube into the GI tract. Enteral feeding is applicable to essentially all patients with intact GI function and should be the first method considered because of increased efficacy. A partial listing of the indications for enteral nutrition include protein-calorie malnutrition, severe anorexia, major full-thickness burns, low-output enterocutaneous fistulas, major trauma, and critical illness. Enteral feeding cannot be used safely in patients with hemodynamic instability, enteric losses of >1,000 ml/24 hr, or massive GI bleeding. Examples of conditions that preclude the use of enteral nutrition are intestinal obstruction and paralytic ileus. Problems due to gastric ileus can be overcome with transpyloric passage of the feeding tube. In the absence of excessively high GI output, abdominal distention, and massive GI bleeding, a trial of enteral nutrition is warranted to determine if the GI tract can be used safely for feeding.

Enteral Formulas

Before delivery of enteral nutrition, the appropriate diet must be selected on the basis of the patient's nutrient requirements. Most liquid formula diets are either polymeric or chemically defined. Balanced polymeric diets contain carbohydrates, proteins, and fats in complex forms in proportions similar to those of a regular Western diet, with ~30% of the calories supplied by fat. In general, they are isotonic, lactose free, and inexpensive.

Chemically defined or modified diets generally contain monomeric or short-chain hydrolysate products of protein and carbohydrate macronutrients, with the predominant calorie source as carbohydrate. The fat-to-carbohydrate ratio varies depending on the purpose of the modification. These formulas are hyperosmolar, unpalatable, expensive, and poorly tolerated in the glucose-intolerant patient. They are indicated for patients with partial intestinal function as may occur in inflammatory bowel disease, pancreatitis, short-bowel syndrome, radiation enteritis, bowel resection, and severe burns.

Finally, in addition to polymeric and chemically defined diets, there are modular formulas that provide one or two macronutrients only, with no micronutrients. Protein, carbohydrate, and fat modules are available to customize shelf products.

There are also disease-specific formulas for use in patients with glucose intolerance, hepatic failure, or renal insufficiency. New immunomodulary formulas have been developed that contain increased amounts of glutamine, arginine, omega-3 fatty acids, and nucleic acids. These formulas are quite expensive and need further evaluation to determine indications for their use.

Assessment of Feeding Tolerance and Feeding Regimens

The selected formula may be started at isotonicity and delivered continuously at 25 to 30 ml/hr for the first 12 to 24 hr as feeding tolerance is assessed. Poor tolerance is indicated by vomiting and severe abdominal cramps, gastric residual of >200 ml, abdominal distention, and worsening of diarrhea. If the residual volume is large, as is the case with gastric atony, a nasoduodenal or nasojejunal tube should be placed. If the patient develops diarrhea, the loose stools may be controlled with antidiarrheals. When crampy pain or distension is present, tube feedings should be discontinued and parenteral nutrition initiated.

Patients fed into the stomach may receive an isotonic balanced formula. The rate of delivery is advanced each 12 to 24 hr. Patients fed into the small intestine should initiallly receive an elemental formula at full strength delivered with the aid of a peristaltic pump. Tube feedings may be started at a rate of 20 to 30 ml/hr initially and then gradually increased every 12 to 24 hr.

Feeding Access

In critically ill patients, access for enteral feeding is most commonly via the stomach, duodenum, or jejunum. If there is no evidence of intolerance, the patient is assessed for risk of aspiration. If the risk of aspiration is minimal, intragastric feedings are preferred. Methods of access for intragastric feeding include small caliber nasogastric tubes and feeding gastrostomies placed endoscopically or during laparotomy. The major advantages of gastric feedings are that the stomach tolerates higher osmolar loads and permits bolus feeding. The higher risk of aspiration is the major disadvantage.

Patients with feeding tubes placed into the small intestine have a reduced risk of aspiration, can be fed distal to a fistula or obstruction, and can be fed despite gastric atony. Disadvantages to small bowel feedings include low tolerance to high osmolar loads and intolerance to bolus feeding. These feedings require the use of a peristaltic pump and frequent irrigation of the feeding tube with water to maintain patency. This method is preferred in acutely ill patients and and in patients receiving nocturnal feedings.

Monitoring and Prevention of Complications

In patients receiving enteral nutrition, particular attention must be directed to the patient's metabolic status, GI function, and fluid and electrolyte balance. A typical protocol for monitoring includes physical examination of the abdomen, the recording of input and output, weights, and laboratory studies including electrolytes, magnesium, calcium, phosphorus, albumin, and prealbumin.

There are four major classifications of complications that are related to enteral nutrition: metabolic, GI, mechanical, and infectious. Metabolic complications include hyperglycemia, hypoglycememia, hyperosmolar nonketotic coma, undernutrition, overfeeding, sodium imbalance, and hypophosphatemia. Hyperglycemia may occur with low-fat formulas and is most easily treated by changing to formulas that provide 40% to 50% of the calories as fat. It may also be necessary to add insulin to the patient's regimen. Hypoglycemia may occur with sudden cessation of tube feedings. Hyperosmolar nonketotic coma may occur in patients who are fed with hyperosmolar formulas and have an unappreciated volume loss, usually secondary to glycosuria. Sodium imbalance is most commonly seen when there is either free water excess or depletion and is adjusted with correction of the free water imbalance. Serum phosphorous should always be measured and repleted in those patients with severe malnutrition who are initiated on enteral or parenteral feedings.

The most frequent GI complication is diarrhea, which may occur in as many as 75% of critically ill patients receiving enteral nutrition. Diarrhea is defined as >300 g/day of stool or more than three large, loose bowel movements daily. The stools should initially be checked for *Clostridium difficile* toxin. Patients with *C. difficile* colitis may also present with leukocytosis and abdominal pain or distention. One week of oral metronidazole is usually curative. In the absence of *C. difficile*, the desired

therapeutic approach is initially to treat with an antidiarrheal agent and adjust the enteral regimen accordingly. Osmolarity, volume, rate, and type of diet may be altered with subsequent observation for improvement.

Enteral feedings may prevent peptic ulcerations and bleeding. Patients who are fed directly into the stomach should not require H_2 blockers, since the liquid formula provides a physiologic means of buffering acid. However, this effect has also been reported in jejunal feedings. The amino acid glutamine may also be administered to prevent mucosal ulceration of the upper GI tract.

The most common mechanical complications that are related to enteral nutrition are tube dislodgment, clogging of the tube, and leakage of enteric contents around the exit site of the tube onto the skin. Tube dislodgement is catastrophic and is associated with peritonitis and occasionally the development fistulae. Tubes that are displaced should be replaced immediately with radiographic confirmation of appropriate placement prior to use. Another catastrophic complication of jejunostomy tubes is intestinal volvulus and infarction. This should be suspected whenever abdominal distention occurs in a patient receiving jejunostomy tube feedings. Clogging or plugging of the feeding tube is reduced by routine irrigations with normal saline or water. The injection of a small volume of carbonated beverage into a plugged tube will sometimes clear the blockage. Leakage around the tube can usually be treated by replacing it with a smaller catheter that allows for contraction. The skin should be protected with powders and paste.

Aspiration is a major infectious complication in patients receiving enteral nutrition. The propensity to aspirate enteral feedings is often related to the patient's primary disease, neurologic status, the site of GI access, and the method of delivery. Important factors in assessing risk for aspiration include depressed sensorium, increased gastroesophegal reflux, and history of previously documented episodes of aspiration. Nasogastric intubation may render the upper and lower esophageal sphincter incompetent and prone to reflux. For most enterally fed patients, safety demands that the head be elevated at feeding time and for some period thereafter to prevent regurgitation. Gastric residuals should be measured and feedings held if they >200 ml. Aspiration of liquid formulas can be verified if a bit of food coloring or methylene blue is included in the feeding mixture and subsequently detected in pharyngeal or tracheal secretions.

PARENTERAL NUTRITION

In general, parenteral nutrition is administered to patients who require nutritional support but in whom the GI tract is nonfunctional. Parenteral nutrition allows for the infusion of high osmolar solutions in low volumes and creates a state of precise control of daily nutrient intake. However, these advantages must be balanced by the need for central venous catheter placement, the high cost of both materials and personnel, the high incidence of complications, and the nonphysiologic delivery of nutrients bypassing intestinal and hepatic metabolism.

Indications for Total Parenteral Nutrition

Clinical settings in which parenteral nutrition is indicated as a part of routine care include patients with an inability to absorb nutrients due to radiation enteritis, severe inflammatory bowel disease, diarrhea, and intractable vomiting. An additional indication for total parenteral nutrition (TPN) is severe malnutrition in the face of a nonfunctional GI tract as may occur in association with high-dose chemotherapy, bone marrow transplantation, moderate to severe pancreatitis, and high-output enterocutaneous fistulas. Patients with intestinal failure may require long-term parenteral nutrition at home as nocturnal cyclic feedings. Any patient who requires nutritional support and fails enteral feedings should have parenteral nutrition instituted promptly, but parenteral feedings should never be utilized as a substitute for enteral feedings in patients with GI function. However, once initiated, parenteral feedings should not be discontinued until adequate enteral caloric intake and absorption is documented.

Parenteral Solutions

Standard parenteral solutions are combinations of 50% dextrose solutions with a caloric density of 3.4 kcal/g and 10% amino acid mixtures with a caloric density of 4 kcal/g. These are mixed in varying amounts, and electrolytes, vitamins, and trace elements are added. New computerized systems permit a wide variety of dextrose and amino acid concentrations. Each day, from 1 to 4 L of solution can be infused via a central venous catheter.

Sodium and potassium salts are added as chloride or acetate, depending on the acid-base status of the patient. Sodium bicarbonate is incompatible with the nutrient solutions, thus acetate is administered when additional base is required. Trace elements are given routinely to all patients except those with renal failure or severe liver disease. Alcoholics and patients with malabsorption may require additional zinc supplementation. Although the main excretory route for zinc and chromium is via the feces, renal excretion will minimize dangers from modest excesses of these elements. In patients with renal insufficiency, daily zinc and chromium administration may be contraindicated. Copper and manganese are excreted primarily via the biliary tract; therefore, they should be avoided in patients with biliary tract obstruction. Iron is

contraindicated in patients with sepsis due to its support of bacterial growth. Selenium affects lipid peroxidation of polyunsaturated fatty acids in cell membranes and should be administered in all patients with severe malnutrition or long-term parenteral support.

Administration of fat emulsion daily or twice weekly meets essential fatty acid requirements and provides additional kilocalories at 9 kcal/g. No more than 30% of the daily caloric requirement should be supplied as lipid. Lipid is available in either 10% or 20% emulsions and should be infused over 12 hr.

Slightly hypertonic nutrient solutions can be prepared for peripheral venous infusion. These commonly consist of 4.5% amino acids and 7% to 10% dextrose with additional calories supplied by the administration of fat emulsion. This system is capable of supplying 550 to 2,000 kcal/day. With mild stress, body protein mass is somewhat preserved, although the patient continues to be catabolic. Peripheral venous feeding provides minimal nutrition temporarily during periods of decreased or absent enteral intake. Indications for peripheral feeding include short periods of mild stress and starvation (<10 days), temporary support following an episode of catheter sepsis prior to insertion of a new central catheter, and as supplementation while increasing to full enteral support.

Benefits of peripheral parenteral nutrition include less complicated monitoring protocols and the lack of risk associated with central venous catheter insertion and maintenance. However, due to the moderate nitrogen load and caloric concentration, patients must tolerate 2 to 3 L/day of fluid. Patients rarely receive maximum caloric intake due to peripheral venous access problems that occur with rapid infusion. Peripheral venous solutions are contraindicated in patients with fluid restriction such as those with renal failure or hepatic insufficiency.

General Guidelines for Metabolic Monitoring

Patients receiving central venous feedings should be weighed daily, and have accurate intake and output records maintained. Urinary glucose and ketones should be monitored every 6 hr. Persistent glycosuria indicates hyperglycemia and may be associated with a concomitant osmotic diuresis and dehydration. Hyperglycemia should be treated with a sliding scale of regular insulin. Half to two-thirds the quantity of insulin administered should be added to the next day's bag of solution. Laboratory studies, including electrolytes, liver function tests, prealbumin levels, and calcium, phosphorous, and magnesium levels, should be measured frequently at first and then weekly. In stable home TPN patients, they may be evaluated monthly.

Nitrogen balance should be calculated weekly, and a 24-hr urinary creatinine should be measured in those patients who are on an anabolic regimen. Nitrogen balance reflects the extent of catabolism that is ongoing, while the creatinine height index reflects the extent of erosion or increase in lean body mass. A repeat nutritional assessment at weekly intervals should be performed in hospitalized patients.

The quantity of energy administered should maintain lean body mass and adipose tissue. If sustained weight loss occurs, or the creatinine height index decreases, caloric intake may be inadequate, and an additional 500 kcal should be administered. However, if there is an excessive weight gain of >1 lb/week despite a stable fluid balance, caloric support should be decreased.

Complications of Parenteral Nutrition

Complications of parenteral nutrition include those related to line placement, indwelling lines, metabolic disturbances, and GI derangements. The most common complications related to line placement are arrythmias and pneumothorax. However, during line placement, any adjacent structure may be injured and result in arterial laceration, brachial plexus injury, hemothorax, hydrothorax, chylothorax, and subclavian vein thrombosis. Another complication that may occur either during line placement or removal is air embolus. The risk is minimized by hydrating the patient and performing the procedure in the Trendelenberg position.

The most serious problem associated with indwelling central venous catheters is sepsis, and the incidence is between 4% and 5% in hospitalized patients. Primary catheter sepsis is diagnosed when there are signs and symptoms of infection and the indwelling catheter is found to be the only anatomic focus. After removal of the catheter, the symptoms usually attenuate. Cultures of the intracutaneous segment with semiquantitative techniques yield >15 colony-forming units per milliliter. The most common bacterial organisms causing catheter sepsis are the skin contaminants *Staphyococcus epidermis* and *S. aureus, Klebsiella pneumoniae,* and *Candida albicans.* Secondary catheter infection is associated with a separate infectious focus that causes bacteria and seeds or contaminates the catheter.

A wide variety of metabolic complications may occur during parenteral feeding. The most common are hyperglycemia, glycosuria, and nonketotic hyperosmolar coma. Although vitamin D levels are usually normal, hypercalciuria may accompany amino acid infusions. Other metabolic complications include deficiencies of vitamins, minerals, electrolytes, trace metals, and essential fatty acids. Hepatic dysfunction and fatty infiltration are commonly seen with overfeeding. Liver function tests are elevated secondary to amino acid imbalance or to excessive deposition of glycogen or fat in the liver. Cholestasis, cholelithiasis, or acalculous cholecystitis may develop in as many as one-third of

long-term TPN patients. These complications may be avoided by the administration of ursodeoxycholic acid or by the maintenance of a slow infusion of enteral feedings. Concomitant enteral feedings will also prevent the development of gut mucosal atrophy, which occurs in patients on parenteral feedings.

SUMMARY

Early fasting is characterized by increased catabolism due to a significant requirement for glucose as substrate, while prolonged starvation is characterized by adaptation, increased utilization of adipose tissue, and protein sparing. This adaptation does not occur in the presence of stress or sepsis. Despite the increased utilization of lipid substrate, protein catabolism proceeds at a rapid rate in order to expand the amino acid pool to provide building blocks for acute-phase proteins, immune functions, and wound healing. The mediators of these processes include corticosteroids, catecholamines, and cytokines.

Patients at risk for malnutrition due to periods of inadequate nutrient intake or increased metabolic rate need detailed nutritional assessment along with the institution of rapid and aggressive nutritional therapy. During the last decade, it has been increasingly clear that enteral support, when feasible, is far more efficacious than parenteral support. This may be due to the presence of glutamine in enteral feedings and its absence in parenteral solutions. Nevertheless, in patients with intestinal failure, TPN is life-saving and may be necessary for weeks, months, or years. Regardless of the nutritional support administered, the prescriber must perform ongoing monitoring and be aware of the inherent complications associated with therapy.

STUDY QUESTIONS

1. Discuss your plan of nutritional support for the following patients: (a) 25-year-old male with acute pancreatitis; (b) 32-year-old female following a car accident with a closed head injury; (c) 72-year-old female admitted with biliary pancreatitis and scheduled for a laparoscopic cholecystectomy in 3 or 4 days.
2. Discuss the adaptation of carbohydrate, protein, and fat metabolism during mediastinitis from an esophageal anastomotic leak.
3. A 54-year-old alcoholic presents with anemia, dermatitis, mucositis, and altered mental status. Discuss the possible nutritional etiology of these symptoms.
4. Discuss the risks and benefits of perioperative TPN.
5. A patient who is receiving tube feeds begins to have diarrhea. How would you evaluate and treat this common problem?

SUGGESTED READING

Askanazi J, Carpentier YA, Elwin DH, et al. Influence of total parenteral nutrition on fuel utilization in injury and sepsis. *Ann Surg* 1980;191:40.

Cahill G Jr. Starvation in man. *N Engl J Med* 1970;282:668.

Mainous MR, Dietch EA. Nutrition and infection. *Surg Clin North Am* 1994;74:659.

Moore FD. *Metabolic care of the surgical patient.* Philadelphia: Saunders, 1959.

Rombeau JL, Rolandelli RH, Wilmore DW. Nutrition support. *Sci Am* 1994.

Wolman SL, Anderson GH, Marliss EB, et al. Zinc in total parenteral nutrition: requirements and metabolic effects. *Gastroenterology* 1979;76: 458.

CHAPTER 5

Fluids and Electrolytes in the Surgical Patient: The Basics

John H. Armstrong, Eduardo Parra-Davila, and Danny Sleeman

The paths of physiology and surgery cross in the discussion of fluids and electrolytes. The surgical disease processes themselves, as well as the body's response to the stress of anesthesia and surgery, make this management essential for the care of surgical patients. Understanding begins with a description of the normal fluid physiology defined by functional fluid compartments separated by membranes.

FUNCTIONAL FLUID COMPARTMENTS

The body is a compartmentalized water sac: roughly half of body weight is comprised of water, 60% of kilogram body weight in males and 50% in females. In infants, 75% of body weight is water, decreasing to the adult percentage by 1 year of age. Fat contains little water; thus, an obese person has less proportionate water than a

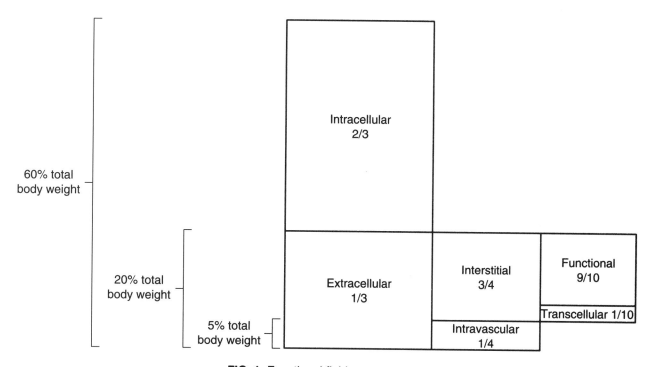

FIG. 1. Functional fluid compartments.

41

lean individual. Fluid compartments are described as percentages of body water or body weight, and have been defined through a variety of fluid dilution techniques.

Body water is divided into two-thirds intracellular and one-third extracellular fluid compartments, or 40% (two-thirds of 60%) and 20% (one-third of 60%) of body weight, respectively. The extracellular fluid compartment is further subdivided into interstitial (extravascular) and plasma (intravascular) fluid compartments, which translates into 15% and 5% of body weight, respectively. The interstitial compartment volume includes a functional space of 90%, which equilibrates rapidly between cells and capillary membranes, and a nonfunctional (transcellular) space of 10%, made up of connective tissue, and cerebrospinal and joint space fluids (Fig. 1).

COMPARTMENT COMPOSITION

Fluid compartments are bordered by cell membranes, which are completely permeable to water but vary in solute permeability and active transport mechanisms. Thus, fluid spaces have different ionic compositions. The principal intracellular cations (positively charged ions) are potassium and magnesium, with proteins and phosphates comprising the dominant intracellular anions (negatively charged ions). Sodium is the principal extracellular cation and best reflects the body's water balance; chloride and bicarbonate are the extracellular anions.

Electrical neutrality is maintained within each specific fluid compartment, meaning that the sum of the cations must equal the sum of the anions. This is commonly expressed using the term "milliequivalents," which refers to the chemical combining activity of electrolytes (number of electrical charges per liter). In any fluid compartment, the number of milliequivalents of cations equals the number of milliequivalents of anions. However, across fluid compartments, the concentrations of an individual ion do not need to be the same, and electrical neutrality does not need to be maintained: selective permeabilities and transport properties of membranes determine composition. For example, across the capillary membrane (which separates the interstitial fluid compartment from the plasma compartment), plasma proteins (anions) are not freely permeable. The resolution of concentration gradients (equilibrium) results in relatively greater plasma concentrations of cations and decreased plasma concentrations of diffusible anions. Electrical neutrality is maintained across capillary membranes. In contrast, an electrical potential difference is generated across cell membranes based on electrolyte concentration differentials between the intracellular fluid compartment and the interstitial compartment and is maintained by the Na^+–K^+ ATPases. This preserves intracellular electrical neutrality.

COMPARTMENT VOLUME

Osmolality refers to the number of osmotically active particles in solution and accounts for solute dissociation. For example, 1 mmol of sodium chloride dissociates into sodium and chloride, and contributes 2 mOsm to fluid osmolality. Water is freely permeable across cell membranes and equilibrates osmolality between compartments (normal osmolality = 290 to 310 mOsm/L). Thus, the volume of each compartment reflects the content of osmotically active particles, including electrolytes, proteins, and sugars. Substances within a compartment that fail to pass through the semipermeable membrane create an effective osmotic pressure that draws water into that compartment. Plasma proteins (colloid) are nonpermeable, and effect a colloid osmotic pressure between the plasma and interstitial extracellular fluid compartments. Sodium regulates an effective oncotic pressure between the extracellular and intracellular fluid compartments. Again, because water follows the osmotic gradients freely between compartments, the effective oncotic pressure is equal within these compartments. Plasma osmolality (P_{osm}) can be calculated from serum sodium (Na^+), glucose, and blood urea nitrogen (BUN) as follows:

$$P_{osm} = 2[Na^+] + glucose/18 + BUN/2.8$$

REGULATION OF FLUIDS AND ELECTROLYTES

To achieve fluid and electrolyte balance, the output of water and electrolytes must match (and will reflect the composition of) intake (Fig. 2). Regulation of this output occurs predominantly via the kidney, interacting with the neuroendocrine and circulatory systems. So first, let's take a look at the world according to the kidney.

The kidney developed through evolution first to conserve salt for the internal saltwater milieu, then to excrete free water in the form of hypotonic urine, and finally to conserve free water. The path of urine through the nephron follows this evolution of purposes. Fluid and electrolyte balance is maintained by reabsorption of a large quantity of glomerular filtrate by the renal tubules prior to excretion. Urine is plasma-based, an ultrafiltrate that is then further processed through the tubular pathway of the nephron to reflect the fluid needs of the body.

It leaves the glomerular capillary tuft into Bowman's capsule as an ultrafiltrate and undergoes isosomotic fluid reabsorption in the proximal tubule. Sodium is actively transported with chloride, bicarbonate, glucose, and amino acids; water accompanies sodium. The rate of delivery of ultrafiltrate, known as glomerular filtration rate (GFR), and the rate of proximal tubule reabsorption determine the rate of sodium and water delivery to the distal nephron: decreased GFR or increased proximal

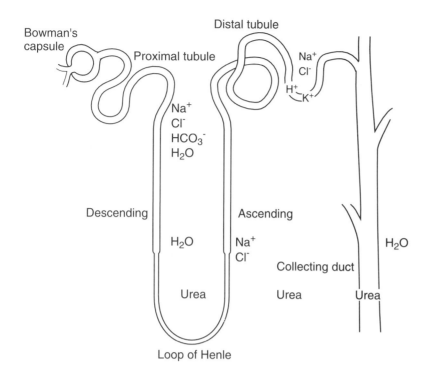

FIG. 2. The journey of urine through the kidney, with reabsorption of sodium and water, and secretion of acid and potassium. Substances reabsorbed are shown outside the tubule; those secreted are inside.

tubular reabsorption reduces the delivery of tubular fluid to the distal diluting segments of the nephron.

Next on its journey is the loop of Henle, which concentrates the urine. This occurs because of the differential permeabilities and transport characteristics of the descending versus ascending limbs of the loop, coupled with the medullary concentration gradient that results from the concentration scaffolding of the hairpin vasa recta. The descending limb is permeable to water but not to sodium; on the other hand, the ascending limb actively transports sodium chloride. Urea plays an essential role in maintaining the medullary concentration gradient, this gradient being trapped by the countercurrent mechanism of the vasa recta. In the descending limb, water is extracted through osmosis by this urea gradient, and when the urine enters the ascending limb, now relatively rich in sodium chloride, sodium chloride moves passively down its concentration gradient without water, leaving tubule fluid relatively hyposmotic to the surrounding interstitium.

The distal tubule further dilutes the tubular fluid by reabsorbing sodium without water. By the time the tubular fluid has reached the distal tubule, >90% of sodium has been reabsorbed; thus, the distal tubule is the fine regulator of sodium reabsorption, influenced by aldosterone and done initially with chloride and then in exchange for potassium or hydrogen (note that acid secretion generates bicarbonate). This illustrates the principle of electroneutral exchange, either through co-transport of cation/anion or through cation exchange. Aldosterone is secreted in response to the renin-angiotensin system,

adrenocorticotropic hormone (ACTH), and increased plasma potassium. Renin is secreted by the renal juxtaglomerular apparatus in response to tubular fluid flow as well as sodium and chloride sensed by the macula densa receptor of the distal tubule. A vascular stretch receptor and B-adrenergic receptor on the juxtaglomerular apparatus also promote renin secretion. Renin cleaves angiotensinogen from the liver into angiotensin I; this, in turn, is converted by angiotensin-converting enzyme to angiotensin II. In addition to stimulating aldosterone release, angiotensin II is a potent vasoconstrictor.

The last part of the tubular fluid journey is the collecting duct, which ultimately regulates urine tonicity by modulating water reabsorption under the direction of antidiuretic hormone (ADH), also known as vasopressin. Urine osmolality varies between 50 and 1,200 mOsm. ADH is secreted from the posterior pituitary under neural control by two mechanisms: more sensitive osmotic regulation via osmoreceptors that reflect cell volume in the hypothalamus, and more potent nonosmotic regulation via automotic neural tone, which reflects volume. Potassium secretion occurs in the collecting duct as well and is augmented by high tubular flow rates and alkalosis.

BODY'S ASSESSMENT OF VOLUME STATUS

The kidney is the major volume and electrolyte regulator of the body. It avidly retains sodium, usually in exchange for potassium or acid to maintain electrical

TABLE 1. *Differentiation of oliguria (low urine output)*[a]

Index	Prerenal	Renal
Urine sodium	<20 meq/L	>30 meq/L
Urine osmolality	>500 mOsm/L	<350 mOsm/L
Fractional excretion of sodium		
Urine[Na^+]/plasma[Na^+] × 100	<1	>1.5
Urine[creatinine]/plasma[cr]	—	—
BUN/serum creatinine	>20	<10

[a]The most common differentiation of oliguria is between prerenal and renal causes. Analysis of urine sodium, creatinine, and osmolality, in comparison with serum values, can be very helpful.

neutrality across the renal tubular membrane. Sodium is regulated neurohormonally by the renin-angiotensin-aldosterone system through the juxtaglomerular apparatus. Plasma osmolality is monitored by osmoreceptors near the hypothalamic ventricles in the CNS; an increase results in the secretion of ADH and stimulation of thirst. Intravascular volume is also monitored by baroreceptors in the carotid arteries, aorta, and atria.

CLINICAL ASSESSMENT OF VOLUME STATUS

The adequacy of fluid replacement is assessed predominantly by hemodynamic profile (pulse, blood pressure) and by evidence of adequate tissue perfusion. Urine output reflects renal perfusion and should be 0.5 cc/kg/hr in the adult. It can be easily measured by collecting bottles or indwelling catheter collecting systems (e.g., Foley catheter). Low urine output (oliguria) is defined as <400 cc of urine/day. Causes may be inadequate renal perfusion, due to hypovolemia or low cardiac output (prerenal), nonfunctional renal parenchyma (renal), or renal outlet obstruction, such as bladder neck or urethral obstruction (postrenal). This differentiation is imperative for fluid management: for example, prerenal hypovolemia requires further fluid administration, whereas acute renal failure requires fluid restriction. Differentiation of prerenal from renal failure can be made using a variety of diagnostic indices that are obtained or calculated using measurements of serum and urine (Table 1). These values reflect the underlying pathophysiology: in prerenal oliguria, the kidneys respond appropriately to the reduction in circulating volume by retaining sodium and water; thus, the urine is concentrated, and the urine sodium concentration is low. In contrast, the renal tubules do not function in renal failure, and a marked reduction in glomerular filtration occurs. Therefore, any urine that is formed has not been modified and reflects plasma osmolality and an inability to retain sodium. Many physicians send urine electrolytes only to find that they are uninterpretable. Urine electrolytes are useful for volume assessment only in oliguric patients, not in patients with normal urine values.

BODY FLUID CHANGES

Disorders in fluid and electrolyte balance can be grouped into three categories: volume, concentration, and composition.

1. Volume: Pure volume change occurs when fluid isotonic with body fluids is either added or lost. There is no osmotic gradient created; the compartmental fluid volumes simply increase or decrease, and there is no fluid shift between compartments.
2. Concentration: Pure free water loss or addition to the extracellular compartment changes the concentration of osmotically active particles, prominently sodium. This creates an effective osmotic gradient that forces water out of or into the intracellular compartment until osmolality is equal between the two compartments.
3. Composition: Alterations in the concentration of extracellular ions beyond sodium occur without significantly altering the number of osmotically active particles. The most common example relates to elevated or lowered potassium concentrations.

VOLUME AND INTRAVENOUS FLUIDS

Assessment of volume status is the essential first step in managing fluids. Fluid therapy must cover normal

TABLE 2. *Normal fluid and electrolyte losses per day in 70-kg adult*[a]

	Water (ml)	Na^+ (meq)	K^+ (meq)
Sensible			
Urine	700–1,500	10–80	50–80
Sweat	0–50	10–60	0–10
Stool	0–250	0–20	1–2
Insensible			
Skin	350	0	0
Lung	350	0	0
Average total	1,700	100	80

[a]Urine, sweat, and stool constitute the normal sensible losses. Insensible losses represent evaporative free water losses from the skin (not sweat) and lungs.

TABLE 3. *Approximate electrolyte content of body fluids and intravenous fluids (meq/L)[a]*

	Na$^+$	Cl$^-$	K$^+$	HCO$_3^-$	H$^+$	Ca^{2+}
Body fluid						
Serum	140	100	4	27	—	9
Sweat	50	50	5	—	—	—
Stomach	60	90	10	—	90	—
Pancreas	140	70	5	90	—	—
Ileum	130	110	10	30	—	—
Colon	50	40	30	20	—	—
Intravenous fluid						
D5W (free water)	0	0	—	—	—	—
Normal saline (0.9%)	154	154	—	—	—	—
Half NS (0.45%)	77	77	—	—	—	—
Quarter NS (0.21%)	34	34	—	—	—	—
Hypertonic saline (3%)	513	513	—	—	—	—
Lactated Ringer's	130	109	4	28[b]	—	2.7
5% albumin	140	140	1	—	—	—

[a]The choice of replacement fluids for deficits and ongoing losses requires matching the electrolyte content of the lost body fluid to that of the replacement intravenous fluid.
[b]Present in solution as lactate, which is converted to HCO$_3^-$

maintenance requirements of the patient, correction of previous losses (deficit), and replacement of ongoing losses.

Normal loss of fluid includes measurable (sensible), through urine, stool, and sweat, and unmeasurable (insensible), via lungs and skin, routes (Table 2). Insensible losses are relatively fixed, whereas sensible losses vary with environmental temperature, fever, activity, and fluid intake.

Daily maintenance fluid requirements can be met using the following rate scale, additive based on weight: (a) first 10 kg, 4 cc/kg/hr (100 cc/kg/day); (b) second 10 kg, 2 cc/kg/hr (50 cc/kg/day); (c) each additional kg, 1 cc/kg/hr (20 cc/kg/day); and (d) average adult, 30 to 40 cc/kg/day. To provide free water for insensible losses, sodium for renal regualtion of serum osmolality, and potassium for fixed renal losses, a hypotonic solution, half normal saline (NS) plus 20 meq KCl/L, is the usual maintenance fluid for adults. This is coupled with 5% dextrose in water for its protein-sparing effect.

The volume and composition of deficit and ongoing losses must be assessed (Table 3). Blood loss occurs with trauma. Urine constitutes the major source of potassium loss, though significant loss can also occur

with diarrhea. Acid and chloride are deficient with gastric loss from vomiting, and sodium and bicarbonate are lost with pancreatic fistula.

The fluid being lost is then matched with potential replacement fluids in volume and electrolyte (occasionally protein) content. Lactated Ringer's solution is the initial fluid of resuscitation in situations associated with metabolic acidosis, such as hypovolemia from trauma (Table 4).

Sources of ongoing losses include those responsible for deficit (e.g., osmotic diuresis from hyperglycemia, vomiting, diarrhea, ileostomy, pancreatic fistula), as well as those related to the progression of a disease process or the process of surgery. Third-space loss denotes fluids of extracellular composition that shift into a pathologic space which cannot be regulated, such as the retroperitoneum (e.g., pancreatitis), interstitium (systemic inflammatory response syndrome), or enteric lumen (e.g., bowel obstruction). In adults, 1 L of fluid is lost to this third space for each quadrant of the abdomen that is explored, injured, or inflamed. Fever adds 2 cc/kg/day to sweat losses for each degree above 37°C. Fluid from surgical drains or new fistulae can also be significant.

TABLE 4. *Suggested replacement intravenous fluids for a variety of lost body fluids*

Body fluid lost	Replacement intravenous fluid
Gastric emesis	NS + 40 meq KCl/L
Pancreatic fistula	Lactated Ringer's + 44 meq NaHCO$_3$/L
Ileostomy	Lactated Ringer's
Colonic diarrhea	fi NS + 20 meq KCl/L + 25 meq NaHCO$_3$/L
Blood (acute loss)	Lactated Ringer's versus blood
Third-space	Lactated Ringer's (acidosis) versus NS (alkalosis)

DISORDERS OF CONCENTRATION

Sodium

As the dominant osmotically active electrolyte in the extracellular fluid compartment, the serum sodium concentration reflects the body's water balance more than the absolute amount of sodium in the body. Therefore, the clinical assessment of volume status is critical to any interpretation of sodium concentration. One can find hypo- or hypernatremia with a hypovolemic, euvolemic, or hypervolemic state. The kidney regulates volume through sodium retention, and urine sodium concentration can serve as a window into the kidney's function and view of volume. The daily requirement for sodium intake is 1 to 2 meq/kg/day due to irretrievable loss, and the normal serum sodium ranges from 135 to 145 meq/L.

Low Na⁺ (Hyponatremia): Serum Sodium of <135 meq/L

Causes

The most common cause of hyponatremia is relative dilution of sodium by overhydration, and because sodium reflects the plasma osmolality, hyponatremia is usually equivalent to hypotonicity (Table 5). However, an increase in lipids or proteins in plasma (creating a reduced volume of water in plasma that distorts the concentration calculation, thus creating a fictitious hyponatremia) or an increase in osmotically active solutes in the plasma (such as glucose and mannitol, which attract water to plasma) can create a pseudohyponatremia that is hyper- or isotonic. In fact, the serum sodium concentration is reduced by 1.6 meq/L for every 100 g/dl rise in glucose above 150

TABLE 5. *Abnormalities of sodium*^{a}

Top five causes of hyponatremia
  Overhydration
    Iatrogenic administration of hypotonic intravenous fluids
    Congestive heart failure
    Liver failure
  Dehydration
    Gastrointestinal and third-space losses
  Euhydration
    SIADH
Top five causes of hypernatremia
  Dehydration
    Burns and granulating wounds
    Hypotonic gastrointestinal losses
  Freewater deficit
    Diabetes insipidus
    Iatrogenic salt intake
  Overhydration
    Primary hyperaldosteronism

^{a}The hydration status of the patient is essential for the differentiation of causes.

mg/dl. Thus, it is important to include serum osmolality with urine sodium concentration and osmolality in the laboratory evaluation. The main question to answer in evaluation of hyponatremia is the following: Is the patient overhydrated, dehydrated, or euhydrated?

1. Overhydration (relative free water excess): Hypotonic hyponatremia can occur in any volume status, though the most common setting in surgical patients is overhydration due to the administration of hypotonic fluids. The stimulus of surgery, with its attendant hypovolemia, pain, and anxiety, leads to the increased secretion of ADH and aldosterone. These hormones then cause the reabsorption of more water relative to sodium (because hypotonic fluids provide more water than sodium), and hyponatremia results. Urine sodium is low (<20 meq/L), and urine osmolality is high, reflecting renal conservation of sodium and water appropriately. Severe hypovolemia may also produce hyponatremia via the same hormonal mechanisms, as volume is conserved before regulation of osmolality.

Congestive heart failure, liver failure (with ascites), and nephrotic syndrome all are perceived by the kidney as a relatively low circulatory volume, thus resulting in avid proximal renal sodium and water retention as the baroreceptors and kidneys perceive a decrease in arterial volume and attempt to restore intravascular volume (aldosterone mechanism). The increase in proximal reabsorption results in less delivery of sodium to the distal tubule and thus in diminished ability to produce dilute urine (and excrete free water). The extracellular fluid compartment expands, leading to edema. The overall result is an increased total body sodium and water. At the same time, the ADH receptors in the atria sense a low-volume state and thus stimulate ADH release. This causes water reabsorption. Since aldosterone causes increased sodium and water retention, while the increased ADH causes further water retention, the net effect is hyponatremia. Thus, two mechanisms promote water retention, while only one promotes sodium reabsorption. Urine sodium is low (<20 meq/L) and osmolality high.

2. Dehydration (relative free water deficit): Loss of fluid with sodium can occur with gastrointestinal (GI) losses (vomiting or nasogastric tube drainage, diarrhea, fistulas) or renal losses (chronic diuretic use, salt-losing nephritis, adrenal insufficiency). With GI losses, the kidneys respond by conserving sodium and water. Thus, urine sodium is low (<20 meq/L) and osmolality high. Renal losses, on the other hand, are characterized by sodium wasting (urine sodium, >20 meq/L) and an inability to dilute urine (elevated urine osmolality). The hypovolemia stimulates water and sodium reabsorption, but because of impaired sodium reabsorption, water is reabsorbed in excess of sodium, leading to hyponatremia.

3. Euhydration (isovolemic): The syndrome of inappropriate antidiuretic hormone secretion (SIADH) occurs

when ADH is produced without known appropriate stimuli. It results from CNS disorders (head trauma, tumors, infections, stroke), pulmonary diseases (infections, tumors), and other malignancies with ectopic production. Renal function is normal, and thus in response to ADH, the urine is concentrated (elevated urine osmolality) and urine sodium increased (>20 meq/L). A free water challenge fails to lower urine osmolality.

Symptoms and Signs

Most patients with mild to moderate hyponatremia are asymptomatic; severe hyponatremia (sodium, <120 meq/L) produces neuropsychiatric symptoms and findings, including lethargy, disorientation, agitation, seizures, and coma. The severity of symptoms is dependent not only on the absolute level of hyponatremia, but also on the rate at which it developed. Acute decreases are more serious and relate to rapid development of cerebral edema.

Treatment

Understanding the cause of the hyponatremia leads to appropriate therapy. Again, the importance of assessing the volume status cannot be overemphasized. Overhydration under conditions of appropriate ADH secretion is corrected by eliminating the administration of hypotonic fluids; normal saline and diuretics are used as needed. The overhydration of the edematous states, however, is best corrected by restricting sodium and water intake and correcting the underlying cause (e.g., in congestive heart failure, improving contractility with digoxin and reducing preload with diuretics). Dehydration hyponatremia responds to volume replacement with normal saline; adrenal insufficiency is corrected with mineralocorticoid and corticosteroid replacement. The treatment of SIADH is strict fluid restriction (>500 cc/day) and correction of the underlying process.

Severe hyponatremia that develops acutely or is symptomatic requires urgent treatment with hypertonic saline (3% NaCl), with the goal of correcting the sodium to 130 meq/L (or to resolution of symptoms) at a rate no faster than 1 meq/L/hr. Careful monitoring is essential: rapid correction may cause neurologic injury (central pontine myelinolysis—particularly in young women, seizures, and permanent brain damage) and flash pulmonary edema. Therapy is guided by calculating a body sodium deficit, which equals the difference in serum sodium from normal multiplied by the total body water,

$$[\text{Normal serum Na}^+ - \text{actual serum Na}^+]$$
$$\times [0.6 \text{ L/kg} \times \text{kg body weight}],$$

and then dividing by the concentration of 3% NS (0.5 meq/ml) to yield the necessary replacement volume with hypertonic saline. Usually less than half of this calculated volume is used in replacement. The rate is then determined by this :

$$\frac{[1 \text{ meq/L/hr} \times \text{normal body water volume (L)}]}{0.5 \text{ meq/ml}} = \text{ml/hr of 3\% NaCl}$$

High Na⁺ (Hypernatremia): Serum Sodium of >145 meq/L

Causes

Hypernatremia is always associated with hyperosmolality in the extracellular fluid compartment, but can exist in any volume setting. It has two main causes: free water deficit, as seen in patients who are given isotonic solutions with little free water, and dehydration. Both can exist in the same patient and result from loss of free water or hypotonic body fluids, either from extrarenal (skin: sweating from fever, evaporation from burns and granulating wounds; GI: hypotonic diarrhea; or pulmonary: insensible evaporation) or renal (osmotic diuresis, central or nephrogenic diabetes insipidus) sources. Extrarenal loss stimulates the kidney to retain fluid, and because volume preservation predominates over osmolar correction, the urine sodium is low (<20 meq/L) and the osmolality is high. Renal losses represent a loss of renal concentrating ability, and thus, the sodium is high (>20 meq/L) and the osmolality is low.

A rare cause of hypernatremia is an excess of body sodium and consequent hypervolemic state: this occurs with retention of sodium from adrenal disorders (primary hyperaldosteronism, Cushing's syndrome), as well as from iatrogenic salt intake. Typically, the urine sodium is normal, and the osmolality is variable.

The hyperosmolality that occurs with an increase in serum sodium normally triggers an increase in thirst (with consequent increase in water intake), an increase in the secretion of ADH, or an increase in renal conservation of water. Central and nephrogenic diabetes insipidis represent failure of the later two mechanisms, respectively. Persistent hypernatremia can only occur, then, when hypotonic or free water fluid losses combine with inadequate water replacement.

Symptoms and Signs

As with hyponatremia, neuropsychiatric symptoms predominate, with restlessness, hyperreflexia, and weakness progressing to delirium. Fluid shifts from the intracellular to the extracellular fluid compartment result in cellular and cerebral dehydration, which eventually can cause tearing of cerebral vessels with intracerebral and subarachnoid hemorrhage. The rate of development of hypernatremia and volume status affect the presentation. Core temperature elevation can occur, and with the more common dehydration state, signs of volume depletion are manifest by dry mouth and swollen tongue, as well as tachycardia and oliguria in the later stages. At its onset, patients with diabetes insipidus will have a copious urine output.

Treatment

The cause of the hypernatremia dictates the treatment, as illustrated in two examples. First, consider a stable patient who has been receiving large quantities of normal saline with hypotonic fluid losses and no free water (D_5W) administration. This patient's Na^+ is 160. Treatment consists of D_5W administration and Na^+ restriction.

Now, examine an 80-year-old patient who has been vomiting for a number of days. At presentation to the emergency room, the blood pressure is 70/40, pulse is 160, urine output is absent, and Na^+ is 160. The patient is dehydrated and in shock, and treatment will be completely different from the first case. The top priority is to stabilize the patient by administering isotonic solutions, preferably lactated Ringer's or normal saline (recall that all physiologic isotonic fluid solutions are relatively hypotonic when serum sodium exceeds 145 meq/L), depending on acid-base status. With improvement of the patient's volume status, urine will be produced, and a solute diuresis (i.e., brisk elimination of Na^+) will occur. After adequate resuscitation, if the patient remains hypernatremic, free water is then administered. Though a sodium deficit exists initially in this case, there is a larger free water deficit.

A free water deficit should be corrected so that the serum value of Na^+ is corrected no faster than 1 meq/hr. Faster correction can result in cerebral edema, intracerebral bleeding, and death. The free water deficit calculation serves as a useful guideline:

Normal total body water $\times$ [normal serum Na^+] = Current total body water $\times$ [current serum Na^+]

Solving for current total body water and substituting this in the equation,

Water deficit = current - normal total body water = $(0.6 \times$ kg body weight) [(current serum $Na^+/140) - 1$],

where normal serum Na^+ is 140. For example, a 70-kg man with a Na^+ of 160 will have a free water deficit of

$$[0.6 \times 70] \times [(160/140) - 1] = 6 \text{ L}$$

The serum Na^+ should not be lowered at a rate faster than 1 mOsm/hr. Thus, in order to lower the Na^+ safely from 160 to 140, 40 hr are required (a 20 meq/L Na^+ difference equals a 40-mOsm difference including the accompanying anions). The rate at which D_5W should be administered, then, is 6,000 ml/40 hr, or 150 ml/hr.

Central diabetes insipidus leads to hypernatremia with free water deficit. Not only is D_5W fluid administra-

tration required, but also replacement of ADH with 1-deamino-8-D-arginine vasopressin (DDAVP) (5 U s.c. every 4 hr) or with an intravenous pitressin drip, titrated to reduce urine output to 100 cc/hr. Nephrogenic diabetes insipidus will not respond to DDAVP and requires sodium restriction with augmented water intake.

The patient with hyperaldosteronism needs removal of excess sodium, which can be accomplished with a loop diuretic (e.g., lasix) coupled with free water administration.

Chloride

Chloride is the forgotten anion, always reported with electrolyte panels but often ignored. Its importance lies in the maintenance of tonicity, renal reabsorption of sodium, and acid-base regulation. Chloride provides only a share of anion tonicity with bicarbonate and varies with acid-base change; thus, sodium is a more convenient reflection of serum osmolality.

Renal sodium reabsorption requires anion accompaniment to maintain electroneutrality, and both chloride and bicarbonate fulfill this role depending on availability and acid-base status. Chloride and bicarbonate maintain an inverse relationship: low chloride leads to elevated bicarbonate, and vice versa. Adequate chloride is essential to allow normal renal regulation of acid and correction of alkalosis.

Chloride is a component of the anion gap and thus assists in the detection of unmeasured acids. Its renal handling can be analyzed by determining urine electrolyte concentration: in the absence of acid-base changes, chloride and sodium move in parallel fashion, and thus urinary chloride can validate the urinary sodium concentration. A discrepancy may be due to an underlying acid-base disorder. Urinary chloride measurement is an essential part of the evaluation of metabolic alkalosis; again, it demonstrates how the kidney is attempting to correct the situation and whether or not more chloride is needed. Normal serum chloride is 95 to 105 meq/L.

Low Chloride (Hypochloremia): Serum Chloride of <95 meq/L

Greater chloride loss relative to sodium loss is seen with loss of gastric juice (such as protracted vomiting with pyloric stenosis or gastric outlet obstruction) or renal failure to reabsorb chloride (Bartter's syndrome). The urinary chloride concentration is low (<20 meq/L) in the former situation and high in the latter. The treatment of the hypochloremic, hypokalemic (acid-base effect) metabolic alkalosis (loss of gastric acid) is normal saline volume repletion with potassium, followed by correction of the underlying cause.

High Chloride (Hyperchloremia): Serum Chloride of >105 meq/L

Hyperchloremia represents serum hyperosmolality when the acid-base status is normal. Its correction parallels that for hypernatremia. Renal tubular acidosis produces a hyperchloremic acidosis because of defective acid excretion; again, renal acid excretion (with bicarbonate reabsorption) depends on chloride excretion, and the urinary loss of bicarbonate leads to marked chloride reabsorption. Loss of bicarbonate with diarrhea or pancreatic fistula can also lead to a hyperchloremic metabolic acidosis, again because of renal reabsorption of chloride in the absence of bicarbonate.

DISORDERS OF ELECTROLYTE COMPOSITION

Potassium

Potassium is an intracellular cation, totalling 4,200 meq in a 70-kg individual. This intracellular pool equilibrates with the extracellular concentration across the cellular membrane that enforces a concentration gradient with the Na-K ATPase pump. The normal value is 3.5 to 4.5 meq/L. Thus, the serum concentration of potassium is the tip of the iceberg of total body potassium (Fig. 3).

Potassium homeostasis is dependent on adequate intake to replace daily losses, roughly 30 to 40 meq/day, and on adequate renal function. Because potassium is the intracelluar portion of membrane potential, abnormalities are manifest in the cardiovascular, GI, and musculoskeletal systems.

Low K⁺ (Hypokalemia): Serum Potassium of <3.5 meq/L

Causes

Hypokalemia results from potassium loss, inadequate intake, or intracelluar displacement. Sources of loss

include augmented renal excretion, such as that which occurs with diuretics causing increased distal tubule delivery of sodium or that accompanies volume depletion; GI loss from vomiting, diarrhea, or fistula; and hyperaldosteronism. Inadequate intake is less usual but may occur in patients with inadequate nutrition. Finally, potassium is driven intracellularly by alkalosis, with a 0.6-meq/L drop for each 0.1 pH unit increase, and by hyperinsulinism. A second mechanism by which alkalosis causes hypokalemia occurs in the kidney: in the distal tubule, where Na⁺ is reabsorbed in exchange for K⁺ and H⁺, K⁺ replaces H⁺ when H⁺ concentration is low (i.e., alkalosis). This also illustrates why hypokalemia itself can cause alkalosis.

Symptoms and Signs

These do not begin usually until the K⁺ is <3.0 meq/L. The most common manifestations are demonstrated by electrocardiogram (EKG) abnormalities, which progress from low-voltage tracings, flattened T waves, and prominent U waves, to a prolonged P-R interval and QRS widening. Weakness and lethargy, as well as ileus, reflect the electrophysiologic dysfunction and are most often experienced at K⁺ of <2.5 meq/L.

Treatment

The etiology provides the clue for treatment. Initial analysis should include an assessment of the acid-base balance and glycemic state of the patient, as well as current potassium intake; correction of these underlying causes will then produce a eukalemic state. Losses should be replaced, first noting deficits and then correcting for ongoing losses and daily maintenance. These are guidelines for potassium repletion: serum K⁺ 3 to 4 meq/L, 100 to 200 meq deficit; K⁺ 2 to 3 meq/L, 200 to 400 meq deficit; K⁺ 1 to 2 meq/L, 400 to 800 meq deficit. In most circumstances, oral replacement is preferred because it rarely produces overshoot hyperkalemia; seemingly small, yet rapid changes in plasma potassium concentration can result in large changes in neuromuscular irritability. However, with potassium of <3 meq/L or clinical symptoms or EKG signs, intravenous replacement must be instituted. Potassium can be added to the intravenous fluid for mild deficits, administered intermittently, or initiated as an infusion. The maximum safe replacement rate is 20 meq/hr under electrocardiographic monitoring.

High K⁺ (Hyperkalemia): K⁺ of >5.0 meq/L

Causes

Hyperkalemia results from poor renal excretion, as in renal failure, hypoaldosteronism, or use of potassium-

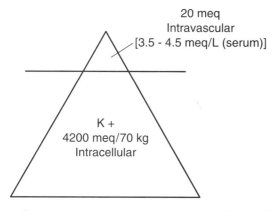

20 meq
Intravascular
[3.5 - 4.5 meq/L (serum)]

K +
4200 meq/70 kg
Intracellular

FIG. 3. Serum potassium represents the tip of the total body

sparing diuretics, from the release of potassium from the intracellular to the extracellular compartments, which occurs with cell death (burns, crush injury); or from extracellular shift in acidosis. Beware of pseudohyperkalemia due to hemolysis of the blood sample.

Symptoms and Signs

As with hypokalemia, the clinical effects of hyperkalemia are found in the cardiovascular, neuromuscular, and GI systems. Effects are usually not seen until the potassium is >6 meq/L. The EKG reveals peaked T waves and shortening of the QT interval, the opposite initial manifestations of hypokalemia. These progress to QRS widening and ST segment depression, progressing to the sine wave tracing and cardiac arrest. Lethargy and weakness are similar to hypokalemia, but the GI symptoms relate to hyperactivity with vomiting and diarrhea.

Treatment

First, verify that hyperkalemia is indeed present by reviewing the clinical situation and the specimen for hemolysis. Stop potassium administration (in either intravenous fluids, penicillin antibiotics, or enteral feeds). Then, protect against the cardiac dysfunction produced by hyperkalemia by administering calcium gluconate slowly if EKG changes are present (calcium lowers the threshold potential needed for electrical excitation). Therapy next involves driving potassium intracellularly, which can be accomplished acutely by giving insulin (10 U) and glucose (1 ampule of $D_{50}W$), as well as bicarbonate (recall that alkalosis shifts potassium intracellularly). Finally, the excess potassium must be removed; if renal function is normal, diuretics can do this. However, the usual clinical situation is renal failure. Thus, potassium binding resins, such as kayexalate, are given with sorbitol (to prevent constipation) either orally or rectally to use the gut as an eliminator. Ultimately, hemodialysis may be necessary for ongoing removal (in the setting of renal failure, recalcitrant hyperkalemia, volume overload, metabolic acidosis, and uremic pericarditis constitute the four indications for emergent hemodialysis).

Calcium

The major calcium reservoir is bone mineral (calcium phosphate), where most of the 1,200 g total resides. Normal daily intake is 1 g, some of which is absorbed in the proximal small bowel (under guidance from vitamin D), but most of which is excreted through the GI tract. Less than 200 mg is excreted in the urine. The normal plasma calcium is 9.0 to 10.5 mg/dl, half of which is not ionized and is bound to proteins (80% to albumen). Thus, for every 1 g/dl decrease in albumen of <4.0 g/dl, the normal cal-

cium range should be adjusted by subtracting 0.8 mg/dl. The remaining half of plasma calcium is ionized and responsible for neuromuscular and cardiovascular stability. Serum calcium levels are increased by parathormone.

Low Calcium (Hypocalcemia): Calcium of <8 mg/dl

Causes

Causes of hypocalcemia are poor absorption, related to vitamin D deficiency (including renal failure, which reduces conversion to vitamin D_3, and fat malabsorption); tissue binding, as in acute pancreatitis with saponification; hypoparathyroidism; and severe hypomagnesemia (causing parathyroid dysfunction).

Symptoms and Signs

Neuromuscular findings predominate, with perioral numbness and tingling of fingertips and toes as the earliest symptoms. Hyperactive tendon reflexes, Chvostek's sign (ipsilateral facial twitching with tapping over the facial nerve), Trousseau's sign (carpopedal spasm), muscular and abdominal cramps, tetany, and convulsions follow. On EKG, the Q-T interval is prolonged.

Treatment

It is essential that hypomagnesemia be diagnosed and treated prior to intervention for hypocalcemia. Symptomatic hypocalcemia is best handled acutely with intravenous calcium gluconate, either intermittently or as an infusion in a monitored setting. Long-term hypocalcemia is managed with oral calcium and vitamin D, which address deficiencies in absorption or regulation.

High Calcium (Hypercalcemia): Calcium of >10.5 mg/dl

Causes

The most common underlying cause is the increased release of calcium from bone as a result of hyperparathyroidism and metastatic cancer (breast, lung, kidney, colon, thyroid, myeloma). Other causes are far less common and listed in Table 6.

Symptoms and Signs

Weakness, vomiting, and fatigue lead to somnolence, stupor, and coma with increasing levels of calcium. Other symptoms include headaches, back pain, and polyuria (accompanied by thirst and polydipsia).

TABLE 6. *Most common causes of deficiency and excess of potassium, calcium, magnesium, and phosphate*

Abnormalities of potassium
    Top three causes of hypokalemia
        Diuretics
        Gastrointestinal loss
        Alkalosis
    Top three causes of hyperkalemia
        Renal failure
        Cell death (burns, crush injury, tissue necrosis)
        Acidosis
Abnormalities of calcium
    Top five causes of hypocalcemia
        Renal failure
        Fat malabsorption
        Acute pancreatitis
        Iatrogenic hypoparathyroidism
        Hypomagnesemia
    Top five causes of hypercalcemia
        Metastatic breast cancer
        Metastatic lung cancer
        Metastatic renal cancer
        Hyperparathyroidism
        Sarcoidosis
Abnormalities of magnesium
    Top three causes of hypomagnesemia
        Chronic alcoholism
        Absence of magnesium in nutritional support
        Starvation
    Top three causes of hypermagnesemia
        Renal failure
        Magnesium-containing antacids
        Acidosis
Abnormalities of phosphate
    Top three causes of hypophosphatemia
        Absence of phosphate in nutritional support
        Hyperparathyroidism
        Diarrhea
    Top three causes of hyperphosphatemia
        Renal failure
        Hypoparathyroidism
        Cell death (tumor lysis, tissue necrosis)

Treatment

Calcium levels above 12 mg/dl become increasingly concerning, reaching a critical level at 15 mg/dl. The first priority is to correct the extracellular volume deficit that occurs because of hypercalcemia-induced vomiting and diuresis. This is best accomplished with normal saline, which dilutes the calcium level and increases urinary calcium excretion. Once hydrated, the patient can then receive nonthiazide diuretics (note that thiazide diuretics retain calcium) to maximize renal clearance of calcium. With diuresis, the serum potassium and magnesium must be closely monitored.

When the acute situation is corrected, attention is focused on the subacute management: mithramycin directly inhibits calcium release from bone; corticosteroids reduce reabsorption of calcium from bone and reduce intestinal absorption of vitamin D; and calcitonin modestly pushes calcium into bone. Hyperparathyoidism is a surgically correctable disease.

Magnesium

Of the 2,000 meq of magnesium in the body, most is intracellular. The normal serum concentration is 1.5 to 2.5 meq/L. Normal dietary intake is 20 meq/day, with excretion in the feces and urine (though magnesium conservation is a role of the kidney).

Magnesium is an essential cofactor for many metabolic energy processes.

Low Magnesium (Hypomagnesemia): Mg^{2+} of <1.5 meq/L

Causes

Deficiency is most commonly due to inadequate intake, occurring with starvation, chronic alcoholism, and prolonged parenteral nutrition without addition of magnesium. Excessive loss of GI fluid and renal wasting, either from renal disease or diuresis, are further causes, as is chronic extracellular volume expansion (e.g., hyperaldosteronism).

Symptoms and Signs

These are similar to hypocalcemia, which again emphasizes the linkage between calcium and magnesium.

Treatment

Magnesium deficiency is best treated by intravenous administration of magnesium sulfate or magnesium chloride, with dosage and timing dependent on renal function and symptoms. Renal insufficiency requires much lower doses, and asymptomatic patients can be repleted over a longer period of time. Repletion of severe hypomagnesemia requires a monitored setting and is accomplished initially with up to 80 meq of magnesium over 4 hr, to a total dose of 2 meq/kg/day. Decreased deep tendon reflexes can be monitored for clinical evidence of hypermagnesemia during repletion. Because magnesium is predominantly an intracellular cation, it can take several weeks to replenish magnesium stores fully.

High Magnesium (Hypermagnesemia): Mg^{2+} of >2.5 meq/L

Causes

Continued intake of magnesium in the setting of renal failure will lead to hypermagnesemia. Magnesium-containing antacids and laxatives are often the culprits. Magnesium and potassium levels change in parallel fashion, with acidosis pushing magnesium out of cells.

Symptoms and Signs

Progressive loss of deep tendon reflexes remains the cardinal sign, accompanied by lethargy and weakness. Cardiac conduction abnormalities are similar to those with hyperkalemia. Symptoms become increasingly more prominent at levels of >4.0 meq/L and end with coma and cardiopulmonary failure.

Treatment

Initially, calcium gluconate is given to antagonize the effect of magnesium on nerve and muscle membrane potentials, as well as correction of any acidosis and replenishment of any extracellular volume deficit. Magnesium administration is stopped, and further management may require dialysis.

Phosphate

Phosphate is an essential substrate for cellular energy (ATP) and the major intracellular anion in the body. The majority of the 800 g body store is contained in bones, and serum phosphate varies inversely with calcium. Roughly 1 g is required daily, with efficient intestinal absorption and dominant renal excretion. The normal serum level is 2.5 to 4.5 mg/dl.

Low Phosphate (Hypophosphatemia): Phosphate of <2.5 mg/dl

Causes

Nutritional support without phosphate will rapidly use up intracellular phosphate and shift serum phosphate intracellularly. Hyperparathyroidism results in mobilization of calcium and phosphate from bone stores, with renal excretion of phosphate. Finally, diarrhea and phosphate-binding antacids will result in GI losses.

Symptoms and Signs

These reflect the essential role of phosphate in metabolic processes and are neuromuscular (weakness, hyporeflexia, numbness, fatigue, seizures) and cardiorespiratory (decreased cardiac contractility, diaphragmatic failure). Remember, lack of phosphate means lack of energy and global cellular dysfunction (e.g., membrane systems fail, leading to rhabdomyolysis).

Treatment

Identification of the underlying cause and appropriate phosphate repletion are the goals. Serum calcium should be checked (if elevated, calcium may precipitate when phosphate is given), and phosphate-binding antacids should be stopped. Mild hypophosphatemia (>1 mg/dl) can be repleted with either enteral or intravenous phosphorus, but severe hypophosphatemia (<1 mg/dl) requires intravenous replacement (1.5 to 2.0 mmol/hr) and a monitored setting. Once the phosphate level is >2.0 mg/dl, then the enteral route (neutraphos 500 mg bid) can be used.

High Phosphate (Hyperphosphatemia): Phosphate of >4.5 mg/dl

Causes

Reduced renal excretion (renal failure, hypoparathyroidism), increased intake from phosphate-containing laxatives or enemas, or release of intracellular phosphate into the extracellular compartment (cell death from tumor lysis or tissue necrosis).

Symptoms and Signs

Given the reciprocal relationship between calcium and phosphate, and the tighter regulation of calcium, the clinical features of hyperphosphatemia reflect hypocalcemia and calcium precipitation (ectopic calcification in muscles and organs).

Treatment

Again, as with the other hyperelectrolyte disorders, therapy consists of finding the underlying cause and eliminating the excess phosphate. Intake is eliminated, and in patients with normal renal function, renal excretion is promoted by using normal saline and diuretics. Phosphate-binding antacids can be used to encourage elimination via the intestines, and ultimately, dialysis is quite effective in removing phosphate in the setting of renal failure.

NORMAL ACID-BASE PHYSIOLOGY

The normal pH of blood is between 7.35 and 7.45. The pH reflects the hydrogen ion concentration. This concentration has to be maintained within a certain range to maintain life. The amount of H^+ present in the body fluids at any given time is only an infinitesimal fraction of the daily intake and output. Intake of H^+ is actually not dietary intake, but rather, a byproduct of cellular metabolism. The cells produce undesirable waste products, which include sulfuric and phosphoric acids (from the breakdown of proteins), and lactate (from the incomplete breakdown of sugar). Ionization of these acids liberates H+ at a rate of 60 mmol/day.

Obviously such intake has to be matched by an equal output and thus, the kidneys eliminate some 60 mmol/day of H+. Every second, we produce a little more than the total amount of H+ in all of our extracellular fluid; three times the normal concentration of H+ is the maximum compatable with life, which means that we produce more than enough H+ to kill ourselves every 3 sec. There is not enough time to carry all that poison to the kidney for elimination, so additional rapid mechanisms for the disposal of H+ are required: the buffers. They dispose of unwanted H+ from a strong acid, by combining with that acid to create an inactive salt and weak acid. The same total amount of H+ is still present, but it is largely rendered inactive as a weak acid.

In the blood there are several main buffers. The plasma and red cells contain bicarbonate, plasma proteins, and inorganic phosphates, but the red cells also contain organic phosphates and hemoglobin. At normal physiological temperatures, bicarbonate and hemoglobin are the most important blood buffers. The buffering capacity of the blood is further backed by extracellular fluid and intracellular buffers.

The serum concentration of H+ is only 40 nmol/L (1 nmol = 10^{-9} moles, 1 million times less than a millimole) because most H+ is combined with a weak acid. The kidney extracts the H+ from the molecule of the weak acid, excretes it in the urine, and returns the original buffer to the circulation. The urinary H+ is captured by combining with ammonia (NH_3) for conversion to ammonium (NH_4^+), yielding a urinary pH of 4.5.

Carbonic acid is another source of H+ that is constantly produced, buffered in transit, and eliminated. CO_2 and water may combine to produce carbonic acid (H_2CO_3), particularly when catalyzed by the enzyme carbonic anhydrase. Fortunately, not all the CO_2 becomes carbonic acid. The majority of the CO_2 is carried as a gas dissolved in plasma, and at the normal concentrations of CO_2, only one of every 800 molecules actually becomes carbonic acid. Furthermore, it is a very weak acid, of which only one of every 1,000 molecules is ionized to H+. Still, the total daily contribution of H+ from this source is relatively great, requiring constant excretion as well as buffering in transit. The lungs eliminate the dissolved CO_2 gas, thereby indirectly diminishing the amount of H_2CO_3, and hemoglobin provides the buffering. Acid is regulated by two pathways, metabolic (renal) and respiratory. The former buffers acid in the blood and eliminates it through the kidneys, whereas the latter buffers carbonic acid with hemoglobin and eliminates CO_2 through the lungs.

The respiratory component of H+ homeostasis handles carbonic acid so efficiently that the process can respond instantly to very rapid increases in acid production, preserving balance by increasing pulmonary ventilation and excreting CO_2. On the other hand, the metabolic (renal) system is a very slow one: it takes the kidney several days to adjust itself to the higher rate of acid production. Thus, the cushioning effect of buffers like bicarbonate (creating the weak carbonic acid) is quite important. Normally, the kidney breaks the carbonic acid, eliminating the H+ and

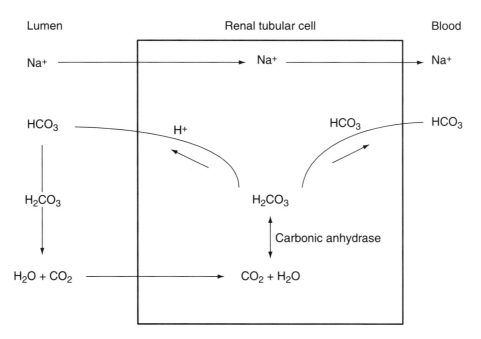

FIG. 4. Renal acid secretion and bicarbonate reabsorption are linked through carbonic acid (H_2CO_3) and depend on the enzyme carbonic anhydrase. This process, in turn, supports reabsorption of tubular sodium.

TABLE 7. *Primary and compensatory acid-base disorders[a]*

Primary disorder	Compensatory response
Metabolic acidosis: ↓ HCO_3^-	↓ pCO_2: Respiratory alkalosis
Metabolic alkalosis: ↑ HCO_3^-	↑ pCO_2: Respiratory acidosis
Respiratory acidosis: ↑ pCO_2	↑ HCO_3^-: Metabolic alkalosis
Respiratory alkalosis: ↓ pCO_2	↓ HCO_3^-: Metabolic acidosis

[a]Rule: HCO_3^-/pCO_2 is constant. Each primary acid-base disorder has a corresponding compensatory response, which tends to bring the pH closer to 7.40 but does not correct completely. This reflects the body's tendency to maintain a nearly constant HCO_3^-/pCO_2 ratio.

returning the bicarbonate to the circulation. However, if the amount of the carbonic acid is too large, the lungs play an important role eliminating the acid, but with an acute price for this rapidity: bicarbonate is lost in the process of CO_2 elimination. Fortunately the kidney can later regenerate bicarbonate, as seen in the following equation and Fig. 4.

$$H_2O + CO_2 \leftrightarrow H_2CO_3 \leftrightarrow H^+ + HCO_3^-$$

The hydrogen ion concentration in blood is determined by the balance between carbon dioxide (PCO_2) and the serum bicarbonate (HCO_3^-). This relationship is expressed as the modified Henderson-Hasselbach equation:

$$pH = 6.1 + \log \{[HCO_3^-]/(0.03 \times PCO_2)\}$$

Knowing any of the two variables in the Henderson-Hasselbach equation can result in calculation of the third variable. H^+ concentration is inversely related to pH: a 1 mmol/L increase in H^+ equals a decrease in pH of 0.01. Serum H^+ changes in the same direction as the PCO_2 and in the opposite direction from the serum HCO_3^-. Four primary and compensatory acid-base disorders evolve from an understanding of the Henderson-Hasselbach relationships, as shown in Table 7. The goal of compensation is to keep the HCO_3^-/PCO_2 ratio constant. When one of the two components becomes abnormal, adjustments are made to change the other component in the same direction.

ACID-BASE ASSESSMENT

Assessing a patient's acid-base status begins with the measurement of the arterial pH, partial pressure of CO_2, and bicarbonate. Blood gas analyzers directly measure the pH and PCO_2. The bicarbonate value is calculated from the Henderson-Hasselbach equation.

TABLE 8. *Normal arterial and venous pH, pCO_2, and HCO_3^- values*

	pH	pCO_2 (mm Hg)	HCO_3^- (meq/L)
Arterial	7.37–7.43	36–44	22–27
Venous	7.32–7.38	42–50	23–28

If the pH is less than normal (<7.35), the patient is acidemic. If the pH is greater than normal (>7.45), the patient is alkalemic. Normal ranges are listed in Table 8.

If the PCO_2 is lower than normal (<35 mm Hg) and this is a primary process, then a respiratory alkalosis present. If the PCO_2 is higher than normal (>45 of mm Hg) and this is a primary process, than a respiratory acidosis is present.

If the arterial bicarbonate level is less than normal (<22 mmol/L) and this is a primary abnormality, a metabolic acidosis is present. If the bicarbonate level is higher than normal (>27 mmol/L) and this is a primary process, a metabolic alkalosis is present.

Respiratory compensation for metabolic disorders is rapid. Full metabolic compensation for respiratory disorders, however, requires renal adjustment and takes 3 to 5 days. The primary disorder dictates the pH. The body does not overcompensate for the primary disorder: a primary acidosis will not be corrected to an alkalotic pH.

Steps in Acid-Base Analysis

1. Determine whether the patient is acidemic or alkalemic based on measurement of arterial pH.
2. Determine whether the acid-base disturbance is due to a primary respiratory or metabolic disorder by measuring PCO_2 and bicarbonate levels (Fig. 5).
   A. A primary metabolic disorder is present if the pH and PCO_2 change in the same direction or the pH is abnormal but the PCO_2 is normal; e.g., if the pH and PCO_2 are low, then a metabolic disorder (acidosis) is present.
   B. A primary respiratory disorder is present if the pH and the PCO_2 change in opposite directions; e.g., if the pH is low and the PCO_2 is high, then a respiratory disorder (acidosis) is present.
   C. A mixed disorder is present if pH is normal and PCO_2 is abnormal. A high PCO_2 and pH normal indicates a mixed respiratory acidosis/metabolic alkalosis. A low PCO_2 and pH normal indicates a mixed respiratory alkalosis metabolic acidosis. A normal PCO_2 may indicate normal acid-base status but does not rule out a combined metabolic acidosis/metabolic alkalosis.

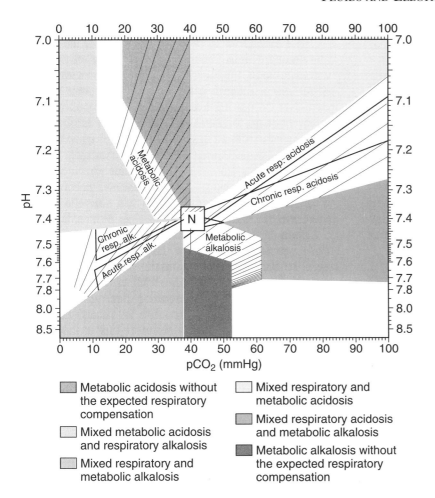

Metabolic acidosis without the expected respiratory compensation

Mixed metabolic acidosis and respiratory alkalosis

Mixed respiratory and metabolic alkalosis

Mixed respiratory and metabolic acidosis

Mixed respiratory acidosis and metabolic alkalosis

Metabolic alkalosis without the expected respiratory compensation

FIG. 5. Acid-base nomogram, illustrating acid-base disturbances by region on a pH × pCO_2 grid.

3. Calculate the anion gap (particularly when a metabolic acidosis is present).

Anion Gap = Serum Na^+ − Serum Cl^- + Serum HCO_3^-

The normal anion gap is 12, ranging from 10 to 14. One of the hidden anions is protein, particularly albumen. When albumen is decreased by 1 g/dl, the adjusted normal anion gap is reduced by 4.

Arterial Versus Venous Acid-Base Values

Acid-base values between arterial and venous blood (Table 8) can be similar in stable patients. Venous blood should be a closer approximation of the acid-base status at the tissue level under normal circumstances, while the arterial blood depicts pulmonary gas exchange. However, values can vary considerably in patients who are hemodynamically unstable. Venous blood may not mirror tissue values in sepsis because of microcirculatory shunts that divert blood away from metabolizing tissues. In low-flow states (hypovolemia, cardiac failure), the venous blood may reveal the tissue acidosis better than an arterial sample because ischemic cells are drained by venous blood. When a patient is hemodynamically unstable, do not assume that arterial blood is an accurate measure of

tissue acid-base status. A venous blood sample should be checked periodically while monitoring the arterial blood gases in unstable patients.

METABOLIC ACIDOSIS

This is defined by a high $[H^+]$ (low pH) and low $[HCO_3^-]$ in plasma. Calculation of the anion gap assists further in finding the cause. A hidden metabolic acidosis may also be detected by finding a wide serum anion gap (>14 meq/L), even without a pH or HCO_3^- change (because of compensation and multiple acid-base disorders). The expected pulmonary response is to lower PCO_2, so that the pH fall is minimized. The renal response is to excrete H^+ as NH_4^+, so that new HCO_3^- is generated. Normally, the kidneys excrete 40 mmol NH_4^+/day; during metabolic acidosis, this should be at least as large as dietary acid production (1 mmol/kg/day) and ideally as high as 300 mmol/day.

Causes and Treatment

Metabolic acidoses are separated into two groups by the anion gap. High anion gap acidoses are characterized by the addition of a fixed acid (e.g., lactic acid), while the nonanion gap acidoses are characterized by loss of bicarbonate buffers (e.g., diarrhea). In the latter condition, chloride replaces the loss of bicarbonate for electrical neutrality and the increased serum chloride produces a hyperchloremic metabolic acidosis. Thus, there are two major categories, acid gain and HCO_3^- loss.

Acid Gain

Acid gain is recognized by finding a widened plasma AG (>14 meq/L). In quantitative terms, the rise in the anion gap should equal the fall in the plasma $[HCO_3^-]$ due to the increase in fixed acids.

The major acids are (a) l-lactic acid (tissue hypoxia); (b) ketoacids (insulin deficiency); (c) d-lactic acid (GI ischemia or altered GI flora, e.g., blind loop syndrome); and (d) intoxicants which are or become acids, including methanol to formic acid, ethylene glycol to glyoxalic acid, paraldehyde to acetic acid, and salicylates (aspirin) (also triggers central hyperventilation). Furthermore, (e) in renal failure (uremia), decreased GFR leads to retention of acid metabolites, and renal tubular dysfunction limits excretion of NH_4^+.

Treatment

The treatment priority is to stop the rate of production of H^+ by identifying and correcting the underlying cause. In surgical patients, the most common cause is lactic acidosis from inadequate tissue perfusion associated with volume loss or sepsis. Restoration of oxygen delivery to the tissues is the goal. Acidosis from renal failure may require hemodialysis.

$NaHCO_3$ is given as a temporary expedient when the pH is <7.20 to prevent cardiac arrythmias and improve cardiac contractility. It is not the primary therapy for correction of a metabolic acidosis. Administration of bicarbonate generates CO_2, which is acid, and this acid must be excreted by the lungs. Thus, adequate pulmonary function is essential for use of bicarbonate. $NaHCO_3$ therapy can induce hypernatremia with hyperosmolality (based on the sodium load), fluid overload, and hypokalemia (alkalosis shifts K^+ into cells).

HCO_3^- Loss

1. Loss of HCO_3^- via the GI tract (diarrhea, ileus, fistula): In this case, the urine should contain >80 mmol NH_4^+/day. Treatment requires fluid replacement commensurate in volume and composition with that lost, in addition to addressing the cause of loss.
2. Loss of HCO_3^- in the urine: The most convenient way to detect this loss is to measure a urine pH of >6.

Causes include proximal renal tubular acidosis (defective reclamation of HCO_3^-) and the use of carbonic anhydrase inhibitors. One obvious treatment is cessation of the offending diuretic. For proximal renal tubular acidoses, it is difficult to restore plasma HCO_3^- to normal because of the enormous ongoing bicarbonate loss: 85% of the filtered load of bicarbonate is normally reabsorbed by the proximal tubule.

3. Failure of the kidney to secrete sufficient H^+ (distal renal tubular acidosis): This is characterized by a low rate of excretion of NH_4^+. Treatment/correction is achieved by providing sufficient bicarbonate to restore normal serum acid-base values; normally, 1 to 3 mmol/kg/day is sufficient.
4. Hyperchloremia: Any increase in Cl^- will cause a loss of HCO_3^- in order to maintain electrical neutrality in renal reabsorption of sodium. This increase is usually iatrogenic, such as giving the patient too much normal saline.

METABOLIC ALKALOSIS

This is one of the most common disorders. It is defined as plasma HCO_3^- of >27 mmol/L and pH of >7.45. However, it can still be present with a lower pH and HCO_3^- if there is a widened plasma anion gap. A serum pH of >7.60 is an emergency. Severe alkalosis can cause seizures and refractory cardiac arrythmias. Alkalemia causes the oxyhemoglobin dissociation curve to shift to the left, which increases the affinity of hemoglobin for O_2 and hence reduces the release of oxygen at the tissue level. It can also cause depression of the respiratory center leading to respiratory acidosis.

Causes

1. Loss of H^+: Any loss of H^+ is a gain of HCO_3^-. Vomiting will cause loss of H^+ because of gastric juice acidity.
2. Loss of Cl^-: Any loss of Cl^- is compensated by an increase in HCO_3^- reabsorption with Na^+ to maintain electrical neutrality. Diuretic therapy, vomitting and diarrhea can cause hypochloremia.
3. Loss of K^+: H^+ and K^+ are exchanged in the distal tubule for Na^+. If the K^+ is low, then H^+ is retained. This will result in alkalosis.
4. Volume contraction: Free water loss concentrates HCO_3^- and thus increases the HCO_3^- concentration, and aldosterone release increases Na^+ reabsorbtion with K^+ and H^+ secretion in the distal tubules. Therefore, both alkalosis and hypokalemia result.
5. Massive resuscitation/transfusion: Common sources include lactate (Ringer's lactate) and citrate (blood).
6. Hypercarbia: Metabolic alkalosis is a compensatory response.

TABLE 9. *Random urinary electrolytes in metabolic alkalosis*[a]

	Saline sensitive	Saline resistant
Cl^-	<10 meq/L (no diuretics)	>10 meq/L
Na^+	<20 meq/L (unless recent vomiting)	>20 meq/L
K^+	High due to exchange for Na^+	High due to aldosterone effect

[a]Evaluation of urinary electrolytes assists in the assessment of metabolic alkalosis.

7. Hyperadrenalism (primary hyperaldosteronism and Cushing's disease): The high levels of hormone secretion cause retention of Na^+ and HCO_3^-, with excessive loss of Cl^- in the urine. The extracellular fluid compartment is volume expanded.

The classic cause of metabolic alkalosis is gastric outlet obstruction, such as with pyloric stenosis or peptic ulcer disease. Four contributors to alkalosis are present in this setting (loss of H^+, loss of K^+, loss of Cl^-, and volume contraction).

The expected pulmonary compensation in metabolic alkalosis is small: for every 1.0 mmol/L rise in plasma $[HCO_3^-]$, the PCO_2 should rise by 0.7 mm Hg. Because the causes of metabolic alkalosis involve volume loss, the kidneys respond by expanding the extracellular fluid compartment volume with Na^+ retention. Excretion of bicarbonate is not an option, due to the renal mechanisms for retaining Na^+.

Treatment

The vast majority of causes of metabolic alkalosis are chloride-responsive (Table 9); that is, by replenishing chloride, sodium can be reabsorbed by the kidneys with chloride and not with bicarbonate, and the alkalosis corrects. Urine electrolyte analysis reveals low chloride. Volume replacement with normal saline and potassium is the treatment for chloride-responsive alkalosis. Hyperadrenal disorders do not respond to chloride replacement; the extracellular volume compartment is already expanded, and the kidney is responding to the increased steroid milieu. Acetazolamide (carbonic anhydrase inhibitor, which inhibits reabsorption of bicarbonate) has a role in these chloride-resistent alkaloses, but the primary adrenal disorder must be addressed. The administration of acid as HCl is rarely needed, except in severe metabolic alkalosis, to prevent cardiac dysfunction.

RESPIRATORY ACID-BASE DISORDERS

In respiratory disorders, the PCO_2 is too high or too low and is a consequence of a problem with ventilation. In a normal person, the PCO_2 is close to 40 mm Hg. In respiratory acidosis, there is an increase in PCO_2 secondary to decreased alveolar ventilation. In respiratory alkalosis, there is a decrease in PCO_2 secondary to alveolar hyperventilation.

Physiological Response to PCO_2 Changes

Physiological responses to PCO_2 changes are as follows:

1. In acute respiratory acidosis, the HCO_3^- will remain close to 25 mmol/L and the pH will decrease by 0.1 U for each 10 mm Hg increase in PCO_2.
2. In chronic respiratory acidosis, the HCO_3^- will increase by 3 mmol/L for each 10 mm Hg rise in PCO_2. The pH will correct toward normal, but will remain acidotic.
3. In acute respiratory alkalosis, the changes are almost the same as in respiratory acidosis but in opposite direction. There is almost no change in plasma HCO_3^- and 0.1 pH unit rise for each 10 mm Hg fall in PCO_2.
4. In chronic respiratory alkalosis: The pH remains quite close to normal, but is alkalotic. The plasma HCO_3^- falls 5 mmol/L for each 10 mm Hg fall in PCO_2.

RESPIRATORY ACIDOSIS

Respiratory acidosis represents a failure of ventilation (removal of CO_2 from the alveoli). This can be either acute or chronic.

I. Inhibition of medullary respiratory center
   A. Acute
      1. Drugs (opiates, anesthetics, sedatives, alcohol)
      2. Oxygen administration in setting of chronic hypercapnea (hypoxia, not hypercarbia, is the main stimulus for ventilation in chronic obstructive pulmonary disease)
      3. Cardiac arrest
      4. Central sleep apnea
   B. Chronic
      1. Extreme obesity
      2. CNS lesion
II. Disorders of respiratory muscles
   A. Acute: muscle weakness (crisis in myasthenia gravis, aminoglycosides, severe hypokalemia, Gullain-Barré syndrome, hypophosphatemia)

B. Chronic
   1. Muscle weakness (amoytrophic lateral sclerosis, multiple sclerosis, myxedema)
   2. Kyphoscoliosis
   3. Extreme obesity
III. Acute upper airway obstruction (aspiration of foreign body or vomitus, obstuctive sleep apnea, laryngospasm)
IV. Disorders affecting gas exchange across pulmonary capillary
  A. Acute
   1. Exacerbation of underlying lung disease
   2. Adult respiratory distress syndrome
   3. Acute cardiogenic pulmonary edema
   4. Severe asthma or pneumonia
   5. Pneumothorax or hemothorax
  B. Chronic obstructive pulmonary disease (emphysema, chronic bronchitis)
V. Mechanical ventilation (improper settings, ventilator failure)

Treatment

Therapy focuses on improving alveloar ventilation, initially with aggressive pulmonary toilet and culminating in intubation. Underlying causes are then addressed and corrected. Bicarbonate is contraindicated as a quick fix, because in neutralizing acid it creates CO_2 which must be excreted.

Oxygen must be used cautiously in patients with chronic obstructive pulmonary disease and respiratory decompensation. Ventilatory drive in these patients derives from the hypoxic stimulus to the brainstem, not from the hypercarbic stimulus (reset because of the chronic hypercarbia). Thus, overoxygenation can lead to hypoventilation and exacerbation of the respiratory acidosis.

RESPIRATORY ALKALOSIS

Causes relate to hyperventilation, with consequent removal of greater CO_2. Again, this can represent an acute or chronic process.

I. Acute
  A. Psychogenic hyperventilation
  B. Errors in mechanical ventilation
  C. Acute hypoxemia (pneumonia, pulmonary embolism, pneumothorax, atelectasis, asthma)
  D. Drugs (salicylates)
  E. Fever
  F. CNS (tumor, infection, trauma, cerebrovascular accident [CVA])
  G. Sepsis
II. Chronic
  A. Prolonged hypoxemia (anemia, congenital heart disease, high altitude)
  B. Mechanical hyperventilation
  C. Sepsis
  D. CNS (tumor, infection, trauma, CVA)

Treatment

Treat the underlying disorder. Ventilated patients require ventilator adjustments that decrease ventilation.

CASE STUDY

The patient is a 55-year-old man with severe pancreatitis in renal, GI, and respiratory failure requiring mechanical ventilation. He has large nasogastric losses of >4 L/day. His lab values are as follows: $PO_2 = 60$; $Na^+ = 142$; $PCO_2 = 55$; $K^+ = 3$; pH = 7.21; $CO_2 = 28$; $HCO_3^- = 30$; $Cl^- = 90$. Acid-base analysis reveals the following: (a)

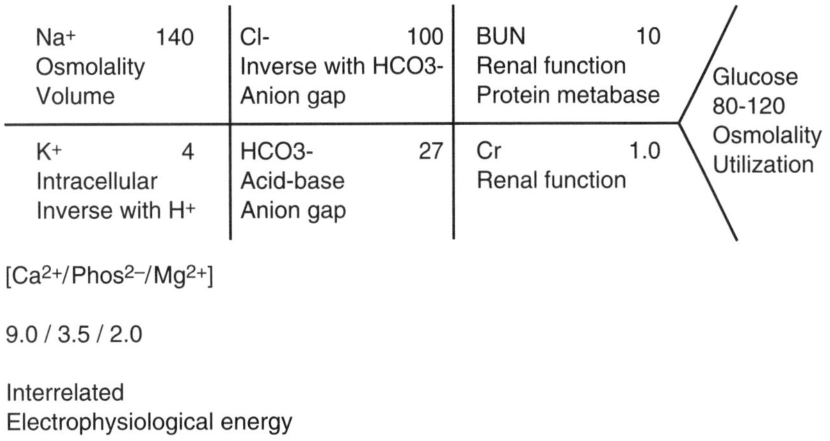

Na^+ 140 Osmolality Volume	Cl^- 100 Inverse with HCO_3^- Anion gap	BUN 10 Renal function Protein metabase	Glucose 80-120 Osmolality Utilization
K^+ 4 Intracellular Inverse with H^+	HCO_3^- 27 Acid-base Anion gap	Cr 1.0 Renal function	

$[Ca^{2+}/Phos^{2-}/Mg^{2+}]$

9.0 / 3.5 / 2.0

Interrelated
Electrophysiological energy

FIG. 6. Shorthand diagram for electrolytes, renal function, and glucose. Normal average values are listed, as well as concepts that underlie each. Na^+, sodium; K^+, potassium; Cl^-, chloride; HCO_3^-, bicarbonate; BUN, blood urea nitrogen; Cr, creatinine; Ca^{2+}, calcium; $Phos^{2-}$, phosphate; Mg^{2+}, magnesium.

respiratory acidosis: pH low, PCO_2 high; (b) metabolic alkalosis: $HCO_3^- = 30$; and (c) metabolic acidosis: on initial glance, this patient seems to have a combined disorder of respiratory acidosis and metabolic alkalosis; however, the patient is also in renal failure and has a hidden metabolic disorder; calculation revealed an increased anion gap of 24; if the anion gap is increased, then a metabolic acidosis must exist.

The respiratory acidosis was treated by increasing ventilation. The metabolic alkalosis, whch was caused by the large gastric losses, was treated by normal saline fluid replacement and K^+ administration. Finally, the metabolic acidosis, secondary to uremia, was treated by dialysis.

Figure 6 illustrates the organizational diagram often used for assessing electrolytes.

STUDY QUESTIONS

1. If the serum Na^+ is 140 meq/L, glucose 180, and BUN 28, what is the calculated plasma osmolality?
2. A 25-year-old male presents to the Emergency Room after being shot in the abdomen. His blood pressure is 70/40, with a pulse of 140. His skin is cool, and he is confused. Describe the appropriate choice and sequence of intravenous fluid replacement.
3. A 50-year-old, otherwise healthy, 50-kg female, 2 days after a sigmoid colectomy for diverticulitis, has a serum Na^+ of 130. She is taking nothing by mouth, and her maintenance intravenous fluid is D_5 half NS + 20 meq KCl/L at 150 cc/hr. Her urine output is 100 cc/hr. What is the most likely cause and most appropriate management of the hyponatremia?
4. Compare and contrast the EKG findings in patients with severe hypokalemia and hyperkalemia; then, find the similarities with disorders of serum calcium and magnesium concentration.
5. A 66-year-old, 70-kg male, previously healthy, presented to the Emergency Room with a 3-day history of severe periumbilical abdominal pain, vomiting, and absence of bowel movements or flatus. His pulse is 135, and his blood pressure is 90/60. Physical examination reveals a protruding, tender umbilicus, consistent with an incarcerated umbilical hernia. Laboratory values were as follows: Na^+ 128, K^+ 2.5, Cl^- 62, HCO_3^- 45, BUN 45, Cr 1.5; arterial blood gas pH 7.65, pCO_2 48. Define the full extent of the patient's fluid, electrolyte, and acid-base disorders, as well as the appropriate correction for each. When, in this patient's clinical course, should the umbilical hernia be repaired?

SUGGESTED READING

Gann D, Amaral J. Fluid and electrolyte management. In: Sabiston D, ed. *Essentials of surgery.* Philadelphia: Saunders, 1987:64–86.

Haber R. A practical aproach to acid-base disorders. *West J Med* 1991; 155(2):146–151.

Lyerly H, Gaynal W. Fluid and electrolytes/acid-base regulation. In: Lyerly H, ed. *Handbook of surgical critical care.* 3rd ed. St. Louis: Mosby, 1992:402–448.

Marino PL. *The ICU book.* Philadelphia: Lea and Febiger, 1991:415–450.

Morganroth M. Six steps to acid-base analysis: clinical applications. *J Crit Illness* 1990;5:81–85.

Pestana C. *Fluids and electrolytes in the surgical patient.* 4th ed. Baltimore: Williams and Wilkins, 1989.

Peterseim D. Fluids, electrolytes, and acid-base management. In: D'Amico T, Pruitt S, eds. *Handbook of surgical intensive care.* 4th ed. St. Louis: Mosby, 1995:472–491.

Schrier R, ed. *Renal and electrolyte disorders.* 3rd ed. Boston: Little, Brown, 1986.

Shires T, Canizaro P. Fluid and electrolyte management of the surgical patient. In: Sabiston D, ed. *Textbook of surgery.* 14th ed. Philadelphia: Saunders, 1991:25–38.

SECTION II

General Surgery

CHAPTER 6

Skin and Soft Tissue

Magesh Sundaram and David S. Robinson

DISEASES OF THE SKIN

Anatomy and Function

Skin is comprised of the epidermis and dermis separated by a basement membrane (Fig. 1). The main cells within the epidermis are keratinocytes that are found in various stages of maturity between the basement membrane and granular layer. Actively dividing keratinocytes line the basal layer, whereas senescent keratinocytes that have lost mitotic activity predominate in the superficial layer. During fetal life, neural crest cells migrate to the epidermis and become melanocytes. Dendritic processes extend from the melanocyte to interact with the many surrounding keratinocytes. Melanosomes within the dendritic processes contain melanin and are taken up by the keratinocytes by phagocytosis. Although all human skin has approximately the same number of melanocytes, individual skin pigmentation differs based on melanin production and transfer as well as melanosome degradation. The basement membrane represents a highly organized protein layer that anchors the epidermis to the dermis. Invasion of skin malignancy beyond the basement membrane defines an invasive cancer. Mechanical or inflammatory disruption of the basement membrane, e.g., toxic epidermolysis, results in epidermal slough and skin loss.

The majority of the skin's structural proteins and framework are found in the dermis. Structural and glandular elements as well as lymphatic channels and blood vessels are located in the ground substance that is composed chiefly of glycosaminoglycans (chondroitin sulfate, heparan sulfate, and hyaluronic acid). Structurally, collagen fibers provide the deep or reticular dermis of the skin with elastic deformability as well as tensile strength. Collagen is produced by the helical cross-linking of three tropocollagen chains composed of hydroxyproline, hydroxylysine, and glysine. Although seven types of collagen have been identified, type I collagen is the major

constituent of nonfetal human skin. Glandular structures of skin include pilosebaceous units and eccrine and apocrine glands. The pilosebaceous unit is composed of a hair follicle arising from a mitotically active germinal center with surrounding sebaceous glands that empty oily sebum into the follicle. Distributed throughout the body, but especially in the axillae, forehead, and palms are eccrine sweat glands that release sweat through pores in the papillary ridges of the dermis. The apocrine sweat glands, found in the axillae, inguinal, perianal, and periareolar regions, produce and release skin lubricants.

The skin is the largest organ in the human body and functions both as a protective barrier and a sensory interface between an individual and the external environment. Over different parts of the body, skin is classified into either glabrous or hairy skin. A thick keratinized epithelial layer of glabrous skin, found primarily in the palms and soles, provides a protective barrier against infectious agents (bacteria, viruses, parasites), noxious stimuli (toxic chemicals, gases), and solar radiation. Additionally, well-developed papillary ridges in the dermis limit shear stress trauma of skin during contact. Mechanical and corpuscular receptors and terminal sensory afferent nerves in the glabrous portion enable the skin to act as an exquisite sensory organ. Pacinian receptors in the deep reticular dermis respond to environmental pressure stimuli, whereas Meissner's corpuscles in the papillary dermis provide vibratory sense discrimination. Fine sensory innervation leading to Merkel cells and Ruffini endings provide fine touch information. Hairy skin provides barrier protection but at the expense of reduction in tactile and mechanical sensing abilities.

Thermoregulation is an important function of skin. Increased blood flow through an extensive capillary plexus within skin allows for rapid dissipation of elevated body heat during periods of fever or intense metabolic activity. Conversely, extreme external cold results in closure of cutaneous precapillary sphincters to mini-

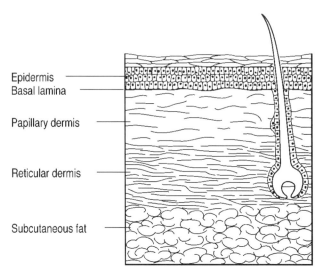

FIG. 1. Skin. Epidermal and dermal layers with hair follicle.

Epidermis
Basal lamina
Papillary dermis
Reticular dermis
Subcutaneous fat

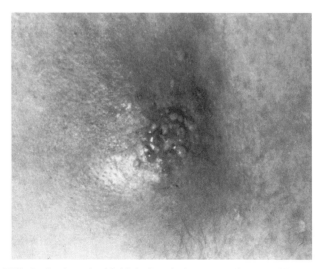

FIG. 2. Carbuncle. Multiple loculations erupting on skin surface with surrounding erythema.

mize heat loss by limiting cutaneous blood flow. The immunologic function of the skin is performed by specialized macrophages (Langerhan cells) that collectively amount to only 4% of the epidermal cell population. As HLA class II immune cells, the Langerhan cells have receptors for activated complement and the F_c component of immunoglobulin and are instrumental in initiating cutaneous immune function by identifying foreign antigens of bacteria and viruses.

DERMATOLOGIC PROBLEMS IN THE SURGICAL PATIENT

Infections

Infection and inflammation of a hair follicle by staphylococcus results in a superficial pustular process known as folliculitis. Obesity with secondary intertriginal folds, poor hygiene, diabetes, and humid weather are predisposing factors to infection. Although recurrence is common, folliculitis is generally self-limiting and will resolve with supportive care and improved hygiene. Untreated folliculitis may progress to a small abscess surrounding a hair follicle (furuncle). Oral antibiotics such as dicloxacillin or erythromycin are effective in treating simple folliculitis and small to moderate sized furuncles. Hexachlorophine soap leaves a residual film that inhibits the process from appearing at other sites.

Carbuncles (Fig. 2) are multiple communicating furuncles and typically grow to very large (>10 cm) multiloculated masses with multiple draining sites on the skin surface. A mature multiloculated carbuncle is invariably refractory to antibiotic therapy alone. Wide excision of the infected tissues and unroofing of sinus tracts are required to ensure complete drainage of infection.

Hidradenitis Suppurativa

Hidradenitis is a cutaneous bacterial infection as a result of occluded apocrine glands. Common skin bacteria, including staphylococcus and streptococcus, are the usual infectious agents. This condition is seen predominantly in areas of highest apocrine gland distribution including axillary (most common), inguinal, perianal, areolar, inframammary, and umbilical skin. After full development of apocrine glands, hidradenitis is usually recognized after puberty and may persist into adulthood.

Early in the course of apocrine gland and follicular occlusion, heightened infiltration by polymorphonuclear leukocytes results in perifolliculitis that manifests as erythematous, tender, subcutaneous nodules. Medical treatment of early hidradenitis consists of warm compresses, improved hygiene, and oral antibiotics. Oral tetracycline or erythromycin over a 2-week period is effective in treating early hidradenitis. Untreated acute hidradenitis will progress to local abscesses requiring surgical incision and drainage.

Persistent or incompletely treated disease results in multiple deep abscesses interconnected by sinus tracts lined with epidermis. The chronic inflammatory and infectious nature of this disease is exhibited by painful, indurated regions with foul-smelling, purulent drainage. Treatment of an acute exacerbation of chronic disease requires antibiotics and surgical unroofing of the draining sinus tracts. The wound is then allowed to heal by secondary intention. Chronic hidradenitis without acute infection may be electively treated with total excision of all affected apocrine gland bearing tissue followed by primary closure or autologous skin grafting. Such therapy is often more successful in the axillae than in the inguinal, perineal, or periareolar regions.

Psoriasis

The psoriasis syndromes are a constellation of dermatologic diseases that usually manifest during early adulthood. Stress, minor trauma, drug interaction, sunlight, and obesity are associated risk factors. Psoriasis often presents as a pruritic rash or irregularly confluent patch of sharply demarcated papular lesions with crusty silver-white scales. There may be associated symptoms of malaise, fever, and nonspecific arthritis. The underlying pathophysiology common to the various psoriatic syndromes includes increased turnover of the keratinocyte maturation cycle within the epidermis in response to inflammatory changes in the dermis. In general, treatment involves prevention of rubbing, scratching, and other minor local trauma to avoid continued stimulation of the psoriasis. Topical corticosteroid creams such as betamethasone and fluocinolone are effective in decreasing the underlying inflammatory process.

Psoriasis vulgaris (Fig. 3) presents as multiple scaly bright pink papular lesions on the trunk and extremities with sharply marginated borders. Exacerbation of this disorder is associated with nervous stress. Topical corticosteroids with or without occlusive dressings are effective. Psoriasis of the scalp may present in isolation or in combination with generalized psoriasis. Flaky white scales cover psoriatic plaques. Initial treatment involves removing the overlying scaling process by applying 2% salicylic acid followed by steroid lotions to plaques. Because pruritis is a self-perpetuating component of this disorder, effective treatment cannot be rendered without a conscious effort by the patient to abstain from rubbing or scratching the affected areas. When the disease appears on the palms and soles, topical steroid treatment is not always effective. Large lesions may require ultraviolet A (UVA) photochemotherapy and oral retinoids.

Keloids and Hypertrophic Scars

A disproportionate overgrowth of fibrous tissue within a healing wound, often occurring 6 months to 1 year after injury, leads to the formation of keloids and hypertrophic scars. These entities are commonly found in ethnic groups with deeper skin pigment (e.g., individuals of African descent). Hypertrophic scars are thickened, raised, or nodular tissue within the borders of the wound whereas keloids are bulky, nodular scars that extend beyond the wound borders (Fig. 4).

Mechanical pressure garments worn by patients beginning immediately upon appreciation of scar hypertrophy and lasting for up to 12 months applies constant local pressure upon the fibrous overgrowth, stimulates scar remodeling, and restores skin deformability. Surgical treatment is reserved for cosmetic revision or excision. Injection of glucocorticoids directly into keloids may reduce their bulk. Surgical excision of keloid formations is rarely undertaken because the very act of excision may stimulate the process with frequent recurrence leading to an unacceptable cosmetic result.

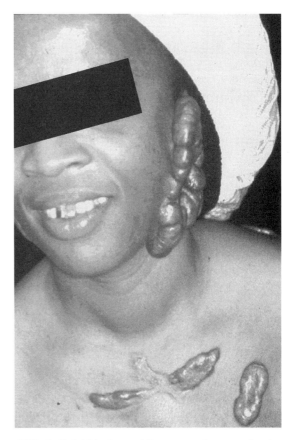

FIG. 4. Keloid lesions of the ear and upper chest.

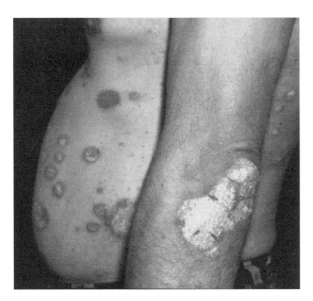

FIG. 3. Multiple psoriasis lesions of the trunk and upper extremity.

BENIGN NEOPLASMS OF THE SKIN

Seborrheic Keratosis

Seborrheic keratosis is a common hereditary (autosomal dominant transmission) skin disorder of older individuals. Lesions typically occur after the age of 30 and grow slowly over a period of months to years, appearing as light brown or yellow raised plaques on the face, trunk, and upper extremities. Seborrheic keratosis is uncommon in individuals of deeper skin pigmentation. The histopathology of these tumors is characterized by a proliferation of immature keratinocytes leading to horn cysts and papillomatosis without dermal extension. Small early lesions have a waxy, greasy surface with a stuck-on appearance. Larger keratoses have a more verrucous texture that is friable and may become secondarily infected. Larger, pigmented keratotic lesions look similar to pigmented basal cell carcinoma (BCC) and malignant melanoma; however, seborrheic keratosis has no premalignant potential. Cosmetic removal of large seborrheic keratotic lesions can be performed by excision or curettage followed by either electrocautery or cryotherapy under local anesthesia. Residual scarring is not a common complication of either treatment.

Keratoacanthoma

Keratoacanthoma (Fig. 5) appear as a solitary nodular lesion in older individuals. These lesions arise in sun-exposed skin such as the face, ears, and hands. Although spontaneous resolution can occur, characteristic rapid proliferation of keratinocytes with metaplasia of adjacent sebaceous glands leads to a nodular growth with a cratered center filled with horn cysts and keratin. Aggressive keratoacanthoma growth has been recognized in the immunocompromised population.

Although keratoacanthoma has no malignant potential, the rapid growth and striking appearance often necessitates a biopsy including a rim of normal adjacent skin to exclude malignancy. Unlike squamous cell carcinoma (SCC), keratoacanthoma does not exhibit invasion of the deep dermis. On occasion, a recurrence of SCC after resection and radiation may be histologically indistinguishable from keratoacanthoma. Surgical excision of the benign, primary lesion or revision of a cosmetically unacceptable scar following regression can be performed under local anesthesia.

Cysts (Epidermal, Dermoid, Pilar)

Epidermal (inclusion) cysts occur on the face, scalp, trunk, and extremities as solitary nodules and are the most common type of intradermal cysts. Dermoid cysts result from trapped epithelium enveloped during healing of a scar or during embryological development. Pilar

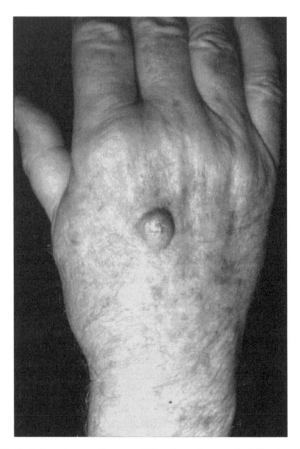

FIG. 5. A keratoacanthoma of the dorsal aspect of the hand.

(trichilemmal) cysts are indistinguishable from epidermal cysts, but are found only in the scalp, and the pilar cyst wall resembles the sheath of a hair follicle. When epidermal inclusion cysts are multiple, they may be associated with familial colonic polyposis syndromes, such as Gardener's syndrome.

These cysts are lined with one complete layer of epidermis. Incorrectly referred to as sebaceous cysts due to the clinical appearance of a creamy center thought originally to be sebum, it is now recognized that the white cheesy material consists of desquamated keratinocytes collected at the cyst center from epidermal maturation. Occasionally, an epidermal cyst becomes infected exhibiting erythema and swelling of the surrounding skin. An infected cyst requires incision and drainage. Upon resolution of the abscess, the cyst wall and surrounding indurated dermal tissues must be excised to prevent disease recurrence of an infection. Asymptomatic epidermal cysts may be excised with a elliptical skin incision. These cysts have no malignant potential.

Nevi (Acquired, Congenital)

Acquired nevi, or moles, are found most frequently in Caucasian individuals. Typically, these small pigmented, maculopapular lesions arise from a benign overgrowth of melanocytes in various parts of the skin. They may be dermal nevi or junctional nevi present in the epidermal-dermal skin junction or compound nevi that have a histologic combination of both junctional and dermal nevi. Although some of these lesions may appear during childhood, acquired nevi occur most commonly in adults and may involute later in life. Generally, no treatment is necessary.

Congenital nevi such as the giant hairy nevus are rare. Commonly described as bathing trunk lesions, these appear over the scalp, back, and trunk and may involve large diffuse segments of skin or scattered discontiguous patches. As with acquired nevi, there is a proliferation of the melanocytic nevus cell in the dermis and subcutaneous fat. Although these lesions primarily pose a cosmetic problem, malignant melanoma may develop within a giant hairy nevus. Consequently, if not removed, such lesions require aggressive surveillance. The treatment of congenital nevi is surgical excision and either skin grafting or tissue expansion and flap advancement. Large congenital nevi encompassing a majority of an infant's skin surface area may require several excisions over a period of years.

Hemangiomas and Vascular Malformations

Hemangiomas are benign lesions that arise from excessive proliferation of mature vascular elements within endothelial channels. The most common hemangioma is the capillary (strawberry) variety; this lesion is often present at birth, but it can develop during the first few weeks of life. These hemangiomas are characterized as lobular, bright red or purple lesions with a spongy texture. Despite some growth during infancy, immediate surgical excision of this hemangioma is not advised because >90% will involute without cosmetic impairment by 6 or 7 years of age. A rapid growth of a giant or cavernous strawberry hemangiomas over a period of weeks may be associated with thrombocytopenia due to platelet sequestration (Kasabach and Merrit syndrome) or high output cardiac failure due to trapping of blood in the vascular channels. If intervention is necessary, corticosteroids usually inhibit the rapid growth and alleviate the systemic consequences. Surgical excision or laser ablation may be used in treating giant hemangiomas, but both may have adverse cosmetic consequences. The former technique typically results in a scar while the latter leaves white hypopigmented skin.

Vascular malformations of the skin include port wine stains, arteriovenous malformations, and glomus tumors. Unlike the actively dividing endothelium of hemangiomas, these lesions are caused by ectasia of normal skin vascular elements with nonproliferating endothelial channels. A progressive ectatic growth of skin capillaries results in the port wine stain. A flat purple-red lesion

appears typically at birth over the trunk and face and grows in proportion with the body. Spontaneous involution is uncommon. Port wine stains presenting in the trigeminal distribution of the face may be a manifestation of Sturge-Weber syndrome or Osler-Weber-Rendu syndrome and should alert clinicians to the possibility of associated glaucoma or intracranial vascular malformations.

Previous treatment of port wine stains, including cryotherapy as well as surgical excision and grafting, was often unsatisfactory resulting in poor cosmesis. Currently, dye lasers are used in the partial or complete excision of port wine stains without significant scarring, but, again, with diffuse hypopigmented areas as the consequence of therapy.

PREMALIGNANT NEOPLASMS OF THE SKIN

Actinic Keratosis

Actinic keratosis, also known as solar or senile keratosis, is a common premalignant lesion arising in previously sun-exposed skin of the elderly. Cumulative skin damage develops from prolonged skin exposure to ultraviolet B (UVB) radiation. The proliferation of neoplastic keratinocytes with cellular anaplasia makes actinic keratosis the earliest form of epidermal cutaneous malignancy; however, there is no propensity for invasion of the basement membrane. SCC may develop in up to 20% of patients with actinic keratosis, but fortunately such lesions rarely metastasize.

Although easily recognized as dry, rough, and scaly papules, the color of an actinic keratotic lesion may vary from bright pink to dark brown. These lesions respond quite well to excision or topical 5-fluorouracil treatment. Larger hypertrophic lesions may be treated with liquid nitrogen cryotherapy. Prevention of actinic keratosis is best accomplished through routine use of UVB sunscreens.

Leukoplakia

Leukoplakia is a premalignant lesion occurring on oral, rectal, or vulvar mucosal surfaces, that the World Health Organization defines as a white spot that cannot be rubbed or stripped away and is not attributable to other causes. Oral leukoplakia is most commonly seen in discrete or confluent patches among users of tobacco products including pipes, cigars, and chewing tobacco. Histologic features of leukoplakia include parakeratosis and hyperkeratosis and in more advanced premalignant stages may also reveal anaplastic basal keratinocytes with dysplasia and abnormal mitosis. A biopsy is often necessary to distinguish leukoplakia from lichen planus or candidiasis. Invasive SCC arises in 5% to 7% of these lesions and may have metastatic potential. Erythroplakia is similar but appears as a pink on red patch. A histologic analysis will demonstrate multiple capillaries in addition to the changes of leukoplakia. In 80% of cases, coexistent squamous cell cancer will be found. Quiescent leukoplakia can be observed. Complete regression of oral disease has been reported when an offending irritant (i.e., tobacco) has been removed. Resection of small lesions can be performed safely without significant post excisional deformity. Large areas of disease, if not resected, mandate careful routine follow up to monitor dysplastic transformation of the plaque. Residual oral leukoplakia showing progressive growth despite withdrawal of carcinogenic agents must be considered clinically suspicious for malignancy and biopsied.

MALIGNANT NEOPLASMS OF THE SKIN

Nonmelanoma malignancies

Epidemiology

Skin cancer is the most common malignancy in the United States. Approximately 800,000 new cases are diagnosed annually. The most common nonmelanoma skin cancer is BCC, followed by SCC. Cancer of the adnexal skin structures (apocrine, eccrine glands) and accessory cellular elements (Merkel cell) are much rarer clinical entities.

The primary risk factor in development of skin cancer is prolonged exposure to solar radiation. The most damaging type of radiation in sunlight is UVB, in the 290- to 320-nm range. Living in equatorial or ozone-depleted regions carries the greatest risk of UVB radiation exposure. Studies have shown that individuals with outdoor occupations are more likely to develop skin cancer than those with indoor occupations. Individuals with less skin pigmentation, including albinos, are more prone to skin cancer than those who are more deeply pigmented.

There are other etiologic factors that raise the risk of skin cancer. Arsenic and nitrogen mustard are recognized chemical carcinogens known to cause basal cell cancer. Ionizing radiation therapy may lead to the development of BCC in the irradiated skin. Chronic viral infection with human papilloma virus and chronic nonhealing skin (e.g., burn wounds, stasis ulcers) may lead to SCC after several years.

Staging

The current staging system for both basal and SCC of the skin has been established by the American Joint Committee on Cancer (AJCC) to include clinical and pathologic evaluation of the tumor, nodal, and metastatic status

TABLE 1. *TNM staging classification of carcinoma of skin (excluding eyelid, vulva, and penis)*

Stage	T	N	M
I	T_1	N_0	M_0
II	T_{2-3}	N_0	M_0
III	T_4	N_0	M_0
	Any T	N_1	M_0
IV	Any T	Any N	M_1

T (primary tumor): T_x, primary tumor cannot be assessed; T_0, no evidence of primary tumor; T_1, tumor >2 cm in greatest dimension; T_2, tumor > 2 cm but >5 cm in greatest dimension; T_3, tumor >5 cm in greatest dimension; T_4, tumor invades deep extradermal structures, i.e., cartilage, muscle bone.

N (regional lymph nodes): N_x, regional lymph nodes cannot be assessed; N_0, no regional lymph node metastasis; N_1, regional lymph node metastasis.

M (distant metastasis): M_0, no distant metastasis; M_1, distant metastasis.

(Table 1). Clinical examination includes physical examination and palpation of the primary tumor and regional lymph nodes. A complete excision of the entire tumor including tissue below its depth is required for pathologic evaluation.

Basal Cell Carcinoma

Basal cell cancers (Fig. 6) are the least aggressive of the skin cancers and grow slowly, often ignored by patients for years. Originally believed to arise from the mitotically active keratinocytes in the basal layer of the epidermis, BCC is now thought to arise from a pluripotent epithelial cell. Histologically, basal cell cancers are comprised of small undifferentiated cells with high nuclear content in a palisading formation. BCC is categorized into five distinct subtypes: noduloulcerative, superficial multicentric, sclerosing (fibrosing morphea-form), pigmented, and fibroepithelioma/carcinoma. Met-

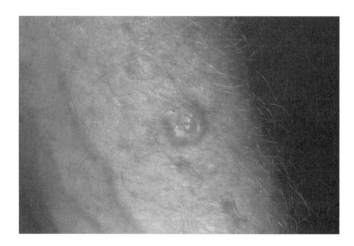

FIG. 6. Basal cell carcinoma of the forearm.

astasis from BCC occurs in <0.1% of cases. While lymphatic spread to regional lymph nodes and hematogenous spread to the lung have been reported, if they occur, the original diagnosis should be reviewed. Local invasion and destruction is a common feature seen with larger BCC. BCC will spread along periosteal, perineural, or fascial planes as the path of least resistance before invading bone or muscle. This feature accounts for the high recurrence rate after surgical excision of basal cell cancers of the central portion of the face and of the periauricular areas.

Treatment

Complete elimination of the cancer with preservation of cosmesis and skin function encompass the major principles of treatment for BCC. Surgical excision should ideally remove the tumor with a 2- to 4-mm edge form the margin to minimize the risk of recurrence. Large superficial multicentric BCC and sclerosing BCC are the subtypes more likely to have incomplete excision with positive margins. The risk of locally recurrent disease can be assessed by evaluating ulceration, tumor thickness, infiltrative radial spread, and anatomic location in cosmetically vital areas. Primary closure, autologous skin grafting, and local flap rotation are all acceptable means of coverage of the surgical defect after excision.

Curettage and electrodesiccation can be used to treat small BCCs. Sharp curettage to the base of the lesion followed by monopolar electrosurgery can excise a small lesion under local anesthesia. Prior to applying this form of treatment, however, the subtype of BCC must be accurately determined as deeply infiltrative tumor may require deeper resection. Cure rates are high with curettage and electrodesiccation, but poor cosmesis may result from repeated therapy for recurrent lesions.

Moh's surgery is an approach employed by dermatologists specializing in this area. The primary advantage of Moh's surgery is intraoperative examination of the radial and deep margins of tumor extent. Following surgical excision of the tumor, serial sections of the underlying and surrounding skin are taken parallel to the surface. The sections are then fixed in the surgical suite and examined for microscopic residual tumor. Once clear deep and radial margins have been appreciated, complete resection of the tumor has been performed. Depending on the defect, its location, and its depth, the wound may be closed surgically or left to close by secondary intent.

Reports describe the removal of multiple small lesions with cryosurgery using liquid nitrogen that causes cell destruction by intracellular ice crystal formation. More importantly it preserves surrounding normal tissue. Cryosurgery is useful in treating small benign warts and keratoses. Complications include inflammatory pigmentation and hypertrophic scarring.

Superficial external beam radiation therapy is an alternative means of treating BCC in elderly patients with comorbid medical disease that prohibits extensive surgical procedures. Radiation therapy is particularly useful in treating BCC of the nose and eyelid to avoid surgical excision. Radiation delivered over multiple sessions in fractionated doses can provide cure rates of >90%, but adverse effects include radiation dermatitis ("sunburn") and involutional scarring.

Squamous Cell Carcinoma

Radiation damage to the skin from chronic sun exposure is the primary predisposing factor for SCC. Cumulative ultraviolet (UV) radiation damages the protective clearance ability of the skin's immune system. Other factors include environmental carcinogens, viral infection, previous irradiation, and premalignant skin lesions such as actinic keratosis. Although uncommon in heavily pigmented people, SCC may still arise in pigmented individuals who have chronically inflamed wounds such as burn wounds (Marjolin's ulcer). SCC will also arise in the sun-exposed skin of immunosuppressed patients (renal transplant, chronic lymphocytic leukemia, and AIDS); UV radiation combined with functional depression of the cutaneous Langerhan cells is postulated to be the etiology.

Squamous cell cancer is usually more aggressive than basal cell cancer because it has a greater tendency to be locally invasive and develop metastatic disease. The biologic behavior of SCC is dependent on tumor thickness and depth of invasion; metastasis of SCC can occur once there is deep dermal or subcutaneous invasion. Intraepithelial SCC without invasion of the dermis is referred to as in situ disease. Bowen's disease is an in situ SCC typically found in the anogenital skin region presenting as a slow-growing erythematous plaque. Erythroplasia of Queyrat refers to in situ disease of the penis, vulva, or anogenital region.

Squamous cell cancer (Fig. 7) presents as a plaque or nodule with superficial ulceration, crusting, or scale formation. The change in appearance of a previously diagnosed premalignant or in situ lesion warrants suspicion. There can be rapid growth over weeks to months. Although often pink or deep red in Caucasian individuals, SCC can be hyper- or hypopigmented in individuals of deeper skin pigmentation.

Metastatic skin lesions are more common in squamous cell cancers arising from irradiated tissue or at mucocutaneous junctions such as the mouth, anus, or vulva. The degree of cellular differentiation appears to influence lymphatic spread with more pernicious tumors exhibiting cellular atypia or anaplasia developing metastatic regional lymph node disease. Hematogenous metastasis to distant organs is seen in only 5% to 10% of SCC.

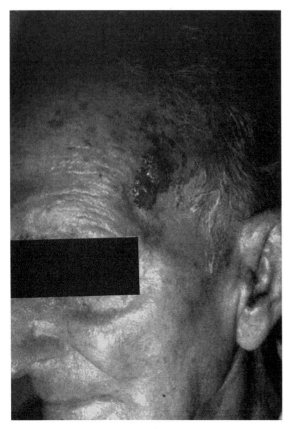

FIG. 7. Sun-exposed areas like the forehead are common sites for the development of squamous cell carcinoma of the skin.

Treatment of SCC involves aggressive, wide surgical excision. Ideally, 1-cm clear margins in noncosmetic and 3- to 5-mm margins in cosmetically vital areas should be obtained. Additionally, lymph node metastases should be aggressively pursued with therapeutic lymphadenectomy. Moh's surgery may be employed in the treatment of recurrent or incompletely excised SCC. As with basal cell cancers, fractionated superficial radiation therapy may also provide an effective treatment alternative.

Uncommon Nonmelanoma Skin Malignancies

Cancer of skin adnexal structures are rare malignancies involving the apocrine, eccrine, sebaceous, and follicular structures of the skin. The malignant potential of these cancers is dependent on the degree of cellular differentiation and atypia. These tumors can be highly invasive and may metastasize to distant organs. Surgical and radiation therapy are possible treatment options. Merkel cell carcinoma is another rare skin cancer derived from the neuroepithelial Merkel cell. While this tumor will usually appear as an independent lesion, there have been reports of SCC associated with this locally aggressive tumor. Surgical resection of Merkel cell carcinoma with regional lymphadenectomy and radiation therapy are recommended.

Malignant Melanoma

Epidemiology

Malignant melanoma is the most aggressive of the skin cancers. Arising from melanocytes, 50% to 60% of malignant melanoma can be attributed to a change in an existing benign nevus, while the remainder appears to evolve in otherwise normal skin de novo. Although most melanoma patients have no known hereditary factors, an apparent genetic link exists in 3% to 6% of patients, and 40% to 50% of those with familial malignant melanoma will develop multiple primary sites of disease. Still others with dysplastic nevus syndrome may manifest a genetic predisposition for malignant melanoma. These individuals have multiple, often unusual appearing nevi.

Malignant melanoma has been linked to excessive sunlight exposure. It is seen most frequently in those of northern European ancestry who have emigrated to areas of greatest sunlight exposure. In that regard, in the southern United States (the so-called sunbelt) there is an increased prevalence of malignant melanoma. While rare in people with deeper skin pigment, melanoma has been found in all peoples. In those of African descent, acral lentiginous melanoma develops on the soles of the feet and the palms of the hands, usually at the interface of pigmented and unpigmented skin.

Clinically, malignant melanoma is divided into four categories. Seventy percent of malignant melanoma is of the superficial spreading (Fig. 8) variety originating from a macular nevus or normal skin and exhibiting a radial (lateral) growth phase. Superficial spreading malignant melanoma is an unfortunately misleading misnomer in that, with development of a vertical growth phase, a large percentage of cases will develop metastatic disease.

Nodular melanoma (Fig. 9) constitutes 10% to 15% of cutaneous malignant melanoma and is characterized primarily by vertical growth. The acral lentiginous (Fig. 10) variant, occuring predominately on the soles of the feet and in subungual locations and on the palms, has both radial and vertical growth phases, but under the nail may simply appear like a splinter hemorrhage.

The least virulent form of the disease is the lentigo maligna variant often occurring in a Hutchinson's freckle on the face of an older individual. Ten percent to 15% of melanomas are of this variety. Often indolent and unchanging for years with an unassuming growth pattern, when patients with lentigo melanomas develop a change such as a nodule (vertical growth) or ulceration, they are just as prone to metastatic disease as the other variants.

Diagnosis

Often it is difficult to determine whether a lesion is a malignant melanoma or some other variant of dermato-

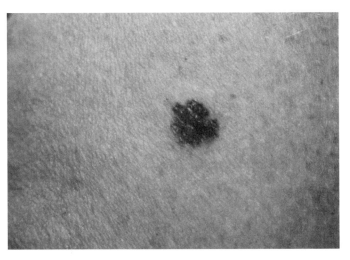

FIG. 8. Superficial spreading malignant melanoma.

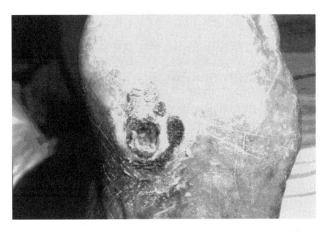

FIG. 10. Acral lentiginous melanoma found on sole of foot.

logic disease. Clinical doubt should indicate the need for biopsy of the lesion including a significant portion of underlying tissue to allow the pathologist to make an appropriate determination of depth of involvement and risk of metastasis. These lesions should never be removed tangentially (shaving) because that will often slice the upper portion of the lesion away while the rest remains behind leaving in question the true depth of the cancer, an important prognostic indicator of potential metastasis. Lesions that are reported after tangential excision showing melanoma still present in the lesions and excised base must be presumed to be deep enough to carry a risk of metastasis until proven otherwise.

Disease Behavior

"Local" metastases consist of satellite lesions described as small clusters of cells trapped in regional lymphatic vessels presenting around the primary site of malignant melanoma. These lesions typically occur within a 2- to 3-cm distance from the primary lesion. More distant, locoregional metastases are subcutaneous sites of intransit disease caught in the lymphatic vessels between the primary site and the regional lymph nodes.

Regional lymph nodes are considered one of the primary deposits of metastatic disease. Whereas the upper extremities drain to the axillary lymph nodes and the lower extremities drain to the inguinal lymph nodes, melanomas of the trunk may show some variability in draining to one or more lymph node basins sometimes crossing the midline or the beltline (Sappey's line: just cephalad to the umbilicus to the L_1-L_2 level). Because of variability in truncal anatomic lymphatic anatomy, lymph shed mapping was introduced in the mid-1970s with the intradermal injection of a radioactive colloid that is picked up by the dermal lymphatics and transported to regional lymph nodes where it is concentrated. Scintiscanning can demonstrate the direction of lymph flow. More recent advances have refined this technique to evaluate patients in the operating room with a sterile hand-held radiation counter to determine the first lymph node(s) that drain the area of concern. Studies of these sentinel nodes are ongoing, using this technique of the injection of a colloid blue dye for visual sighting, to determine if removal of this first node(s) will provide the appropriate information regarding the presence of metastasis.

Therapy

Historically, the treatment of malignant melanoma has involved radical surgical excison with wide margins. In the last decade studies suggest that a 1.0- to 1.5-cm margin around disease may be appropriate for relatively superficial lesions, but lesions of >2.0 mm in depth may require a wider reexcision. For thicker areas such as the back, excision of the underlying muscular fascia has not been shown to be of increased benefit. Primary closure of

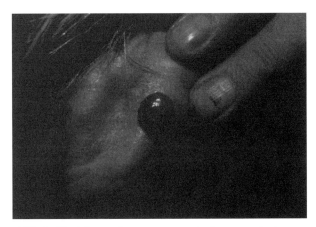

FIG. 9. Nodular melanoma on posterior aspect of ear.

the defect, when possible, is the optimal cosmetic and oncologic maneuver; however, in some anatomic sites, placement of a split-thickness skin graft may be necessary.

The efficacy of resection of regional lymph nodes remains in debate. While advocates of resection have suggested that prophylactic removal of regional nodes may be of benefit, others have reported little or no benefit to this approach. For the selected patient of higher risk (e.g., a male with a deep malignant melanoma of the head-and-neck region), a regional lymph node dissection may be appropriate. While therapeutic lymph node dissection is the only prophylactic approach to surgical therapy beyond local excision for patients at risk, it does not guarantee that the patient will not develop distant metastasis.

Although malignant melanoma is the most aggressive skin malignancy, it is also one of the most protean diseases in terms of its manifestations. Some patients with large bulky disease experience long disease-free intervals after surgical resection. In contrast, other patients with seemingly minimal amounts of melanoma develop widespread metastases to which they succumb in short order. Since outcome cannot be predicted consistently, most surgeons who treat malignant melanoma are aggressive in its care. Given melanoma's idiosyncratic nature, the removal of distant metastatic disease is undertaken in an effort to improve disease-free survival but only rarely will this result in cure. Consequently, large and sometimes unconventional operations are performed because the true natural history of metastatic disease is uncertain. The most common sites of metastases include lungs, liver, peritoneal surfaces, and gastrointestinal tract.

Various nonsurgical modalities have been developed in the treatment of metastatic malignant melanoma, all with little success. The most widely used chemotherapeutic agent in treatment of melanoma has been dacarbazine. Disappointing response rates of 15% to 20% that last <6 months and result in complete remission in <5% of patients have been reported. Newer, multiagent trials with dacarbazine, cisplatin, and tamoxifen have also been used as adjuvant therapy for malignant melanoma. Nonspecific immunotherapy has shown no improval in survival. Postoperative (adjuvant) administration of alpha interferon has shown benefit for patients who have been cleared of local and regional melanoma and who are at risk to develop metastatic disease. Radiation therapy for metastasis has not traditionally been used because doses required to affect known disease are higher than that needed for other types of cancer. Consequently, the higher complication rate restricts this modality for patients with known metastatic disease of a specific site.

Prognosis

Clark, a pathologist, was the first to define the levels of melanoma invasion through the skin (Fig. 11). Clark rec-

ognized that melanoma invasion to deeper levels of skin gave malignant cells greater access to blood and lymphatic vessels with a greater possibility for metastasis. In a similar analysis, another pathologist, Breslow, began to look at the risk of spread of melanoma as a consequence of tumor thickness in fractions of millimeters. While Clark's level are independent of thickness and Breslow's numerical approach is independent of anatomic depth, they correlate well with one another. Both are valid and have their place in determination of risk from the primary site of malignant melanoma (Table 1).

Studies demonstrate that very few patients with lesions of <0.76 mm in depth (Clark's level I or a thin Clark's level II lesion) developed local recurrence, regional recurrence, or distant metastasis. Conversely, in the same report, a majority of patients with lesions of >4.0 mm in depth developed distant metastases beyond the site of locoregional treatment and almost always succumbed to the disease, giving rise to concern that such patients should not be offered extensive therapy with little hope of cure. The presence of ulceration or bleeding from a nevus further increases the risk for the development of metastatic disease. In every circumstance, the depth of disease potential of metastatic disease must be considered against the consequent risks and benefits of therapy.

NEOPLASMS OF THE SOFT TISSUES

Over 50% of the human body consists of muscle, fascia, fat, bone, cartilage, and connective tissue derived from the embryologic mesoderm; this is all collectively termed the "soft tissues." Benign soft tissue tumors generally have the same degree of cellular differentiation as adult tissues. Malignant tumors from these soft tissues

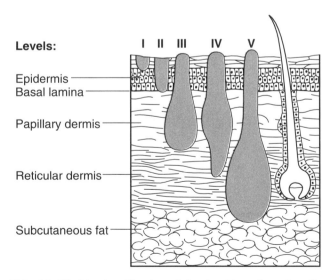

FIG. 11. Clark's classification of depth of invasion of malignant melanoma.

(sarcoma, from the Greek root *sarkoma*, meaning fleshy tumor) are rather uncommon and represent only 1% of all cancers newly diagnosed in the United States; 1996 estimates are that only 6,400 new cases of sarcoma were diagnosed.

Benign Soft Tissue Neoplasms

Benign tumors are much more common than malignant tumors of soft tissues, but the true incidence is not known because the vast majority of these tumors, when small, are not submitted for pathological examination after surgical excision.

Nonaggressive benign tumors show no propensity for local invasion or distant metastasis and once excised with few exceptions do not recur. Lipomas are benign growths of adipose tissue that often present as painless subcutaneous masses. Clinically, they are soft to rubbery and while they are distinct their edges may be difficult to palpably define. At resection they are discrete from the surrounding subcutaneous fat and may be either simple or multilobulated collections of adipose tissue. Simple surgical excision is warranted for larger lipomas or those that are cosmetically or functionally bothersome. If incompletely excised, including the thin outer membrane, they can recur. Dermatofibromas are nodular lesions of the skin arising from a proliferation of dermal fibroblasts. Found commonly on the lower extremities, these benign tumors are generally asymptomatic and can be observed if they are historically unchanged of long duration. Neurofibromas, tumors of Schwann cell origin, often present as multiple small variably sized cutaneous flesh-colored tumors; the association with a hyperpigmented macular cafe-au-lait spot defines von Recklinghausen's disease, a familial disorder that carries an underlying risk of malignancy through degeneration of one of the neurofibromas (~7%). Leiomyomas are tumors of the smooth muscle most commonly seen in the gastrointestinal tract and the uterus. No directed surgical intervention is required for asymptomatic leimyomas; however, those in the stomach of >4 cm should be considered at greater risk of malignant degeneration.

Aggressive benign tumors are notable for their propensity to locally infiltrate and have a high rate of recurrence if inadequately resected. Desmoid tumors arise from fibrous and muscular tissues. When discovered clinically, desmoids may present in the abdominal wall and, in that location, are discovered more often in postpartum women. Resection with surrounding clear margins can be curative. Intraabdominal desmoids growing unobserved until late can become quite large or they may be multifocal. These discrete tumors may invade the intestinal mesentery and surround or invade vascular structures. In those circumstances, aggressive en bloc resection with associated organs is required to

minimize recurrence. An aggressive excision may mean removal of a good deal of small bowel because of the involvement of the mesentery leaving the patient with a short bowel syndrome. Gardner's syndrome is an autosomal dominant disease characterized by colonic polyposis, mesenteric desmoids and fibromatosis, and soft tissue osteomas. In treatign large debilitating desmoids of the extremities, radiation therapy has proved to be effective as a nonsurgical option. Dermatofibrosarcoma protuberans is a progressive and recurrent variant of the benign cutaneous dermatofibroma. This tumor is noted for diffuse infiltration of the dermis & subcutis and is typically seen as a nodular cutaneous mass on the trunk or scalp with slow growth over years. Despite its locally aggressive behavior and local recurrence, this tumor rarely metastasizes, and should not be considered a true sarcoma. The ideal treatment consists of initial wide local resection with clear margins of at least 2 cm.

Malignant Soft Tissue Neoplasms

Sarcomas, malignant mesencyhmal tumors, may arise in any part of the body, but are most common in the extremities, the peritoneum and retroperitoneum. Sarcomas are usually classified by their predominate tissue type (Table 2). For example, a rhabdomyosarcoma is a tumor of a predominate striated muscle cell type. Histologically, they may be difficult to define because of the presence of several mesenchymal tissue types. There is no clear etiologic factor that leads to the development of most sarcomas. The literature does reflect a few instances of causal agents. Environmental factors such as exposure to the herbicide dioxin or the chemical polyvinylchloride have been found to cause sarcoma. Sarcomas can also be traced to antecedent medical therapy or chronic disease. Lymphangiosarcoma is a uncommon sequelae of chronic primary or secondary lymphedema. Previously, exposure to thorotrast, a radiographic contrast, increased patient risk of developing angiosarcoma of the liver. There is no inherited risk for most sarcomas, but a genetic predisposition, the Li-Fraumeni syndrome, has been well documented. Here, family members present with both breast cancer and soft tissue sarcomas.

Clinical Presentation

Soft tissue tumors present with various signs and symptoms depending on location and size of tumor. Sarcomas of the extremities present as a swelling or mass recently noted by the patient over the previous few weeks. One-third will report pain with the swelling. Progressive growth increases the likelihood of a malignant soft tissue tumor. In contrast, intraabdominal or retroperitoneal sarcomas are for the most part, asympto-

TABLE 2. *Clark and Breslow staging of malignant melanoma based on depth of invasion*

Stage	Clark	Breslow
I	*In situ* melanoma confined to epidermal basement membrane	Tumor depth of <0.75 mm
II	Melanoma invasive to the papillary dermis	Tumor depth of 0.75–1.5 mm
III	Melanoma invasive to the junction of the papillary-reticular dermis	Tumor depth of 1.5–4.0 mm
IV	Melanoma invasive to the reticular dermis	Tumor depth of >4.0 mm
V	Melanoma invasive to the subcutaneous tissues	

matic and may grow to massive proportions before causing noticeable symptoms (Fig. 12). Vague, nonspecific abdominal pain of 6 to 8 months duration is typical of these sarcomas. Pelvic sarcomas may lead to symptoms of sciatica or leg edema from nervous or venous entrapment. Sarcomas involving the gastrointestinal tract may present acutely causing bleeding, intestinal obstruction, or perforation.

Diagnosis

Physical examination is directed to the specific body region in question. Careful examination of the abdomen will reveal a palpable mass in a large percentage of patients with abdominal or retroperitoneal sarcomas. With regard to extremity masses, exact size and location, neurovascular status, and attachment to bony structures are important details. Radiologic evaluation by computed tomography (CT) scan or magnetic resonance imaging (MRI) scans should be obtained. A chest radiograph and CT scan of the chest should also be obtained to exclude pulmonary metastases once a tissue diagnosis has been made.

The appreciation of an intraabdominal mass which potentially represents a sarcoma, by standard practice will come to diagnosis with operative excision of the tumor for both a diagnostic and therapeutic event. This is because of the difficulty in obtaining tissue without general anesthesia and laparotomy, and because these tumors often invade organs and vascular structures. Once encountered, the consideration, often, is that additional preoperative treatment will not alter the course of disease. Still, because of the rarity of these tumors a large prospective trial of preoperative chemotherapy has yet to be undertaken.

On the other hand, the actual diagnosis of an extremity sarcoma should be made prior to and not concurrent with treatment. Fine needle aspiration is generally not helpful because cytological exam cannot demonstrate the architectural features necessary for diagnosis. By the same token, core samples may not be adequate to diagnose a sarcoma because of the small sample size. Open biopsy of tumors may be either incisional or excisional. Generally, an incisional biopsy is recommended when a sarcoma is suspected. Enucleation is never acceptable. Very small tumors may be excisionally biopsied but excisional biopsy of larger sarcomas is not recommended because tumor cells may be shed into the wound along tissue planes of dissection. The standard of care in sarcoma surgery is that, when possible, the tumor should be resected with a surrounding cuff of normal tissue; the tumor at resection should not be seen. Consequently, an excisional biopsy may obligate needless radical therapy for complete resection to be certain of completely encompassing the cancer.

The direction of incision of large tumors should be in the longitudinal axis of the extremity, directly over the most superficial, central part of the tumor (Fig. 13). The biopsy should be carried out by cutting straight down to the tumor, without performing lateral dissection along tissue planes. Horizontal dissection should be avoided because resection and closure is far more difficult in that circumstance.

Staging and Prognosis

Staging of soft tissue sarcomas, as determined by the American Joint Committee on Cancer (AJCC), is based on tumor size, lymph node involvement, metastasis, and histopathologic grade (Tables 3 and 4). Histopathologic grade, tumor size, patient age, and the presence of distant metastasis are important factors in predicting overall prognosis. Tumor size is generally assessed preoperatively by

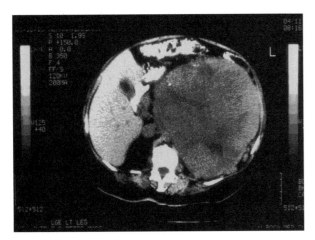

FIG. 12. Computed tomography scan of the abdomen demonstrating a large mass with features characteristic of a sarcoma.

TABLE 4. *TNM staging classification of soft tissue sarcoma*

Stage	G	T	N	M
IA	G_1	T_1	N_0	M_0
IB	G_1	T_2	N_0	M_0
IIA	G_2	T_1	N_0	M_0
IIB	G_2	T_2	N_0	M_0
IIIA	G_{3-4}	T_1	N_0	M_0
IIIB	G_{3-4}	T_2	N_0	M_0
IVA	Any G	Any T	N_1	M_0
IVB	Any G	Any T	Any N	M_1

gle tumor. Fortunately, newer developments in immunohistochemistry and tumor-specific marker stains have improved histopathologic diagnosis. Sarcomas are termed "low-grade" or "high-grade" based on specific features identified by the pathologist, as outlined in (Table 5).

Treatment

Although the treatment of any sarcoma is dictated by its location and tumor type, general principles in the treatment of the cancers have been defined. Surgical resection remains the only treatment modality leading to cure of the disease. Here, the goal is to remove the primary tumor with a wide margin of adjacent normal tissue. There are many options among authorities as to the importance of the additional modalities of chemotherapy and radiation therapy before and after surgical resection. Some would support the idea that the risk of local recurrence may be decreased by administering preoperative (neoadjuvant) chemotherapy and, in some insititutions, in concert with radiation therapy prior to resection. The addition of neoadjuvant therapy may decrease the need for resection of an entire muscle compartment that traditionally has been required for a deep central tumor. In the past, amputation of an involved limb was often considered necessary for curative resection, but studies of neoadjuvant treatment followed by local resection indicates that no improved survival benefit with radical amputations. Microinvasion of tumor along compartment planes, extension beyond the tumor pseudocapsule, and failure to obtain clear surgical margins are the most common causes of local recurrence that may be as high as 65% to 90% after initial surgical therapy. Although

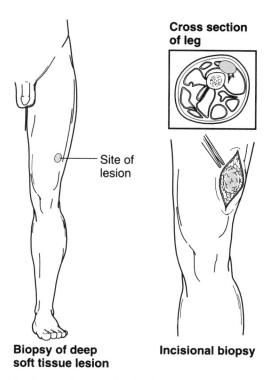

FIG. 13. Appropriate method of performing an incisional biopsy over a suspicious lesion of the extremity.

Cross section of leg — Site of lesion

Biopsy of deep soft tissue lesion — **Incisional biopsy**

clinical and radiological examination. Lymph node status is determined by clinical appreciation of palpable disease; it should be noted that most sarcomas do not metastasize to regional lymph nodes. While local invasion and recurrence are the primary malignant features of sarcomas, distant metastasis often is a greater life-threatening event. Synovial cell sarcoma, osteosarcoma, epithelioid sarcoma, and malignant fibrous histiocytoma have the greatest risk of distant metastasis. Lung is the most common distant site of metastasis. Most practitioners suggest that chest CT scans be obtained before planning a major resection of the primary disease. CT scans may be as much as 15% more revealing of pulmonary nodules than the standard two-view chest radiographs.

Histopathologic grade is the best indicator of recurrence and overall prognosis of sarcomas. Given the heterogeneous histologic nature of these relatively rare cancers, it is often difficult to determine the specific subtype of a tumor. Moreover, more than one tissue type may be seen in a sin-

TABLE 3. *Histologic subtypes of soft tissue sarcomas*

Liposarcoma
Fibrosarcoma
Leiomyosarcoma
Malignant fibrous histiocytoma
Synovial sarcoma
Malignant peripheral nerve tumor
Unclassified

TABLE 5. *Histologic grading soft tissue sarcomas*

Low-grade	High-grade
Good cellular differentiation	Poor cellular differentiation
Hypocellular	Hypercellular
Increased stroma	Minimal stroma
Hypovascular	Hypervascular
Minimal necrosis	Significant necrosis
<5 mitoses per ×10 HPF	>5 mitoses per ×10 HPF

HPF, high-power field.
Adapted from Hadju et al., Memorial Sloan-Kettering Cancer Center.

TABLE 6. *Unfavorable prognostic factors
of soft tissue sarcomas*

Size of >5 cm
Deep location
High-grade histology
Inadequate/incomplete surgical resection
Invasion of bone or neurovascular structures
Spread to contiguous anatomical compartments

patients with unfavorable prognostic factors, as outlined in Table 6, may benefit from adjuvant therapy after surgical resection to reduce the chance of local recurrence, there appears to be no change in survival with such therapy.

Because overall survival and 5-year disease-free survival are equivalent for amputation and limb salvage surgery with adjuvant or neoadjuvant therapy, the traditional concept of radical sarcoma surgery has largely been abandoned. Still, for the patient with a large sarcoma that cannot be locally resected from an extremity with free margins along vascular, neural, and bone and joint planes, an amputation may be preferrable. Radiation, both by high-dose external beam and brachytherapy by interstitial catheters, has been reported effective for local control. Interstitial radiation therapy involves the delivery of a concentrated dose of radiation to the tumor bed by the instillation of radioactive sources, either temporary or permanent, at the time of surgical resection of the tumor. The term "brachytherapy" is applied because of the short—*brachy*—distance of the treatment.

SUMMARY

The skin is the largest organ of the human body, with many different functions. Skin cancer is the most common malignancy in the United States, and, unfortunately, the incidence does not appear to be decreasing. Malig-

nant melanoma, despite being a rare disease compared to BCC and SCC, causes approximately three-fourths of all deaths from skin cancer. The clinician must recognize the importance of early diagnosis, which must begin with a high degree of suspicion in patients with predisposing factors and skin nevi.

Surgical resection of soft tissue sarcomas is the only method of offering cure, though radical surgery is generally not necessary. The addition of chemotherapy and radiation therapy has permitted local resection rather than amputation to be the standard approach. Future development of adjuvant therapy programs may offer improved survival.

STUDY QUESTIONS

1. What is the pathogenesis of hidradenitis suppurativa? What is appropriate treatment for this disease?
2. Characterize the premalignant skin lesions: actinic keratosis, leukoplakia, and erythroplakia.
3. In general, what are the risk factors for the development of nonmelanoma skin cancer?
4. What is Moh's surgery? For which skin malignancies can it be used as therapy?
5. What are the factors that influence survival prognosis from soft tissue sarcoma?

SUGGESTED READING

Beahrs OH, ed. *Manual of staging of cancer/American Joint Commission on Cancer.* 4th ed. Philadelphia: Lippincott, 1992.
Bland K, Karakousis C, Copeland E, eds. *Atlas of surgical oncology.* Philadelphia: Saunders, 1995.
Conlon KC, Brennan MF. Soft tissue sarcomas. In: Murphy GP, Lawrence W, Ledhard RE, eds. *Textbook of clinical oncology.* 2nd ed. American Cancer Society, 1995
Swetter SM, Smoller BR, Bauer EA. Cutaneous cancer. In: Abeloff MD, Armitage JO, Lichter AS, Niederhuber JE, eds. *Clinical oncology.* New York: Churchill-Livingstone, 1995.

CHAPTER 7

Breast

Anthony M. Gonzalez and Frederick L. Moffat, Jr.

The breast is a glandular organ found only in mammals. It develops from ectodermal tissue in response to hormonal fluctuations and undergoes almost continuous morphological change under the influence of puberty, pregnancy, and menopause. In the United States, one out of every two women will consult her physician regarding a breast complaint, one in four women will have a breast biopsy, and one in nine women will develop a form of breast cancer. Breast cancer is among the most common malignant neoplasms in U.S. women and the second leading cause of cancer death. It has been estimated that 1.5 million women will be diagnosed with breast cancer in the United States in the 1990s. Despite extensive ongoing basic and clinical research efforts, one-third of women diagnosed with breast cancer will die of the disease.

ANATOMY AND EMBRYOLOGY

In early fetal life, the human breast develops in the thickened portion of ectodermal tissue known as the milk line, coursing from the axilla to the pubis (Fig. 1). In the first trimester of pregnancy, the milk line atrophies, with the exception of the pectoral region, which thickens, forming a nipple bud. The ductal system develops by invagination of ectodermal cells from the nipple (Fig. 2). The breast parenchyma is cushioned by fat and lies on the deep pectoral fascia that envelops the pectoralis major muscle (Fig. 3). Deep to the pectoralis major muscle is the pectoralis minor muscle enclosed by the clavipectoral fascia that is continuous with the axillary fascia.

The lymphatic drainage of the breast begins in the subareolar plexus and follows a centrifugal pathway along the major lactiferous ducts, and subsequently along the efferent veins to the regional lymph nodes. The major lymphatic drainage basins for the breast are the axillary nodes, the supraclavicular nodes, and the internal mammary lymph nodes.

There is substantial variance in the number of lymph nodes in the axilla. In the context of breast cancer surgery, the axillary lymph nodes have been divided into three levels as described by Berg (Fig. 4). Level I nodes are those found lateral to the lateral border of the pectoralis minor muscle and inferior to the axillary vein. Level II nodes are those posterior to the pectoralis minor

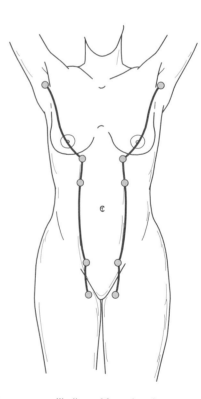

FIG. 1. Mammary milk line. After development of the milk buds in the pectoral area of ectodermal thickening, the milk streak extends from the axilla to the inguinal areas. At week 9 of intrauterine development, atrophy of the bud has occurred except for the presence of the supernumerary nipples or breast.

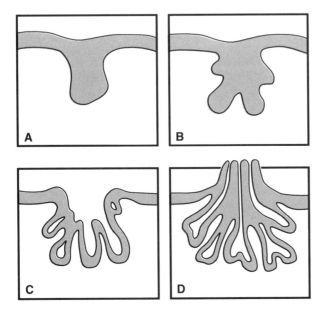

FIG. 2. Sections through evolutionary development and growth of the mammary bud. **(A–C)** Similar sections showing the developing gland at successive stages between the 12th week and birth. The mammary pit develops, and major lactiferous ducts are present at the end of gestation. **(D)** A similar section showing the elevation of the mammary pit by proliferations of the underlying connective tissue forming the nipple soon after birth.

and inferior to the axillary vein. Level III nodes are medial to the pectoralis minor muscle, inferior to the axillary vein, and lateral to Halsted's ligament. Halsted's ligament (the costoclavicular ligament, which is the subclavius muscle invested by the clavipectoral fascia) defines the apex of the axilla. Just medial to Halsted's ligament, at the lateral edge of the first rib, the axillary vein becomes the subclavian vein and enters the thorax. Rotter's nodes, interpectoral nodes, are located in the space between pectoralis major and minor.

While performing axillary lymphadenectomy, a detailed understanding of the anatomy of the axilla is required to avoid inadvertent injury to important structures. The long thoracic nerve of Bell courses along the chest wall on the medial aspect of the axilla, innervating the serratus anterior muscle. Injury to this nerve can result in the "winged scapula" deformity. The thoracodorsal nerve arises from the posterior aspect of the brachial plexus and traverses the axilla on the medial surface of the latissimus dorsi muscle, which it innervates. The lateral pectoral nerve travels along the lateral margin of the pectoralis minor muscle. The medial pectoral nerve courses along the undersurface of the pectoralis major; Rotter's lymph nodes are closely associated with the medial pectoral neurovascular bundle. The intercostobrachial nerves traverse the axillary contents and supply sensation to the skin of the medial aspect of the upper arm, the axillary skin, and the lateral chest wall.

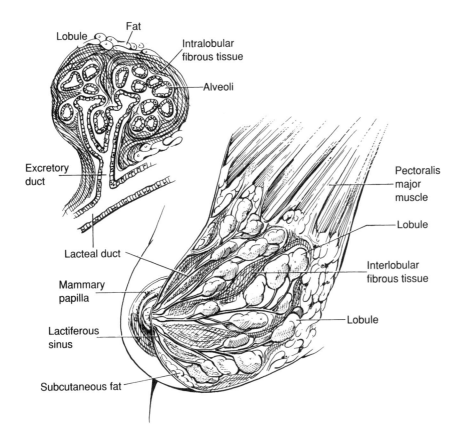

FIG. 3. Internal structure of the breast. The breast is a large apocrine gland. The secreting parenchyma is composed of lobules containing acini, fat, and fibrous tissue. The ducts drain centrally toward large lacunae located directly beneath the nipple. These act as reservoirs until they receive the impetus for ejection. (From Rock JA, Thompson JD, eds. *Te Linde's operative gynecology.* 8th ed. Philadelphia: Lippincott–Raven, 1997:1241)

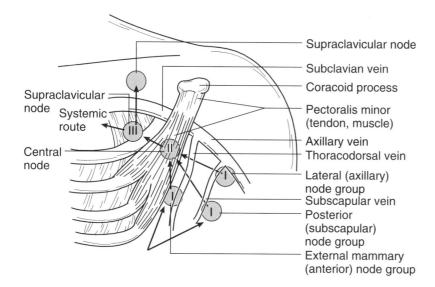

FIG. 4. Major lymph node groups associated with the lymphatic drainage of the breast. The Roman numerals indicate three levels or groups of lymph nodes that are defined by their location relative to the pectoralis minor. Level I includes lymph nodes located lateral to the pectoralis minor; level II, lymph nodes located deep to the muscle; and level III, lymph nodes located medial to the muscle. The *arrows* indicate the general direction of lymph flow. The axillary vein and its major tributaries associated with the pectoralis minor are included.

PHYSIOLOGY

As a secondary sex organ, the breast requires estrogen for functional maturation in the human female. Function and structure of the breast are affected by estrogen and progesterone fluxes associated with puberty, the menstrual cycle, and pregnancy.

The breast is a modified sweat gland. Prior to puberty, the breast consists of rudimentary ducts, a few acini, and specialized connective tissue. The ducts and acini are arranged in lobules. Each lobule empties at the nipple through a separate orifice. At puberty, the ductal elements proliferate and bud, and acinar elements become more profuse. The breast undergoes cyclic histopathological changes related to the menstrual cycle. As estrogen rises, the ductal epithelium becomes hyperplastic and changes from cuboidal to columnar. The progesterone surge results in acinar hyperplasia. Between ovulation and menstruation, the breasts become engorged, resulting in soreness or tenderness. Immediately prior to menstruation, the breasts are most fibrocystic, and after menstruation least so. Ovulatory suppression with oral contraceptives affects the breast in an unpredictable manner. Because the response of the breast to menstrual cycle hormonal changes may not be uniform, the breast tissue often becomes irregular in consistency and texture. This irregularity is the clinical manifestation of fibrocystic mastopathy.

During pregnancy, the duct size and the number of glands increase, with glandular hyperplasia predominating in later stages. As the acini increase, the interlobular connective tissue decreases, the superficial veins dilate, and the areolae become pigmented. After parturition, breast secretion begins and persists as long as breast feeding continues. If nursing is discontinued, the breast will initially engorge, resulting in local discomfort and even systemic symptoms. During postlactational involution, the breast may change shape because most antepartum connective tissue has been replaced by glandular elements; these glands atrophy following cessation of breast feeding. The breast may become smaller and pendulous, and develop striae.

Menopause heralds ovarian hormonal insufficiency, but production of estrogen from the adrenal cortex and from androgenic metabolism continues and is responsible for postmenopausal fibrocystic mastopathy. The breast tissue gradually atrophies, with flattening of ductal epithelial cells and loss of acini.

EVALUATION OF PATIENTS WITH BREAST DISEASE

History, Symptoms, and Breast Cancer Risk Factors

The history obtained from the patient is very important in assessing risk for breast cancer as well as elucidating the nature of a clinical complaint related to the breasts. The age of the patient as well as the menstrual history (age of menarche, menstrual irregularities, and age of menopause) should be obtained. The obstetrical history (age of patient at first childbirth, history of breast feeding), family history, and a history of previous biopsies should also be sought.

A mass in the breast is a common presenting symptom. Sixty-five percent of all breast masses are brought to the physician's attention by the patient. Patients may also complain of breast pain. Pain is common in premenopausal women and is infrequently associated with cancer. In the absence of a mass, pain is usually caused by a benign process. Local pain related to cancer is usually (but not always) due to coincidental benign conditions in the vicinity of the neoplasm.

Nipple discharge is another common complaint. Non-bloody, bilateral multiductal discharge is commonly physiological, benign, or drug-induced. Spontaneous, unilateral, bloody discharge from a single duct, however, is clinically significant and is a classical mode of presentation of intraductal papilloma or, much less often, carcinoma. Cytological examination may be helpful in a minority of cases.

Other less common presenting symptoms of breast cancer include breast enlargement, changes in nipple appearance such as retraction or eczematous rash, alterations in breast symmetry or shape, skin ulceration, erythema, peau d'orange skin changes (Fig. 5), axillary mass, and, infrequently, musculoskeletal discomfort due to metastatic disease.

In taking the history, other breast cancer risk factors should be elicited in order to further guide the management of a breast mass. The relative risk of breast cancer may be increased twofold by a high-fat diet. Total fat, saturated fat, unsaturated fat, and animal fat all contribute to the risk. The quality of the fat may influence the risk, since the consumption of omega-3 fatty acids in marine-derived lipids consumed by Eskimo women may be causally related to a lower incidence of breast cancer. This hypothesis of Western diet influence is corroborated by data of Japanese immigrants, who have a very low incidence of breast cancer. The first- and second-genera-tion offspring born within the United States of Japanese immigrants have the same breast cancer risk as other native-born Americans.

The influence of oral contraceptive usage on breast cancer risk is controversial. Some studies demonstrate no effect on the risk when the oral contraceptive is used in the middle of the reproductive years, whereas others suggest an increased risk is present if contraceptive hormone preparations are used prior to the first pregnancy or over a prolonged period of time. There may exist a slight increase in the risk in use of estrogen replacement in the perimenopausal and postmenopausal patients. This risk may be significantly higher in women with known breast cancer risk factors such as a family history.

Obesity may increase relative risk of breast cancer 1.5- to 2-fold. Late menopause (after age 55) is also associated with higher risk. In contrast, oophorectomy at an early age may mitigate breast cancer risk.

Late first pregnancy (after age 35) and nulliparity are associated with a higher risk of breast cancer. This increased relative risk is thought to be related to long-term unopposed estrogen effect. Breast feeding mitigates the risk, presumably due to suppression of hormonal fluxes associated with the menstrual cycle.

Women with a history of multiple exposures to low-dose radiation or of one high-dose exposure have a greater risk of breast carcinoma. A personal history of

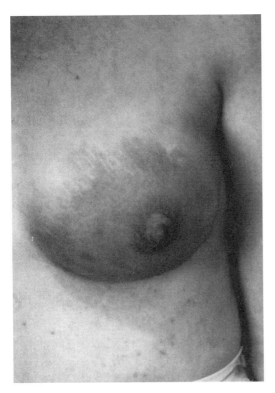
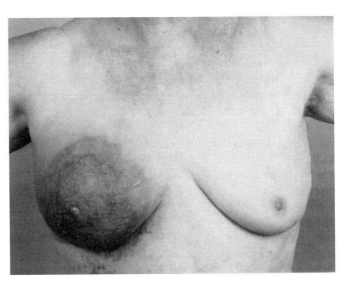

A B

FIG. 5. Primary inflammatory carcinoma. **(A)** Cutaneous erythema predominantly over the dependent part of the breast. **(B)** Most of the swollen breast is involved and there is desquamation of the skin. (From Rosen PP. *Rosen's breast pathology.* Philadelphia: Lippincott–Raven, 1997:587.)

cancer in one breast increases relative risk of contralateral breast cancer by a factor of three. Among women with fibrocystic disease of the breast, only those with hyperplasia, and particularly atypical hyperplasia, have an excess risk for breast carcinoma.

Old age, birthplace in the United States or Northern Europe, family history, and personal history of breast cancer are all strong risk factors for breast carcinoma. The other risk factors discussed above are associated with a less striking increase in relative risk.

Physical Examination

Examination of a patient's breasts should occur in a well-lighted room and include inspection and palpation of the entire breast and axilla. Inspection should be performed with the patient's arms by her side, with her arms straight up in the air, and her hands on her hips with and without pectoral contraction. Size, shape, symmetry, and skin changes of the breast should be documented. Skin retraction can be accentuated by the patient sitting and leaning forward with her arms extended forward. Inspection and palpation of the breast should be performed in the sitting and supine positions. Palpation is performed with the palmar aspect of the fingers, with examination of all four quadrants from the clavicle to the sternum and to the latissimus dorsi laterally. The axillary lymph nodes are palpated with the patient sitting and with the shoulder relaxed in the adducted position. Lymphadenopathy is sought in the axillary, subclavicular, supraclavicular, and parasternal basins.

Edema of the breast skin gives an appearance reminiscent of the skin of an orange; hence, the term "peau d'orange." When this occurs with erythema, tenderness, and warmth, the clinical differential diagnosis includes acute mastitis and inflammatory breast cancer. Mastitis is very rare in the absence of lactation and breast feeding. Peau d'orange and erythema in the context of cancer are caused by obstruction of the dermal lymphatics caused by metastatic carcinoma cells. These findings may not be as readily apparent in dark-skinned individuals.

Involvement of the nipple and areola complex by cancer may cause retraction, flattening, or inversion of the nipple. Tumors located directly beneath the areola may infiltrate the areolar complex. Carcinoma may also present as an eczematoid dermatitis, either moist or dry, of the nipple. This presentation, known as Paget's disease, is caused by intraductal or invasive carcinoma cells permeating the epidermal layer of the skin of the nipple.

Radiological Studies

Mammography has been in use in the United States for >30 years. Mammography delivers 0.2 rad per breast per study, as compared with a chest radiograph, which delivers 0.15 rad per study. The benefits of screening mammography clearly outweigh the breast cancer risk from this low-dose irradiation, because there is no proven increased risk with screening mammography.

The indications for diagnostic mammography include a suspicious breast mass, a mass in a cystic/nodular breast that cannot be examined thoroughly, follow-up examination in a patient with previous history of breast cancer, and routine screening in patients >50 years of age. Fine stippled microcalcifications, branched linear calcifications in a segmental or ductal distribution, and/or a stellate or irregular soft tissue density are all findings suggestive of carcinoma.

A complete mammographic study of each breast involves at least two views, the craniocaudal and the mediolateral view. When read by an experienced radiologist, the false-negative rate for detection of cancer by mammography is ~10%. The American Cancer Society currently recommends that all women initiate breast self-examination at the age of 20 and that a baseline mammogram be done at age 35. Annual mammograms are indicated after age 50. Screening mammograms done between the ages of 35 and 40 are generally indicated no more often than every 2 years. Controversy persists regarding frequency of screening mammography between ages 40 and 50.

Ultrasound is superb for determining whether a mammographic density is cystic or solid. Ultrasound can also be used to localize nonpalpable cysts for aspiration. This modality may also be of value in women under the age of 30, in whom the presence of dense glandular tissue limits the accuracy of mammography. Ultrasound, however, has a very low sensitivity for breast cancer. Microcalcifications are not seen on ultrasound, and this modality is ineffective in evaluation of fatty or senescent breasts.

The primary indication for galactography (ductography) is serosanguinous or bloody discharge from the nipple. Galactograms are performed by injecting contrast into the mammary ducts from which the discharge originates. Sequential mammograms are then performed. Cysts opacify when they communicate with the injected ducts, and papillomas appear as filling defects. Carcinomas may appear as irregular masses or as multiple intraluminal filling defects.

Magnetic resonance imaging (MRI) has proven value in the diagnosis of musculoskeletal pathology and more recently has been used in breast diagnosis. Carcinomas are diagnosed on MRI by criteria comparable to those used in mammography, but the expense of this modality precludes its use for breast cancer screening.

Doppler flow studies are useful in evaluating breast cancer. The multiple arteriovenous shunts, and the redundant and somewhat chaotic pattern of tumor vessels give a characteristic "tumor flow signal" by Doppler examination. Although much more clinical research is needed, this modality might eventually prove useful in the triage of patients with palpable mammographic abnormalities for biopsy.

Digital subtraction angiography of the breast (DSAB) is a new, still experimental technique that utilizes iodinated contrast dyes. The preinjection breast image is subtracted from the postinjection study by a computer, revealing areas of increased uptake. Preliminary studies suggest that DSAB can consistently identify breast cancers by their abnormal vasculature and retention of contrast in neoplastic breast tissue.

Radioimmunoscintigraphy (RIS) using radiolabeled monoclonal antibodies with antitumor specificity can image primary, regional, and metastatic breast cancer. Carcinomas of >0.5 cm can be imaged by this technique. The role of RIS in diagnosis and evaluation of breast cancer is currently under study.

Tissue Diagnosis

Fine needle aspiration cytology (FNAC) is a rapid, simple diagnostic technique widely used in office practice. The biopsy is performed by repeatedly passing a needle back and forth into the mass with continuous negative pressure applied to the syringe. The contents of the syringe are smeared on slides and sent to pathology preserved in 95% isopropyl alcohol. FNAC differentiates cystic from solid breast masses, and simultaneously yields cytological information. Benign cystic fluid is usually green or amber in color. Pathological examination of the fluid is generally not required if the mass disappears entirely with aspiration. Open biopsy of aspirated masses may be indicated if no fluid is obtained, a solid mass is encountered, the cystic fluid is thick or blood-tinged, a mass effect persists despite aspiration of the fluid, or the mass reappears after two aspirations.

It is important to recognize that a negative FNAC does not completely exclude carcinoma. If clinical suspicion is high based on clinical or mammographic findings or if a mass persists 4 to 6 weeks after a negative FNAC, an excisional biopsy should be performed.

Excisional Breast Biopsy

Despite the fact that 75% to 85% of suspicious breast lesions prove to be benign on biopsy, the very low specificity of noninvasive diagnostic modalities often mandates that excisional biopsies be performed in order to maximize the accuracy in diagnosing breast cancer. For nonpalpable mammographic abnormalities, biopsy is indicated for indiscrete or stellate soft tissue mass, architectural distortion, or suspicious microcalcifications in clustered, pleomorphic, or linear/branched distributions. Radiological localization techniques for biopsy of mammographic abnormalities include the use of external skin markers, percutaneous needle localization with a hooked Kopans wire, and stereotactic methods.

Palpable lesions may be biopsied by incisional or excisional techniques. Incisional biopsy is appropriate in a patient with a large breast mass or in whom a mesenchymal neoplasm is suspected. This method provides a histological diagnosis and hormone receptor and flow cytometry data. Small masses are usually excised with a narrow margin of grossly normal breast tissue. Excision of the entire mass avoids the small probability of a diagnostic error related to sampling. Specimens are sent fresh (not in formalin) in order to look for estrogen and progesterone receptors in the specimen. For the same reason, biopsy is best performed with a scalpel rather than electrocautery, because electrocoagulation destroys and disrupts histological features and may result in false-negative receptor assay results.

BENIGN BREAST DISEASE

Infections

Acute mastitis is a generalized cellulitis that often encompasses a large portion of breast tissue. This clinical entity is an ascending bacterial infection beginning in the subareolar ducts and extending outward from the nipple. Physical findings include cutaneous erythema and edema, tenderness, and induration of the underlying breast parenchyma. Commonly, mastitis is a complication of lactation caused by inspissation of milk, ductal obstruction, and secondary Staphylococcus or Streptococcus infection. Conservative treatment consists of application of heat, ice packs, mechanical breast pumping, and broad-spectrum antibiotics. Streptococcus infections tend to produce diffuse cellulitis, whereas *Staphylococcus aureus* tends to localize forming deep abscesses.

The initial treatment of mastitis should be conservative, with oral broad-spectrum antibiotics. If the process does not quickly resolve, the patient may require hospitalization for intravenous antibiotics. Incision and drainage should be performed if the infection does not respond within a short time.

Inflammatory carcinoma must be excluded by close patient follow-up to be certain all signs and symptoms have completely resolved. If there is any question about the diagnosis, incisional biopsy of skin and breast parenchyma must be performed.

Fibrocystic Disease

Approximately 70% to 80% of women in North America have some degree of fibrocystic mastopathy. This group of histological entities encompasses cyst formation, fibrous breast nodularity, stromal hyperplasia, atypical hyperplasia, and sclerosing adenosis. In general, fibrocystic disease implies no increased risk for breast cancer. However, detection of cancer may be more difficult (on mammography and physical examination). Proliferative fibrocystic disease may connote a small excess risk for breast cancer, and atypical ductal and lobular hyperplasia in particular are known risk factors for cancer. Relative risk is increased four- or fivefold, and these lesions are difficult to distinguish from carcinoma in situ on histopathology. Fibrocystic disease is in essence a response of normal breast parenchyma to locally produced and circulating hormones and growth factors.

Patients with fibrocystic disease may present with bilateral breast pain and multiple irregularities on palpation. The pain associated with fibrocystic mastopathy is more pronounced during the second part of the menstrual cycle and diminishes with the onset of menses. Patients with mastodynia (painful breasts) from fibrocystic disease may benefit from scrupulous deletion of caffeine from the diet or the use of vitamin E.

Other Common Benign Breast Pathologies

A knowledge of benign pathology of the breast is important. The three benign lesions that mimic breast cancer clinically and mammographically are mammary duct ectasia, fat necrosis, and sclerosing adenosis.

Ductal ectasia may present as a subareolar induration, masses, and/or nipple discharge. Ductal inflammation leads to scarring, destruction, and dilatation, with eventual periductal fibrosis and ectasia. These lesions are commonly found in premenopausal and perimenopausal patients. Because calcifications may be seen on mammography and the intense cicatricial reaction may result in a stony hard mass, differentiation of this lesion from carcinoma often requires biopsy.

Fat necrosis usually occurs following chest or breast trauma, although the patient may often be unable to recall the inciting trauma. Although it is completely benign, it is frequently indistinguishable from cancer by clinical and mammographic criteria. Histologically, it is similar to fat necrosis found elsewhere.

Sclerosing adenosis is a densely sclerotic proliferative variant of fibrocystic disease that presents as a stony hard mass and may have suspicious microcalcifications on mammography. Sclerosing adenosis may imply a modest increase in breast cancer risk.

BENIGN BREAST NEOPLASMS

Fibroadenomas

Fibroadenomas occur most commonly in the fourth decade of life and are composed of epithelial and stromal elements. African-American women have a greater propensity to develop these lesions. These benign tumors present as rubbery, firm, solitary masses. If the diagnosis can be established with FNAC, the lesions can be followed in patients younger than 35 years of age. Excision is required to exclude carcinoma in older women, in women with breast cancer risk factors, or when the lesion is enlarging over time. As a general rule, fibroadenomas do not have malignant potential, even though a few invasive and noninvasive carcinomas have been discovered in preexisting fibroadenomas. The carcinoma most commonly identified is lobular carcinoma in situ (LCIS).

Giant fibroadenomas are usually >5 cm in diameter and commonly found in juveniles. When encountered in adolescents, they are termed "juvenile fibroadenomas." Benign cystosarcoma phylloides can be confused with giant fibroadenoma.

Phylloides Tumor

Phylloides tumor, or cystosarcoma phylloides, is a common nonepithelial tumor of the breast, with a cystic fish-flesh appearance on cut section. Phylloides is derived from the Greek *phyllon,* meaning "leaf." On gross examination, the cut surface of the tumor has a leafy appearance. Most cystosarcoma phylloides tumors are benign, despite the name, which implies malignancy. The World Health Organization has designated the term "phylloides tumor" to include lesions with both benign and malignant biological behavior.

These lesions occur most often in the fifth decade of life. On mammographic examination, they are large, with smooth borders and areas of calcification. Mammography is not useful in predicting malignant potential. Differentiation from the giant or juvenile fibroadenoma on the basis of histology is difficult, although phylloides tumors tend to have greater cellular activity in the stroma.

Treatment options vary with tumor size and assessment of malignant potential. If clinical behavior and histology suggest a benign lesion, wide local excision is acceptable. When histopathology and/or behavior suggest malignancy, or when the mass is large, mastectomy is advisable. Because axillary metastasis is rare, axillary node dissection is not warranted. Postoperative radiotherapy improves local control for large infiltrative or rapidly growing phylloides tumors.

Recurrences are mostly local, but when metastasis occurs, it is generally to the lung, mediastinum, and bone. When local recurrence is seen following breast-conserving surgery, completion mastectomy and radiotherapy constitute the best treatment. Chemotherapy is indicated for distant metastasis.

Intraductal Papillomas

Intraductal papillomas are epithelial polyps of breast ducts. When centrally located, they are usually solitary.

When peripherally situated, they are more likely to be multiple (papillomatosis) and may connote an increased risk for carcinoma.

Intraductal papilloma presents clinically as bloody or serosanguinous nipple discharge. Although papilloma is the most common cause of bloody nipple discharge, biopsy is often necessary to exclude carcinoma. This is performed after cannulation of the involved duct with a lacrimal probe. A circumareolar incision is made and the probed duct identified. This is then dissected from the surrounding tissues and sent for pathological confirmation. Some of these lesions are associated with epithelial hyperplasia and papillomatosis, and imply increased risk for cancer.

Nipple Adenoma

Nipple adenoma is similar to papilloma, but occurs in the nipple or adjacent to the ductal ampulla. This lesion may be confused with Paget's disease of the nipple. It may develop hyperplastic features and can therefore also be confused with carcinoma.

MALIGNANT NEOPLASMS OF THE BREAST

Epidemiology

In the United States, breast cancer is the most common malignancy in women, comprising 32% of all cancers in women. New breast cancer cases were diagnosed in 183,000 women and ~2,000 men in 1995. In the same year, 46,000 people died of the disease. The incidence of breast cancer has increased steadily since the 1960s.

Breast cancer is the second leading cause of cancer-related death in women in the United States, surpassed by lung cancer in 1985. For women aged 15 to 54 years, breast cancer remains the leading cause of cancer mortality. Despite the increasing incidence of breast cancer, mortality from breast cancer has remained essentially constant for >50 years. Given the high incidence and prevalence of this disease, even modest improvements in treatment outcome would result in many lives saved.

There is a genetic and hereditary predisposition to breast cancer, although truly hereditary cases comprise only a small fraction of patients. If breast cancer is found in a patient with a first- or second-degree relative having a history of breast cancer or with a family pedigree consistent with a highly penetrant autosomal dominant pattern, it is considered hereditary. Other factors that support the diagnosis of hereditary breast cancer are early age of onset, premenopausal bilateral breast cancer, and association with other primary cancers. A patient with a first- or second-degree relative with breast cancer who does not otherwise fit the description of hereditary breast cancer is deemed to have familial breast cancer. A patient with no family history of breast cancer has sporadic breast cancer.

Histopathology

Noninfiltrating (In Situ) Carcinoma

LCIS develops predominantly in premenopausal Caucasian women (mean age 45) and is almost invariably found incidentally in otherwise benign breast biopsies or in association with invasive cancer. LCIS is neither palpable, nor does it have any mammographic characteristics. It arises from the lobular elements of the breast but does not penetrate the basement membrane.

Approximately 10% to 37% of patients with LCIS will develop invasive breast cancer within 20 to 30 years of LCIS being diagnosed, the risk being uniformly distributed over both breasts without regard for the site of the original LCIS. The incidence of multicentricity and bilaterality of LCIS may be as high as 90% at the time of diagnosis. The majority of invasive cancers diagnosed in patients with LCIS are ductal, and these cancers show no predilection for the site of the original lesion. Although some clinicians consider LCIS as purely a histopathological entity, most consider it a marker for breast cancer risk rather than a true breast cancer precursor.

The most appropriate management for patients with LCIS is close clinical and mammographic surveillance only. In the individual with a strong family history of breast cancer, bilateral total mastectomy is a viable option in a willing patient. Subcutaneous mastectomy is no longer an acceptable option in the management of neoplastic breast disease, because 5% to 15% of breast tissue is left in situ. In the future, chemoprevention with medications such as tamoxifen may significantly reduce the risk of invasive cancer in patients with LCIS. Clinical trials are in progress.

In contrast to LCIS, the age profile of patients with ductal carcinoma in situ (DCIS) parallels that of patients with invasive cancer. The lesion is now diagnosed much more frequently because of widespread use of screening mammography. DCIS develops from proliferation of the inner epithelial layer of the lactiferous ducts, which form papillary ingrowths. There are four histological variants: papillary/micropapillary, solid, cribiform, and comedo. Comedo DCIS is associated with a higher incidence of anaplasia and predilection for occult invasion, cancer recurrence, and metastasis.

The risk of metachronous breast cancer associated with biopsied but otherwise untreated DCIS is 30% to 50% over 10 years. DCIS is thought to be a true precursor of invasive breast cancer because, in contrast to LCIS, subsequent invasive cancers are usually in the same breast and quadrant as the original in situ lesion. DCIS is often multifocal or multicentric but less likely to be bilateral than LCIS.

Contemporary treatment of DCIS is a current area of controversy. Total mastectomy remains a reasonable option in the minority of patients with extensive or diffuse DCIS. The National Surgical Adjuvant Breast Project (NSABP) B-17 trial, comparing lumpectomy (with tumor-free margins) to lumpectomy plus breast radiotherapy demonstrated both treatments to be acceptable options. A lower incidence of subsequent ipsilateral in situ or invasive cancer was seen in the irradiated patients. The NSABP B-24 trial, currently maturing, will test whether tumor-free margins are truly necessary when lumpectomy and radiotherapy are undertaken for DCIS and whether tamoxifen is effective for this disease. In general, contralateral mastectomy is not indicated for DCIS.

Infiltrating Breast Malignancies

Infiltrating ductal carcinoma, also called "scirrhous carcinoma," is the most frequent adenocarcinoma of the breast. As its name implies, it is a tumor of ductal epithelium that invades the surrounding breast stroma, unlike noninvasive cancer, which remains confined to the ducts and acini. It usually presents as a solitary, nontender, ill-defined mass in a perimenopausal or postmenopausal woman. Histologically, the tumor has a poorly defined border and may comprise a range of in situ cellular elements to highly anaplastic infiltrating cells. As the tumor grows and becomes more desmoplastic, involvement and foreshortening of Cooper's ligaments results in skin dimpling. When the tumor invades the dermis of the skin and the subdermal lymphatics, peau d'orange skin changes will develop.

Infiltrating lobular carcinoma, a histological subtype, constitutes ~5% of breast carcinoma. Lobular cancer originates in the breast acini and is characterized histologically by small round cells that infiltrate surrounding stromal tissue in a classical "Indian-filing" pattern. The presentation and mammographic features are similar to infiltrating ductal carcinoma. The contention in the past that invasive lobular carcinoma has a greater incidence of bilaterality has been challenged in the recent literature. At present, routine prophylactic contralateral mastectomy is not justified in patients with this type of breast cancer.

Paget's disease of the nipple was first described by Sir James Paget in 1874. This condition presents as an encrusted, scaly, hyperemic eczematoid lesion that occupies most or all of the nipple-areolar complex. It accounts for ~2% of all breast carcinomas and is associated with an underlying intraductal or invasive carcinoma.

Patients present with complaints of itching, burning, and skin changes of the areolar complex, with or without a palpable mass. The pathognomonic histological findings in this disease consist of intraepidermal clear tumor cells with large prominent nuclei (Paget's cells). Paget's disease is distinguished from pagetoid intraepithelial malignant melanoma by immunochemistry for S-100 (positive in melanoma) or for carcinoembryonic antigen (positive in Paget's disease).

Inflammatory carcinoma presents as erythema, edema, and/or warmth of the nonlactating breast. Unfortunately, this lesion is often misdiagnosed as cellulitis or mastitis and treated solely with antibiotics. The clinical signs of inflammatory breast cancer are the manifestation of extensive invasion of the subdermal lymphatics and vascular channels by tumor cells. The diagnosis is made by incisional biopsy that includes skin, subcutaneous tissue, and breast parenchyma.

Inflammatory breast cancer is an extremely aggressive malignant neoplasm, with 75% of patients having axillary metastasis and a high probability of disseminated disease at the time of presentation. Historically, 5-year survival has been anecdotal. More recently, with the use of preoperative multimodality chemotherapy (cyclophosphamide, doxorubicin, and 5-fluorouracil, for example), modified radical mastectomy (MRM), and postoperative chemotherapy with chest wall irradiation, 5-year survival in the range of 30% to 40% has been attained.

Staging

Staging in breast cancer determines extent of disease and therefore assists in predicting outcome. The most important predictor of prognosis by far is the presence or absence of axillary nodal metastasis. Clinical evaluation of the axilla is inaccurate, with false-positive and false-negative rates of 25% to 40%. Therefore, axillary dissection is a necessary part of surgical management of breast cancer.

Prognosis is inversely related to the number of axillary lymph nodes involved. Only 10% to 15% of patients with >10 lymph nodes involved will survive 10 years without adjuvant systemic therapy (Table 1). Clinical or pathological evidence of supraclavicular nodal metastasis is considered stage IV disease, as is the presence of distant metastasis. The most common and widely used staging system for breast cancer is the primary tumor/regional nodes/metastasis (TNM) staging system developed cooperatively by the American Joint

TABLE 1. *Breast cancer prognosis and number of involved lymph nodes*

No. involved nodes	10-year survival	
	NSABP B-04	NSABP B-06
0	67%	75%
1–3	47%	62%
4–9	30%	42%
>10	12%	20%

In NSABP B-04, axillary node–positive patients did not receive postoperative adjuvant systemic therapy. Node-positive patients in NSABP B-06 were treated with a now outdated, relatively ineffective regimen of 5-fluorouracil and melphalan.

TABLE 2. *TNM staging of breast cancer*

Stage	T	N	M
I	T_1	N_0	M_0
II	T_1	N_1	M_0
	T_2	$N_{0,1}$	M_0
	T_3	N_0	M_0
III	$T_{1,2}$	N_2	M_0
	T_3	$N_{1,2}$	M_0
	T_4	Any N	M_0
	Any T	N_3	M_0
IV	Any T	Any N	M_1

T (primary tumor): T_0, no evidence of primary tumor; T_1, tumor is <2.0 cm in greatest diameter; T_2, tumor is >2.0 cm, but <5.0 cm in greatest diameter; T_3, tumor is >5.0 cm in greatest diameter; T_4, tumor of any size with direct extension to chest wall or skin.

N (regional lymph node involvement): N_0, no regional lymph node metastasis; N_1, metastasis to movable ipsilateral axillary lymph nodes; N_2, metastasis to ipsilateral axillary lymph nodes fixed to one another or other structures; N_3, metastasis to ipsilateral internal mammary, supraclavicular, or infraclavicular nodes.

M (distant metastasis): M_0, no distant metastasis; M_1, distant metastasis present.

Simplified breast cancer staging: stage I, small (<2 cm) tumor with no involved regional lymph nodes; stage II, tumor of >2 cm but <5 cm or involved regional lymph nodes; stage III, tumor of >5 cm or feature suggestive of extensive local or regional spread; stage IV, distant metastasis.

Committee on Cancer and the Union Internationale Contre le Cancer (Table 2).

Treatment

Mastectomy

For the first half of this century, breast cancer was treated according to Dr. William Halsted's concept of its biological behavior. Halsted hypothesized that breast cancer remains localized initially, progressing in an orderly, predictable manner from the primary tumor to the regional lymph nodes and on to distant sites. Halsted taught that radical mastectomy, therefore, offered the best chance of cure as the breast cancer was removed en

bloc with the overlying skin, the pectoral muscles, and the axillary lymphatics.

This concept was challenged in the 1940s with the development of the MRM. In this procedure, the breast tissue, overlying skin, and axillary lymphatics are removed. The pectoralis major and the medial and lateral pectoral nerves are spared, providing better function and cosmesis and less morbidity. Only the breast and axillary nodes are resected.

The NSABP B-04 trial confirmed that clinical outcome is the same after total mastectomy (leaving the muscles and lymph nodes) as that following radical mastectomy. This led to the alternate hypothesis of breast cancer biology, which postulates that breast cancer is systemic from the outset or becomes so at a preclinical stage in its development. Cure and disease-free survival are, therefore, not dependent on locoregional treatment (surgery and radiotherapy) but are a function of the host-tumor relationship. However, locoregional treatment remains very important for control of the primary tumor and regional nodal disease. With an exception for extensive locally advanced breast cancer, the Halsted radical mastectomy is rarely performed routinely because of the better cosmetic and functional results of the MRM.

The logical clinical consequence of the alternate hypothesis has been the advent of breast-conserving therapy (breast-conserving surgery and radiotherapy). This has been compared with radical surgery in seven prospective randomized trials worldwide (Table 3). No differences in overall or disease-free survival between conservative surgery and mastectomy was demonstrated. The most important of these trials, NSABP B-06, found no survival differences among mastectomy, breast-conserving surgery, and breast-conserving surgery plus radiotherapy.

If the size of the primary tumor and the size of the breast allow for microscopic tumor-free excision of the cancer with preservation of a cosmetically acceptable breast, conservative treatment is appropriate. Breast-conserving operations have variously been termed "quadrantectomy," "partial mastectomy," "segmental mastectomy," "sector resection," "lumpectomy," and "tylectomy." If the tumor cannot be removed in its entirety with breast-conserving surgery, mastectomy should be performed.

TABLE 3. *Prospective randomized trials comparing breast-conserving therapy and mastectomy*

Trial[a]	Treatment arms
Guy's Hospital	Tylectomy and XRT, vs. radical mastectomy and XRT
Milan NCI	Quadrantectomy and XRT and AND, vs. radical mastectomy
Institut Gustave-Roussy	Tumorectomy and XRT and AND, vs. MRM
NSABP B-06	Segmental mastectomy and AND, vs. segmental mastectomy and XRT and AND, vs. MRM
EORTC 10801	Segmental mastectomy and XRT and AND, vs. MRM
U.S. NCI	Segmental mastectomy and XRT and AND, vs. MRM
DBCG-82TM	Segmental mastectomy and XRT and AND, vs. MRM

[a]For details on the trials, see Early Breast Cancer Trialists' Collaborative Group (1995).
XRT, breast radiotherapy; AND, axillary node dissection; MRM, modified radical mastectomy.

Along with lumpectomy, the ipsilateral axillary lymph nodes should be dissected to determine disease stage and the need for adjuvant chemotherapy, and to provide axillary disease control. Optimal axillary staging surgery encompasses at least Berg's level I and II lymph nodes. The incidence of complications such as arm and breast lymphedema and limitation in shoulder mobility is very low provided the axilla is not irradiated postoperatively.

The indications for lumpectomy, axillary lymphadenectomy, and irradiation of the ipsilateral breast include small (<4 cm) primary tumor size and breast volume of adequate size to allow a cosmetic result. Numerous studies have shown that local recurrence eventuates within 5 years in 25% to 30% of patients treated by breast-conserving surgery without radiotherapy. Adjuvant (postoperative) breast reduces the risk of breast relapse to 5% to 10%. Lumpectomy, axillary lymphadenectomy, and postoperative radiation provide an excellent functional and cosmetic result, with survival equivalent to that observed with radical surgery.

Adjuvant (Postoperative) Therapy

Adjuvant systemic therapy (chemotherapy, hormonal therapy, or both) results in significant improvement in overall and disease-free survival, as well as improved rates of local and distant disease recurrence. Commonly used chemotherapeutic regimens are cyclophosphamide, methotrexate, and 5-fluorouracil (CMF) and cyclophosphamide, doxorubicin (adriamycin), and 5-fluorouracil (CAF). The heterogeneity of the cancer cell population necessitates the use of multiagent chemotherapy to achieve optimal clinical results.

Within the cytoplasm of the breast cancer cell are protein receptors that bind estrogen and progesterone. Well-differentiated tumors and tumors of postmenopausal patients are more likely to exhibit estrogen and progesterone receptor (ER and PR) activity. Because the presence of these receptors implies a better response to hormonal therapy, tumor tissue removed during surgery should be analyzed for ER and PR activity.

The antiestrogen drug, tamoxifen, is used as adjuvant treatment and has been shown to improve survival and local control, reduce the likelihood of metastasis, and reduce the incidence of contralateral breast cancer. It is a tumoristatic drug and is ideally utilized for long-term cancer therapy. The potential side effects of long-term antiestrogen therapy (osteoporosis, coronary atherosclerosis, etc.) as well as a concern of increased development of uterine cancer have been investigated. At the present time, the benefits from the use of tamoxifen in the treatment of receptor-positive breast cancer far exceed the side effects.

General guidelines for postoperative adjuvant systemic therapy are as follows. In the premenopausal patient with axillary nodes that contain metastatic disease, combina-tion chemotherapy is warranted. Tamoxifen is often added for ER-positive tumors. In premenopausal patients with axillary node–negative and hormone receptor–negative breast cancer, CMF or sequential methotrexate and 5-fluorouracil are of proven benefit. In patients with node-negative receptor-positive disease, the use of tamoxifen also decreases the incidence of subsequent primary breast cancer in the contralateral breast (NSABP B-14 trial). The postmenopausal patient with axillary metastasis and positive hormone receptors should be treated with tamoxifen. Combination chemotherapy should be considered for postmenopausal node-positive receptor-negative breast cancer. Tamoxifen is considered appropriate for postmenopausal node-negative disease.

Special Considerations

Clearly, breast-conserving therapy cannot be applied to all cases. In particular, postoperative radiation is contraindicated in patients with concurrent pregnancy and collagen vascular disease. Furthermore, segmental mastectomy with axillary node dissection and adjuvant therapy is not appropriate for patients with multiple ipsilateral primary cancers and locally advanced breast cancer. At present, the only true indication for the radical mastectomy is in patients with locally advanced breast cancer. As a means of achieving better local control of disease, however, neoadjuvant (preoperative) high-dose chemotherapy with or without postoperative autologous bone marrow transplant can reduce the tumor burden in a significant percent of cases. It must be recognized that these neoadjuvant protocols are purely investigational, and no improvement in long-term survival has yet been reported. At this time, mastectomy and appropriate adjuvant therapy remain the standard of care for locally advanced breast cancer.

Metastatic Disease

Once the cancer has spread beyond the breast and axillary lymph nodes, it is no longer curable by surgery. The median survival of patients with stage IV (metastatic) cancer is ~2 years. Treatment is palliative; that is, it is directed at control of pain, improved sense of well-being, improved performance status, and possibly prolongation of life. Patients can be effectively palliated by chemotherapy and tamoxifen, with response rates approaching 50%. A few patients can survive many years with advanced disease. Autologous bone marrow transplantation with high-dose chemotherapy may improve prospects for survival.

In the patient with metastasis to visceral organs, chemotherapy and/or tamoxifen should be employed. If the patient is older and has hormone-sensitive cancer with metastasis to nonthreatening locations, tamoxifen may be used initially. For solitary bony metastasis or for spinal metastasis impinging on the spinal cord, palliative radiotherapy is highly effective in ablating pain and preventing pathological fracture. Bone stabilization may be required with extensive osseous metastasis prior to beginning radioablative therapy, because cancer destruction may create a void resulting in fracture. Rarely, emergent surgical decompression of the spinal canal is necessary to prevent hemiplegia.

Breast Reconstruction

Breast cancer threatens patients' femininity and body image as well as their lives. In the past, breast reconstruction after MRM was usually performed as a delayed procedure, but this is no longer the case. In patients with stage I or II breast cancer, immediate reconstruction usually does not interfere with adjuvant chemotherapy. Reconstruction can be achieved with tissue expanders and breast implants or with autologous musculocutaneous flaps from either the back, abdomen, or buttocks. The most common flap is the transverse rectus abdominis myocutaneous (TRAM) flap, in which the skin, fat, and rectus abdominis muscle are mobilized and fashioned into a new breast. Other flaps include the latissimus dorsi myocutaneous flap and the free gluteus maximus flap with microsurgical anastomosis.

OTHER MALIGNANT NEOPLASMS OF THE BREAST

Sarcomas

Sarcomas that occur in the breast include fibrosarcoma, desmoid tumor, malignant fibrous histiocytoma, liposarcoma, leiomyosarcoma, extraskeletal osteogenic sarcoma, and chondrosarcoma. Breast sarcomas present as a rapidly growing painless mass. Mammography is not especially helpful. Tumor grade is the single most important prognostic variable in sarcomas. The incidence of regional nodal involvement even with large sarcomas tends to be low, the route of metastasis being primarily hematogenous. The most common site of metastasis is the lungs. Wide local excision is the treatment of choice and can usually be performed without radical chest wall excision. Adjuvant radiotherapy may be indicated for high-grade lesions.

Lymphoma

Lymphoma may secondarily involve the breast. Such lesions tend to present as a large mass in a postmenopausal patient. Primary lymphoma of the breast is rare. Breast lymphoma is similar to non-Hodgkin's lymphoma in other parts of the body. Treatment consists of chemoradiation, with surgery reserved for treatment failure.

ADENOCARCINOMA OF THE MALE BREAST

Less than 1% of all breast cancer occurs in men. Male breast cancer has occasionally been associated with Klinefelter syndrome, estrogen therapy, testicular feminization syndromes, irradiation, and trauma. It can masquerade as gynecomastia. The incidence peaks at 60 to 70 years old. The tumor is usually ER-positive. Overall, the neoplasm has the same stage-for-stage survival of breast cancer in women, but the overall prognosis is worse because of more advanced stage at diagnosis. Male breast cancer is always of ductal histology. Because of the lack of stromal and lobular elements, lobular carcinoma does not occur in men. The preferred treatment is MRM, with postoperative radiation for ulcerative or high-grade anaplastic tumors. Orchiectomy and the administration of estrogens may induce remissions of metastatic disease. Tamoxifen and chemotherapy have been utilized for node-positive receptor-positive male breast cancer.

SUMMARY

Complete evaluation of the breast requires a detailed history and thorough physical examination. Common pathologies and the respective treatments have been discussed. The incidence of malignant diseases of the breast appears to be on the rise. Screening involves routine bilateral mammogram in women over the age of 50. Suspicious nonpalpable breast masses detected by mammography require tissue biopsy. Likewise, suspicious palpable masses mandate biopsy. Surgical extirpation of the tumor with staging axillary lymph node dissection remains the cornerstone of therapy. Variations in treatment, including adjuvant and neoadjuvant therapy, have been presented. The treatment that is appropriate for each patient must be individualized to match personal desires with expected and reasonable outcomes.

STUDY QUESTIONS

1. Describe the embryologic development of human breast tissue.
2. Explain in detail the proper method of performing a breast examination.
3. What are consequences and patient limitations following an axillary lymph node dissection?
4. What are factors that influence the choice of surgical therapy for breast?
5. What are the current survival statistics of treated breast cancer?

SUGGESTED READING

Early Breast Cancer Trialists' Collaborative Group. Effects of radiotherapy and surgery in breast cancer—an overview of the randomized trials. *N Engl J Med* 1995;333:1444.

Early Breast Cancer Trialists' Collaborative Group. Systemic treatment of early breast cancer by hormonal, cytotoxic, or immune therapy. 133 randomized trials involving 31,000 recurrences and 24,000 deaths among 75,000 women. *Lancet* 1992;339:71.

Fisher B, Anderson S, Fisher ER, et al. Significance of ipsilateral breast tumor recurrence after lumpectomy. *Lancet* 1991;338:327.

Fisher B, Anderson S, Redmond CK, et al. Reanalysis and results after twelve years of follow-up in a randomized clinical trial comparing total mastectomy with lumpectomy with or without irradiation in the treatment of breast cancer. *N Engl J Med* 1995;333:1456.

Fisher B, Costantino J, Redmond C, et al. Lumpectomy compared with lumpectomy and radiation therapy for the treatment of intraductal breast cancer. *N Engl J Med* 1993;328:1581.

Fisher B, Redmond C, Fisher ER, et al. Ten-year results of a randomized clinical trial comparing radical mastectomy and total mastectomy with or without radiation. *N Engl J Med* 1985;312:674.

CHAPTER 8

Hernia

Carl Schulman and Joseph A. Moylan

All patients should be offered surgery . . . operation is almost mandatory for every case of hernia.

—Nyhus and Condon, 1995

As defined by Stedman, a hernia is a "protrusion of a part or structure through the tissues normally containing it," usually the peritoneum and other intraabdominal contents protruding through the abdominal wall. The majority of hernias are of the inguinal type (75%), followed by incisional and ventral abdominal (10%), femoral (6%), umbilical (3%), and esophageal hiatal (1%). The focus here is on groin hernias. Inguinal hernias are more common in males, whereas most femoral hernias occur in females. There is a relationship with race, as noted by the fact that groin hernias are at least three times more common in African-Americans than in the white population.

Herniorraphy is the most frequent general surgical procedure performed in the United States, accounting for 10% to 15% of all operations. With >700,000 repairs taking place annually, the economic impact of the medical costs and the estimated loss of working days is reported to be upwards of $28 billion.

The history of hernia is the history of surgery.

—Nyhus and Condon, 1995

From an historical perspective, the surgical treatment of hernias has evolved with the major advances in surgery as well as with increased understanding of the complex anatomy of the groin. Early attempts at repair included the routine sacrifice of the spermatic cord and testicle in males. Not until the detailed anatomy was outlined by Astley Paston Cooper (for whom the superior pubic ligament is named) and others were attempts at repair based on sound anatomic and scientific principles. These efforts culminated in the technical advancement by Edoardo Bassini "to restore those conditions in the area of the hernial orifice which exist under normal circumstances." This leap forward heralded a new era of hernia surgery,

with each successive modification providing an anatomically correct, stronger surgical repair.

These developments, along with new techniques in anesthesia, hemostasis and antisepsis, brought about the modern version of herniorraphy.

For the understanding of the etiology, the pathology, the clinical manifestations and, particularly, the surgical repair of an indirect inguinal hernia, a profound knowledge of the anatomy of this region is indispensable.

—F. Netter, 1979

The anatomy of the groin has been a challenge for many students and young surgeons. Its three-dimensional interrelationships and their contributions to the formation and repair of groin hernias require repeated study and in situ visualization in order to comprehend its meticulous design fully. It is best to learn the inguinal anatomy in a series of layers, and then define its borders and more intricate relationships.

The layers of the inguinal region are simply those of the abdominal wall (Fig. 1). Beneath the skin and in the subcutaneous tissue lie the superficial Camper's and Scarpa's fascia. The next layer is the aponeurosis of the external oblique muscle. This can be followed down medially, where the opening known as the external or superficial inguinal ring can be found. Underlying the external oblique aponeurosis is the spermatic cord in males. In the female, the round ligament of the uterus is found in place of the spermatic cord. The cord protrudes lateral to the inferior epigastric vessels, through an opening called the "deep" or "internal inguinal ring." The internal oblique muscle and aponeurosis form an arch over the spermatic cord as it emerges from the deep inguinal ring. The transversalis muscle and its fascia are encountered medial and posterior, making up the posterior wall of the inguinal canal. Therefore, in basic layers, one will encounter, in order from anterior to posterior, the skin, subcutaneous tissues, external oblique aponeurosis, spermatic cord, transversus abdominis aponeurosis and

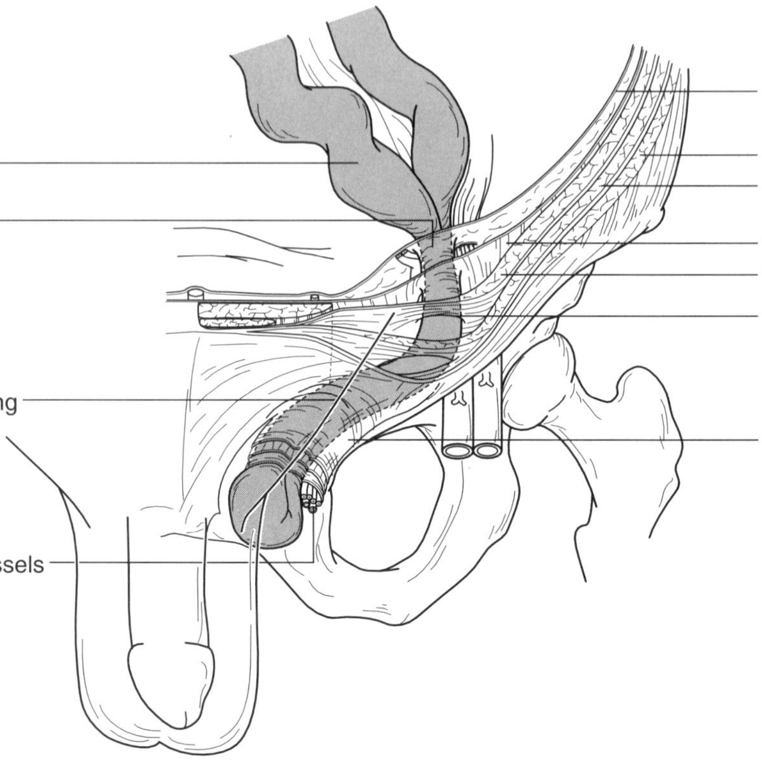

FIG. 1. Anatomy of the inguinal region showing the layers of the abdominal wall and the course of an indirect inguinal hernia.

transversalis fascia, and, finally, the peritoneum. Modern-day repairs are based on the restoration of the normal anatomic relationships.

The spermatic cord is enveloped by the cremasteric muscle fibers, a natural extension of the internal oblique muscle. The contents of the cord are the vas deferens, the testicular vessels, and a plexus of veins, lymphatics, and nerves. Also coursing through the canal, next to the spermatic cord and between the external and internal oblique muscles, lies the ilioinguinal nerve. This supplies cutaneous innervation to the medial thigh and scrotum.

It is also important to know the major landmarks used for reference points when describing the locations of structures and the types of hernias. The inguinal ligament lies along the line connecting the pubic tubercle and the anterior superior iliac spine. An inguinal hernia by definition protrudes from above the inguinal ligament. This is in contrast to a femoral hernia, which by definition protrudes inferior to the inguinal ligament. A femoral hernia protrudes along the femoral sheath in the femoral canal, posterior to the inguinal ligament, anterior to the pubic ramus periosteum (Cooper's ligament), and medially to the femoral vessels. Any hernia palpated below the inguinal ligament should be suspected of being a femoral hernia.

The difference between a direct and indirect inguinal hernia is based on whether the hernia protrudes medial or lateral to the inferior epigastric vessels. One that pro-trudes lateral to the vessels emerges from the internal inguinal ring and is an indirect inguinal hernia. A hernia arising medial to the vessels protrudes directly through the floor of the inguinal canal (the transversalis fascia) and is therefore termed a direct inguinal hernia. It should be noted that a direct inguinal hernia arises from within Hesselbach's triangle, bounded inferiorly by the inguinal ligament, laterally by the inferior epigastric vessels, and superomedially by the lateral border of the rectus sheath. A hernia with direct and indirect components is known as a pantaloon hernia as it tends to be so large as to straddle the vessels on both sides. A sliding hernia is one in which the wall of the hernia sac consists partly of a viscous structure (i.e., colon, bladder). A Richter's hernia occurs when one side of the bowel wall is trapped in the hernia rather than the entire loop of bowel. In this circumstance, it is possible to have intestinal strangulation without complete bowel obstruction.

If I have seen further, it is by standing on the shoulders of giants.

—Sir Isaac Newton, 1643–1727

The exact causative factors of inguinal hernias remain unclear. Even to this day, the congenital predisposition to inguinal hernias is a topic of debate. The testes begin their descent in the third month of fetal life. They are tethered to the scrotum by the gubernaculum testis and follow a retroperitoneal course. At the end of the seventh month, the testes pass through the internal inguinal ring and inguinal canal and, within the next several weeks, descend into the scrotum. The peritoneal fold that is attached to and pulled along with the testes is called the "processus vaginalis." In nearly all pediatric cases and in most adults, the processus vaginalis remains patent, thereby predisposing to inguinal hernia. It normally becomes obliterated during the last month of intrauterine life, but in some remains as a peritoneal sac. This etiology is supported by the fact that 80% to 90% of groin hernias occur in males.

Several predisposing factors to inguinal hernias in adults have been noted. They are all centered around the premise that an increase in intraabdominal pressure causes weakening of the floor of the inguinal canal and its supporting structures. They include such common problems as chronic cough (COPD), prostatic hypertrophy, and constipation or other causes of colonic obstruction. Strenuous physical activity is thought to be a risk factor, and trauma to the inguinal region can serve as another contributing factor.

Two physiologic mechanisms have been proposed that prevent the development of groin hernias. One is the shutter mechanism, produced by the transversus aponeurotic arch, which when tensed moves in apposition to the iliopubic tract and reinforces the floor of the inguinal canal (Fig. 2). The second is the sphincter mechanism. It refers to the transversalis fascial sling, which, when

pulled superiorly and laterally, closes the internal inguinal ring around the cord structures. Therefore, the shutter and sphincter mechanisms serve to prevent direct and indirect hernias, respectively.

Several classification schemes have been proposed in an effort to standardize the description and severity of inguinal hernias as well as provide a more structured approach to the indications and need for the various types of repairs. The classification proposed by Nyhus is based on anatomic criteria and is presented in Table 1. They are classified according to severity of damage to the internal inguinal ring or the defect in Hesselbach's triangle. Initially confined to the internal inguinal ring (type I), they enlarge medially (type II) and then through the posterior inguinal wall (type III). Recurrent hernias are designated type IV.

The doctor may also learn more about the illness from the way the patient tells the story than from the story itself.

—James B. Herrick, 1861–1954

Diagnosis is often made on the basis of history and physical examination alone. This is almost always the case when dealing with hernias. In many cases, the diagnosis is obvious, but for those less clear, it is important to delineate the relevant information. A common complaint is pain in the groin. This must be investigated further to determine the exact nature of the pain, its location, duration, and any alleviating or aggravating factors. A typical

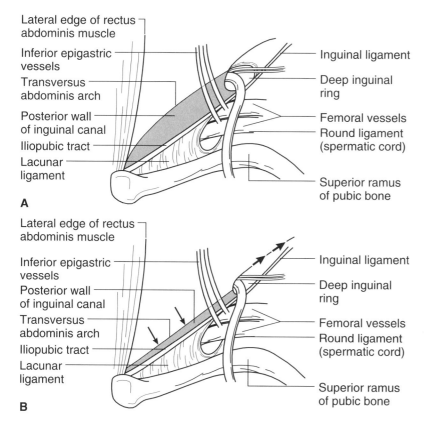

Lateral edge of rectus abdominis muscle
Inferior epigastric vessels
Transversus abdominis arch
Posterior wall of inguinal canal
Iliopubic tract
Lacunar ligament

Inguinal ligament
Deep inguinal ring
Femoral vessels
Round ligament (spermatic cord)
Superior ramus of pubic bone

A

Lateral edge of rectus abdominis muscle
Inferior epigastric vessels
Posterior wall of inguinal canal
Transversus abdominis arch
Iliopubic tract
Lacunar ligament

Inguinal ligament
Deep inguinal ring
Femoral vessels
Round ligament (spermatic cord)
Superior ramus of pubic bone

B

FIG. 2. Posterior view of the lower right anterior abdominal wall. The drawings show how the two most important factors that protect against inguinal hernia operate. **(A)** The abdominal muscles are in the relaxed position. **(B)** What happens when the internal oblique and transversus abdominis muscles contract. Shutter mechanism: when the internal oblique and transversus abdominis muscles contract, they partly cover the posterior wall of the inguinal canal. Closure (sphincter) mechanism: contraction of the transversus abdominis muscle results in cranial-lateral displacement and narrowing of the deep inguinal ring.

TABLE 1. *Classification of groin hernias*

Type I: indirect inguinal hernia
    Internal inguinal ring normal (e.g., pediatric hernia)
Type II: indirect inguinal hernia
    Internal inguinal ring dilated but posterior inguinal wall intact; inferior epigastric vessels not displaced
Type III: posterior wall defects
    A. Direct inguinal hernia
    B. Indirect inguinal hernia: internal inguinal ring dilated, medially encroaching on or destroying the transversalis fascia of
       Hesselbach's triangle (e.g., massive scrotal, sliding, or pantaloon hernias)
    C. Femoral hernia
Type IV: recurrent hernia

Adapted from Nyhus LM, Klein MS, Rogers FB. Inguinal hernia. *Curr Probl Surg* 1991;28:401–450.

history will be that of a middle-aged man who says he first felt the pain when lifting a heavy object or straining. The pain is usually sharp in nature and can radiate to the inner groin or scrotum. It is short-lived and subsides as quickly as it began. Often, the pain can be reproduced by having the patient strain (a Valsalva maneuver).

Another presenting feature that can be easily elicited during the history is the presence of a mass. Exact location of the mass can determine if it is in fact a hernia as well as determining which type of hernia may be present. Scrotal swelling, which may be seen most commonly in indirect inguinal hernias, must be delineated from other causes of scrotal enlargement such as epididymal enlargement, a varicocele, a spermatocele, or a hydrocele. It is also important to note when the mass first appeared and whether it changes size with different positions. An inguinal hernia is often seen while standing erect and can spontaneously or manually be reduced while supine. As stated previously, femoral hernias should be suspected with a mass palpable below the inguinal ligament.

It is of tantamount importance to ask for any possible causative factors regarding urologic, colonic, or pulmonary pathology. One should define any treatable causes of increased intraabdominal pressure to determine if further testing and correction is needed prior to or shortly after repair of the hernia.

Don't touch the patient—state first what you see; cultivate your powers of observation.

—Sir William Osler, 1849–1919

The first step in the examination for hernia is inspection. With the patient standing, have him turn his head and cough while you look for any bulges in the groin region, comparing both sides. The exact location of a mass may be determined during this maneuver. Palpation is performed by placing the index finger in the scrotum above the testicle and invaginating the scrotal skin to reach to the external inguinal ring. The pad of the finger should be facing inward. The finger should follow the spermatic cord laterally into the inguinal canal and upward toward the internal inguinal ring (Fig. 3). At this point, the patient should be asked once again to cough or perform a valsalva maneuver. A hernia will be felt as an

impulse against either the tip or the pad of the finger. If a hernia is detected, the patient should be asked to lie down to insure the hernia is easily reducible. This procedure is then duplicated to examine the other side. If a large scrotum is noted, auscultation is sometimes helpful to determine the presence of bowel sounds, indicative of a large indirect inguinal hernia with bowel contents. Figure 4 and Table 2 illustrate the major differences in the diagnosis of hernias.

Once diagnosed, suitable candidates should be offered surgery to prevent potential complications. The complications associated with unrepaired inguinal hernias are those of intestinal obstruction and strangulation. In an elderly male with a large, easily reducible hernia and in patients who are poor operative risks, the benefits of surgery must be weighed against the morbidity and mortality related to the risk of obstruction and strangulation. As the contents of the hernia become unable to traverse the hernial orifice easily, they may become unreducible and are termed incarcerated. When the blood supply to

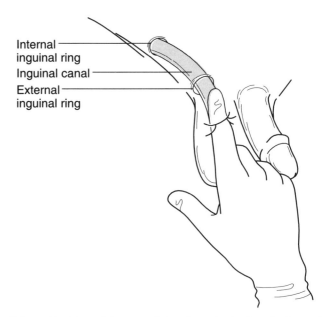

Internal inguinal ring
Inguinal canal
External inguinal ring

FIG. 3. Position of the examining finger in the inguinal canal.

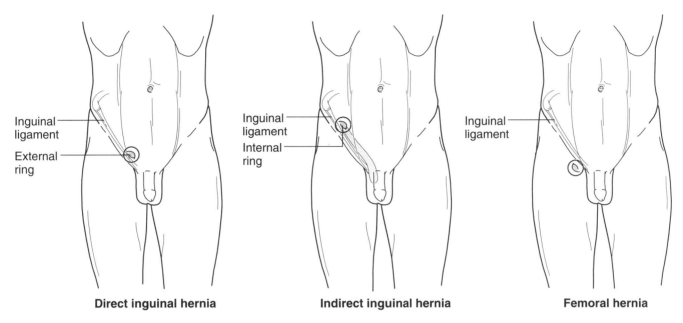

Direct inguinal hernia **Indirect inguinal hernia** **Femoral hernia**

FIG. 4. The location of direct, indirect, and femoral hernias in the inguinal region.

this segment of bowel becomes compromised, strangulation occurs with resulting intestinal ischemia. Statistically, the risk of strangulation is 0.3%/year or 4% over the lifetime of an older individual. Incarceration is a surgical emergency; therefore, it is preferred to repair all hernias electively to avoid this complication. Femoral, indirect inguinal, and umbilical hernias are more likely to cause strangulation of bowel because they have narrower necks and tend to be surrounded by rings of rigid tissue, whereas direct inguinal hernias usually have a broader neck. Although prevention of complications by elective repair has decreased the mortality rate, hernia remains a cause of significant morbidity and mortality worldwide.

Preoperative preparation is usually minimal in hernia surgery. Comorbid medical conditions should be optimized prior to elective surgical repair. Standard preoperative testing in healthy patients includes a hemoglobin/hematocrit for those <6 months or >40 years of age, men-

struating females, and those with a history of anemia, abnormal bleeding, renal disease, or anticoagulant use; urinalysis for those suspected of having a urinary tract infection, especially in women; electrocardiogram for those >40 years of age; and radiographs in those with cardiovascular disease, respiratory disease, a >20-pack/year history of tobacco use, and those >60 years of age. In those patients with constipation, the routine use of colonoscopy prior to hernia surgery is a subject of debate and probably not an effective screening method for colonic neoplasm.

Preoperative bowel preparation is not routinely done. Prophylactic antibiotics should be given if the use of synthetic materials is anticipated. The types of anesthesia used for inguinal hernia repair differ with the preferences of both the surgeon and the patient and should be an informed, mutual decision. Local anesthesia allows the patient to bear down during the operation, helping to

TABLE 2. *Characteristics of groin hernias*

Feature	Direct inguinal	Indirect inguinal	Femoral
Occurrence	Middle-aged and elderly men	All ages	Least common: more frequent in women
Bilaterality	55%	30%	Rarely
Origin of swelling	Above inguinal ligament; directly behind and through external ring.	Above inguinal ligament. Hernial sac enters inguinal canal at internal ring and exits at external ring.	Below inguinal ligament
Scrotal involvement	Rarely	Commonly	Never
Impulse location	At side of finger in inguinal canal	At tip of finger in inguinal canal	Not felt by finger in inguinal canal inguinal; mass below canal

Adapted from Swartz M. *Textbook of physical diagnosis.* Philadelphia: Saunders, 1989.

identify a small hernia and test the adequacy of the repair. It is favored in patients at increased risk of complications from general anesthesia. In addition, costs are reduced, and operative turnover is facilitated. Regional or block anesthesia requires greater effort on the part of the anesthesiologist but affords greater relaxation of the abdominal musculature during repair. Epidural and spinal anesthesia are popular in some ambulatory surgery settings but can be complicated by postoperative urinary retention. Good relaxation and comfort during the procedure are afforded by general anesthesia, but general anesthesia eliminates straining down during the procedure to test the repair. Following anesthesia, the patient should be positioned in the Trendelenburg position, allowing easier reduction of the hernia. The skin overlying the incision is shaved immediately prior to the operation. The operative field, including the genitalia, is cleansed in the usual fashion.

Fit your operation to your patient—not your patient to your operation.

—J. M. T. Finney

As mentioned previously, the goal of inguinal hernia repair is to restore the anatomic relationships that exist normally. This means reduction of the hernia, ligation and removal of the hernia sac, and reconstruction of the layers of the abdominal wall. The type of hernia repair is varied among surgeons and should be dictated by the overall clinical picture, including the patient's age, medical condition, level of strenuous activity, type and size of defect, and the risk of recurrence over the lifetime of the patient.

An incision is made following the skin crease just above the inguinal ligament, starting slightly above and medial to the pubic tubercle and continuing for 6 to 8 cm toward the anterior superior iliac spine. This is carried down to the aponeurosis of the external oblique, which is opened from and including the external inguinal ring in the direction of the fibers of the external oblique aponeurosis. The spermatic cord is identified, bluntly dissected free, and encircled with a rubber drain for easy manipulation (Fig. 5). Some advocate the identification and preservation of the ilioinguinal nerve, while others routinely sever it to avoid entrapment and postoperative neuralgia.

An indirect hernia is found by carefully dissecting the cremaster muscle off the spermatic cord to identify the hernia sac. An indirect hernia usually lies anterior and medial to the cord at the level of the internal ring. The sac is dissected free to the level of the abdominal wall and

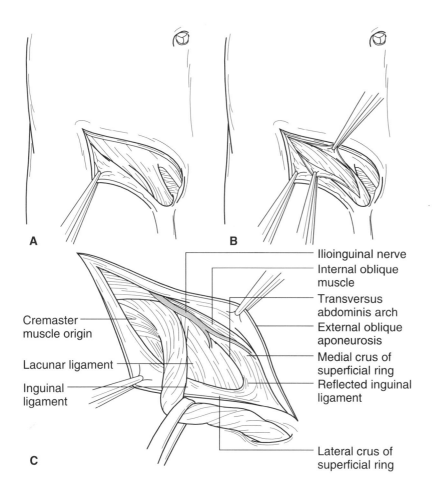

Cremaster muscle origin

Lacunar ligament

Inguinal ligament

Ilioinguinal nerve
Internal oblique muscle
Transversus abdominis arch
External oblique aponeurosis
Medial crus of superficial ring
Reflected inguinal ligament

Lateral crus of superficial ring

A

B

C

FIG. 5. Dissection of the inguinal canal. **(A)** The intact external oblique muscle and aponeurosis are depicted. **(B)** The external oblique aponeurosis has been incised in the direction of its fibers, toward the superficial inguinal ring. **(C)** The external oblique aponeurosis is opened widely and the spermatic cord mobilized.

opened; any intestinal contents are reduced, and the neck of the sac is ligated at the level of the abdominal wall. The remaining distal sac is amputated. A direct hernia will be found medial to the inferior epigastric vessels. Most direct hernias can be reduced without opening the sac. Combined indirect and direct sacs are joined by dividing the inferior epigastric vessels and closing the sacs as one peritoneal defect. In indirect hernias where the internal ring is intact and admits only the tip of a finger, high ligation of the sac alone may be adequate.

The Bassini (inguinal ligament) repair is often performed for simple, indirect and direct hernias. It involves approximating the transversalis fascia to the iliopubic tract (shelving portion of the inguinal ligament). A transition stitch is placed at the junction of the inguinal ligament and the symphysis pubis (at Cooper's ligament) to ensure closure of the medial aspect of the repair. A new internal ring is created laterally. The spermatic cord is then returned to its normal anatomic position, and the external oblique fascia is reapproximated over the cord down to the level of the previous external ring. The wound is then closed in two layers using subcutaneous and subcuticular sutures.

The McVay (Cooper's ligament) repair can be performed for primary or recurrent hernias, femoral hernias, and large mixed hernias. The hernia is identified similar to the Bassini repair. In addition, a relaxing incision is made at the line of fusion of the external oblique aponeurosis and the rectus sheath just above the pubic symphysis. This allows the repair to be done with less tension on the structures being approximated, providing a more secure repair. The repair begins by approximating the transversus abdominis arch to Cooper's ligament. This extends from the pubic tubercle to as far laterally as the medial edge of the femoral vein. The femoral canal is closed by approximating the anterior femoral fascia to Cooper's ligament. The repair is continued laterally, placing sutures between the transversus abdominis arch, the anterior femoral fascia, and the inguinal ligament until a new internal inguinal ring has been created. The ring should be snug enough to admit only the tip of a finger or a large kelly clamp. The external oblique and remaining layers are closed as in the Bassini repair. The McVay repair provides greater reinforcement for the posterior wall of the inguinal canal as well as repair of any defects that may contribute to a femoral hernia.

Yet another era of hernia surgery was heralded by the technique pioneered by Shouldice. He emphasized a six-layer closure with running sutures. Other caveats included the use of local anesthesia and early ambulation and exercise the day after surgery. Shouldice also insisted on preoperative weight loss for obese patients, making the tissues easier to identify, permitting a more stable closure, and thus reducing the recurrence rate. The hernia is identified, and the transversalis fascia is incised as in the McVay repair. The Shouldice repair, however, advocates

the imbrication of the transversalis fascia. The lateral (or inferior) edge of the transversalis fascia is sutured medially to the undersurface of the internal oblique. The medial superior edge is sutured to the inguinal ligament. The conjoined tendon (the terminal portion of the internal oblique aponeurosis and the transversus abdominis aponeurosis) is then sutured to the inguinal ligament. The spermatic cord is then placed in its normal anatomic position, and closure of the external oblique aponeurosis and subcutaneous tissues is performed in the standard fashion.

Laparoscopic hernia repair is now advocated by some. It can be performed via a transperitoneal or completely preperitoneal approach. The preperitoneal approach avoids contact with the intraabdominal contents and allows direct visualization of the pubis symphysis and Cooper's ligament. The transperitoneal approach allows easy visualization of the contralateral side, where an occult hernia may be found, as well as direct visualization of any viscera that may be contained within the sac. While return to work and normal activity is often as quick or quicker than following an open repair, laparoscopic repair requires general anesthesia. While similar recurrence rates have been shown compared to open techniques, further long-term studies and proven cost and patient-related benefits are needed before this approach can be fully endorsed.

The use of biosynthetic materials is also gaining increasing popularity. The most commonly employed is a polypropylene mesh. Lichtenstein pioneered the use of biosynthetic material in his tension-free hernia repair. The mesh is sutured in place below the spermatic cord to reinforce the posterior wall of the inguinal canal and create a new internal ring. It is felt to be beneficial in the elderly, in large defects, and in recurrent hernias where the strength of the remaining tissues is in question. There has been no documented increase in the rates of infection following its use, but once again long-term effects and recurrence rates warrant further study.

In the modern era, most hernia repairs are performed on an outpatient basis. Patients can return to normal activities (limited to those that do not produce pain) the day following surgery. A full range of strenuous activities is usually permitted by the second to fourth postoperative week. Instructions to the patient should detail the most common sequelae, including scrotal swelling and ecchymoses. A mild laxative should be used in the event of constipation. The signs and symptoms of infection should be made clear prior to release. A single postoperative evaluation to inspect the wound is usually all that is required.

While most of the complications of hernia repair are fairly minor, significant morbidity may result from poor attention to technique and detail. The mortality rate from elective hernia surgery is <0.01%. Thromboembolic complications are also extremely rare due to short operative duration and early mobilization following surgery. Postoperative hematoma is found in 5% to 7% of cases and is largely dependent on the extent of spermatic cord dissection, the difficulty of repair, and the skill of the surgeon. The frequency of wound infection has been documented to be 1% to 2% for all repairs.

Rarely, damage of the nerves and vessels associated with the spermatic cord occurs. Entrapment of the ilioinguinal or genitofemoral nerve cause either pain or paresthesias (i.e., neuralgia) in the inguinal region with extension to the scrotum and upper thigh. This may become apparent immediately following surgery or may be delayed for years. Diagnosis consists primarily of nerve blocks which, if successful, should be followed by exploration and neurectomy. These syndromes can be caused by poor surgical technique or unpredictable variations in patients' scar-forming physiology.

Compression of the cord and testicular blood supply can lead to the development of ischemic orchitis. It presents as painful swelling of the testes, sometimes with fever and leukocytosis, usually within 1 to 2 days following the operation. Expectant management is the treatment of choice; spontaneous remission occurs in 60% of cases. The remaining cases subside over time, with development of varying degrees of testicular atrophy. This complication occurs in 0.03% to 0.5% of elective primary repairs. Frequency is greater with large and sliding hernias where extensive dissection of the sac from the cord is required. Reproductive capability is thought to be unaffected by unilateral atrophy, but extreme care must be taken with any procedures involving the contralateral side.

Absence of tension in the completed hernia repair is essential to success.

—Nyhus and Condon, 1995

Hernia recurrence depends largely on the technique employed and the skill of the operative surgeon. Recurrence rates vary widely in the reported literature, from 1% to 3% at many clinics specializing in herniorraphy to as high as 5% to 10%. Those who do large numbers of hernias in an efficient, standardized fashion can usually obtain recurrence rates of >2%. A trend toward ambulatory surgery in centers specializing in herniorraphy may contribute to further reduction in the rate of recurrence. Most agree, however, that true recurrence rates are hard to determine because most studies are flawed with respect to length or lack of follow-up (most recurrences occur >5 years after surgery) and the difference in techniques. Recurrences can be classified into two broad categories. Early (mechanical) recurrences develop within the first 2 years and are felt to be due to tension on the suture line. Late (physiologic) recurrences develop many years after the initial operation and are felt to be due to a disorder of collagen metabolism. This age-related decreased collagen content of the groin tissue has led some to advocate permanent replacement of the floor of the inguinal canal with synthetic material, producing a tension-free repair.

Pediatric hernias have several special considerations that merit attention. Repair of congenital inguinal hernia is the most common operation in the pediatric age group. As many as 5% of full-term infants may be born with an inguinal hernia, and the incidence is substantially increased in premature infants. The processus vaginalis is patent in 90% of all newborn infants. The pediatric hernia is almost always indirect and carries a high risk of incarceration, usually within the first 6 months. Pediatric hernias are more common on the right side and are frequently bilateral. Often, the mother will have noticed a lump that is not obvious on physical examination. Due to the high risk of incarceration, a thorough physical exam should be performed to demonstrate the hernia so that prompt repair can be undertaken. An undescended testicle is a frequent finding in association with an inguinal hernia and can be repaired simultaneously if warranted. The repair performed depends on the size and nature of the defect, but in general very little repair is necessary after ligation of the sac. Some surgeons advocate routine exploration of the contralateral side due to the high incidence of bilateral inguinal hernia.

There are several other types of hernias that are encountered infrequently. A Littre's hernia is simply the incarceration or strangulation of a Meckel's diverticulum. Spigelian hernias, also known as spontaneous lateral ventral hernias, protrude through the spigelian fascia. They occur along the semilunar line (the lateral edge of the rectus muscle) below the umbilicus at the semicircular line of Douglas (where the transversus abdominis and internal oblique aponeuroses change to pass anterior to the rectus muscle). An obturator hernia passes through the obturator foramen or canal. It cannot be seen or palpated in the usual fashion; hence, diagnosis is difficult. Pain in the medial aspect of the thigh produced upon extension, adduction, or medial rotation of the thigh is the Howship-Romberg sign. It is caused by pressure by a hernia on the obturator nerve and felt to be pathognomonic for an obturator hernia. Umbilical hernias, more common in women, occur at the umbilicus and are thought to be related to a congenital defect where the umbilical structures passed through the abdominal wall. It is common in children and usually closes by 2 years of age, with only 5% persisting until adulthood. Treatment of small umbilical hernias (fascial defect of <1.5 cm) can be delayed at least until the age of 5 years in anticipation of spontaneous closure. An obvious protuberance, a large defect, or a tender hernia should be repaired earlier to prevent complications and psychological damage to the child. Given enough time, it is possible all umbilical hernias would resolve; therefore, those patients with a small defect and no protuberance can be observed until the age of 9 or 10 years, or even longer. Acquired umbilical hernias in adults tend to incarcerate and strangulate, do not resolve spontaneously, and therefore necessitate expedient operative repair. Incisional hernias are often the result of a wound infection, but can also be caused by advanced age, obesity, malnutrition, or a postoperative increase in intraabdominal pressure such as ascites. Lumbar hernias, some of which are known as Petit's hernia, are extremely rare. They represent any defect in the lumbar region of the torso and vary widely in size, anatomic location, and contents. Repair is difficult, and mesh repair is gaining increasing favor. Epigastric hernias are those that occur in the midline, through the linea alba, above the umbilicus. Many are small and asymptomatic, and remain undiagnosed. If symptomatic, repair is simple. A peristomal hernia occurs adjacent to or surrounding a colostomy or ileostomy. It makes fitting the stoma appliance difficult, is a potential site for infection, and can cause obstruction of the bowel traversing the abdominal wall.

You can judge the worth of a surgeon by the way he does a hernia.

—Fairbank

Hernias represent a large segment of the operations performed in general surgery. As such, one must be aware of the potential morbidity and mortality and the indications for repair. Once diagnosed, the surgeon and the patient must discuss the risks and benefits to determine the appropriate course of action. Surgical repair is possible in many different fashions. The type of repair is generally decided by the type of defect found at operation and the familiarity of the surgeon with a particular style of repair. Newer techniques, such as laparoscopic repair and the use of biosynthetic materials, will undoubtedly be the focus of much attention in the future of hernia surgery. It should be the goal of all surgeons to become proficient at this very common operation to provide the best possible repair for the lifetime of the patient.

STUDY QUESTIONS

1. Describe the work-up required for a patient undergoing elective inguinal hernia repair, including the predisposing factors thought to contribute to inguinal hernia formation.
2. Would you operate on a 70-year-old man with a large, easily reducible direct inguinal hernia who is completely asymptomatic? Discuss your reasoning.
3. What type of repair would you choose for a young, athletic 30-year-old man with a painful, indirect inguinal hernia? Discuss the use of synthetic mesh, antibiotics, and postoperative care.
4. Describe the layers of the abdominal wall in the inguinal region, their relation to the spermatic cord, and the general method for repair of an inguinal hernia.
5. Describe the typical history, physical examination, and differentiation of a direct from an indirect inguinal hernia.

SUGGESTED READING

Carbonell JF, Sanchez JL, Peris RT, et al. Risk factors associated with inguinal hernias: a case control study. *Eur J Surg* 1993;159:481–486.

Laws HL. Groin hernia: a current perspective. *Ala Med* 1995;64:15–17.

Lichtenstein IL, Shulman AG, Amid PK. The cause, prevention, and treatment of recurrent groin hernia. *Surg Clin North Am* 1993;73:529–544.

Nyhus LM, Condon RE. *Hernia.* Philadelphia: Lippincott, 1995.

Nyhus LM, Klein MS, Rogers FB. Inguinal hernia. *Curr Probl Surg* 1991;28:401–450.

Pollak R, Nyhus LM. Complications of groin hernia repair. *Surg Clin North Am* 1983;63:1363–1371.

Rutkow IM, Robbins AW. Demographic, classificatory, and socioeconomic aspects of hernia repair in the United States. *Surg Clin North Am* 1993;73:413–426.

Sabiston D. *Textbook of surgery.* Philadelphia: Saunders, 1991.

Schumpelick V, Treutner KH, Arit G. Inguinal hernia repair in adults. *Lancet* 1994;344:375–379.

Skandalakis JE, Colborn GL, Androulakis JA, Skandalakis LJ, Pemberton LB. Embryologic and anatomic basis of inguinal herniorraphy. *Surg Clin North Am* 1993;73:799–836.

CHAPTER 9

Esophagus

Cristina Lopez and Alan S. Livingstone

ANATOMY

The esophagus is a long muscular tube that extends from the pharynx to the stomach for a distance of ~25 cm. It begins in the midline at the level of the sixth cervical vertebra and terminates in the gastroesophageal (GE) junction or cardia at the 11th thoracic vertebral level. It is divided into cervical, thoracic, and abdominal segments. In the neck, it is a midline structure and enters the superior mediastinum between the trachea and the vertebral column. The thoracic esophagus enters the posterior mediastinum and curves slightly to the left passing behind the left mainstem bronchus. It then deviates somewhat to the right for a short distance and then returns to the left of midline as it courses posterior to the pericardium and anterior to the thoracic aorta. Its position to the left or right of midline influences surgical accessibility. The cervical and lower thoracic portions of the esophagus are best approached from the left side, whereas the subcarinal esophagus is more accessible through a right thoracotomy. Distally, it enters the abdomen through the esophageal hiatus in the diaphragm, where it travels for a distance of several centimeters before joining the stomach. Several supporting structures are found in the area of the cardia and include the diaphragmatic crura and the phrenoesophageal membrane. This membrane is a continuation of the transversalis fascia of the abdomen and circumferentially attaches the esophagus to the diaphragm. The normal esophagus has three predictable areas of narrowing. These constrictions occur at the levels of the cricopharyngeus muscle (the narrowest point of the esophagus), the left bronchus and aortic arch, and the diaphragm. They are of clinical interest because they indicate where swallowed foreign bodies are likely to lodge.

The esophageal wall is composed of a mucosal and muscular layer, and, unlike the remainder of the gastrointestinal tract, lacks a serosal layer. Squamous epithelium lines the majority of the esophagus with a few areas of columnar epithelium being present distally at the GE junction. The outer longitudinal and inner circular muscle layers are striated in the upper third of the esophagus and smooth in the lower two-thirds.

The arterial blood supply and venous drainage of the esophagus are segmental and come from various sources. The superior and inferior thyroid arteries supply the cervical esophagus. The blood supply to the thoracic esophagus comes from the aorta and bronchial arteries. Intercostal, inferior phrenic, and left gastric arterial collaterals supplement the main arterial supply. Venous blood is drained from the cervical, thoracic, and abdominal esophagus by the inferior thyroid and vertebral veins, the azygous and hemiazygous veins, and the left gastric vein, respectively.

The esophagus is innervated by both sympathetic and parasympathetic systems. The sympathetic innervation comes from cervical sympathetic ganglia, thoracic and splanchnic nerves, and the celiac ganglion. The recurrent laryngeal branch of the vagus nerve supplies parasympathetic innervation to the cervical esophagus. In the thorax, the two vagus nerves supply the esophagus and form a large plexus around it. At the hiatus, they join to form a left vagal trunk which courses anterior to the esophagus and a right, posterior trunk.

There is a rich lymphatic drainage that may extend longitudinally in the esophageal wall before exiting to regional lymph nodes. This is of clinical importance when performing esophagectomy for malignant disease.

PHYSIOLOGY

The esophagus functions as a muscular conduit for the passage of food from the pharynx to the stomach. An upper and lower esophageal sphincter lie at either end to help regulate this function. The upper esophageal sphincter (UES), or cricopharyngeus muscle, is ~3 cm long. It relaxes with swallowing, allowing the food bolus to enter the espha-

TABLE 1. *Factors affecting lower esophageal sphincter tone*

	Increase tone	Decrease tone
Hormonal	Gastrin	Secretin
	Motilin	Cholecystokinin
	Glucagon	Progesterone
	Prostaglandin $F_{2\alpha}$	Prostaglandins E_1, E_2, A_2
		Vasoactive intestinal polypeptides
Drugs	α-Adrenergic agonist	α-Adrenergic antagonist
	Norepinephrine	Phentolamine
	Phenylephrine	Anticholinergics
	Anticholinesterase	Atropine
	Edrophonium	Theophylline
	Cholinergic agents	β-Adrenergic agonist
	Bethanechol	Isoproterenol
	Methacholine	Nitroglycerin
	Metoclopramide	Nicotine
		Ethanol
Foods	Protein meal	Fatty meal
		Chocolate
Miscellaneous	Gastric alkalinization	Gastric acidification
	Gastric distention	Gastrectomy

Adapted from Castell DO. The lower esophageal sphincter: physiologic and clinical aspects. *Ann Intern Med* 1975;83:390.

gus, and then promptly contracts. This swallowed bolus initiates a primary peristaltic wave that propels the bolus, in a coordinated and progressive fashion, down the esophageal body and into the stomach. If the entire bolus of food fails to reach the stomach, local distention of the esophagus activates a secondary peristaltic wave to continue the emptying process. Tertiary contractions are simultaneous, nonprogressive waves that result from chaotic contractions of the circular muscle. They are depicted as a "cork-screw" esophagus on barium swallow.

The lower esophageal sphincter (LES) is not an anatomic sphincter, but, rather, a physiologic sphincter. Manometrically, it is represented by a 3- to 5-cm area of high pressure in the distal esophagus. The resting pressure within this high-pressure zone varies from 10 to 20 mm Hg. Like the UES, it too relaxes with swallowing, allowing the food bolus to enter the stomach. Once the peristaltic wave has passed, the sphincter contracts in order to prevent reflux of gastric contents. Various factors are known to affect LES tone (Table 1).

ESOPHAGEAL MOTILITY DISORDERS

Achalasia

Achalasia is the most common esophageal motility disorder with an incidence of six per 100,000 population. It is primarily a motility abnormality of the LES characterized by incomplete relaxation with resultant abnormal peristalsis in the esophageal body. Its pathogenesis is incompletely understood, but is postulated to be a neuro-

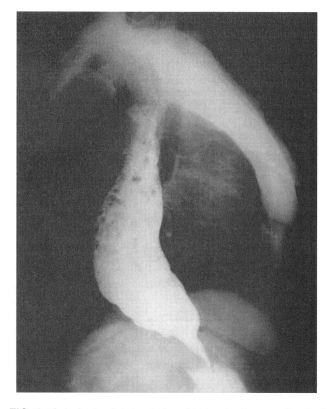

FIG. 1. Achalasia. A lateral view (during barium swallow) of a dilated esophagus containing large particles of undigested food. Note in the distal esophagus the classic "bird's beak" deformity of the lower esophageal sphincter.

genic degeneration of infectious or idiopathic etiology. The degeneration is presumed to be in the vagus nerve and the ganglia of Auerbach's plexus.

Achalasia typically presents with the classic triad of dysphagia for both liquids and solids, regurgitation of undigested food, and weight loss. With progression of the disease, the esophagus dilates due to retained food and can lead to regurgitation of foul-smelling contents. Pulmonary complications can also occur and result from chronic aspiration.

The diagnosis is readily made radiographically by contrast esophagram. The barium swallow typically demonstrates a dilated esophagus with a "bird-beak" tapering distally. The narrowing at the cardioesophageal junction is always subdiaphragmatic, in contrast to a reflux stricture, which is often at or above the diaphragm. Retained food, as well as the presence of an air-

fluid level in the esophagus, can also be illustrated (Fig. 1). Manometry will also confirm the diagnosis by documenting the classic features of the disorder: failure of the LES to completely relax with swallowing, elevation of intraluminal esophageal pressure, and lack of progressive peristalsis in the esophageal body characterized by low-amplitude, simultaneous contractions (Figs. 2–4). This abnormal peristalsis is the result of the outflow obstruction caused by the nonrelaxing LES and can occasionally normalize after dilatation or esophagomyotomy. The pattern of high-amplitude, simultaneous contractions associated with incomplete relaxation of the LES on manometry is known as vigorous achalasia.

The management of achalasia is directed at relieving the resistance from the noncompliant LES. Both operative and nonoperative forms of treatment are available and include dilatation and surgical myotomy. Pneumatic

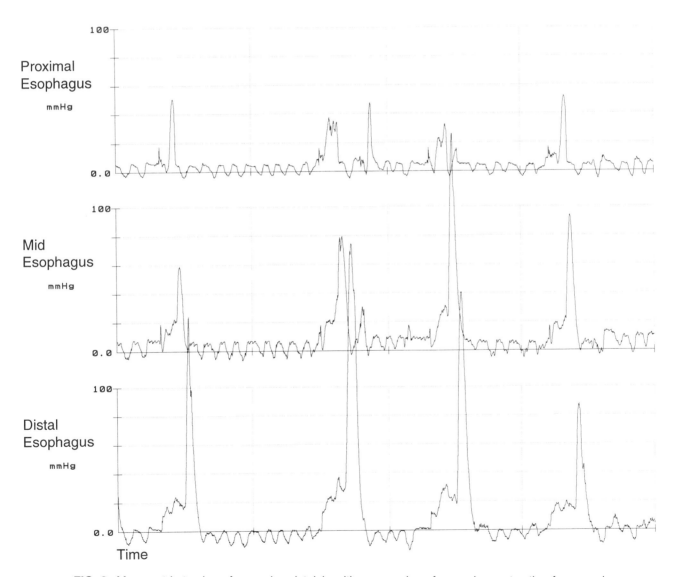

FIG. 2. Manometric tracing of normal peristalsis with progression of muscular contraction from proximal to distal.

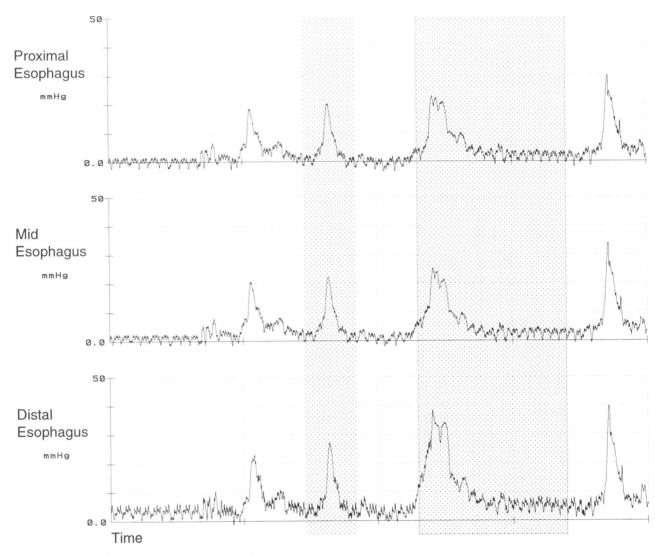

FIG. 3. Manometric tracing in a patient with achalasia revealing nonperistaltic, simultaneous contractions of the esophageal body.

or hydrostatic dilatation is performed endoscopically and involves forceful dilatation of the high-pressure LES by rapid inflation of a balloon. Okike and others from the Mayo clinic reported a 65% success rate with hydrostatic dilation. This, however, is not without risk and can result in perforation. Esophagomyotomy, as first proposed by Heller in 1913, can be performed through an abdominal or thoracic approach and involves division of the esophageal muscle. It is safer than dilation, with a 1% risk of perforation versus 4% for dilatation, and more successful, with 85% of the patients obtaining good to excellent relief of their dysphagia (Table 2). Csendes and associates showed that surgical myotomy resulted in a greater reduction of LES pressure. This was associated with a resultant improvement in the amplitude of esophageal contractions and return of peristalsis in 28% of patients versus 13% in the dilatation group. At 5 years, 95% of the patients treated with myotomy were doing

well versus 54% of patients undergoing dilatation. Of the patients who were dilated, 16% needed a second dilatation and 22% required a myotomy to obtain relief of their dysphagia.

Controversy exists regarding the distal extent of the myotomy and the need for an accompanying antireflux procedure. Carrying the myotomy onto the stomach for 1 to 2 cm will ensure relief of the obstruction by making the LES incompetent, but can result in GE reflux. Therefore, a concomitant partial fundoplication should be performed to prevent reflux and its complications if such an extended myotomy is performed. Thoracoscopic or laparoscopic myotomies appear to be equally efficacious to the traditional open approach, and are attendant with much less morbidity and better cosmesis.

Another nonoperative technique whose role has yet to be defined is the endoscopic injection of botulinum toxin into the LES. The benefit tends to disappear by 6 months,

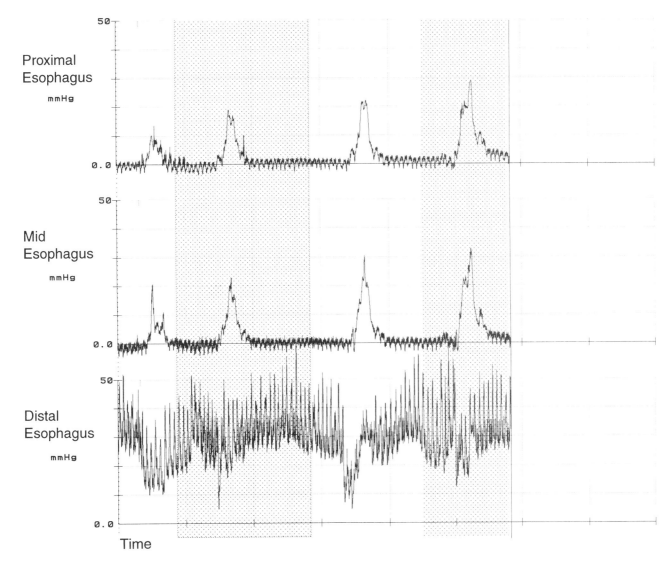

FIG. 4. Manometric tracing in a patient with achalasia revealing incomplete relaxation of the lower esophageal sphincter with swallowing.

but repeat injections are readily performed even in high-risk patients.

Diffuse Esophageal Spasm

Diffuse esophageal spasm (DES) is a hypermotility disorder of unknown etiology. Clinically, patients experience intermittent pain, dysphagia, or both. The pain may be postprandial or may occur spontaneously, and may be difficult to differentiate from cardiac pain. Patients with spasm are typically anxious and have their symptoms exacerbated by stress or ingestion of cold liquids.

Because of the intermittent nature of the disorder, the esophagram is frequently normal. Classic findings, however, include a corkscrew esophagus caused by segmental contractions of the circular muscle of the esophagus (Fig. 5). The presence of a pulsion diverticula may also be

seen. Manometry is the diagnostic test of choice, but will only be helpful if the patient is experiencing spasm at the time of the study. The manometric features of DES include simultaneous, high-amplitude contractions that occur both spontaneously and after swallowing. "Nut-cracker" esophagus is a variant of the esophageal spasm syndrome and is characterized by high-amplitude, normal peristaltic contractions.

Medical therapy for DES with sublingual nitroglycerin or calcium channel blockers constitutes the initial form of treatment. Mechanical dilatation with Hurst-Maloney bougies may cause temporary relief of dysphagia and chest pain. Surgery is reserved for patients with incapacitating symptoms that are refractory to medical therapy. It involves an extended thoracic esophagomyotomy and is less effective than when performed for achalasia. The proximal extent of the myotomy is defined by esophageal

TABLE 2. *Hydrostatic dilatation versus esophagomyotomy for treatment of achalasia*

	Dilation	Esophagomyotomy
No. of patients	431	468
Follow-up (years)	1–18	1–17
Response		
Good–excellent	65%	85%
Perforation	19(4%)	5(1%)
Mortality	2(0.5%)	1(0.2%)

Adapted from Okike N, Payne WS, Neufeld DM, et al. Esophagomyotomy versus forceful dilation for achalasia of the esophagus: results in 899 patients. *Ann Thorac Surg* 1979; 28:119.

motility studies and may extend up the esophagus to the level of the aortic arch. Distally, if the myotomy is carried through the cardia because of a hypertonic LES, a concurrent antireflux procedure should be added. If the LES pressures are normal, the myotomy does not need to extend across this region. With the advent of minimally invasive surgery, a long myotomy is now being performed thoracoscopically. This obviates a thoracotomy and its associated morbidity. Pellegrini and others have reported a 90% success rate with this technique.

Scleroderma

Scleroderma, or progressive systemic sclerosis, is a multisystem disorder of unknown etiology. It affects the esophagus by causing atrophy of the esophageal muscle with subsequent fibrotic replacement. With progresssion of the disease there is reduced motility of the lower two-thirds of the esophagus and the LES becomes hypotonic. This leads to dysphagia from slow emptying and GE reflux. Patients may complain of the need to ingest large volumes of water to force down their food. Manometry reveals aperistaltic, low-amplitude contractions in the lower two-thirds of the esophagus. A barium contrast study may demonstrate a dilated esophagus with GE reflux. Treatment is largely medical and focused on control of the reflux with antacids and prokinetic agents, elevation of the head of the bed, and avoiding meals at bedtime. Medical treatment should be initiated prophylactically at the time of diagnosis even if the patient has no symptoms of reflux. Although there is no cure for scleroderma, a palliative antireflux operation should be considered for patients with persistent symptoms of severe esophagitis. A loose, partial wrap is preferred in all patients with motility disturbances to avoid dysphagia from partial esophageal obstruction. Once a stricture develops secondary to reflux, dilatation may be tried. If unsuccessful, a transhiatal esophagectomy with gastric pullup may be the only solution.

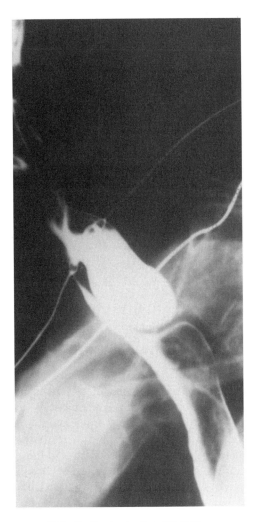

FIG. 6. Zenker's diverticulum.

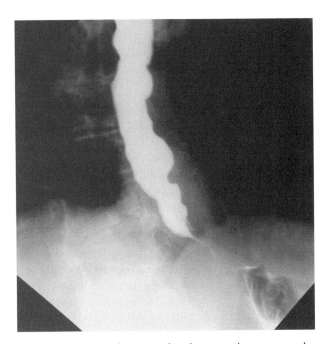

FIG. 5. Barium esophagram showing a corkscrew esophagus of diffuse esophageal spasm.

ESOPHAGEAL DIVERTICULA

Diverticula are acquired esophageal outpouchings that are classified as pulsion or traction depending on their mechanism of formation. Increased pressure within the lumen of the esophagus results in herniation of the esophageal mucosa through a defect in the muscle giving rise to pulsion diverticula. Traction diverticula occur when inflammation in the adjacent parabronchial lymph nodes pulls the entire esophageal wall towards them as they heal and contract. Diverticula are further categorized as true if the wall of the diverticulum contains all the layers of the esophagus, as in traction diverticula, and false if the diverticulum consists of only mucosa and submucosa, as in pulsion diverticula. Diverticula occur at the cervical (pharyngoesophageal), mid (parabronchial), and distal (epiphrenic) esophagus.

Cervical or pharyngoesophageal diverticula, also known as Zenker's diverticula, are the most common type. They are false diverticula of the pulsion variety related to incoordination of the swallowing mechanism with pharyngeal contraction occurring after cricopharyn-geal closure. They tend to arise in the midline posteriorly in Killian's triangle. This area of potential weakness lies between the oblique thyropharyngeal portion of the inferior constrictor and the more horizontal cricopharyngeus muscle. Regurgitation of undigested food, halitosis, dysphagia, choking, and aspiration are some of the symptoms associated with Zenker's diverticula. The severity of symptoms is related to the degree of cricopharyngeal dysfunction and not to the size of the diverticulum. The diagnosis is readily made with a barium esophagram which demonstrates its posterior location (Fig. 6). Therapy is directed at the underlying cricopharyngeal motor disorder responsible for formation of the diverticula. Cricopharyngeal myotomy with or without excision (diverticulectomy) or suspension (diverticulopexy) of the pouch is the treatment of choice and is associated with a low morbidity and mortality. Diverticulectomy alone results in at least a 20% recurrence rate.

Midesophageal or parabronchial diverticula are true diverticula associated with mediastinal granulomatous disease such as tuberculosis or histoplasmosis (Fig. 7). Inflamed adjacent paratracheal nodes scar and contract, causing retraction of the esophageal wall and thus giving rise to traction diverticula. They are usually asympto-

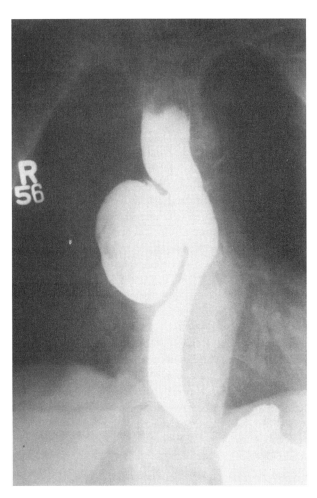

FIG. 7. Parabronchial diverticulum.

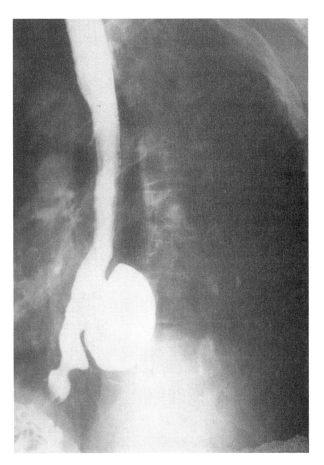

FIG. 8. Epiphrenic diverticulum.

matic and, therefore, require no treatment. In the rare instance of tracheo- or bronchoesophageal fistula formation, treatment is indicated with excision of the pouch, and division of the fistula.

Epiphrenic diverticula are pulsion diverticula that arise in the distal esophagus above the diaphragm as a result of an associated motor disturbance. They are usually asymptomatic but may be associated with complaints of dysphagia, chest pain, and regurgitation. Although the diagnosis is established with a barium swallow, esophageal manometry can aid in defining the underlying motor abnormality and directing subsequent therapy (Fig. 8). Diverticulectomy and esophagomyotomy are performed through a left thoracotomy.

PERFORATION OF THE ESOPHAGUS

Esophageal perforation carries a high risk of morbidity and mortality because of failure to recognize the diagnosis early and institute prompt therapy. Most perforations are iatrogenic, resulting from instrumentation with an endoscope, dilatation, or passage of a nasogastric tube. Forceful vomiting can produce a spontaneous perforation just above the cardia, as in Boerhaave's syndrome, and accounts for 15% of all such cases. Other less common causes of esophageal disruption include rupture from a swallowed foreign body, trauma, and surgical dissection. The lack of a serosal covering makes the esophagus more susceptible to rupture than the remainder of the gastrointestinal tract.

A high index of suspicion is required to make an early diagnosis. Classic findings of chest pain, fever, subcutaneous emphysema, and pneumothorax may be absent in early cases. In perforations limited to the mediastinum, Hamman's crunch can be heard as the crackling of air in the mediastinum synchronous with each heart beat, while violation of the pleura can lead to a hydropneumothorax. In 90% of patients, extravasation of contrast on esophagram establishes the diagnosis and documents the level of perforation. Some authorities recommend using water-soluble gastrograffin to prevent mediastinal contamination, but if the patient aspirates this material, it is similar to salt water aspiration. However, barium is inert in the tracheobronchial tree and gives better detail.

The treatment is primarily surgical and depends on the cause and site of the perforation and on the time interval between diagnosis and intervention. Patients with cervical perforations have the best prognosis, with a survival of 90%. The disruption is handled with transcervical drainage and closure of the perforation if possible, antibiotics, and hyperalimentation. Nonoperative management can be utilized selectively in patients with limited extravasation and no evidence of thoracic involvement. Outcome of intrathoracic esophageal perforations depends on the time elapsed between perforation and

TABLE 3. *Mortality rates of esophageal perforation based on time of diagnosis*

Author (year)	No. of patients	<24 hr	>24 hr
Goldstein (1982)	44	25%	44%
Tilanus (1991)	59	28%	30%
Skinner (1993)	47	9%	29%

Adapted from Cameron JL. *Current surgical therapy.* 5th ed. Philadelphia: BC Decker, 1995:6.

surgery. The longer the diagnosis and treatment are delayed, the greater the mortality (Table 3).

Early perforations can be successfully managed by thoracotomy, primary repair, and drainage. The primary closure should be reinforced with a pleural flap, a patch of diaphragm, or a gastric fundoplication. Although primary closure is the treatment of choice in early cases, the management of delayed perforations with mediastinal sepsis is controversial. Late perforations in septic patients require more aggressive control of the septic focus with either esophageal exclusion or esophagectomy. Because extravasation of bacteria and digestive juices can lead to mediastinitis, Urschel has advocated esophageal exclusion by ligation of the cardia to prevent reflux, and diversion in continuity by cervical esophagostomy. Orringer, however, advocates esophagectomy in patients with delayed perforations and intrinsic esophageal disease because it eliminates the perforation, the source of sepsis, and the underlying esophageal abnormality. Salo concludes that esophagectomy is superior to primary repair alone in the management of delayed perforation with mediastinal sepsis because the latter often leads to mediastinal leakage, continued sepsis, and death (Table 4). Conservative management has been used selectively in patients with contained esophageal perforations. Cameron 's proposed criteria for nonoperative therapy include: disruption contained within the mediastinum with drainage of the cavity back into the esophagus, mild symptoms present, and minimal evidence of clinical sepsis.

CAUSTIC INJURIES OF THE ESOPHAGUS

Ingestion of caustic substances can lead to acute and chronic esophageal injury. Ingestion can be accidental as seen in young children or intentional in adults attempting suicide. Some of the agents responsible for caustic burns of the esophagus include acids such as hydrochloric, sulfuric, and nitric acids present in battery acids and various cleaners and disinfectants, and alkaline compounds such as sodium hydroxide, the active ingredient in lye and drain cleaners such as Drano and Liquid-plummer. Alkali can lead to significant damage because they produce a full-thickness esophageal burn and liquefactive necrosis. Acid chemicals, however, rarely injure the esophagus severely because of its relatively resistant squamous

TABLE 4. *Mortality of esophagectomy versus primary closure for esophageal perforation*

Author (year)	No. of patients	Closure and drainage	Esophagectomy
Orringer (1990)	24	—	13% (3/24)
Salo (1993)	34	68% (13/19)	13% (2/15)

Adapted from Cameron JL. *Current surgical therapy.* 5th ed. Philadelphia: BC Decker, 1995:6.

epithelium, but can cause pylorospasm with gastric pooling of the compound resulting in coagulation necrosis or even perforation of the stomach.

During the initial assessment of the patient it is important to identify the type of agent swallowed, and whether this was an accident or a suicidal gesture. The latter tend to be much more serious. One should make an effort to find the container in order to check the pH of the ingested substance. Once the etiologic agent is identified, the depth and extent of injury must be determined. This is accomplished endoscopically after patency of the airway is established. The oropharynx and larynx are examined for evidence of burns; although lack of involvement of these areas does not exclude esophageal injury. Symptoms of hoarseness, stridor, or dyspnea suggest laryngeal edema and mandate intubation or close observation to ensure a patent airway during the period of maximal edema. These patients should be admitted and started on steroids and antibiotics immediately. Since esophagoscopy is contraindicated in this group of patients, the esophagus should be evaluated by an esophagram within 24 hrs of injury.

If neither impending airway obstruction nor perforation is suspected, esophagoscopy should be performed in the first 12 to 24 hrs. This will identify the presence or absence of a caustic burn and allow estimation of its severity if present. If there is no injury past the mouth, the patient can be discharged or transferred to the care of a mental health professional. Esophageal injuries are graded according to their depth and classified as superficial or deep. If a deep burn is visualized, the endoscope must not be passed beyond the proximal point of injury to avoid perforation. The distal extent of injury can be evaluated with a gastrograffin swallow.

Management of a patient with a confirmed esophageal corrosive injury is tailored to the depth of the burn. After several days, once the edema has subsided, patients with superficial burns are started on a clear liquid diet, advanced as tolerated, and discharged. Oral intake provides the simplest method of achieving esophageal dilatation. Although superficial burns usually heal without residual scarring, deeper burns result in deformities that can progress to stricture formation. With deep, transmural burns, patients are placed on hyperalimentation and antibiotics (for the potential of translocation) and monitored for the development of strictures or perforation. The clinical picture along with the endoscopic findings are critical in directing initial therapy. Early surgical

intervention can be life saving in some patients. Mediastinitis after lye ingestion, particularly if there is perforation, indicates full-thickness injury and is best treated by esophagectomy. An acute abdomen after liquid lye ingestion strongly suggests gastric necrosis or perforation. These patients usually require a total gastrectomy and esophagectomy, as the esophagus is routinely more severely damaged than the stomach by alkali. An acute abdomen after acid ingestion implies gastric perforation, and surgical exploration is mandatory. A total gastrectomy may be required, but the extent of the proximal resection will be directed by endoscopy. With acid, the esophagus may be spared.

The use of steroids is controversial and is confined to deep injuries. Steroids are thought to prevent strictures by modifying the inflammatory response; however, they are contraindicated in patients with suspected perforation or acid ingestion. In the latter group, the stomach is more frequently injured, and the addition of steroids may increase the risk of hemorrhage.

A common complication of caustic injury is the development of strictures. Strictures can be dilated in an antegrade fashion or retrograde through a gastrostomy. If strictures are persistent and refractory to multiple dilatations, surgery should be considered. Esophageal resection can be technically demanding and dangerous secondary to mediastinal scarring, and sometimes it is more prudent to leave the esophagus in situ and perform a bypass. Bypass alone will not obviate the potential of malignant degeneration. There is at least a 100-fold increased risk of developing esophageal cancer in patients with esophageal burns, and they should, therefore, be followed indefinitely with yearly endoscopy.

GASTROESOPHAGEAL REFLUX DISEASE

Reflux of acidic gastric contents can occur normally after a large meal. It becomes pathologic, however, when it occurs frequently with each meal and between meals. The etiology for this abnormal regurgitation is multifactorial. Factors responsible for pathologic GE reflux include an incompetent LES and an ineffective esophageal pump resulting in impaired clearance of refluxed acid. Most cases of gastroesophageal reflux disease (GERD) are caused by a defective LES. A low resting pressure, short length, and abnormal position lead to a faulty sphincter. Normally, the intraabdominal LES is under positive pressure and provides the necessary barrier against abnormal reflux. Motor disorders can cause abnormal peristalsis, which, in turn, affects the ability of the esophagus to clear refluxed acid. In addition, the resistance of the LES can be overcome by abnormalities of the gastric reservoir that result in elevated intragastric pressure.

Patients with pathologic reflux complain of heartburn, or a burning epigastric pain that is worsened by leaning over or assuming the recumbent position, and improved by standing upright. They may also experience dysphagia as the result of an induced motor disorder or the development of a stricture. Respiratory symptoms from chronic aspiration may predominate.

The diagnosis of reflux can be made clinically based on the patient's history and their response to empiric medical therapy. Failure to respond or the onset of atypical symptoms should prompt a more comprehensive evaluation. Intially, a barium swallow and upper endoscopy should be performed. Although a barium swallow can be diagnostic, it will only demonstrate reflux in 40% of patients. An upper endoscopy is useful in identifying GERD if any of its complications can be observed. The effects of gastric acid on the esophageal mucosa may lead to esophagitis, stricture formation, or Barrett's esophagus which can all be detected by this procedure. The use of 24-hr esophageal pH monitoring, however, is the gold standard for diagnosing GERD, and this approach should be utilized when the above tests have failed to document the presence of reflux in a patient with typical symptomatology. Esophageal manometry is an important adjunct to the workup of these patients because it will detect a mechanically defective sphincter and assess the effectiveness of esophageal peristalsis. This is a vital piece of information prior to antireflux surgery because it allows the surgeon to identify the precise abnormality responsible for the reflux.

Once the diagnosis has been established, the first-line of therapy is medical. This includes elevation of the head of the bed at least 6 in.; weight loss if obese; avoidance of tight clothing and stooping which increase intraabdominal pressure; elimination of coffee, tobacco, alcohol, and meals before bedtime; and the use of antacids, H_2 blockers, or prokinetic agents. About two-thirds of patients will respond to medical therapy, and one-third will require surgery. The indications for surgical intervention include failure of medical therapy, aspiration resulting from reflux, the presence of bleeding, stricture, grade II esophagitis, or Barrett's esophagus despite adequate medical therapy. The goal of surgery is to prevent reflux by correcting the mechanically defective LES. This is accomplished by restoring an intraabdominal esophageal segment, plicating the stomach around this segment, and tightening the esophageal hiatus to prevent the wrap from slipping into the chest. Various antireflux procedures have been described to accomplish these goals. The most common of these is the Nissen fundoplication, described in 1955, which involves a 360-degree wrap of fundus posteriorly around the distal esophagus (Fig. 9). This can be performed via an abdominal or thoracic approach. Although the abdominal approach is less morbid, the transthoracic approach is preferred in patients with a shortened esophagus. Because it is a total wrap, it may be associated with postoperative dysphagia or "gas-bloat syndrome," especially in patients with impaired esophageal peristalsis. To reduce these complications, the wrap should be short (2 cm) and loose. Other antireflux operations involving partial fundoplications have been developed in an effort to minimize these problems. These include the Belsey Mark IV partial fundoplication and the Hill posterior gastropexy. The Belsey operation, performed through a thoracic approach only, utilizes a 270-degree anterior gastric wrap as well as diaphragmatic crural approximation (Fig. 10).

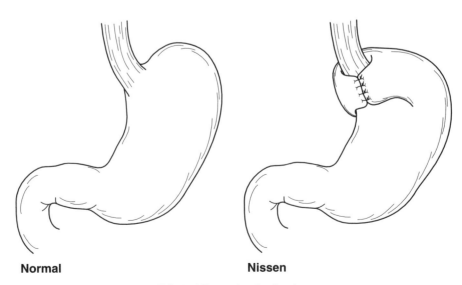

Normal　　　　　　　　**Nissen**

FIG. 9. Nissen fundoplication.

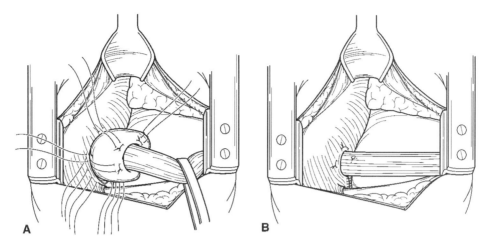

FIG. 10. (A, B) Belsey Mark IV fundoplication.

The Hill posterior gastropexy is performed through an abdominal incision and entails anchoring of the anterior and posterior portions of the GE junction to the arcuate ligament, as well as tightening of the esophageal hiatus (Fig. 11). Each of these repairs has comparable success rates and relieves symptoms in up to 90% of patients. Dysphagia ad the gas-bloat syndrome with the inability to belch or vomit are the major complications of antireflux surgery. Other problems include slipping of the wrap into the chest, vagal injury, and esophageal or gastric perforation. Recently, minimally invasive surgery has become a popular modification to standard open approaches for antireflux operations. Current literature supports that laparoscopic antireflux procedures are safe, provide comparable results in terms of reflux control, are associated with similar complication rates, and have shorter hospital stays.

BARRETT'S ESOPHAGUS

The end result of severe GERD may be columnar metaplasia of the normal esophageal squamous epithelium, a condition known as Barrett's esophagus. This occurs in ~5% to 10% of patients with GERD. Although this is usually acquired as a result of chronic acidic reflux, it can rarely be congenital. The columnar lining may be continuous or discontinuous with the gastric epithelium, and while it is usually in the distal esophagus, it can migrate proximally to the thoracic inlet.

Complications of Barrett's esophagus include ulceration, with subsequent bleeding or perforation, stricture formation, and the development of dysplasia or cancer. The exact risk of developing adenocarcinoma is unknown, but it is estimated to be a 7% to 10% lifetime risk. Because of this, frequent screening with upper endoscopy and multiple biopsies is recommended.

Barrett's esophagus is diagnosed endoscopically and confirmed histologically by multiple biopsies. The presence of mild, moderate, or severe dysplasia bears important consequences in terms of subsequent management. The propulsive force of the esophageal body should also be evaluated with manometry to determine if a total fundoplication will be acceptable.

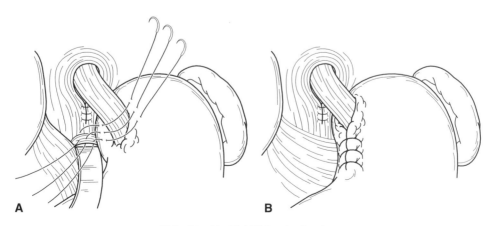

FIG. 11. (A, B) Hill fundoplication.

The indications for surgical intervention are similar to those for GERD. Antireflux surgery may halt progression of the columnar metaplasia and reverse the esophagitis, but it will not predictably cause regression of the Barrett's epithelium or prevent malignancy. Therefore, patients undergoing fundoplication for Barrett's esophagus still require routine screening to identify the development of malignancy in the metaplastic tissue. When severe dysplasia or carcinoma in situ is demonstrated on biopsy, esophagectomy is recommended because as many as 50% of those patients will have underlying invasive carcinoma.

HIATAL HERNIA

A hiatal hernia occurs when the stomach herniates into the chest through the esophageal hiatus in the diaphragm. It has been classified into four types. A type I, or sliding hernia, is the most common type, and is characterized by the stomach and GE junction sliding into the mediastinum through the hiatus. The endoabdominal fascia and phrenoesophageal membrane remain intact. A type II, or paraesophageal hernia, is seen when the stomach herniates alongside the esophagus through a defect in the phrenoesophageal membrane. The GE junction remains in its normal subdiaphragmatic location, while the body and even the antrum of the stomach roll up into the chest. The true type II paraesophageal hernia is rare. More commonly, a combined sliding and paraesophageal hernia is present. In these type III hernias, both the GE junction and the stomach herniate into the thorax. When other abdominal organs such as the small intestine, colon, or spleen enter the hernia sac, a type IV hiatal hernia is present.

Sliding hiatal hernias, in and of themselves, are of little clinical significance. It is when they are associated with reflux that they become symptomatic. Most patients with sliding hiatal hernias do not have symptomatic GE reflux. However, most patients with significant reflux can be shown to have a sliding hiatal hernia. Type II paraesophageal hernias are usually asymptomatic. When the stomach does not easily reduce into the peritoneal cavity or is compressed by the esophageal hiatus, symptoms may occur. Entrapment of food and air in the intrathoracic portion of the stomach will lead to esophageal compression and epigastric fullness. Patients may experience postprandial pain, dysphagia, and regurgitation. These obstructive symptoms are not only caused by gastric compression by the hiatus, but also by torsion of the stomach. The intrathoracic stomach can volvulize by undergoing rotation in a counterclockwise direction. If this volvulus is not detorsed spontaneously it can progress to incarceration, strangulation, necrosis, and perforation. The patient presents with retching and an inability to vomit, epigastric pain, and an inability to pass a nasogastric tube, known as Borchardt's triad. Although

gastric volvulus carries a high morbidity and mortality, the most frequent complication of paraesophageal hernias is anemia from occult gastrointestinal bleeding. This results from ischemic gastritis or linear gastric erosions, and is usually asymptomatic.

The diagnosis of hiatal hernia may be suggested by a chest radiograph if one sees an air-fluid level in the mediastinum posterior to the heart. A barium swallow, however, is the diagnostic test of choice and defines the type of hernia. Once the diagnosis is established, treatment is tailored to the type of hernia present. No treatment is required for an asymptomatic type I sliding hiatal hernia. If the hernia is associated with reflux, then appropriate therapy for GERD is instituted. Because of its association with bleeding and volvulus, type II paraesophageal hernias are repaired surgically regardless of symptoms. The operation can be approached aparoscopically or through an abdominal incision and entails reducing the herniated stomach, excising the hernia sac, and reapproximating the crura to tighten the hiatus. A posterior and/or anterior gastropexy is then performed to prevent a recurrent volvulus. A fundoplication is only performed if the patient has concomitant reflux.

ESOPHAGEAL TUMORS

Benign Tumors

Benign tumors of the esophagus are rare making up less than 1% of all esophageal neoplasms. Leiomyomas are the most common type, and usually arise from the smooth muscle of the lower or middle thirds of the esophagus. These tumors are rarely symptomatic but can produce dysphagia, occasional bleeding, nausea and vomiting, and vague pain if large. Characteristically, they appear as a smooth defect with intact mucosa on barium swallow. This is confirmed by endoscopy which reveals extrinsic compression of the lumen with overlying intact mucosa. Transesophageal ultrasonography will also suggest the diagnosis if a hypoechoic area is seen beneath intact mucosa. Surgical therapy is indicated for symptomatic leiomyomas and to exclude cancer from malignant conversion to leiomyosarcoma (rare). Enucleation of the tumor from the muscular wall can be accomplished via a thoracotomy or more recently through a thoracoscopic approach.

Esophageal Carcinoma

Incidence and Etiology

Cancer of the esophagus accounts for ~1% of all malignant tumors in the United States, and in 1994, there were 11,000 new cases. The incidence, however, varies widely, with geographic location being significantly higher in China, Japan, the Caspian Littoral of Iran, Russia, and among the native Bantu of South Africa. Esophageal carcinoma is primarily a disease of men in the sixth and seventh decades of life, with a male-to-female ratio of 3:1. It is also more commonly seen in blacks than in whites. An interesting and poorly understood phenomenon has been the remarkable increase in adenocarcinoma of the esophagus in white males over the past 20 years. In 1975, 16% of esophageal cancers in this group were adenocarcinoma, but by 1990 this had increased to 50%.

Although the exact etiology of esophageal carcinoma is unknown, various factors have been implicated. With the exception of tylosis (familial keratosis palmaris et plantaris), a condition inherited as an autosomal dominant trait, genetics does not appear to be causative. Dietary factors thought to play a significant role include nitrosamines, alcohol, and tobacco. This is supported by the high incidence of esophageal carcinoma in the Linksien province of North China, where the food and water are known to contain high concentrations of nitrosamines. The importance of alcohol and tobacco consumption in the occurrence of esophageal carcinoma in the United States is well established. In addition, several premalignant esophageal lesions have been recognized: achalasia, caustic burns of the esophagus, esophageal diverticula, leukoplakia, radiation esophagitis, Paterson-Kelly (Plummer-Vinson) syndrome, Barrett's esophagus, and ectopic gastric mucosa.

Symptoms and Diagnosis

The most common clinical manifestation of esophageal carcinoma is progressive dysphagia. This is initially noted with solid foods, but ultimately progresses to liquids and saliva. As the tumor enlarges, weight loss, regurgitation, and aspiration pneumonitis may also occur. The complaint of painful swallowing or odynophagia is suggestive of malignancy. Signs of advanced local disease include back pain due to vertebral involvement; coughing, wheezing, hemoptysis, and choking after eating secondary to a tracheobronchial fistula; and hoarseness due to recurrent laryngeal nerve involvement.

The diagnosis of esophageal carcinoma can be made with a barium esophagram, which should be performed in any patient complaining of dysphagia. This study will usually demonstrate the characteristic "apple-core" lesion in the esophagus (Fig. 12). Esophagoscopy with biopsy for tissue and brushings for cytology is essential in all patients to establish a diagnosis. Bronchoscopy is also necessary for lesions involving the upper or mid esophagus to detect tumor invasion of the adjacent tracheobronchial tree. The patient can be staged clinically with a computed tomography scan of the chest and abdomen, which will evaluate the mediastinum for invasion, and the lungs and liver for metastatic disease. It is

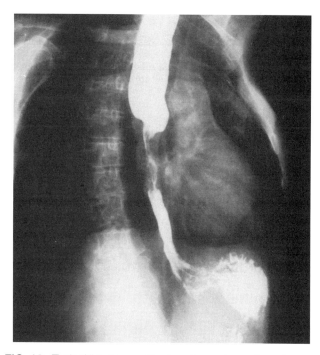

FIG. 12. Typical "apple-core" lesion of esophageal carcinoma.

not always, however, a reliable indicator of nonresectability. Endoscopic esophageal ultrasound is currently the best preoperative staging technique, accurately defining the depth of esophageal wall invasion and regional node involvement. The value of routine laparoscopy to detect regional or hepatic metastases has yet to be defined.

Classification: Pathology and Staging

Squamous cell carcinoma is the most common form of malignancy of the esophagus, accounting for two-thirds of cases and occurring most frequently in the upper two-thirds of the thoracic esophagus. The second most common type is adenocarcinoma. It can arise denovo, from the columnar metaplasia of Barrett's esophagus, or from a tumor in the fundus of the stomach that extends upward into the distal esophagus. Adenocarcinomas occur more commonly in the distal third and account for one-third of all malignancies of the intrathoracic esophagus. Sarcomas (including fibrosarcomas, leiomyosarcomas, and rhabdomyosarcomas) and melanomas are rare and represent the remainder of the malignant tumors of the esophagus.

Currently, esophageal carcinoma is staged according to the American Joint Committee for Cancer (AJCC) primary tumor/regional nodes/metastasis (TNM) staging system (Tables 5 and 6). This is a pathological staging system based on surgical exploration and on examination of the surgically resected esophagus and associated lymph nodes.

TABLE 5. *TNM staging for carcinoma of the esophagus: American Joint Committee on Cancer*

Primary tumor (T)
  T_X, primary tumor cannot be assessed
  T_0, no evidence of primary tumor
  T_{is}, carcinoma in situ
  T_1, tumor invades the lamina propria or submucosa
  T_2, tumor invades the muscularis propria
  T_3, tumor invades adventitia
  T_4, tumor invades adjacent structures
Regional lymph nodes (N)
  N_X, regional lymph nodes cannot be assessed
  N_0, no regional lymph node metastasis
  N_1, regional lymph node metastasis
Distant metastasis (M)
  M_X, presence of distant metastasis cannot be assessed
  M_0, no distant metastasis
  M_1, distant metastasis

TABLE 6. *Staging for carcinoma of the esophagus: American Joint Committee on Cancer*

Stage	Description		
0	T_{is}	N_0	M_0
I	T_1	N_0	M_0
IIA	T_2	N_0	M_0
	T_3	N_0	M_0
IIB	T_1	N_1	M_0
	T_2	N_1	M_0
III	T_3	N_1	M_0
	T_4	Any N	M_0
IV	Any T	Any N	M_1

Treatment

About 20% of patients present with early (stage I or II) disease and 80% with advanced (stage III or IV) disease. Because the majority of patients present with local tumor invasion of adjacent structures or distant metastases, cure becomes impossible. The goal then becomes palliation, in particular relief of dysphagia. Currently, the treatment modalities available to accomplish this are endoscopic palliative techniques, radiation therapy, chemotherapy, or surgery, alone or in combination.

Transoral intubation of the tumor with intraesophageal tubes (expandable metallic stents are currently popular) has been performed to palliate dysphagia in patients with nonresectable tumors. This has been associated with complications, including esophageal perforation, hemorrhage, migration or obstruction of the tube, and even death. In addition, although the patient's ability to swallow saliva is improved, they are usually unable to tolerate a regular diet. The average survival after palliative intubation is a few months, and this has been most useful for patients with malignant tracheoesophageal fistulas. In these cases the esophageal stent not only restores swallowing, but also occludes the fistula. Coagulation of the obstructing esophageal tumor with a neodymium/ yttrium-aluminum-garnet (Nd:Yag) laser has also been used as palliative therapy.

Squamous cell carcinoma of the esophagus is a radiosensitive tumor and, therefore, potentially curable with radiation therapy. Clearly, the presence of tumor outside the irradiated field precludes cure. Radiation alone produces an overall 5-year survival of 6% to 10%, but can be associated with significant complications including radiation pnuemonitis, stricture formation, perforation, tracheoesophageal fistula, and pericarditis. More often, radiation therapy plays a palliative role in patients with incurable disease. Although morbidity is acceptable, swallowing is restored in only about half the patients and often 4 to 6 weeks is required before relief is noted. Some physicians believe radiotherapy should be the mainstay of treatment of cervical and hypopharyngeal carcinomas. This is predicated on concerns for laryngeal preservation and the complexity of earlier techniques for esophageal reconstruction. With modern techniques, the stomach can usually be mobilized and brought up to the neck for a one-stage reconstruction. However, if a patient with such a tumor refuses to consider a laryngectomy, radiation can be employed. Unfortunately, if the tumor relapses, the only option for cure or palliation may be a pharyngo-laryngoesophagectomy.

Over the past decade, there has been considerable interest in chemoradiation alone for adenocarcinoma as well as squamous cell carcinoma of the esophagus. This has produced 2-year survival rates of up to 40%, but swallowing improves in only 60% of patients.

In appropriate patients, surgery provides the most rapid and permanent relief of dysphagia, as well as the best chance for cure. Current controversies surround the extent of surgery and the role of neoadjuvant therapy.

Skinner and Demeester are proponents of en bloc resections. This includes very wide margins of stomach and esophagus, radical lymphadenectomy, and mediastinal dissection, including the thoracic duct, pleura, and adjacent pericardium. The operative mortality is 5% to 10%, and one-third survive 2 years. An alternative approach is the transhiatal esophagectomy, where the operation is done through the abdomen and neck. This avoids a thoracotomy in these patients who often have chronic obstructive pulmonary disease. Orringer's initial experience resulted in a 3-year survival of 22% (similar to en bloc resection). In an effort to improve outcomes, neoadjuvant therapy has been added. This consists of preoperative chemotherapy (often 5-fluorouracil and cisplatin) and radiation therapy (4,500 cGy). With neoadjuvant therapy followed by transhiatal esophagectomy, Orringer has reported 5-year survival of 34%. Although the optimum regimen has yet to be defined, it would appear that a team approach with a medical, surgical, and radiation oncologist is the best way to manage esophageal cancer.

SUMMARY

There are a variety of esophageal motor disorders that can be differentiated based on symptomatology, contrast radiography, and manometric findings. With the advent of minimally invasive surgery, symptomatic relief can now be provided for some motility disorders as well as symptomatic GERD via the laparoscopic or thoracoscopic routes. Recent advances in the management of esophageal cancer have included a greater variety of treatment options, decreased surgical morbidity and mortality, and the addition of more effective adjuvant therapy. However, esophageal cancer remains an aggressive malignancy with a poor survival. Close surveillance of patients at risk for developing esophageal carcinoma leads to earlier diagnosis, which may improve cure rates.

STUDY QUESTIONS

1. How are the motility disorders distinguished radiographically and manometrically?
2. Describe the workup of a patient with suspected GERD. What is the role for barium swallow, endoscopy, 24-hr pH probe study, and manometry? Are they all necessary?
3. Discuss the management of GERD. When is surgical intervention necessary, and what are the surgical options?
4. Describe the diagnostic approach to a patient with dysphagia and its management depending on etiology.
5. Discuss the differences in management of esophageal perforation depending on site of perforation, etiology, and time interval between perforation and diagnosis.

SUGGESTED READING

Beahrs OH, Henson DE, Hutter RVP, Kennedy BJ, eds. *American Joint Committee on Cancer handbook for staging of cancer.* 4th ed. Philadelphia: JB Lippincott, 1993.

Cameron JL, Kieffer RF, Hendrix TR, Mehigan DG, Baker RR. Selective nonoperative management of contained intrathoracic esophageal disruptions. *Ann Thorac Surg* 1979;27:404–408.

Csendes A, Braghetto I, Henriques A, et al. Late results of a prospective randomized study comparing forceful dilatation and oesophagomyotomy in patients with achalasia. *Gut* 1989;30:299.

Okike N, Payne WS, Neufeld DM, et al. Esophagomyotomy versus forceful dilation for achalasia of the esophagus: results in 899 patients. *Ann Thorac Surg* 1979;28:119.

Pellegrini CA, Leichter R, Patti MG, et al. Thoracoscopic esophageal myotomy in the treatment of achalasia. *Ann Thorac Surg* 1993;56:680–682.

Talbert JL. Corrosive strictures of the esophagus. In: Sabiston DC, ed. *Textbook of surgery: the biologic basis of modern surgical practice.* 13th ed. Philadelphia: Saunders, 1986:767.

Warwick GP, Harrington JS. Some aspects of the epidemiology and etiology of esophageal cancer with particular emphasis in the Transkei, South Africa. *Adv Cancer Res* 1973;17:81.

CHAPTER 10

Stomach and Duodenum

Orlando Morejon and Alan S. Livingstone

STOMACH

General Anatomy and Physiology

The stomach is a hollow viscus located in the epigastrium. It receives foodstuffs from the esophagus through the lower esophageal sphincter and empties them into the duodenum by way of the pylorus. The stomach consists of four divisions: the cardia (most proximal), fundus, body, and antrum (most distal). The linea incisura generally marks the border between the body and antrum. The lesser and greater curvatures provide attachments for the gastrohepatic ligament superiorly and the gastrocolic ligament inferiorly. The main trunks of vascular supply and innervation for the stomach are also found along the lesser and greater curvatures. The stomach is closely related to the spleen at its left and to the pancreas posteriorly. It forms the anterior boundary to the lesser sac, which may be accessed surgically via the epiploic foramen of Winslow (behind the hepatoduodenal ligament) or by incising the gastrohepatic ligament.

The stomach is lined by several different kinds of cells, each responsible for one of its functions and contributing to the composition of gastric juice, which may total from 500 to 1,500 cc/day. Mucus is an alkaline glycoprotein secreted by the mucous cells to provide mucosal protection and lubrication for the passage of food. Chief (zygomatic) cells in the fundic area secrete pepsinogen, which is broken down to pepsin for the digestion of proteins. Parietal (oxyntic) cells in the fundus and body are stimulated by gastrin to produce hydrochloric acid, and they also produce intrinsic factor. Parietal cells also maintain the electrolyte balance in gastric juice by secreting K^+, H^+, Na^+, and Cl^-. When gastric distention occurs, G cells in the antrum (and also in the duodenum) release gastrin, which stimulates secretion of acid and pepsin.

Gastric acid secretion is influenced by three modulators (Fig. 1). During eating, secretion is divided into three phases. The cephalic phase is vagally mediated in response to the thought or presence of food. The gastric phase occurs with gastric distention by food. As the food passes through the pylorus, the intestinal phase of gastric acid secretion is thought to take place under the influence of cholecystokinin.

Vascular Anatomy

Arterial Blood Supply

The stomach receives its blood supply from four main arteries which course along its lesser and greater curvatures (Fig. 2). The lesser curvature is supplied by the left gastric artery (from the celiac axis) and the right gastric artery (usually a branch of the common hepatic artery). The greater curvature is supplied by the right gastroepiploic artery (a branch of the gastroduodenal artery) and the left gastroepiploic artery (a branch of the splenic artery). Additionally, the fundus is supplied by the short gastric arteries, which are fed by the splenic and left gastroepiploic arteries. A further fairly constant collateral is a posterior gastric artery that comes off the splenic artery and supplies the back of the fundus of the stomach.

The copious and varied sources of blood to the stomach allow many approaches to partial resections of the organ and versatility in its use in reconstructive procedures. Usually, any three of the four main arteries may be sacrificed with little threat to the viability of the remaining stomach. For example, following an esophagectomy, the lesser curve is partially resected to maximize the working length of the esophageal replacement conduit, and the right gastroepiploic artery serves as the sole source of arterial blood to the mobilized stomach.

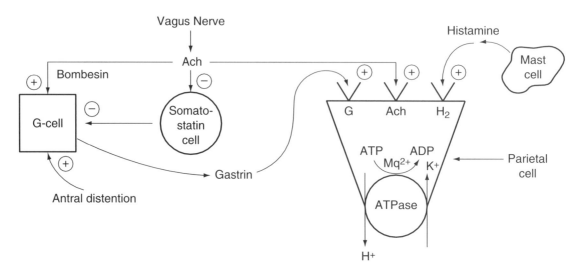

FIG. 1. Neuroendocrine control of acid secretion.

Venous Drainage

The venous drainage pattern generally parallels the arterial supply (Fig. 3). The right and left gastric veins and the right and left gastroepiploic veins all drain into the portal system. The left gastric vein also empties into the azygous system (leading to the inferior vena cava) by way of a lower esophageal venous plexus. This portosystemic collateral network develops into the esophagogastric varices in patients with portal hypertension. In patients with bleeding esophagogastric varices who have failed sclerotherapy, gastric devascularization procedures can be performed to ligate and divide these portosystemic collateral vessels.

Lymphatic System

The lymphatic drainage of the stomach (Fig. 4) generally follows the course of its blood supply. The lymph node groups are dividd into numbered "zones." Zones I and II on the greater curvature and zones III and IV on the lesser curvature represent the earliest drainage sites for

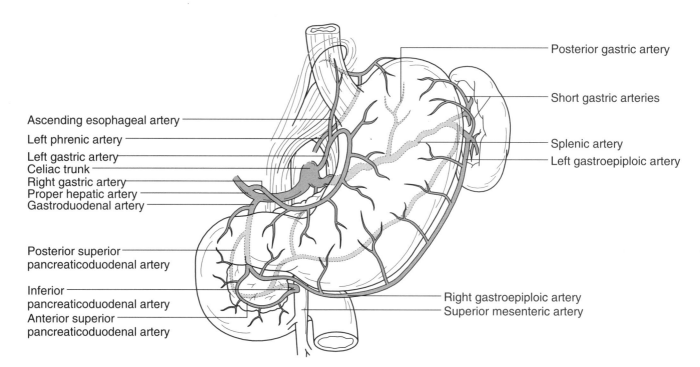

FIG. 2. Arterial supply of the stomach.

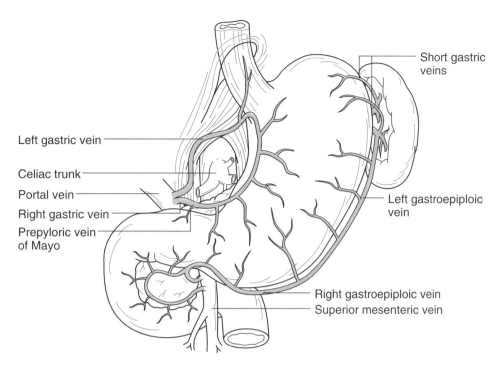

FIG. 3. Venous drainage of the stomach.

gastric lymph, and these are the nodes that would be resected in an "R 1" dissection for gastric cancer. Zones V through VII represent the next level of lymphatic drainage, and these would be removed with an "R 2" dissection. The most radical operation would be an "R 3" dissection and would encompass the lymph nodes in the porta hepatis as well as along the aorta and inferior vena cava.

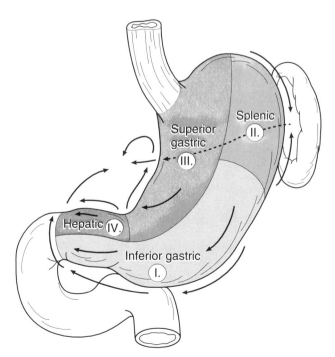

FIG. 4. Lymphatic drainage of the stomach.

Innervation

During embryologic development, the right and left vagus nerves rotate around the esophagus and lie posterior and anterior to the cardia, respectively (Fig. 5). The stomach is innervated by anterior and posterior branches of the vagus nerves, which course along the lesser curvature and terminate in fine individual branches. The antral branches are called the "crow's foot" due to their characteristic appearance.

The lesser curvature branches are divided in a highly selective vagotomy, with sparing of the hepatic and pyloric channel branches (Fig. 6). One branch of the posterior vagus is referred to as the criminal nerve of Grassi due to its culpability in cases of recurrent peptic ulcers following therapeutic vagotomies. Due to its inconsistent presence behind and to the left of the lower esophagus, this branch may evade the surgeon's dissection and remain intact to reproduce the patient's ulcer symptoms postoperatively.

Pathology of the Stomach

Gastritis

Erosive gastritis (acute hemorrhagic gastritis, stress ulceration) is the most common cause of upper gastrointestinal bleeding. It is caused by a breakdown of the protective mechanisms which normally neutralize H$^+$ ions on the mucosal surface of the stomach. These include mucus and alkaline buffers secreted by the gastric epithelium.

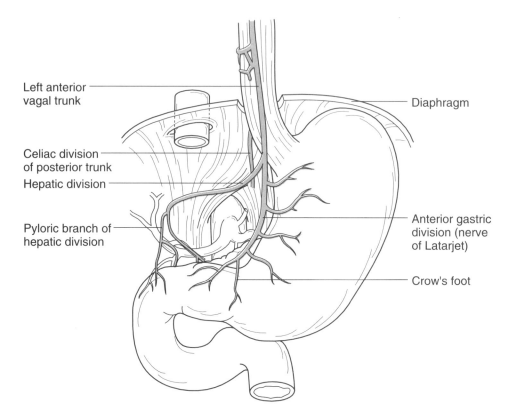

Left anterior vagal trunk

Diaphragm

Celiac division of posterior trunk

Hepatic division

Pyloric branch of hepatic division

Anterior gastric division (nerve of Latarjet)

Crow's foot

FIG. 5. Vago enervation of the stomach.

Alterations in mucosal blood flow will also interrupt the delivery of necessary nutrients and buffers to the gastric epithelium, and patients who experience prolonged or repeated episodes of hypoxia or hypotension are at high risk for developing erosive gastritis.

Patients with gastritis suffer from painless hematemesis or bloody nasogastric tube output, in contrast to those who present with a painful, bleeding peptic ulcer. They may have sepsis or multiple organ system failure, or they may be recovering from major trauma, a major operative procedure, or extensive burns ("Curling's ulcer"). The diagnosis can usually be made on a clinical basis by combining the typical setting with the finding of small amounts of bloody or "coffee-ground" material in the vomitus or nasogastric tube output. If there is a large amount of bleeding or if it persists despite conservative measures, upper endoscopy is indicated as a diagnostic and potentially therapeutic measure.

Blood and clots in the stomach promote fibrinolysis and acid secretion due to gastric distention. Therefore, the first step in management is placement of a nasogastric tube and gastric lavage with room temperature saline. Most patients will respond acutely to this measure alone. Intravenous replacement of lost volume as well as monitoring of the hematocrit, platelets, prothrombin time, partial thromboplastin time, and electrolytes in these patients is essential. The gastric lumen

pH is then neutralized with antacids administered through the nasogastric tube or with H_2-receptor antagonists intravenously.

When bleeding persists or recurs, gastroscopic evaluation with coagulation or sclerotherapy of the bleeding point(s) is indicated. Failure to respond to these measures constitutes an indication for operative intervention. The procedure of choice should include direct control of the bleeding combined with a vagotomy to reduce acid production. An opening in the stomach wall (gastrotomy) is made and the gastric mucosa inspected to identify all bleeding points. A decision is then made as to the need for simple suture ligation of the bleeding points or for a formal gastric resection. A truncal vagotomy (division of vagus nerve) (Fig. 6) is then performed, followed by a drainage procedure (such as a pyloroplasty) if the pylorus has not been resected. Poor operative candidates may undergo an attempt at selective infusion of pitressin or embolization of the left gastric artery.

Atrophic gastritis (chronic gastritis) is diagnosed by gastric biopsy demonstrating an inflammatory infiltrate in the lamina propria and an atrophy of the tubules. The gastric mucosa becomes thin, and parietal cells are lost. The production of gastric acid ceases (achlorhydria), and it is associated with an increased risk of gastric carcinoma. These patients should be followed closely with regular upper endoscopic examinations. The secretion of

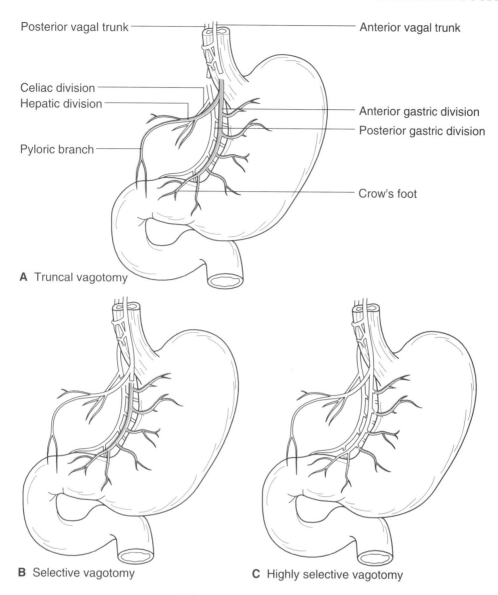

Posterior vagal trunk
Anterior vagal trunk
Celiac division
Hepatic division
Anterior gastric division
Posterior gastric division
Pyloric branch
Crow's foot

A Truncal vagotomy

B Selective vagotomy

C Highly selective vagotomy

FIG. 6. Types of vagotomy.

intrinsic factor is also lost, necessitating monthly intramuscular injections of vitamin B_{12} to obviate the development of pernicious anemia.

Gastric Ulcers

Classification

Gastric ulcers are less common than duodenal ulcers. Their characteristic locations define their behavior pattern and treatment alternatives. Most gastric ulcers occur in the body or in the transitional zone between the body and antrum of the stomach, and they are termed "type I ulcers." When they are associated with duodenal ulcers, they are called "type II ulcers." Ulcers in the distal antrum or in the pyloric channel behave more like duodenal ulcers than gastric ulcers, and they are called "type III ulcers." Type IV ulcers occur high on the lesser curvature of the stomach near the gastroesophageal junction. Type II and III ulcers, unlike type I and IV ulcers, behave pathophysiologically like the peptic ulcers that occur in the duodenum.

Etiology

The etiology of gastric ulcers has been poorly understood but felt to be multifactorial, including bile reflux, local ischemia, and drugs that lower the gastric mucosal barrier to H^+ ions, particularly alcohol and nonsteroidal antiinflammatory drugs (NSAIDS). In contrast to duodenal and type II and III gastric ulcers that develop in an environment of increased acid production, the usual gastric ulcer (types I and IV) is associated with low or normal acid production. Recently, it has become evident that *Helicobacter pylori* is a causative agent in most cases of gastric ulcer not caused by NSAIDS.

Diagnosis

A patient with gastric ulcer disease will typically complain of a burning or gnawing pain in the epigastrium which is relieved with the ingestion of food. An upper gastrointestinal series with swallowed barium contrast will demonstrate about two-thirds of all gastric ulcers. The gold standard for diagnosis is upper endoscopy, during which mucosal samples are taken to test for *H. pylori*. Lesions suspicious for malignancy are also biopsied; at least six biopsies are taken to increase the diagnostic yield.

Medical Treatment

Initial conservative management of gastric ulcers focuses on the avoidance of irritants to the gastric mucosa through cessation of alcohol ingestion and smoking. The pharmacologic mainstay of ulcer treatment includes the administration of cytoprotective agents (sucralfate), H_2-receptor antagonists (cimetidine, ranitidine, or others), or a proton pump inhibitor (pantoprazole or omeprazole). Proton pump inhibitors have demonstrated quicker healing and symptomatic relief of gastroduodenal ulcers than H_2-receptor antagonists. Antibacterial drugs (usually two or three together) such as bismuth subsalicylate, metronidazole, tetracycline, amoxicillin, or clarithromycin are added to the treatment regimen in cases of *H. pylori*. Because *H. pylori* has been described in familial clusters, screening the patient's symptomatic family members is indicated. Misoprostol, a prostaglandin analog, improves the cytoprotective barrier and can prevent the development of gastric ulcers in patients on chronic NSAID therapy. Most benign gastric ulcers will heal with appropriate medical management in 8 weeks. After a 6- to 8-week period of medical treatment, patients with lesions suspicious for malignancy should have follow-up endoscopy with additional biopsies taken of any remaining lesions. Patients with nonhealing ulcers or with any remaining suspicion of malignancy should be referred for surgical intervention.

Complications of Gastric Ulcers

Apart from the problems of intractability and relapse, common complications of gastric ulcers include gastric outlet obstruction, perforation and hemorrhage. The management of gastric outlet obstruction is almost always surgical. Recent evidence indicates that perforated peptic ulcers in stable patients may be treated conservatively if

an upper gastrointestinal series at the time of presentation demonstrates that the perforation is sealed, but this is an uncommon scenario. Patients diagnosed with a bleeding gastric ulcer should be placed in a monitored setting for fluid resuscitation, hemodynamic monitoring, and regular labwork. Upper endoscopy is performed to confirm the diagnosis and as a therapeutic maneuver to sclerose or coagulate any identified bleeding vessels. Coagulopathies should be corrected, and surgery is indicated in any patient requiring transfusion of 4 to 6 U of blood in a 24-hr period.

Surgical Treatment

The indications for operating on a patient with a gastric ulcer are failure to heal or recurrence, gastric outlet obstruction, perforation, massive bleeding (4 to 6 U of blood in 24 hr), suspicion of cancer, and (less commonly) intractable abdominal pain. These patients have usually failed a course of medical management and typically present in a debilitated state. Preoperative planning in elective cases should include measures to restore the patient to an anabolic state with either oral protein supplements or parenteral alimentation through a central venous catheter. In emergency cases, preoperative planning should focus on intravascular volume replacement and correction of electrolyte abnormalities (resulting from prolonged emesis), placing a nasogastric tube to evacuate the stomach and a urinary catheter to monitor urine output (adequate urine output is the key indicator of successful intravascular resuscitation in this setting), checking the hematocrit and transfusing blood if necessary, verifying that coagulation studies are normal, administering intravenous antibiotics, and reserving an intensive care unit bed for postoperative management.

The surgical treatment depends on the type of ulcer and is tailored to the anatomic location and underlying pathophysiology. A fundamental principle, however, is always to biopsy (if not excise) the ulcer to exclude malignancy. For type I ulcers, an antrectomy, hemigastrectomy, or subtotal gastrectomy is indicated, depending on the extent and precise location of the lesion (Fig. 7). The resection is followed by a reconstructive procedure such as a Billroth I, Billroth II, or a Roux-en-Y gastrojejunostomy (Fig. 8) to restore functional anatomy to the gastrointestinal tract. Type IV ulcers behave like type I ulcers, but their surgical approach differs drastically because of their precarious location near the gastroesophageal junction. The Csendes procedure is one of several gastric resections designed specifically to deal with this technical challenge, and the reader is referred to the suggested reading for a detailed description of these advanced techniques.

Type II and III gastric ulcers behave like peptic ulcers of the duodenum, and a vagotomy should be a part of the

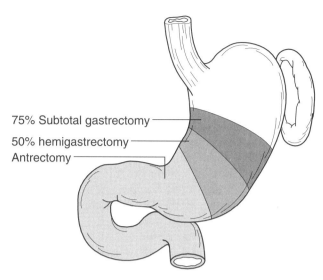

FIG. 7. Levels of stomach resection—antrectomy, 50% hemigastrectomy, and 75% subtotal gastrectomy.

planned procedure for these patients. Resection of the ulcer alone (as part of a wedge resection) will result in an unacceptably high recurrence rate. The procedure of choice is a vagotomy and antrectomy (including the ulcer in the resected specimen). If the ulcer has eroded posteriorly onto the pancreas, closure of the duodenal stump following an antrectomy will be more difficult and at higher risk for leakage postoperatively. If a vagotomy and antrectomy may not be safely undertaken due to a technical factor such as this, or if the patient is hemodynamically unstable (in emergency cases), a vagotomy and drainage procedure (e.g., pyloroplasty, gastrojejunostomy) is a reasonable alternative procedure. In general, any vagotomy other than a highly selective or parietal cell vagotomy should be accompanied by a drainage procedure to prevent postoperative gastric outlet obstruction.

Surgical Outcomes

The surgical treatment of classic gastric ulcers (I and IV) gives excellent results with a <2% recurrence rate. This contrasts with the often higher failure rates after duodenal ulcer surgery. The operative mortality with elective surgery is ~2%, but climbs to 5% to 10% for emergency operations.

Gastric Neoplasms

Patients with gastric neoplasms may present with anorexia and weight loss, acute or chronic hemorrhage, a mass effect, or (less commonly) pain in the epigastrium. Malignancy should be suspected with the presence of a palpable left supraclavicular lymph node (Virchow's node), hepatomegaly, palpable umbilical mass (Sister

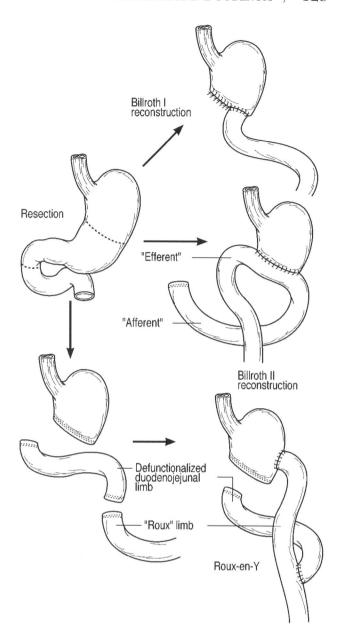

FIG. 8. Roux-en-Y reconstruction. Defunctionalized duodenojejunal limb and "Roux" limb.

Mary Joseph's sign), palpable or radiologically detected metastatic disease in the ovaries (Krukenberg tumor), pelvic cul-de-sac (Blumer's shelf), or the presence of ascites. Although an upper gastrointestinal series may be helpful in visualization, gastroscopy with biopsy is the procedure of choice because it provides tissue diagnosis.

Benign Gastric Neoplasms

Leiomyomas, although unusual, are the most common benign gastric neoplasm. A leiomyoma usually becomes symptomatic when it grows to >4 cm in diameter, at which time it may result in a mass effect or gastric bleeding. Less common benign gastric neoplasms include fibromas, neurofibromas, and angiomas. Most of these lesions can be treated with limited gastric resections.

Gastric polyps may be small and amenable to endoscopic excision, or they may be large enough to require a wedge resection. Most gastric polyps are hyperplastic polyps and are not premalignant. Adenomatous polyps, however, have a high association with carcinoma of the stomach, with ~20% of lesions of >2 cm being malignant.

Malignant Gastric Neoplasms

Conditions that are associated with gastric malignancies include smoking, alcohol abuse, chronic gastric ulcer, achlorhydria, blood group A, Japanese heritage, megaloblastic anemia, and low socioeconomic status.

Over 90% of all gastric neoplasms are malignant, and ~95% of these are gastric adenocarcinomas. They may be fungating, ulcerating, or diffusely infiltrating (linitis plastica). In situ carcinoma is confined to the gastric mucosa. Stage I disease has penetrated the muscularis mucosa and is present in the submucosa. Stage II disease has invaded the muscularis propria. Tumor at any of these levels with lymph node involvement is stage III disease. Tumor that has penetrated the serosa or which is associated with distant metastases is stage IV.

Patients with potentially curable lesions require a subtotal or total gastrectomy with wide margins of resection, as these neoplasms tend to infiltrate extensively in the submucosa. The omentum and surrounding lymph nodes are resected routinely in curative procedures for gastric carcinoma. The goal of an adequate lymph node dissection is to achieve one level of disease-free nodes as the margin of resection. For example, an "R 1" dissection is adequate if the lymph nodes in zones I through IV are disease-free, and an "R 2" dissection is indicated when nodes in zones I through IV contain metastatic disease and nodes in zones V through VII are disease-free. Lesions of the cardia or fundus may also require an esophagogastrectomy or a splenectomy. Unfortunately, only about one-third of gastric carcinomas are potentially curable by the time they become symptomatic. Patients with unresectable lesions that are symptomatic (hemorrhagic or obstructive) are potential candidates for palliative resection or for gastrojejunal bypass. The role of chemotherapy and radiation therapy is in evaluation. Although trials have demonstrated a modest benefit in the adjuvant setting, it is hoped that neoadjuvant (preoperative) chemotherapy will prove to be even more beneficial. With metastatic disease, occasional patients get meaningful palliation with chemotherapy.

The stomach is the most common site for primary intestinal lymphoma. Gastric lymphoma and leiomyosarcoma are usually bulky lesions amenable to partial gastrectomy and tend to have a better prognosis than adenocarcinomas. Treatment options for gastric lymphoma include radiation and usually chemotherapy.

Prognosis

Cure rates correlate closely with stage for gastric adenocarcinoma, and stage for stage the results of treatment are comparable in the United States and Japan. However, aggressive Japanese screening programs detect many in situ or stage I tumors, where the cure rate can be well over 50%. Unfortunately, in the United States cancers are more likely to be stage III or IV, with 5-year salvage of <10%.

Other Gastric Disorders

Gastric outlet obstruction usually presents with abdominal pain, epigastric fullness, and vomiting. The etiology is usually a prepyloric ulcer with a scarred, contracted pyloric channel. The initial treatment is decompression with a nasogastric tube and fluid replacement with correction of electrolyte abnormalities. Definitive treatment, once malignancy is excluded, entails a vagotomy combined with an antrectomy or a drainage procedure.

Gastric volvulus may occur in an organoaxial (around the cardiopyloric axis) or mesentericoaxial (perpendicular to the cardiopyloric axis) orientation. It is commonly seen in association with paraesophageal hiatal hernias. Classically, patients present acutely with Borchardt's triad: severe epigastric pain, nausea and retching without vomiting, and the inability to pass a nasogastric tube. Surgery is almost always indicated and should include reducing the torsion, performing a gastropexy in an anatomic orientation, and repairing the diaphragmatic hernia if one is present. An antireflux operation such as a Nissen fundoplication is not routinely added, but should be included when coincident reflux is suspected.

Mallory-Weiss tears are linear mucosal tears at the cardioesophageal junction caused by forceful or repeated retching or vomiting. Patients present with hematemesis, which may be massive, and the diagnosis is confirmed by upper endoscopy. Bleeding usually ceases with conservative management, but endoscopic injection, left gastric artery embolization, and pitressin infusion may be useful. The few cases that continue to bleed respond to surgical intervention with oversewing of the mucosal tear through a gastrotomy.

Bezoars represent collections of undigested materials in the stomach. The patients are usually infants or mentally deranged patients presenting with vague upper abdominal complaints or nausea and vomiting. The three main types of bezoars are trichobezoars (hair), phytobezoars (fruit and vegetable fibers), and trichophytobezoars (a combination). These may be treated by endoscopic fragmentation or dissolved with various enzyme solutions. Small objects may be followed radiographically. If the object is sharp or too large to pass through the ileocecal valve, it may require endoscopic or surgical extraction.

Hypertrophic gastritis (Menetrier's disease) represents a polypoid-type thickening of the gastric glandular epithelium and submucosa, usually more prominent in the proximal stomach. Its inflammatory etiology is believed to have an autoimmune component. The diagnosis is made by gastroscopy or by contrast radiography. Mild cases may be treated with symptomatic relief and followed endoscopically or radiographically, due to an associated higher risk of gastric cancer. In advanced cases, massive protein loss may lead to kwashiorkor and should be treated with parenteral alimentation followed by total gastrectomy.

Perforated crack ulcer. Drug abusers may present with an acute abdomen within 24 hr of using crack cocaine. The diagnosis of a perforated pyloric channel ulcer is made by the combination of a history of recent ingestion and pneumoperitoneum noted on an upright abdominal film. Management of these patients entails fluid resuscitation in the emergency room followed by emergent laparotomy. The perforation is typically a 1- or 2-mm-wide punched out ulceration located at the antimesenteric border of the pyloric channel. Operative management consists of an omental patch repair of the defect followed by peritoneal lavage. The etiology of these lesions is believed to be ischemic, due to vascular spasm caused by the ingested drug. Therefore, a peptic ulcer operation is not indicated in these patients, unless they have a past history consistent with peptic ulcer disease and are hemodynamically stable intraoperatively.

DUODENUM

General Anatomy and Physiology

The duodenum is continuous with the stomach by way of the pylorus, and it leads into the jejunum at the ligament of Treitz. Unlike the stomach or the rest of the small bowel, the duodenum is predominantly a retroperitoneal organ. It is generally C-shaped and curls around the pancreas, which is also retroperitoneal. It measures ~25 to 30 cm and consists of four portions. The duodenal bulb is the first portion and compromises the first 5 cm distal to the pylorus. The common bile duct and pancreatic duct empty separately or as a common channel into the second portion of the duodenum, which is ~7 cm long and oriented craniocaudally. The third portion is ~12 cm long and lies transversely between the superior mesenteric artery and the aorta, an anatomic relationship referred to as the "nutcracker." The fourth portion represents the ter-

minal 2 or 3 cm, which turns cephalad to end at the ligament of Treitz. During surgery, the ligament of Treitz is easily found to the left of the superior mesenteric artery after lifting the transverse mesocolon cephalad.

Brunner's glands are found exclusively in the proximal duodenum. They produce the alkaline secretion, which serves as a mucosal protective agent.

Vasculature and Lymphatics

The duodenal blood supply consists of the superior and inferior pancreaticoduodenal arteries, branches of the hepatic artery and the superior mesenteric artery, respectively (Fig. 9). The pancreaticoduodenal veins drain into the portal system. The significance of the shared blood supply between the duodenum and pancreas comes to light during planning of pancreatic resections. During a Whipple procedure for a pancreatic neoplasm, the duodenum must be resected because its arterial supply is sacrificed during removal of the target organ. The lymphatic drainage of the duodenum follows the vasculature.

Pathology of the Duodenum

Duodenal Ulcers

Classification

Duodenal ulcers are characteristically peptic in nature and are more common than gastric ulcers. Over 90% are located in the first portion of the duodenum, with those in the second and third portions referred to as postbulbar ulcers.

Etiology

Increased gastric acid production is the leading cause of duodenal ulcers. Patients with blood group O are more likely to have duodenal ulcers than patients with other blood types. As with some gastric ulcers, alcohol and salicylate ingestion may lower the mucosal barrier to gastric acid, thereby increasing the risk of peptic ulcer development. Also, caffeine ingestion and smoking have been associated with an increased incidence of duodenal ulcers. Patients with the Zollinger-Ellison syndrome may suffer from severe duodenal ulcer disease as a result of their gastrin producing tumors.

More recently, infection with *H. pylori* has been implicated as an environmental factor in ulcer pathogenesis. Over 90% of duodenal ulcers are associated with *H. pylori* infection of the antral mucosa. Eradication of *H. pylori,* in combination with a standard medical regimen for duodenal ulcer disease, has resulted in decreased recurrence rates.

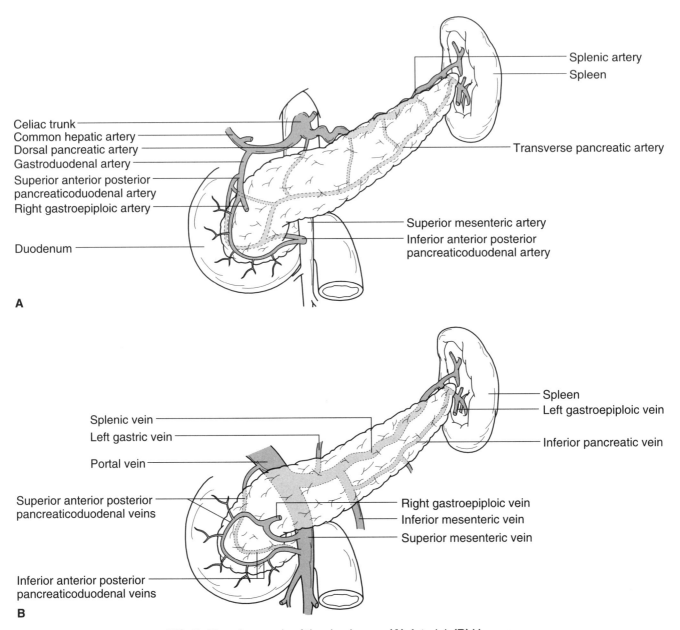

FIG. 9. Vascular supply of the duodenum. **(A)** Arterial. **(B)** Venous.

Diagnosis

A gnawing or burning epigastric pain that radiates to the back characterizes a duodenal ulcer. The pain is often experienced at night and is typically relieved by food. A scarred duodenal ulcer may result in gastric outlet obstruction, which presents as intolerance to solid food or vomiting. The presence of bile in the vomitus will depend on the site of the obstruction, and the patient will usually have a large, flaccid stomach due to the chronicity of the obstruction. If the ulcer is perforated, the patient will complain of severe abdominal pain and an acute abdomen will be present on physical exam. If the ulcer has eroded posteriorly, the gastroduodenal artery may be involved. Significant or even life-threatening hemorrhage may develop.

The initial workup of a duodenal ulcer varies according to the specific complication and the presenting signs and symptoms. An upper gastrointestinal series is the cheapest test for an uncomplicated duodenal ulcer or to confirm a gastric outlet obstruction. However, upper endoscopy has greater sensitivity and specificity. The diagnosis of an anteriorly perforated ulcer may be confirmed by correlating the clinical findings with a pneumoperitoneum on an upright plain abdominal film. The patient who vomits blood must have upper endoscopy to localize the site of bleeding.

It is well recognized that the upper intestinal tract is the source of bleeding in a small minority of patients presenting with bright red blood per rectum (hematochezia). A diagnostic gastric lavage through a naso gastric tube is performed. It is the presence of heme negative bile rather than the absence of blood that excludes gastroduodenal pathology as the primary source of lower gastrointestinal bleeding. If suspicion of a bleeding ulcer is high, upper endoscopy is performed as a diagnostic and potentially therapeutic maneuver. Often, an exposed vessel is seen in the ulcer bed, and it may be sclerosed endoscopically to arrest or prevent further bleeding. Any lesion suspicious for malignancy should be biopsied.

If the ulcer disease is severe or if the patient has a history of recurrent ulcer disease, the serum gastrin level should be checked. If the level is >200 pg/ml, the patient should be evaluated for the Zollinger-Ellison syndrome.

Medical Treatment

Medical management of duodenal ulcers is based on gastric acid reduction strategies and parallels the treatment of type II and type III peptic ulcers of the stomach. Cessation of smoking and alcohol ingestion combined with antacids, H_2-receptor antagonists, or proton pump inhibitors are the mainstays of conservative management. A treatment regimen for an *H. pylori* infection might also include antimicrobials, including various combinations of amoxicillin, metronidazole, tetracycline, clarithromycin, and bismuth subsalicylate. Over 90% of acute peptic ulcers will heal with medical management and not require surgical intervention.

Complications of Duodenal Ulcers

The three most common complications of duodenal ulcers requiring surgery are hemorrhage, perforation, and gastric outlet obstruction. These occur with an incidence of ~30%, 10%, and <10%, respectively. The approach to a bleeding duodenal ulcer parallels that of a bleeding gastric ulcer. Antacid therapy, volume resuscitation, and endoscopy for diagnosis, and possible therapy proceed simultaneously. Surgical intervention is necessary if bleeding persists after 4 to 6 U of transfusions.

Gastric outlet obstruction secondary to an acute duodenal ulcer may respond to acute medical therapy and nasogastric decompression. Chronic scarring requires surgical resection or bypass.

If a perforated ulcer seals spontaneously, medical therapy is an option. Most patients, however, will need an emergency operation.

Surgical Treatment

Failure of medical management or the development of one of the above complications may require operative intervention. The surgical approach varies with the clinical presentation of the disease, but the goal of every pro-

cedure should be acid reduction. Before proceeding to the operating room with a patient who has a complication, gastric decompression with a nasogastric tube and aggressive volume resuscitation must be initiated. An indwelling urinary catheter facilitates the monitoring of the adequacy of resuscitation.

An actively bleeding duodenal ulcer is approached through a pylorotomy to identify and oversew the bleeding vessel within the ulcer bed. Once the hemorrhage is controlled and if the patient stabilizes, a definitive acid-reducing procedure can be done. If the patient has a history or operative findings consistent with chronic or severe ulcer disease, a vagotomy and antrectomy is the procedure of choice. If the patient is older, a poor risk, or hemodynamically unstable, a vagotomy and pyloroplasty may be performed as a quicker, safer procedure. Postoperative rebleeding and recurrence rates are lower in patients treated with vagotomy and antrectomy than in those treated with pyloroplasty.

Patients with a perforated duodenal ulcer may be treated with an omental patch repair of the defect (a Graham patch). If the patient has a history of previous ulcer disease, a proximal gastric vagotomy should be performed as part of the operative plan. A vagotomy and pyloroplasty is an alternative procedure. These additional procedures should only be undertaken if the patient has been adequately resuscitated and has remained stable during the initial part of the operation. Unstable patients should undergo only an omental patch repair of the perforated ulcer with irrigation of the peritoneal cavity to remove any soilage present.

Gastric outlet obstruction may occur as a consequence of repeated ulceration leading to scarring and narrowing of the duodenal bulb. The strategy of treatment must anticipate the handling of the duodenum. If scarring and inflammation is severe, a vagotomy and gastroenterostomy may be the most prudent procedure. If local factors permit, a vagotomy and antrectomy with either a Billroth I or II reconstruction would have the lowest incidence of ulcer recurrence.

Intractability, or failure to heal an ulcer with medical therapy, is now a much less common indication for operative intervention. Proximal gastric vagotomy is the procedure of choice in this setting. If the ulcer is located in the prepylorus or in the pyloric channel, however, a truncal vagotomy with antrectomy or pyloroplasty is the indicated procedure.

Surgical Outcomes

In contrast to the excellent results with gastric ulcers, surgical outcomes for duodenal ulcers are less assured. Highly selective vagotomy, and vagotomy and pyloroplasty have a recurrence rate of ~1%/year (i.e., ~10% after 10 years), but a mortality rate of <1%. Vagotomy and antrectomy has a low long-term recurrence rate of ~2%, but an increased mortality of 2% to 4%.

Duodenal Diverticula

Diverticula of the duodenum are relatively common and usually asymptomatic. Most of these are single and located at or near the ampulla of Vater. Their etiology is unknown. Pulsion diverticula are usually multiple and located in the antimesenteric wall of the duodenum, opposite the ampulla of Vater. These often occur along with diverticulosis throughout the remaining small intestine and colon, and might then be associated with a bacterial overgrowth syndrome. With a single diverticulum, treatment is indicated only in the face of a complication such as perforation, bleeding, or ampullary obstruction. Treatment is consists of excision of the diverticula with primary duodenal closure. Management of periampullary diverticula can be quite complex and may require a biliary bypass or reimplantation of the biliary and pancreatic ducts.

Duodenal Neoplasms

Small bowel tumors are rare. The most common benign small bowel tumors include leiomyomas, lipomas, and adenomas, and they are usually amenable to local resection. Frozen sections should be checked if there is any question of malignancy. Villous adenomas of the small bowel occur most commonly in the duodenum, and although they are premalignant lesions, they can reach very large sizes and still remain benign. Malignant tumors of the duodenum include adenocarcinoma, leiomyosarcoma, carcinoid, and (rarely) lymphoma. Surgical resection is dependent on location. With exception for the second portion of duodenum, duodenal resection and primary reanastomosis is appropriate. Tumors of the second portion of the duodenum generally require a pancreaticoduodenectomy (Whipple procedure). Unresectable disease should undergo a palliative gastrojejunostomy. The prognosis for duodenal carcinoma is in general better than that for pancreatic carcinoma, with 5-year survival in resectable lesions of up to 40%.

Obstructive Disorders

Duodenal obstruction may be due to a primary duodenal disease or secondary to pathology in surrounding organs. Thus, the differential diagnosis of duodenal obstruction includes a diversity of etiologies such as peptic ulceration, annular pancreas, webs, duodenal or pancreatic neoplasm, pancreatitis, or compression by the superior mesenteric artery. Treatment is individualized and can range from duodenojejunostomy, to gastrojejunostomy, to pancreaticoduodenectomy.

Other Diseases

Crohn's disease, adult celiac disease, and polyposis syndromes affect the small or large bowel preferentially and are discussed in their respective chapters.

TERMINOLOGY OF GASTRIC AND DUODENAL SURGERY

Gastric Resections

Gastric resections (Fig. 7) are described by the amount and area of tissue resected, with the extent and type greatly influencing postoperative function. Key factors to be anticipated following a gastrectomy include loss of reservoir capacity, loss of specific cell types that pertain to the resected portion of stomach, loss of the pylorus, and the effects of vagotomy. An antrectomy refers to a resection of the antrum. A hemigastrectomy and subtotal gastrectomy describe removal of one-half to about three-fourths of the stomach, respectively. Complete removal of the organ is termed "total gastrectomy." Each of these includes the pylorus as the distal margin of resection.

Small gastric lesions may not require a formal resection. A wedge resection describes the resection of a small wedge-shaped portion of the stomach with primary closure and usually will not alter the normal gastric physiology. Wedge resections, which are amenable to a laparoscopic approach, are reserved for diagnostic purposes and for resection of small benign lesions.

Postgastrectomy Reconstructive Procedures

The three most common reconstructions following a formal gastric resection (except for a total gastrectomy) are the Billroth I, Billroth II, and the Roux-en-Y gastrojejunostomy (Fig. 8). Familiarity with these is important in order to understand the potential sequelae of the altered anatomy. The Billroth I procedure is a gastroduodenostomy in which the gastric remnant is anastomosed directly to the first portion of the duodenum. The Billroth II procedure is a gastrojejunostomy in which the gastric remnant is anastomosed end-to-side to the proximal jejunum and the duodenal stump is oversewn.

The Roux-en-Y gastrojejunostomy procedure entails creating a Y configuration with the jejunum. The jejunum is first divided a short distance past the ligament of Treitz. The distal end of the divided jejunum is then anastomosed to the gastric remnant, creating a gastrojejunostomy. The proximal end of the divided jejunum is anastomosed distal to the gastrojejunostomy by creating an end-to-side jejunojejunostomy. The jejunal limb, which leads from the gastrojejunostomy to the jejunojejunostomy, should measure at least 40 cm in length to prevent bile and pancreatic juice from refluxing into the gastric remnant.

Drainage Procedures

Drainage procedures describe an alternate means of emptying the stomach in the face of anatomic or functional obstruction of the stomach or duodenum. The two most common kinds of drainage procedures are gastrointestinal bypass and pyloroplasty.

When duodenal obstruction is due to an unresectable tumor mass in the periampullary region, a gastrojejunostomy may be performed to circumvent the obstructed duodenum. If the obstruction results from a scarred ulcer, a gastrojejunostomy or a pyloroplasty may be performed to facilitate gastric emptying. The most common pyloroplasty (Heineke-Mikulicz pyloroplasty) is created by incising the pylorus longitudinally and reapproximating it transversely. The reader is referred to the suggested reading for a more detailed discussion of the various kinds of pyloroplasty.

When a truncal or selective vagotomy is performed, the dennervated stomach will become atonic, the pylorus will not relax, and the stomach will not empty properly. A functional gastric outlet obstruction will develop, and a prophylactic drainage procedure is mandatory at the time of the vagotomy.

Gastrojejunostomy

Gastrojejunostomy may be performed in an antecolic (anterior to the transverse colon) or retrocolic (through a window in the transverse mesocolon) location. The former approach is advocated following a resection for malignancy, to position the gastrojejunostomy as far from the bed of tumor resection as possible to prevent potential obstruction from tumor recurrence. Advocates of the retrocolic approach state that it results in better gastric emptying. No conclusive evidence exists to support the superiority of either approach.

Vagotomy

A truncal vagotomy refers to the division of all fibers of both vagus nerves around the distal esophagus (Fig. 6). A selective vagotomy dennervates the stomach completely but spares the hepatic branch of the anterior (left) vagus nerve and the celiac branch of the posterior (right) vagus nerve. A highly selective vagotomy (proximal gastric vagotomy, parietal cell vagotomy) denotes division of the lesser curvature branches of the vagus nerves, with preservation of the nerves of Latarjet and the innervation of the distal antrum and pylorus.

Kocher Maneuver

The Kocher maneuver is a division of the lateral peritoneal attachments to the second portion of the duodenum. This allows medial reflection of the duodenum and facilitates inspection of the head of the pancreas.

PERIOPERATIVE CONSIDERATIONS

Informed Consent

As with all operations, there must be a discussion of the general risks and anticipated benefits of surgery, along with the unique complications related to gastroduodenal surgery. This should include an explanation of the physiologic consequences of the procedure, such as the higher risk for a patient with a proximal hemigastrectomy to develop vitamin B_{12} deficiency anemia due to lack of intrinsic factor production. Other sequelae might include alterations in transit time due to a dumping syndrome or postvagotomy diarrhea.

Nasogastric Suction

A postoperative ileus usually results after abdominal surgery, particularly if there has been a difficult or prolonged dissection. The length of time a nasogastric tube should be used is often a matter of surgeon's preference, but also depends on the presence of a fresh anastomosis and the extent of intraabdominal dissection. The timing of nasogastric tube removal is based on evidence of a resolving ileus, such as the presence of bowel sounds, decreased abdominal distention, and reduced amounts of nasogastric tube output. Passage of flatus is also an indication of returning bowel function, whereas belching is not. In fact, eructation is suggestive of an obstruction or ileus, and it is indicative of a malfunctioning nasogastric tube if one is in place.

Patients undergoing nasogastric suctioning for prolonged periods of time are at risk for developing fluid depletion and electrolyte abnormalities. Large hydrochloric acid losses in these patients may lead to a hypokalemic metabolic alkalosis. Thus, a plan to replace the nasogastric output should include not only volume replacement, but also a regular schedule for checking and repleting low levels of electrolytes. The suction apparatus should be set to aspirate intermittently or, preferably, to low continuous suction with a sump channel. These methods prevent the tip of the drain from becoming occluded by aspirating the gastric wall and creating a focus of ischemic necrosis in the gastric mucosa.

In recent years, there has been a distinct trend to eliminating altogether or markedly shortening the length of time that nasogastric tubes are used. Even with a fresh anastomosis, most patients do better with this approach, and the complications attendant with nasogastric tube usage are obviated.

COMPLICATIONS OF GASTRIC AND DUODENAL SURGERY

Patients who are nutritionally depleted, those with comorbid diseases, or those with an acute complication such as perforation or bleeding are at higher risk for developing the usual postoperative complications than healthy patients undergoing elective surgery. There are also complications that relate specifically to the complexities of gastric surgery, and these may be grouped together as postgastrectomy or postvagotomy syndromes.

Gastric atony or delayed gastric emptying is probably the most common problem following gastric resections. It is seen more commonly with Roux-en-Y gastrojejunostomies than with the other reconstructive procedures. Prokinetic agents such as metaclopramide or cisapride may be useful, although most cases resolve in several weeks and the medication may then be discontinued.

Alkaline reflux gastritis is a common problem after gastrectomy with a Billroth I or Billroth II reconstruction, although most patients are minimally symptomatic. When the gastritis is severe, the patient usually presents with epigastric pain, nausea, and vomiting after meals. The diagnosis is made by upper endoscopy, which reveals erythematous, atrophic gastric mucosa and bile reflux into the gastric remnant (from the duodenum in the case of a Billroth I or from the afferent limb of a Billroth II). It may be quite difficult to determine if there is an element of recurrent peptic ulceration, and it is usually expedient to medically treat these patients with sucralfate and H_2-receptor antagonists or proton pump inhibitors. Rarely, surgical intervention is necessary and consists of converting the Billroth I or II to a Roux-en-Y gastrojejunostomy.

Afferent loop syndrome is seen following gastrectomy with a Billroth II reconstruction. The patient complains of severe, postprandial epigastric pain and delayed vomiting of old bile, which alleviates the pain. Eating stimulates secretion of bile and pancreatic juice into the duodenum, and if the afferent limb is kinked, it becomes distended and painful. The patent efferent limb efficiently empties the gastric contents (ingested food) distally. When the obstruction is intermittently relieved, the vomitus contains the malodorous contents of the afferent limb, but no food. Treatment consists of conversion of the Billroth II to a Billroth I gastroduodenostomy or to a Roux-en-Y gastrojejunostomy.

Efferent loop syndrome is also seen following gastrectomy with a Billroth II reconstruction. The patient complains of postprandial pain and vomiting. The vomitus includes the recently ingested meal (unlike afferent loop

syndrome) mixed with bile and pancreatic juice, because the obstructed efferent loop prevents drainage of both the stomach and afferent limb. The treatment can be the same as that of an afferent loop syndrome, or as simple as relieving the efferent limb obstruction.

Blind loop syndrome may be seen after a Billroth II procedure. It is due to bacterial overgrowth in the afferent limb, with resultant deconjugation of bile salts, steatorrhea, and abnormal metabolism of vitamin B_{12} and folate. Medical management relies on antibiotics to eradicate the bacteria. These efforts are often unsuccessful, and conversion to a Billroth I may be necessary.

Following an extensive gastric resection, a small gastric pouch or small capacity syndrome manifests itself by early satiety. It results in dramatic weight loss and may lead to malnutrition. A similar clinical picture may follow gastric stapling procedures for morbid obesity. Remedial operations are aimed at restoring the lost reservoir capacity of the stomach. This is usually achieved by mobilizing a segment of jejunum in an antiperistaltic fashion or as a loop and anastomosing it to the stomach.

Dumping syndrome following gastrectomy is relatively common but usually mild. Due to the absence of the stomach's digestive role as well as the loss of regulation of emptying by the pylorus, hypertonic chyme is dumped as a large bolus into the small intestine. The large, sudden fluid shifts into the bowel lumen in response to the meal result in epigastric pain, nausea, dizziness, and diarrhea. The patient also becomes diaphoretic and tachycardic. Several hormones, including insulin, glucagon, vasoactive intestinal peptide, neurotensin, and pancreatic polypeptide, are elevated in these patients.

Conservative management is usually successful and relies on educating the patient regarding diet modifications. A postgastrectomy diet consists of six small meals each day high in fat, moderate in protein, and low in carbohydrates. The patient is advised to avoid drinking liquids with meals, and lying down for a half hour after eating may be helpful. Cyproheptadine tablets or somatostatin analog injections may mitigate the hormonal effects and alleviate the distressing symptoms. The surgical approach to dumping syndrome relies on slowing down gastric emptying by placing an antiperistaltic segment of jejunum between the stomach and duodenum. The length of this segment must be <10 cm to prevent a functional obstruction. If dumping follows a pyloroplasty, preliminary experience with pyloric reconstruction has been promising.

The pattern of postvagotomy diarrhea is such that it is not associated with meals, thus differentiating it from the typically postprandial dumping syndrome. Patients with this syndrome suffer from sporadic and explosive bouts of diarrhea numerous times daily. Severe weight loss and malnutrition may result. Postvagotomy diarrhea has been attributed to dysfunction of the denervated stomach, small bowel, pancreas, and biliary system. High bile salt excretion and bacterial colonization of the small bowel have been implicated, as well. Conservative management consists of cholestyramine administration to bind the bile salts and antibiotics to eradicate bacterial overgrowth. Opiates and octreotide may slow gastrointestinal transit. In the rare instances that are severe and persistent, surgical management is aimed at prolonging small bowel transit by placing an antiperistaltic segment (10 cm long) of jejunum 100 cm from the ligament of Treitz.

Following a Billroth II gastric resection, a potentially serious complication is leakage from the oversewn duodenum—or duodenal stump leak. The factors that predispose to development of a duodenal stump leak include nutritional depletion, hemodynamic instability, the presence of tumor or inflammation at the suture lines, technical error, and distal intestinal obstruction. Any closure that is considered to be at risk for leak should have a drainage catheter placed next to the duodenal stump. If a leak occurs, the result is a controlled fistula rather than bile peritonitis. An omental flap may also be placed over a duodenal stump to help seal the suture line and prevent a leak.

No matter how technically proficient a surgeon is, there will be operative failures and recurrent peptic ulcers. Ironically, the operation with the highest incidence of recidivism is the highly selective vagotomy, but this is counterbalanced by the lowest incidence of all the other complications associated with ulcer surgery.

Initial treatment of recurrent ulcers is medical, including searching for *H. pylori*. This may be unsuccessful,

necessitating further surgery. A Zollinger-Ellison syndrome must be ruled out, but the most common technical problem is an incomplete vagotomy, and a missed vagus nerve must always be sought. Treatment strategies for failures involve converting a highly selective vagotomy to a vagotomy and pyloroplasty, or vagotomy and antrectomy; and a vagotomy and pyloroplasty to a vagotomy and antrectomy. If a missed vagal branch is not found after a failed vagotomy and antrectomy, then a higher gastric resection is undertaken.

STUDY QUESTIONS

1. Describe the pathogenesis of peptic ulcer disease.
2. What are risk factors for development of gastric cancer?
3. How can the gastroduodenal area be excluded as the source of hematochezia?
4. What is the arterial supply of the stomach?
5. What comprises the pancreatico-duodenal arterial arcade?

SUGGESTED READING

Cameron JL, ed. *Current surgical therapy.* 5th ed. St. Louis: Mosby, 1995.
Nyhus MN, Baker RJ, Fischer JE, eds. *Mastery of surgery.* 2nd ed. Boston: Little, Brown, 1992.
O'Leary JP, ed. *The physiologic basis of surgery.* Baltimore: Williams and Wilkins, 1993.
Schwartz SI, Shires GT, Spencer FC, eds. *Principles of surgery.* 6th ed. New York; McGraw-Hill, 1994.

CHAPTER 11

Small Intestine

Hector Pombo and Joe U. Levi

ANATOMY

The jejunum and ileum comprise approximately three-fifths the length of the gastrointestinal tract, ~260 cm. The jejunum begins at the ligament of Treitz. There is no clear demarcation between the jejunum and ileum, although the proximal two-fifths are considered jejunum. Luminal diameter progressively decreases. The small intestine is supported by its mesentery, a large fold of peritoneum originating in the posterior abdominal wall to the left of the second lumbar vertebrae. The mesentery contains blood vessels, nerves, lymphatics, and fat. The blood supply to the midgut is from the superior mesenteric artery. The superior mesenteric artery supplies the pancreas, duodenum, jejunum, ileum, and the ascending and transverse colon. The intestinal branches of the superior mesenteric artery form a series of arcades within the mesentery, entering the small intestine along its mesenteric border. Venous drainage of the small intestine is via the superior mesenteric vein, which joins the splenic vein to form the portal vein. The small bowel, particularly the ileum, is rich in lymphatic aggregates (Peyer's patches) located in the intestinal submucosa. Lymphatic drainage of the small intestine is via superior mesenteric preaortic lymph nodes, which drain into the cisterna chyli. Autonomic innervation to the small intestine is both sympathetic and parasympathetic. Sympathetic innervation from preganglionic fibers arising from the lower thoracic spinal cord segments synapse with postganglionic fibers in the superior mesenteric ganglia. Parasympathetic innervation from preganglionic fibers arising from the vagus nerves increases tone and enhances motility.

The small intestinal mucosa is composed of an epithelium, a lamina propria, and a muscularis mucosae. The mucosa is lined with columnar epithelium and also contains goblet cells, argentaffin cells, Paneth cells, and endocrine cells of the amine precursor uptake and decarboxylation (APUD) system. The small intestinal mucosa contains numerous circular folds called "plicae circulares" or "valves of Kerckring," which consist of mucosa and submucosa. The villi are finger-like lumenal projections with columnar epithelium, each containing a lymphatic vessel, artery, and vein. At the base between villi are the crypts of Lieberkuhn or intestinal glands. The absorptive cells are characterized by a specialized surface called the "brush border." This brush border is composed of microvilli with a glycocalyx surface coat rich in digestive enzymes, particularly disaccharidases. The plicae circulares, villi, and microvilli exponentially increase the small intestinal absorptive surface area.

PHYSIOLOGY

The major function of the small intestine is to prepare food for assimilation and the absorption of water, electrolytes, minerals, and other nutrients. Approximately 5 to 8 L of fluid, consisting of ingested nutrients and salivary, gastric, biliary, pancreatic, and small intestinal secretions, enters the small intestine daily; however, only 1 to 1.5 L reaches the iliocecal valve, which testifies to the tremendous absorptive capacity of the small bowel. The movement of water across the epithelial membrane occurs as a result of electrolyte exchange and the development of an osmotic gradient. Movement of electrolytes across epithelial membranes occurs via active and passive mechanisms. The active transport mechanisms involve a membrane bound sodium-potassium ATPase pump. Active transport of sodium across epithelial membranes is coupled with transport of organic solutes such as L-amino acids, D-hexoses, diglycerides, triglycerides, vitamins, and bile salts.

Carbohydrates represent ~50% to 60% of the average diet. Digestible carbohydrates include sucrose, lactose, starches, and their constituents. The human intestine is incapable of digesting cellulose. Complex sugars and

133

starches are digested into their constituent monosaccharides by digestive enzymes along the microvilli brush border and amylase, respectively. These monosaccharides are then transported into the cell via a sodium ATPase active transport mechanism.

Dietary proteins are derived from meat and vegetables. The average requirement is 0.5 to 0.7 g/kg/day. The absorption of protein in the small intestine is extremely efficient, with <10% of total protein being excreted. Protein digestion is initiated in the stomach via pepsin hydrolysis, resulting in short-chain polypeptides. The major portion of protein hydrolysis in the small bowel results from activated pancreatic secretions. Pancreatic proteolytic enzymes include trypsin, chymotrypsin, elastase, carboxypeptidases, and aminopeptidases. Additional digestion of peptides occurs in the lumenal brush border. There, intestinal peptidases hydrolyze peptides into single amino acids, dipeptides, and tripeptides. Amino acid and peptide absorption across a concentration gradient involves a carrier-mediated active transport mechanism that requires energy in the form of ATP and sodium. Once inside the cytoplasm, amino acids then cross the basolateral membrane to access the circulation. Maximal absorption of peptides occurs ~30 to 90 min after a meal and is usually completed in 3 hr.

Dietary fats are derived from animal fats and vegetable. Digestion of fats begins in the stomach, where 10% to 30% of dietary fat is hydrolyzed by gastric lipase and acid. In the duodenum, dietary fat, in the form of triglycerides, mixes with biliary and pancreatic secretions. Pancreatic lipase hydrolyzes triglycerides into two molecules of fatty acids and one molecule of a 2-monoglyceride. These fatty acids and monoglycerides are then solubilized by bile salts into micelles. The bile salt/monoglyceride micelle then solubilizes cholesterols, phospholipids, and fat-soluble vitamins. Dietary fat is absorbed in the jejunum. Micelles diffuse across the epithelial membrane, releasing fatty acids and monoglycerides into the cytoplasm and releasing the bile salts into the lumen. Approximately 95% of intestinal bile salts are reabsorbed by a carrier-mediated active transport mechanism in the distal ileum. These bile salts are returned to the liver via the portal circulation, where they are then resecreted into bile. Inside the cytoplasm, fatty acids and monoglycerides are reconverted into triglycerides. There, triglycerides, cholesterols, and phospholipids are processed into lipoproteins. These lipoproteins (HDL, LDL, VLDL) are then transported out of the mucosal cell through the basolateral membrane and gain access to lacteals. These lipoproteins ultimately enter the venous system via the thoracic duct.

Water-soluble vitamins and folic acid are absorbed in the proximal intestine via active and passive transport mechanisms. Vitamin B_{12}, complexed to intrinsic factor, is absorbed through a mostly active transport mechanism in the distal ileum. Calcium is absorbed mostly in the duodenum, although some absorption does occur in the jejunum. Magnesium is absorbed passively in the ileum. Iron is absorbed throughout the small intestine.

The small bowel, particularly the ileum, is rich in lymphoid tissues. These tissues are found predominantly in Peyer's patches, intraepithelial lymphocytes, and lamina propria lymphoid tissues. The lymphoid tissues of the small intestine function similarly to systemic lymphoid tissues with their constituent cells being T and B lymphocytes. T lymphocytes can differentiate into several effector cell types, including T cytotoxic cells, T suppresser cells, and T helper cells, which mediate induction of B lymphocytes to create humoral antibodies. Once induced, B lymphocytes transform into plasma cells, which secrete mucosal IgA, which binds antigens and limits their absorption.

Mucosa of the small intestine plays a major role in the development of endocrine peptides. The best-studied intestinal hormone is secretin. Secretin is produced by mucosal S cells within the duodenal mucosa in response to luminal acid. The primary physiologic action of secretin is to stimulate water, electrolyte, and protein secretion from the pancreas and biliary tract. This provides a pH level suitable for digestion of fats within the small bowel. Cholecystokinin is a small peptide produced by the duodenum. The physiologic stimuli for its release are peptides and fats that are delivered to the duodenum. Once stimulated, duodenal release of cholecystokinin into the circulation stimulates gallbladder contraction and relaxation of the sphincter of Oddi, thus increasing bile flow into the duodenum. Vasoactive intestinal peptide (VIP) is a 28–amino acid peptide secreted by nerves found in all layers the gastrointestinal tract. VIP stimulates water and bicarbonate secretion from the pancreas, thus mimicking vagal stimulation on pancreatic function. Hypersecretion of VIP produces Verner-Morrison syndrome or watery diarrhea/hypokalemia/achlorhydria syndrome.

CROHN'S DISEASE OF THE SMALL INTESTINE

Crohn's disease is a chronic, nonspecific inflammatory disorder of unknown etiology that may affect any portion of the gastrointestinal tract. Crohn's disease occurs at a rate of six to seven per 100,000 individuals. It affects males and females equally, with a peak age of onset between the second and fourth decades. The most commonly afflicted groups include Western whites of North-Northeastern European descent and North American and European Jews. Whites are affected more commonly than blacks. Although no etiologic agent has been identified, infectious, genetic, and immune mechanisms or a combination thereof are suspected.

Isolated jejunal-ileal Crohn's disease occurs in 10% of cases. The most common distribution of Crohn's disease is ileocolonic, accounting for ~30% to 50% of cases. Crohn's disease isolated to the colon occurs in ~15% to 25% of cases. Hallmark to the gross presentation of the disease is the presence of "skip lesions" or affected segments with intervening normal segments. The earliest recognizable pathologic change is the development of the aphthoid ulcer. These ulcers may become stellate and coalesce to form a cobblestone appearance. Also typical are linear ulcers that form "railroad track" scars. Macroscopically, the bowel appears thickened where transmural involvement is present. Transmural inflammation is characterized by lymphoid aggregates expanding the submucosa and extending through the muscularis propria and subserosa. The presence of granulomas is common though not constant. Granulomas in Crohn's disease are noncaseating aggregates of epithelioid histiocytes, most commonly found in the submucosa. Additionally, serositis is seen in affected segments of small bowel. Typical changes along the involved mesentery include fat wrapping or "creeping fat." The most common symptoms include crampy abdominal pain, diarrhea, distention, flatulence, fever, malaise, nausea, and vomiting. Poor oral intake and malabsorption result in weight loss, anemia, and other nutritional deficiencies. Extraintestinal manifestations occur in ~30% of patients and include erythema nodosum, pyoderma gangrenosum, iritis, uveitis, ankylosing spondylitis, arthritis, stomatitis, and occasionally pericholangitis. The course of the disease is one of exacerbations and remissions, although the disease remains progressive.

Diagnosis is based on history, physical examination, and confirmatory studies. Physical examination should include a thorough perineal exam to assess for fissures, abscesses, or fistula. Diagnostic studies include computerized tomography (CT) with oral contrast, air-contrast small bowel series, and enteroclysis. CT is beneficial in the diagnosis of abscesses that may also be percutaneously drained. Small bowel contrast series are beneficial in identifying ulcerating lesions, narrowed thickened segments "string sign," and obstruction. Fiberoptic endoscopy via esophagogastroduodenoscopy, enteroscopy, and colonoscopy reveals chronic inflammation with intervening normal segments. Endoscopic biopsies may be difficult to interpret, as only mucosa and superficial submucosa are sampled (Fig. 1).

The medical therapy for Crohn's disease has been extrapolated from clinical experience with ulcerative colitis. As such, steroid therapy remains the mainstay of treatment. Corticosteroid administration at maximum dosages without appreciable response represents failure of medical management and remains a significant indication for operative management. Sulfasalazine has been useful in the treatment of mild to moderate iliocolitis where the effective moiety, 5-aminosalicylic acid, is delivered to the inflamed ileum and colon. More recently, mesalamine compounds have proven beneficial in treating mild to moderate disease. Immunosuppressive thera-

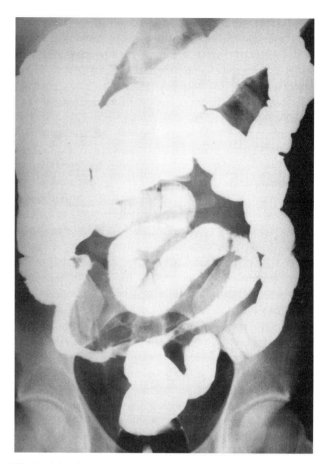

FIG. 1. A barium enema performed in a patient with Crohn's disease. Reflux of contrast through the ileocecal valve demonstrates the "string sign" of luminal anrrowing of the terminal ileum.

pies, including azathioprine and 6-mercaptopurine, once reserved for refractory disease or steroid dependency, have now become more accepted as long-term maintenance therapy with variable response. Metronidazole has also been proven effective when combined with other modalities. Symptoms associated with Crohn's disease may be treated independently with acid-reducing agents, antidiarrheals, bile salt sequestrants, and antispasmodics. Additionally, nutritional interventions have a favorable impact on disease presentation. These include elemental diets and hyperalimentation with bowel rest. Although medical management can alleviate disease, it is estimated that ~50% of patients with Crohn's disease will require surgical intervention within their lifetime, and failure of medical management remains a prime indication for surgical intervention.

Surgical intervention in Crohn's disease is indicated when medical management becomes futile or when complications of the disease are manifest. These include obstruction, inflammatory masses, and abscesses. Paramount to surgical approach is bowel conservation, as multiple resections may render a patient nutritionally crippled with a short bowel syndrome. Surgery is most commonly performed for chronic progressive obstruction, although acute obstruction does occur and represents a surgical emergency. Surgical management for obstructing bowel segments is resection with primary anastomosis, resection with proximal diverting ostomy, or stricturoplasty. Stricturoplasty is reserved for obstructing segments of <12 cm in length and involves a longitudinal full-thickness incision along the bowel wall with a transverse closure. Pneumatic dilatation of obstructing segments has poor success. Long-standing strictures have been implicated in the development of small bowel carcinoma. Inflammatory masses usually result in segmental obstruction and are approached in a similar manner. Intraabdominal abscesses can be drained percutaneously with ultrasound or CT guidance, provided that peritonitis and sepsis are not present. If these abscesses are not amenable to percutaneous drainage, laparotomy is indicated for drainage and resection of the affected bowel segment. The development of fistulae in Crohn's disease is common. These include entero-enteric, entero-colonic, entero-vesical, enterovaginal, entero-biliary, entero-pleural, and entero-cutaneous fistulas. These fistulas may be treated surgically when medical management fails. Bleeding and free perforation in Crohn's disease is seen infrequently and is another indication for surgery.

It should be noted that all of the above modalities represent treatment options and not cures. Medical management palliates disease, and surgical management palliates complications of disease. With this in mind, surgical management should be judicious with regard to bowel conservation therapy, as recurrence rates for small bowel disease are as high as 40% and recurrent resections are the leading cause of short bowel syndrome.

BENIGN SMALL BOWEL NEOPLASMS

Adenomas represent ~35% of all benign small bowel neoplasms. They may be solitary or multiple and are frequently associated with familial adenomatous polyposis (FAP) syndrome and Gardner's syndrome. Adenomas may be classified histologically as tubular, tubulo-villous (intermediate), and villous. Tubular adenomas have a very low potential for malignant conversion and may be managed with endoscopic removal. Malignant degeneration in villous adenomas approaches 50%, particularly with larger tumors (>2 cm). Villous adenomas may occur sporadically, are rare, and are most frequent in the duodenum. The clinical presentation is most frequently bleeding and obstruction via luminal compromise or intussusception. Treatment is wide-margin resection for larger and invasive tumors; endoscopic removal may suffice for smaller biopsy proven noninvasive tumors.

Leiomyomas account for ~20% of all benign small bowel neoplasms. They arise from smooth muscle in the intestinal wall and are most frequent in the jejunum and ileum. Their potential for malignant transformation is low and directly proportional to size. Most leiomyomas eventually become symptomatic, usually presenting with bleeding and varying degrees of obstruction. Diagnostic studies with barium show a typical ovoid filling defect with smooth overlying mucosa or central ulceration. Treatment consists of segmental intestinal resection.

Lipomas are the third most common benign small bowel neoplasms. They are most common in the ileum and duodenum, particularly in older men. Diagnosis is made by small bowel contrast series or CT. Lipomas usually present with varying degrees of obstruction or are found incidentally at surgery. Smaller lesions may be excised locally; larger ones may require segmental resection.

Peutz-Jeghers syndrome is a rare autosomal dominant disorder manifested by multiple intestinal hamartomas and mucocutaneous pigmentation. The polyps are a result of an abnormal overgrowth of the muscularis mucosa, resulting in a proliferation of epithelial elements supported by a stalk of smooth muscle fibers. The hamartomatous polyps are found most frequently in the jejunum and ileum, but may also be found in the stomach and colon. Diagnosis and follow-up is with endoscopy and enteroclysis. Symptomatic patients present with intestinal obstruction and occult bleeding. Treatment is endoscopic removal for small polyps and segmental resection for larger or obstructing lesions. Malignant conversion is low.

Other less frequently encountered benign small bowel neoplasms include the schwannoma, composed of nerve elements, and neurilemomas, which originate from Auerbach's and Meissner's plexi. Both are associated with von Recklinghausen's disease. Hemangiomas occur throughout the gastrointestinal tract and are considered developmental malformations rather than neoplasms.

MALIGNANT SMALL BOWEL NEOPLASMS

Adenocarcinomas account for ~35% to 50% of all malignant small bowel neoplasms. They are most frequently found in the duodenum, jejunum, and ileum in descending order. Adenocarcinomas of the small bowel are associated with FAP syndrome, Gardner's syndrome, and celiac sprue. Clinical presentation includes vague abdominal pain, weight loss, nausea, vomiting, obstruction, and bleeding. Barium contrast study is diagnostic in up to 90% of cases. Treatment is wide-margin excision or intestinal bypass to palliate extensive metastatic disease. Overall 5-year survival is ~15% to 20%.

Carcinoid tumors of the small bowel are most frequent in the appendix and ileum. They are the most common endocrine tumor of the gut. All carcinoids should be considered malignant because they have the capacity of local invasion and distant metastasis. They are multicentric in 20% to 30% of patients.

The malignant potential for small bowel carcinoids is greater than appendiceal carcinoids. An array of neoplasms with endocrine potential are similar to carcinoids and are thought to be derived from neural crest cells. These include medullary carcinoma of the thyroid, oat cell carcinoma, pancreatic islet cell carcinoma, and pituitary tumors. Pearse noted that these tumors have a high amine content in their cytoplasm, are capable of amine precursor uptake, and are able to decarboxylate these precursors to produce amines or peptides that are physiologically active and therefore coined the term "APUDomas." Carcinoid tumors have an incidence of 0.2% to 1.1% in autopsy series. The male/female ratio is 1.5:1.0, and the tumors are seen in all age groups. Carcinoids of the small bowel are usually incidental findings at laparotomy or present with varying degrees of obstruction. Due to its slow insidious course, symptomatic patients usually have locally invasive disease or distant metastasis, usually to the liver, bone, or lung. Local invasion is usually manifested as a severe desmoplastic reaction involving the ileum and its mesentery. Carcinoid tumors of the small bowel should be resected regardless of the presence of metastasis, since growth is slow and obstruction may ensue. In general, the larger the primary tumor (>2 cm), the worse the prognosis. Small (<2 cm) tumors that are noninvasive and nonmetastatic have 5-year survival rates above 90%.

The carcinoid syndrome develops in ~10% of patients with carcinoid tumors. Carcinoid tumors secrete multiple neuroendocrine mediators (serotonin, prostaglandins, substance P, kallikrein, histamine, bradykinin, and VIP), which are responsible for the systemic effects of carcinoid syndrome. The carcinoid syndrome occurs when hepatic metastasis has overwhelmed the liver's detoxifying capabilities, when metastatic disease has attained systemic venous drainage, or when the primary carcinoid tumor is outside the gastrointestinal tract, e.g., bronchial, ovarian, and testicular carcinoids. The classic symptoms of carcinoid syndrome are vasomotor, cardiopulmonary, and gastrointestinal. Chronic watery diarrhea, cutaneous flushing of the head and trunk, valvular heart lesions, and asthma are most common. Increased urinary serotonin metabolite 5-hydroxyindoleacetic acid (5-HIAA) is diagnostic. Medical therapy using subcutaneous somatostatin analogue octreotide is helpful in alleviating the symptoms of carcinoid syndrome. Surgery is standard treatment for resection of primary tumor and known metastasis. Subtotal removal of metastatic disease has been shown to prolong survival and diminish the systemic effects of the carcinoid syndrome. Five-year survival for metastatic disease is ~20% to 40%.

Malignant lymphoma may occur as a primary small bowel neoplasm or secondarily as a systemic disease process. The ileum is the most common location for small bowel lymphomas, due to the abundant lymphatic tissue. Patients usually present with fatigue, weight loss, malaise, abdominal pain, and obstruction. Treatment is surgical resection for local disease and chemotherapy for advanced disease or residual disease after resection. Five-year survival is ~60% for resectable intestinal lymphoma and <25% for advanced disease.

Sarcomas originating from the small bowel are leiomyosarcomas, fibrosarcomas, angiosarcomas, and liposarcomas. They account for ~25% of primary malignant small bowel neoplasms and arise from tissues of mesodermal origin. These tumors may become quite large and outgrow their blood supply and become necrotic. They are usually radioresistant, and treatment involves surgical resection with combination chemotherapy. Five-year survival is ~30% to 40%.

SMALL BOWEL DIVERTICULI

Diverticuli of the gastrointestinal tract may be defined as true or traction diverticuli and false or pulsion diverticuli. True diverticuli are defined as those which contain all wall layers. False diverticuli usually contain only mucosa, submucosa, and some investing fibrous tissues. True diverticuli include Meckel's diverticuli and traction diverticuli, usually as a result of an inflammatory adhesion. False diverticuli include Zenker's and epiphrenic diverticuli of the esophagus, jejunoileal diverticuli, and colonic diverticuli. False diverticuli are thought to result from a pulsion phenomenon secondary to increased intraluminal pressure. In this setting, mucosal and submucosal herniation occurs via points of weakness along the mesenteric border where blood vessels and nerves enter the intestinal wall.

Meckel's diverticuli represent the most common congenital anomaly of the small intestine. They occur as a result of failure of obliteration of the vitelline or omphalomesenteric duct in utero. A simple "rule of two's" may be applied to their presentations. These diverticuli occur in 2% of individuals, they are located within 2 ft of the ileocecal valve, they are usually ~2 in. long, and most symptoms present within the first 2 years of life. These diverticuli are found on the antimesenteric border and are true diverticuli. In the pediatric age group, their most frequent complication is bleeding. This occurs because ~50% contain ectopic mucosa, usually gastric or less frequently pancreatic. Those containing gastric mucosa can be diagnosed noninvasively by means of a technetium pertechnetate scan. In the adult age groups, typical presentations are obstructive, usually as a result of adhesions or as a leading point for an intussusception. Acute diverticulitis has also been described. Although the above are typical presentations, it must be noted that most are asymptomatic and are usually found incidentally at laparotomy or autopsy.

Treatment is reserved for symptomatic diverticuli only. Surgical treatment consists of wedge resection or segmental intestinal resection.

Jejunoileal diverticuli are false or pulsion diverticuli found in the mesenteric border. They are usually multiple and most common in the proximal jejunum. Most patients are asymptomatic. Presenting features include bleeding, diverticulitis, perforation, obstruction, or bacterial overgrowth resulting in malabsorption. Surgical treatment involves segmental intestinal resection with primary anastomosis. Oral metronidazole will usually suffice for malabsorption.

SMALL BOWEL OBSTRUCTION

Intestinal obstruction occurs when luminal contents are prevented from passing distally along the gastrointestinal tract. Small bowel obstructions are classified as mechanical or paralytic. Mechanical causes can be further classified as those resulting from luminal compromise, extrinsic compromise, or intrinsic compromise. Luminal compromise resulting in intestinal obstruction is seen with polypoid tumors, which obliterate the intestinal lumen. Other causes include intussusception and bezoars, and, infrequently, gallstones. Extrinsic causes of small bowel obstruction include adhesions, hernias, volvuli, neoplasms, and abscesses. Adhesions of postoperative, congenital, or postinflammatory origin are the most common cause of small bowel obstruction in the Western world. Intrinsic causes of small bowel obstruction are usually congenital or acquired. Congenital causes include stenosis, atresia, and duplications. Acquired causes are usually inflammatory, which lead to fibrotic strictures, as seen in Crohn's enteritis and postradiation enteritis. Paralytic ileus may progress to obstruction if the underlying cause is not corrected. Paralytic ileus is caused by neural, humoral, or metabolic abnormalities, which are frequently seen in postoperative patients, traumatic injuries, sepsis, chronic debilitating diseases, electrolyte disturbances, spinal injuries, or intestinal ischemia. In this disorder, continuity of intestinal flow is obviated by lack of forward motility rather than mechanical obstruction.

Mechanical obstruction of the small intestine results in a large accumulation of fluids and gas proximal to the point of obstruction, which results in distention. As distention progresses, increased luminal pressure impedes venous drainage from the intestinal wall with resultant bowel wall edema. As edema worsens, large volumes of fluid and electrolytes are secreted into the bowel lumen, which lead to severe dehydration and electrolyte disturbances. If severe distention is not relieved, bowel wall ischemia and perforation will ensue. The metabolic consequences of small bowel obstruction are a profound dehydration and a hypochloremic, hypokalemic, metabolic alkalosis. The systemic effects are oliguria, azotemia, hemoconcentration, reduced central venous pressure, and reduced cardiac output, which may lead to hypotension and hypovolemic shock.

Presenting features include nausea, vomiting, distention, crampy intermittent abdominal pain, and obstipation. As obstruction progresses, pain becomes more diffuse and constant. Localized pain is usually indicative of ischemia or gangrene. Fever and leukocytosis are usually later findings. Acidosis represents intestinal ischemia.

Diagnostic studies are an adjunct to a good history and physical examination. Classic findings on plain radiograph of the abdomen include distended loops of small bowel with air-fluid levels and absent air distal to the point of obstruction (Fig. 2). Water-soluble contrast fluoroscopy and CT with oral contrast are usually confirmatory, though not required to make a clinical diagnosis. Free subdiaphragmatic or retroperitoneal air represent perforation and warrant urgent laparotomy.

Initial therapy is geared toward restoration of the intravascular volume deficit. Volume deficits in long-standing obstruction may be in excess of several liters and should be corrected prior to surgery. Urinary output should be monitored hourly with Foley catheter. Diuretics should be avoided. Patients with cardiorespiratory disease may require central venous pressure and pulmonary artery pressure monitoring to guide fluid resuscitation. Nasogastric tubes are vital in preventing aspiration of gastric contents and removing accumulating gastric fluid and air, which contribute to further distention. Broad-spectrum antibiotics are given prior to surgery.

Patients with partial small bowel obstructions and relatively benign physical findings may be given an initial trial of nonoperative therapy with nasogastric decompression, fluid resuscitation, and electrolyte correction. Partial small bowel obstructions are denoted as those having incomplete obstructions with some colonic gas on abdominal roentgenogram and intermittent passage of flatus or watery diarrhea. Observation of these patients requires repeated physical examination by the same examiner to identify a deteriorating course. Approximately 15% to 25% of patients respond to nonoperative management, although as many as 20% to 30% return within a few years with recurrent small intestinal obstruction.

Operative management is considered when there is no history of previous surgery, when there exist a deteriorating course on nonoperative therapy or failure to improve, or when there is suspicion of ischemic bowel or evidence of perforation or peritonitis. Operative strategies include correction of obstructing culprit, i.e., lysis of adhesions or reduction of hernia, bypassing obstructed segments as in peritoneal carcinomatosis, bypassing an obstruction with a proximal ostomy to relieve the fecal stream, and excision of the offending lesion and restoration of intestinal continuity. It is estimated that 5% to 15% of patients operated on for small bowel obstruction secondary to adhesions will develop obstruction in the future.

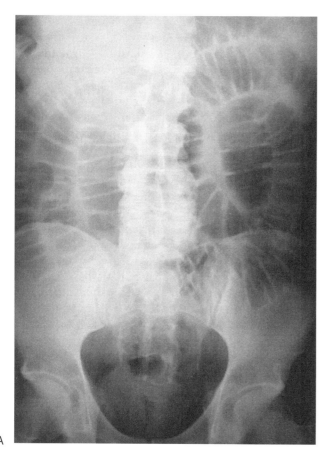 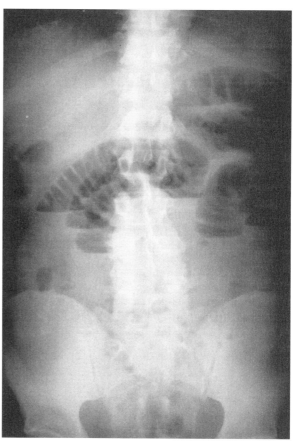

A B

FIG. 2. (A) A supine plain abdominal radiograph in a patient suspected of having small bowel obstruction. Note the distended loops of small bowel with plicae circularis defined throughout and an absence of gas in the large bowel. **(B)** An upright view of the abdomen in the same patient demonstrating multiple "air-fluid levels" isolated to the small bowel and again a virtual absence of gas in the distal bowel.

SHORT BOWEL SYNDROME

Short bowel syndrome occurs when substantial portions of small intestine are resected, resulting in too small an intestinal surface area available for absorption of nutrients, electrolytes, and fluids. Although absolute length of bowel varies from patient to patient, short bowel syndrome usually develops when only 90–100 cm of jejunoileum remain. Jejunal resections are tolerated better than ileal resections. Presence of an intact ileocecal valve is beneficial as jejunoileal exposure to succus is prolonged. The most frequent causes of short bowel syndrome are superior mesenteric arterial or venous thrombosis, multiple resections due to Crohn's disease or abdominal malignancies, mesenteric volvuli, and internal herniations. Currently, the best treatment for short bowel syndrome remains prevention and surgical conservation therapy in order to salvage intestinal length.

Many metabolic derangements are encountered in patients with short bowel syndrome—evidence of the metabolic importance of the small intestine (Table 1). Resection of the distal ileum results in loss of intestinal absorption of vitamin B_{12}, resulting in megaloblastic anemia. Additionally, bile salt reabsorption through the enterohepatic circulation occurs in the distal ileum; thus, resection of this portion may result in massive losses of the bile salt pool with resultant malabsorption of fats or steatorrhea. This steatorrhea results when bile salts are depleted through intestinal losses and fatty acids are not solubilized into micelles. As fatty acids are delivered to the distal ileum and colon, they are bound by calcium, thus making calcium unavailable for binding oxalates. Oxalate, a byproduct of glycine metabolism, is usually conjugated with luminal calcium and excreted in feces.

TABLE 1. *Metabolic derangements in short bowel syndrome*

Electrolyte imbalances
Fat malabsorption/steatorrhea
Calcium oxalate urinary stones
Cholesterol gallstones
Gastric acid hypersecretion
Diarrhea

Thus, when steatorrhea is present and luminal calcium is preferentially bound to fatty acids, oxalate is reabsorbed in the colon and excreted in the urine, where it may precipitate as calcium oxalate urinary stones. Failure of reabsorption of bile salts in the distal ileum results in extensive colonic mucosal irritation, with subsequent outpouring of fluids and electrolytes and subsequent diarrhea. Finally, as the bile salt pool becomes depleted, the concentration of bile salts is insufficient to solubilize cholesterol, and cholesterol gallstone formation is increased. Acid hypersecretion is commonly seen in short bowel syndrome, although its mechanism has not been fully elucidated.

Treatment of short bowel syndrome is based on nutritional support, correction of electrolyte and fluid losses, and symptomatic relief of symptoms. Nutritional support is provided via total parenteral nutrition (TPN). Electrolyte and fluid losses are controlled with repletion, antidiarrheals, bile salt sequestrants, and H-2 blockers or proton pump blockers to minimize acid hypersecretion. In patients with limited tolerance to enteral feedings, bulking agents may be helpful.

Long-term TPN has significant metabolic sequelae. Sepsis remains a significant problem, as prolonged vascular access undoubtedly will result in catheter sepsis and venous thrombosis. Additionally, long-term TPN will lead to fatty infiltration of the liver or cholestasis. This cholestasis may subsequently result in liver failure. Recent advances in intestinal transplantation may be a foreseeable alternative.

MALABSORPTION

Malabsorption is a broad, encompassing entity associated with varying degrees of impaired absorption of fats, carbohydrate, protein, vitamins, electrolytes, minerals, and water. It may manifest itself as a primary medical impairment or a surgical/postsurgical complication.

Clinical manifestations include weight loss, steatorrhea, diarrhea, anemia, bleeding, dermatitis, neuropathies, glossitis, weakness, fatigue, and edema. Once clinical suspicion is aroused, a variety of clinical tests are available to confirm its presence. Screening tests include gross and microscopic inspection for stool fat and protein, D-xylose absorption, radiographic bowel studies, and endoscopy with biopsies. Radioisotope labeling techniques allow for detection of malabsorption for specific compounds that may be easily radiolabeled. Other specific tests include lactose intolerance test and the Schilling test for vitamin B_{12} malabsorption.

As mentioned previously, malabsorption is seen in a variety of surgical and postsurgical scenarios. Varying degrees of malabsorption are seen following extensive or total gastric resections. Nutritional deficiencies, no doubt, are associated with reduced intake. Additionally,

loss of gastric storage capacity and processing, and inadequate mixing of foods with digestive enzymes lead to varying degrees of malabsorption. Pernicious anemia and vitamin B_{12} deficiencies are seen secondary to loss of intrinsic factor. Postvagotomy states are also implicated with malabsorption. Vagal denervation alters to some degree the normal gastric, pancreatic, biliary, and small bowel physiology. Troublesome diarrhea is seen in ~5% of patients following vagotomy. This diarrhea is thought to occur as a result of food stasis in the stomach and small bowel, resulting in bacterial overgrowth, uncontrolled gastric emptying with dumping, and rapid small bowel transit time secondary to denervation. Fistulas remain a significant cause of malabsorption syndromes. Malabsorption occurs as result of bypassed intestinal segments or loss of ingested foodstuffs, fluids, and electrolytes. Pancreatic exocrine insufficiency, whether secondary to intrinsic pancreatic disease or pancreatic resection, can result in the inability to emulsify fats and subsequent steatorrhea. Biliary tract disease may result in malabsorption of fats and fat-soluble vitamins as a result of inadequate bile delivery into the intestinal tract or intrinsic hepatic insufficiency. Extensive small bowel resections may result in insurmountable loss of cross-sectional surface for absorption of nutrients, fluids, and electrolytes. Blind loop obstructions may lead to intestinal bacterial overgrowth with resultant malabsorption. Other disorders associated with malabsorption syndromes include Crohn's enteritis, infectious enteritis, and radiation enteritis, to name a few.

Obviously, correction of malabsorption states involves control of the underlying process. Additionally, nutritional, fluid, and electrolyte support are paramount in order to prevent further metabolic decline.

RADIATION ENTERITIS

Cumulative doses of ionizing radiation to the gastrointestinal tract pose severe early and late complications. The cells of the gastrointestinal tract can tolerate only a finite amount of radiation. Maximal tolerance for the intestine is ~50 to 60 Gy or 5,000 to 6,000 rads. Conditions such as diabetes mellitus, hypertension, previous surgery, sepsis, and ongoing chemotherapy may precipitate complications. Ionizing radiation interacts with intracellular water, releasing free radicals, damaging DNA, causing breakage and point mutations, and causing abnormal production of macromolecules.

In acute intestinal injury, villi become flattened and the mucosal barrier is breached, releasing fluids into the intestinal lumen and allowing translocation of luminal bacteria into the circulation. The ileum is most sensitive due to its high lymphoid tissue content. Nearly all patients receiving abdominal radiation exhibit some degree of early injury, manifested as nausea, vomiting, diarrhea, and crampy abdominal pain.

Late intestinal injury occurs as a result of a progressive vasculitis, fibrosis, and collagen deposition. Late complications may take weeks, months, or years to manifest, and occur in 5% to 25% of patients.

Sequelae of radiation enteritis include malabsorption and diarrhea resulting in significant nutrient, electrolyte, and fluid losses, partial or complete obstruction, perforation and abscess, fistula, and ulceration. Diagnosis is made by careful history of radiation exposure and dose, contrast small bowel series or barium enema, and endoscopy with biopsy. Medical management is directed to nutrient, electrolyte and fluid correction, bowel rest, control of sepsis, and abscess drainage. Surgical intervention is warranted when medical management fails, or when peritonitis or obstruction develops. Caveats for improved surgical outcome include nutritional optimization, strict mechanical and antibiotic bowel preparation, systemic antibiotics, avoiding irradiated bowel for anastomosis, avoiding bypasses, avoiding excessive adhesiolysis, and delaying postoperative enteral feedings. Despite the above and meticulous technique, morbidity and mortality remain high. Patients usually succumb to sepsis or recurrence of primary disease.

SMALL INTESTINAL FISTULA

A fistula is an abnormal communication between two epithelialized surfaces. Fistulae can exist between internal organs and body cavities as well as internal organs and the body surface. Primary fistulae occur spontaneously, while secondary fistulae are due to interventions or instrumentations. Etiologies include complications from operative, interventional, or endoscopic procedures, penetrating or blunt trauma, abscess formation, inflammatory processes, postirradiation, presence of cancer, and severe systemic disease. Enteric fistulae occur most frequently following abdominal surgery.

Diagnosing an enteric fistula may be obvious by observing enteric contents or air from a body surface or sometimes difficult as in internal fistulae. Enterocutaneous fistulae occur most commonly at drain or incision sites. Diagnostic studies to identify enteric fistulae include water-soluble contrast studies of the gastrointestinal tract and/or fistulogram using water-soluble contrast via the cutaneous opening. Contrast studies should help define the fistula and identify communication with the bowel, underlying inflammatory conditions, distal bowel obstruction, abscesses, foreign bodies, or cancer (Fig. 3).

Once an enteric fistula has been identified, initial therapy should include resuscitation and control of sepsis. Depending on the fistula location in the gastrointestinal tract, large volumes of fluids, nutrients, and electrolytes may be lost. Proximal fistulae are noted for their high vol-

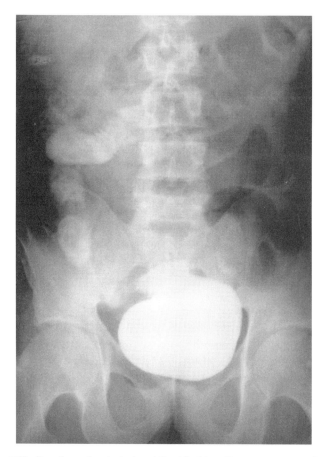

FIG. 3. A contrast study of the bladder. Cystogram reveals an abnormal communication between the bladder and the small bowel (opacified in the right abdomen).

umes, fluid and electrolyte abnormalities, and pancreaticobiliary fluid content. Enterocutaneous fistulae are further classified according to their daily volumes of drainage. A high-output fistula drains >500 ml/day of fluid, whereas a low-output fistula drains <500 ml/day. High-output fistulae are associated with the greatest morbidity and mortality, and a decreased likelihood of spontaneous closure. Correction of fluid and electrolyte disturbances should be addressed first. Control of sepsis should include systemic antibiotics, and identification and drainage of any abscesses. Intraabdominal abscesses may be identified and drained percutaneously with CT scan guidance. Skin breakdown at a stoma site may lead to a focal sepsis with resultant abscess formation. Early skin protection from enteric content exposure is vital. Following resuscitation and sepsis control, attention should be directed at nutritional support. Traditionally, TPN with central hyperalimentation and no oral intake has been the mainstay of therapy. In recent years, elemental feedings have been used in selected patients, particularly those with distal fistulae, to supplement nutrition. Combination nutrition with central hyperalimentation and elemental oral feedings offers the greatest nutritional support. Additionally, H-2 blockers and somatostatin may decrease gastric and pancreaticobiliary secretions respectively.

The likelihood of spontaneous fistula closure depends on its location, accompanying inflammatory component, and the patient's nutritional status. The spontaneous rate of closure for low-output fistulae may reach 80%. If, after a 6-week period, no significant decline in output has occurred, then surgical correction may be contemplated. Surgical correction requires a thorough mechanical bowel preparation. At laparotomy, attention should focus on avoidance of enterotomies, evacuation, and drainage of all abscesses, identification of foreign materials, and identification and correction of any distal obstruction. High-output fistulae are most problematic and do not usually close spontaneously within a reasonable period of time.

SUMMARY

The small bowel is a dynamic organ with a variety of physiologic functions, including processing, absorption, and digestion of nutrients, production of secretory immunoglobulins, and production of neuroendocrine peptides. Due to its large size, it appears vulnerable to many pathologic states. Intestinal obstruction remains a frequently encountered problem, particularly in patients with previous surgeries. Additionally, inflammatory or neoplastic conditions may initially manifest as intestinal obstructions. Crohn's disease of the small bowel remains a common affectation occurring at a rate of six to seven per 100,000 individuals. Crohn's disease remains one of the leading causes of short bowel syndrome due to multiple resections. Treatment is aimed at medical control of disease and surgical control of complications. Both benign and malignant neoplasms are found primary to the small intestine, although their frequency is overall low. The absorptive function of the small intestine may be altered by systemic disease as well as by disorders primary to the small intestine, biliary tract, and pancreas, and control of malabsorption is usually directed at the underlying process.

STUDY QUESTIONS

1. Discuss the metabolic consequences of the short bowel syndrome.
2. Describe the origin and function of the major gut-derived neuroendocrine peptides.
3. Describe the pathophysiology of hemodynamic and acid-base abnormalities in small intestinal obstruction.
4. Describe the role of medical and surgical management in Crohn's disease.
5. Describe the pathophysiology and presentation of early and late radiation enteritis.

SUGGESTED READING

Ashley SW, Wells SA Jr. Tumors of the small intestine. *Semin Oncol* 1988; 15:116–128.
Block GE, Michelassi F, Tanaka M, Riddell RH, Hanauer SB. Crohn's disease. *Curr Probl Surg* 1993;30:2.
Cameron JL. *Current surgical therapy.* 5th ed. St. Louis: Mosby–Year Book, 1995.
Michelassi F, Balestracci T, Chappell R, et al. Primary and recurrent Crohn's disease: experience with 1379 patients. *Ann Surg* 1991;214:230–240.
Pickleman J, Lee RM. The management of patients with early postoperative small bowel obstruction. *Ann Surg* 1989;210:216.
Sabiston DC. *Textbook of surgery: the biological basis of modern surgical practice.* 14th ed. Philadelphia: Saunders, 1991.
Schwartz SI, Shires GT, Spencer FC, eds. *Principles of surgery.* 5th ed. New York: McGraw-Hill, 1989.
Stewardson RH, Bombeck CT, Nyhus LM. Critical operative management of small bowel obstruction. *Ann Surg* 1978;187(2):189–193.
Zuidema GD, ed. *Shackelford's surgery of the alimentary tract.* Vol. 5. 3rd ed. Philadelphia: Saunders, 1991.

CHAPTER 12

Colon, Rectum, and Anus

Rodolfo Martinez and Rene Hartmann

Diseases of the colon, rectum, and anus are common clinical problems that will be encountered regardless of what specialty of medicine is practiced. Knowledge of anatomy, physiology, and pathogenesis of diseases of the colon, rectum, and anus will allow understanding of diverticular disease, inflammatory bowel disease of the colon, anorectal pathology and neoplasms of the colorectal and anal regions, as well as other disease processes that are presented here. If basic concepts are understood regarding these issues, appropriate treatment can be rendered or timely consultation can be obtained.

ANATOMY OF THE COLON

The colon and rectum comprise the majority of the hindgut and are collectively located in the right abdomen, epigastrium, left abdomen, and pelvis (Fig. 1). Three anatomic characteristics help the surgeon distinguish a loop of colon from the small intestine. Taenia coli are three long muscular bands that extend from the tip of the cecum to the rectosigmoid. They are situated equidistant from one another along the surface of the colon (two antimesenteric and one mesenteric). They form the longitudinal layer of muscle fibers of the colon. Haustral sacculations occur on the walls of the colon. Appendices epiploicae are small, fatty appendages of serosal fat studding the external surface of the colon. They are most numerous along the taeniae and are relatively flat on the proximal colon but elongated and pedunculated on the sigmoid colon.

The colon is segmentally divided into the cecum and appendix, ascending colon, transverse colon, descending colon, and sigmoid colon. The rectum is ~15 to 20 cm long and bridges the intraperitoneal colon with the extraperitoneal rectal vault. The cecum is usually located in the right iliac fossa but may be found elsewhere. Its three longitudinal taeniae converge at the tip and serve as a guide in locating the appendix.

The ascending colon occupies the right abdominal "gutter" and terminates at the hepatic flexure at the inferior surface of the right lobe of the liver. Most of the ascending colon is retroperitoneal as it is covered by parietal peritoneum on the lateral, medial, and anterior surface. The "white line of Toldt" represents the lateral attachment of the colon to the abdominal wall.

The transverse colon extends across the abdomen from the hepatic flexure to the splenic flexure. The transverse mesocolon forms a horizontal partition across the abdominal cavity and separates the cavity of the omental bursa and supramesocolic structures from the inframesocolic compartment. It poses a barrier to the spread of infection between these areas. The greater curvature of the stomach is attached to the transverse colon by the gastrocolic omentum. The greater omentum is draped anteriorly along the entire length of the transverse colon.

The descending colon extends from the splenic flexure to the brim of the pelvis, at which point the sigmoid colon begins. Similar to the ascending colon, the anterior, lateral, and medial surfaces of the descending colon are covered by parietal peritoneum which fixes it to the lateral abdominal wall ("white line of Toldt").

The sigmoid colon begins at the brim of the pelvis and ends at the level of the third sacral vertebra, the rectosigmoid junction, where peritoneal investment and mesentery of the sigmoid cease. The rectosigmoid junction is characterized by six anatomic features: (a) narrowing of the diameter of the bowel; (b) lack of the peritoneal investment of the gut below that point; (c) disappearance of a true mesentery below the rectosigmoid; (d) divergence of the three longitudinal taeniae at the rectosigmoid junction to form a continuous longitudinal coat from the rectum; (e) the absence of appendices epiploicae below the rectosigmoid junction; and (f) internally, a gross morphologic change in the mucous membrane that can easily be seen by sigmoidoscopy. The rectal mucosa is smooth and flat, but the mucosa of the sigmoid is seen to form prominent rugal

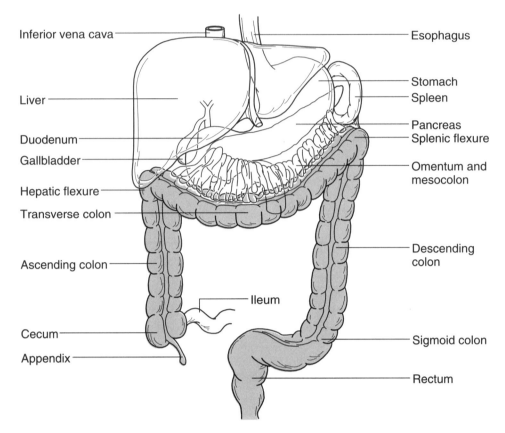

FIG. 1. Anatomy and spatial relations of the colon.

folds. A sharp angulation is invariably encountered at this level during sigmoidoscopy, and the caliber of the bowel lumen is markedly reduced.

ANATOMY OF THE RECTUM AND ANUS

The anal canal extends from the hairy skin of the anal verge to the anorectal ring (Fig. 2). It is bounded by the coccyx posteriorly, the ischiorectal fossa laterally, and the urethra and the lower vagina and perineal body in men and women, respectively. Approximately 2 cm proximal to the anal verge lie the anal valves, also termed the "dentate line." Above each valve is an anal crypt; connected to the crypts are a variable number of glands that traverse the submucosa to terminate either in the submucosa, the internal anal sphincter, or the intersphincteric plane. The anal transition zone is the area of transition from continuous rectal epithelium to uninterrupted squamous epithelium (dentate line) below.

The internal anal sphincter is the continuation of the inner circular muscle of the rectum. The external anal sphincter is continuous with the puborectalis muscle superiorly and becomes subcutaneous inferiorly. It is divided into deep and superficial compartments. The levator ani plate consists of three muscles—the iliococcygeus, pubococcygeus, and puborectalis.

The rectum begins at the sacral promontory and descends caudally, following the curve of the sacrum for a distance of 13 to 15 cm, to end at the anorectal ring. The valves of Houston are located at the intraluminal aspects of the rectum. At the rectosigmoid junction, the transverse folds characteristic of the sigmoid colon give way to the smoother rectal mucosa. Externally, at the same junction, the three taeniae coli diverge to encircle the rectum as the longitudinal muscle layer.

Posteriorly, the rectum is related to the sacrum, coccyx, levator ani muscles, medial sacral vessels, and roots of the sacral nerve plexus. Anteriorly, in males, the extraperitoneal rectum is related to the prostate, seminal vesicles, vas deferens, and urinary bladder. In females, the extraperitoneal rectum lies behind the posterior vaginal wall.

Blood Supply

The proximal one-half of the colon is considered the distal segment of midgut and derives its blood supply from the superior mesenteric artery (SMA) system (Fig. 3). The ileocolic artery, right colic artery, and middle colic artery are all branches of the SMA, and supply the cecum, ascending, and transverse colon, respectively.

The distal one-half of the colon and the rectum comprise the hindgut and receive its arterial blood supply from branches of the inferior mesenteric artery (IMA). The left colic artery divides into ascending and descending branches that supply the splenic flexure and descending colon, respectively. The sigmoid artery and the superior hemorrhoidal arteries are branches of the IMA and supply the sigmoid colon and the superior one-third of the rectum.

From the ileocecal region to the rectosigmoid region, a continuous mesenteric arterial arcade, known as the "marginal artery of Drummond," is formed from the uniting of all arterial supply of the colon. This provides collateral blood flow should arterial supply from a particular artery be decreased or eliminated.

The major arterial blood supply to the rectum and anal canal (Fig. 4) is derived from the superior and inferior hemorrhoidal arteries, whereas the middle hemorrhoidal artery (branch of the internal iliac artery) has a variable contribution. The superior hemorrhoidal artery is a direct continuation of the IMA. The inferior hemorrhoidal arteries are branches of the internal pudendal artery, which in turn is a branch of the internal iliac artery.

The venous drainage of the colon corresponds to the arterial supply. The proximal one-half of the colon drains ultimately to the superior mesenteric vein, while the distal hindgut drains ultimately to the inferior mesenteric vein. The distal two-thirds of rectum drains ultimately to the inferior vena cava (IVC) via the middle and inferior hemorrhoidal veins (Fig. 5).

The arrangement of the lymphatic is uniform throughout the colon (Fig. 6). Submucous and subserous lymphatic plexuses in the wall of the colon communicate through the muscular layer and drain into the epiploic lymph nodes, which lie on the wall of the bowel beneath the serosa and in the epiploic appendices. These nodes are particularly numerous in the sigmoid colon. The lymph drainage sequentially travels from the epiploic nodes to the paracolic nodes then to the intermediate nodes which lie along the arterial arcade supplying the segment of bowel involved. From there, the lymph from the right side of the colon proximal to the splenic flexure eventually drains into the main (principal) nodes around the origin of the SMA, and the lymph from the left colon distal to the splenic flexure eventually drains into the main nodes located at the origin of the IMA. In both instances, ultimate lymphatic drainage is into the iliolumbar chain of lymphatic, which empties into the thoracic duct.

Lymphatic drainage of the anorectal area likewise follows the vascular supply (Fig. 7). Drainage from the upper two thirds of the rectum reaches the inferior mesenteric nodes. The lower third of the rectum drains not only into the inferior mesenteric nodes but also into the internal iliac nodes. Lymphatic drainage of the anal canal drains either to the internal iliac nodes or the superficial inguinal nodal basin.

Physiology of the Colon

The colon and rectum absorb nutrients from intestinal contents and propel, store, and allow a socially acceptable pattern for elimination of feces. Those functions depend on close coordination of neural, hormonal and muscular interactions at both local and central levels.

Colonic contractions can be divided into nonpropulsive segmental contractions and propulsive contractions. Nonpropulsive segmental contractions are isolated random circular muscle contractions that occur predominantly in the right colon. Although these contractions do not propel food distally, the forward and backward motion of lumen contents permits mixing and promotes absorption of water and electrolytes by increasing the exposure time between the liquid colonic contents and the colon mucosa. Propulsive contractions can be divided into those progressing over short lengths of bowel and those migrating rapidly over long lengths of bowel (mass movements). Propulsive activity that progress for short distances and result in caudal or cephalad movement of bowel contents is seen chiefly in the right colon. Mass movements often begin in the transverse colon and occur three to four times per day, stimulated by food intake or physical activity.

A multitude of factors affect motility of the colon. Eating increases colon activity as a result of the "gastrocolic reflex." The gastrocolic response is characterized by an increase of colon propulsive activity beginning 15 to 30 min after ingestion of a meal, which may result in an urge to defecate. Mediators of this colonic response may be neural mechanisms, hormonal mechanisms, or a combination of both. Gastrin, cholecystokinin, and gastric inhibitory polypeptide have been shown to be the predominant humoral factors as the blood levels of these hormones increase in parallel with increases of colonic motility after feeding.

A number of clinical disorders are believed to originate from perturbations of bowel motility. Abnormalities of colonic motility appear to be important in the pathogenesis of irritable bowel syndrome, diverticular disease, idiopathic megacolon, and constipation or diarrhea.

The colon receives ~1,500 ml of chyme during a 24-hr period. Under normal conditions, the colonic mucosa absorbs the majority of water, sodium, and chloride while secreting potassium and bicarbonate and leaves <100 ml of fluid and only 1 meq of sodium and chloride to be lost in the feces.

More specifically, sodium and water are absorbed primarily in the ascending and transverse colon. Active sodium absorption is a process involving electrogenic transport, neutral sodium chloride absorption, or a combination of these mechanisms. The net flux of sodium into and out of the lumen of the colon is regulated mainly by the intraluminal and intracellular sodium concentrations and by aldosterone activity. Chloride absorption in the colon is

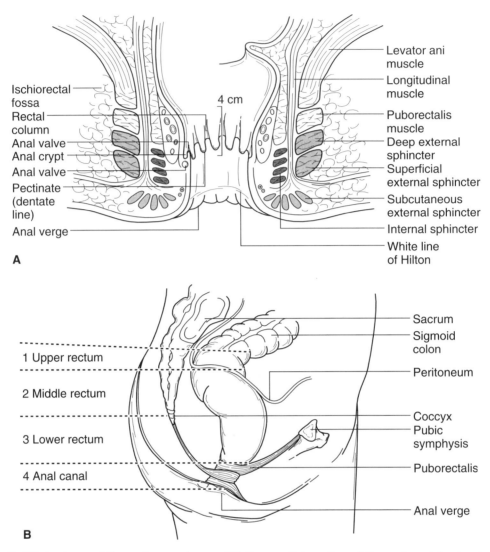

Ischiorectal fossa
Rectal column
Anal valve
Anal crypt
Anal valve
Pectinate (dentate line)
Anal verge

4 cm

Levator ani muscle
Longitudinal muscle
Puborectalis muscle
Deep external sphincter
Superficial external sphincter
Subcutaneous external sphincter
Internal sphincter
White line of Hilton

A

1 Upper rectum
2 Middle rectum
3 Lower rectum
4 Anal canal

Sacrum
Sigmoid colon
Peritoneum
Coccyx
Pubic symphysis
Puborectalis
Anal verge

B

FIG. 2. (A) Anatomy of the rectum and anus. **(B)** Paramedial section of the male pelvis showing the components of the external anal sphincter (triple-loop system of Shafik).

the result of passive transport along favorable electro-chemical gradients as well as active neutral chloride-bicar-bonate exchange or neutral sodium chloride absorption.

A number of heterogeneous agents can stimulate fluid and electrolyte secretion in the colon, including bacteria, enterotoxins, hormones, neurotransmitters, and laxatives. Shigellosis and salmonellosis prohibit normal absorption and increase secretion of water, sodium, and chloride, resulting in diarrhea.

Anorectal Physiology

Extrinsic innervation of the rectum and anal canal is both sympathetic and parasympathetic in origin. Sympathetic tone inhibits contraction of smooth muscle of the rectum when the internal anal sphincter contracts. Para-sympathetic innervation contracts the rectal wall and relaxes the internal sphincter. The high-pressure zone of

the anal canal at rest is due to the internal sphincter and acts as a barrier to prevent leakage of mucus and gas. The external sphincter contributes to anal pressure only when a bolus of stool is present within the anal canal.

Sympathetic supply to the upper rectum arise from L-1 to L-3. The lower rectum is innervated by the presacral nerves. Branches from the pelvic plexus innervate the lower rectum, upper anal canal, bladder, and sexual organs. Parasympathetic innervation originates from the anterior roots of S-2, S-3, and S-4. Other parasympathetics are distributed from the pelvic plexus to the bladder, genitals, and internal anal sphincter. An important subdivision of the pelvic plexus is the periprostatic plexus that supplies parasympathetic and sympathetic input to the prostate, seminal vesicles, corpora cavernosum, vas deferens, urethra, ejaculatory ducts, and bulbourethral glands damage to this nerve plexus results in sexual impotence or dysfunction.

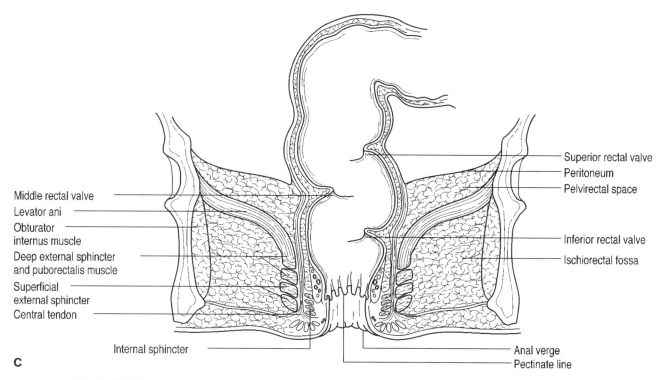

Middle rectal valve

Levator ani

Obturator
internus muscle

Deep external sphincter
and puborectalis muscle

Superficial
external sphincter

Central tendon

Superior rectal valve

Peritoneum

Pelvirectal space

Inferior rectal valve

Ischiorectal fossa

Internal sphincter

Anal verge

Pectinate line

C

FIG. 2. (C) View of rectum and anus in relation to pelvis. (A,B: Adapted from Gray JW, Skandalakis JE. *Atlas of surgical anatomy for general surgeons.* Baltimore: Williams and Wilkins, 1985.)

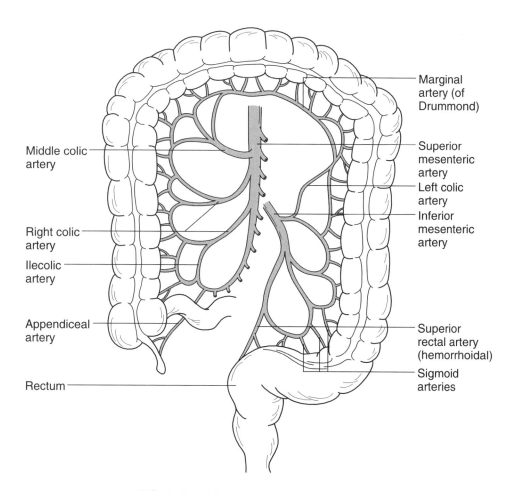

Middle colic
artery

Right colic
artery

Ilecolic
artery

Appendiceal
artery

Rectum

Marginal
artery (of
Drummond)

Superior
mesenteric
artery

Left colic
artery

Inferior
mesenteric
artery

Superior
rectal artery
(hemorrhoidal)

Sigmoid
arteries

FIG. 3. Arterial supply of the colon and rectum.

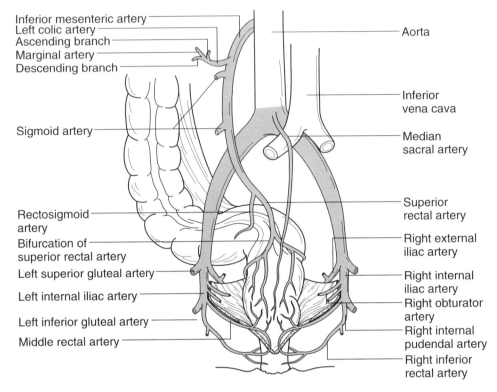

FIG. 4. Close-up of blood supply of the rectum. (Adapted from Gray JW, Skandalakis JE. *Atlas of surgical anatomy for general surgeons.* Baltimore: Williams and Wilkins, 1985.)

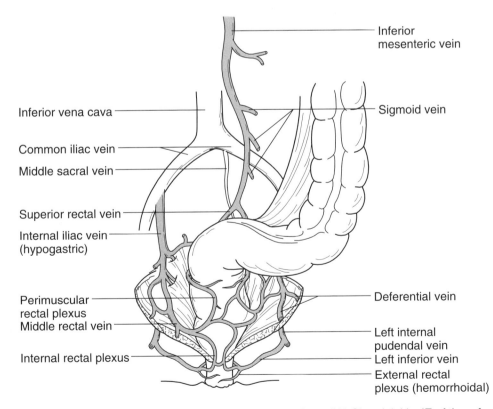

FIG. 5. Venous supply to rectum and anus. (Adapted from Gray JW, Skandalakis JE. *Atlas of surgical anatomy for general surgeons.* Baltimore: Williams and Wilkins, 1985.)

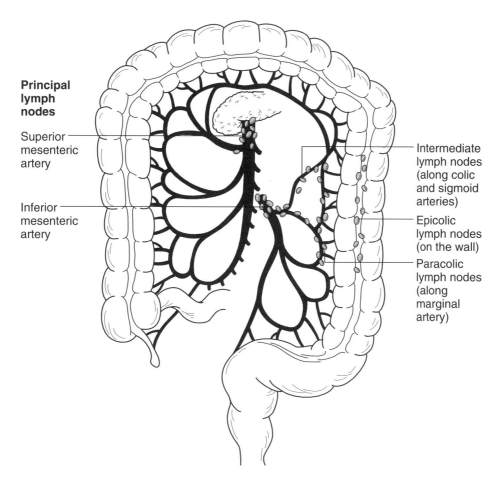

Principal lymph nodes

Superior mesenteric artery

Inferior mesenteric artery

Intermediate lymph nodes (along colic and sigmoid arteries)

Epicolic lymph nodes (on the wall)

Paracolic lymph nodes (along marginal artery)

FIG. 6. Lymphatic drainage of the colon. (Adapted from Gray JW, Skandalakis JE. *Atlas of surgical anatomy for general surgeons.* Baltimore: Williams and Wilkins, 1985.)

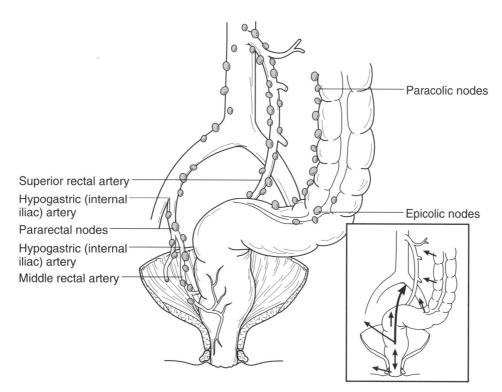

Superior rectal artery

Hypogastric (internal iliac) artery

Pararectal nodes

Hypogastric (internal iliac) artery

Middle rectal artery

Paracolic nodes

Epicolic nodes

FIG. 7. Lymphatic drainage of the rectum and anus. (Adapted from Gray JW, Skandalakis JE. *Atlas of surgical anatomy for general surgeons.* Baltimore: Williams and Wilkins, 1985.)

Motor supply to the external anal sphincter travels in the pudendal nerve (S-2, S-3) and the perineal branch of S-4. The motor supply to the internal anal sphincter is sympathetic (L-5) and parasympathetic (S-2, S-3 and S-4). The tone of the internal sphincter is mediated by both parasympathetic and sympathetic fibers.

Complete anal continence cannot be achieved unless the subject can sense the presence of material in the rectum and can discriminate the quality of the material (feces or gas). The receptors responsible for the appreciation of rectal fullness and impeding evacuation lie within the levator ani muscle. Stool accumulates in the rectum for a variable period of time before the urge to defecate is experienced. Continence is favored by the influence of pelvic muscles on rectal shape. The anal canal is pulled forward by the puborectalis muscle which, as a U-shaped sling, creates an angle of 80 to 90 degrees to the rectum. This anorectal angle (Fig. 2), maintained by the continuous tonic activity of the puborectalis is effective in preventing stool in the rectum from entering the anal canal.

When the rectum is distended, the internal sphincter relaxes (rectoanal inhibitory reflex). This relaxation allows the rectal content to move down the anal canal. In contrast when the rectum is distended, the external sphincter contracts. Reflex contraction of the external sphincter prevents rectal content from leaking through the anus. Although volitional contraction of the external sphincter can only be sustained for short periods, it is the most important mechanism of voluntary continence.

Defecation. The act of evacuating fecal material from the rectum, is a complex process that involves both a reflex response and a voluntary performance. When a fecal bolus enters the rectum, the stretch receptors, register a sensation and a urge to defecate. If rectal distention is maintained, the rectal musculature adapts to decrease the rectal pressure, the accommodation response. The act of defecation proceeds with the subject assuming the squatting or sitting position to straighten out the angle between the rectum and anal canal. Expulsion of the feces is accomplished by contraction of the rectum and by increased intraabdominal pressure by the Valsalva maneuver.

EVALUATION OF PATIENTS WITH COLORECTAL DISEASE

The diagnosis of diseases of the colon and rectum is based on a history and physical examination. Laboratory tests and radiographic studies and certainly endoscopic procedures should be directed by information obtained.

Common Colorectal Symptoms

Altered bowel habits, including constipation, diarrhea, tenesmus (urgency), or a combination, are associated with benign and malignant diseases. Bleeding per rectum may be sudden, dramatic, and life-threatening, or it may be occult. The amount of blood, its color (maroon or bright red), the presence of clots, and the relationship with defecation are important details of patient history. Similarly, mucus secretion may be a predominant part of patient history. Neoplasms, especially villous tumors and carcinoma, and inflammatory diseases can cause excessive mucus production.

The assessment of risk factors for neoplastic disease is important. Age, sex, and family history of neoplasms or inflammatory bowel disease should be noted. Familial adenomatous polyposis and other polyposis syndromes should be sought. Other cancers that are associated with familial colon cancer or cancer family syndromes include cancer of the endometrium, ovaries, and the breasts.

Physical Examination

Beyond the complete physical examination, particular attention should be directed to abdominal and rectal examinations. A mass is palpable in 50% of patients with carcinoma of the cecum, whereas only 10% of patients with cancer of the left colon have a palpable mass. Hepatomegaly may signify metastatic disease. On digital rectal examination, nearly half of rectal neoplasms are appreciated on valsalva maneuver. Gross blood or guaiac positive stool deserves evaluation to exclude malignancy of the colon and rectum.

Endoscopic Examination

Patient history and physical examination may be very suggestive of colorectal malignancy and endoscopy is a very sensitive method of detection. Anoscope allows inspection of the anal canal and distal rectum. Rigid proctosigmoidoscopy allows evaluation of up to 25 cm of combined rectum and sigmoid colon (Fig. 8); flexible sigmoidoscopy allows up to 65 to 70 cm of colon and rectum to be visualized. Both procedures are well tolerated by patients and can be performed in a clinic setting with minimal morbidity.

Colonoscopy permits examination of the entire colon from the anus to the cecum and often into the distal ileum as well. It is diagnostic and in certain conditions therapeutic. Polypectomy, control of bleeding, decompression of obstruction, removal of foreign bodies, and dilatation of strictures are among the therapeutic applications. Contraindications to colonoscopy include fulminant colitis, suspected acute diverticulitis, suspected colonic perforation, or recent colonic anastomosis.

Radiographic Evaluation of the Colon and Rectum

Barium enema (Fig. 9) has been the mainstay of diagnosis of diseases of the colon and rectum for nearly a cen-

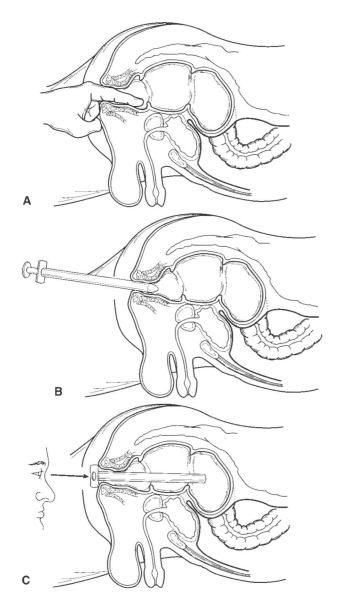

FIG. 8. Endoscopic examination. This figure shows performance of a rigid proctosigmoidoscopy. **(A)** Digital-rectal examination. **(B–C)** Insertion and proper placement of the scope. (Adapted from Gray JW, Skandalakis JE. *Atlas of surgical anatomy for general surgeons.* Baltimore: Williams and Wilkins, 1985.)

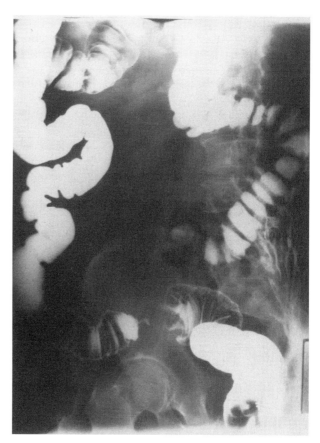

FIG. 9. Barium enema. Note apple core lesion. (Adapted from Gray JW, Skandalakis JE. *Atlas of surgical anatomy for general surgeons.* Baltimore: Williams and Wilkins, 1985.)

tury. Compared to colonoscopy, barium enema is safer, more often complete to the cecum, and less expensive. When properly performed, a barium enema is sensitive in detecting carcinoma in 94% of cases. Single-contrast barium enema uses a low density barium suspension. Double-contrast barium enema combines a viscous barium sulfate suspension of moderate high density and intraluminal insufflation with gas to displace the contrast to the mucosal surface. This technique visualizes colonic lesions as small as 1 cm in diameter. Computed tomography (CT) can stage colonic malignancy, detect recurrent cancer, diagnosis abscesses, and provide therapeutic options regarding drainage of pericolonic fluid collections.

DISEASES OF THE COLON

Ulcerative Colitis

Ulcerative colitis (UC) is a chronic inflammatory bowel disease of unknown etiology affecting the large intestine. The annual incidence of UC has risen worldwide during the past decade, affecting four to six per 100,000 individuals. Although uncommon, UC is not rare. With medical treatment, many patients suffering from UC can maintain good health. In a substantial number of patients, however, the medical treatment fails or an acute exacerbation in disease supervenes necessitating an operation. It should be recognized as well that there is a cumulative risk of the development of colon cancer in patients with UC. Approximately 12% of patients develop colon cancer after 25 years of disease and 30% after 35 years of disease.

Other factors may be important in the pathogenesis of UC. Recently, evidence for genetic heterogeneity has emerged from studies of antineutrophil cytoplasmic anti-bodies (ANCA) in UC; additionally, there is an associa-tion with HLA-DR2. Environmental factors, including infectious agents, may trigger disease activity by altering the target tissue, or more likely, by stimulating the mucosal immune system. Cigarette smoking may be the cause of these effects mentioned.

Pathology

UC, for the most part, is a disease confined to the mucosal and submucosal layers of the colonic wall. The entire colon or a segment of colon can be affected by UC. The rectum is typically involved. Usually, there are no normal segments of colon that bridge between dis-eased segments. Occasionally, with severe pancolitis, the terminal ileum may develop secondary inflammation and dilatation, termed "backwash ileitis." On gross inspection, the colonic mucosa demonstrates healed granular superficial ulcers superimposed on a friable and thickened mucosa with increased vascularity. Patients may also demonstrate superficial fissures and small and regular pseudopolyps. In its earlier stage, the typical lesion consists of infiltration of round cells and poly-morphonucleocytes into the crypts of Lieberkuhn at the base of the mucosa, forming crypt abscesses. As the lesions progress, there is a coalescence of crypt abscesses and desquamation of overlying cells to form an ulcer. Collagen and a luxurious growth of granulation tissue occupy the areas of ulceration, which extend down to, but rarely through, the muscularis.

Clinical Manifestations

Bloody diarrhea, abdominal pain, and fever are typi-cal presenting symptoms. Sixty percent of patients pre-sent with a relatively mild attack that occurs as a seg-mental colitis involving the distal colon (80%) or as a pancolitis (20%). Five percent to 15% of patients with disease limited to the rectosigmoid area show eventual progression to involve most, if not all, of the length of the colon.

Physical findings are directly related to the duration and presentation of the disease. In the active phase, the abdomen in the region of the colon is tender to palpation. During acute attacks or in the fulminant form of the dis-ease, there may be signs of an acute surgical abdomen accompanied by fever, and decreased bowel sounds. In patients with toxic colitis, abdominal distention may indicate colonic distention.

Extraintestinal manifestations of UC include ocular lesions (e.g., uveitis, iritis, conjunctivitis) and peripheral joint disease. Ankylosing spondylitis is seen in 1% to 6% of patients, and sacroiliitis is observed in 4% to 18% of patients. Lesions of the oral cavity and skin are fre-quently observed in patients with UC. Aphthous stom-atitis and gingivitis and erythema nodosum are typical pathologies. Up to 80% of patients, especially patients with pancolitis, demonstrate histologic evidence of peri-cholangitis on liver biopsy. Sclerosing cholangitis is observed in 1% to 4% of patients; the development of biliary cirrhosis is infrequent though not rare.

Diagnosis

A presumptive diagnosis of UC is one of exclusion. An infectious etiology must be excluded in all patients presenting with diarrhea or bloody diarrhea. Stool sam-ples and biopsy specimens should be evaluated for Campylobacter, Salmonella, pathogenic *Escherichia coli,* Aeromonas, amebic colitis, and *Clostridia difficile.*

Flexible sigmoidoscopy is appropriate because UC involves the distal colon and rectum in 90% to 95% of cases. Mild cases may only show a loss of normal vas-cular pattern, a granular texture, and microhemorrhages when the friable mucosa is touched or wiped. In severe cases, there is macroulceration with profuse bleeding and purulent exudate. In advanced disease, areas of ulceration may surround areas of heaped-up granulation tissue and edematous mucosa, so-called pseudopolyps.

Barium enema examination of the colon is useful in most patients with quiescent disease, although con-traindicated in those patients with acute fulminant dis-ease. A mild case of acute UC may be manifested by a diffusely granular appearance, which is best seen on air-contrast barium enema. End stage UC is characterized by shortening of the colon, loss of normal redundancy of the sigmoid colon and at the splenic and hepatic flexures, disappearance of the haustral pattern, and narrowed cal-iber of the bowel (Fig. 10, "lead-pipe colon").

Medical Therapy of UC

Drug therapy for UC consists of antiinflammatory or chemotherapeutic agents. Sulphasalazine (an aminosali-cylate) was the first drug found to have proven therapeu-tic efficacy in patients with quiescent or mild UC. It was developed with the aim of delivering a compound con-sisting of an antibacterial, sulfapyridine, attached to an antiinflammatory agent (5-aminosalicylic acid; 5-ASA), to the connective tissue of joints in patients with rheuma-toid arthritis and the mucosa of patients with UC. Sul-phasalazine is metabolized by colonic bacteria and azo-reduction to produce the sulpha and salicylate moieties in the colonic lumen. Most sulphapyridine is absorbed, acetylated by the liver, and excreted by the kidneys. Most of the 5-ASA, however, remains within the lumen and is excreted mainly in the feces.

Alternative delivery methods include direct colonic luminal applications (enema, suppository, foam), substi-

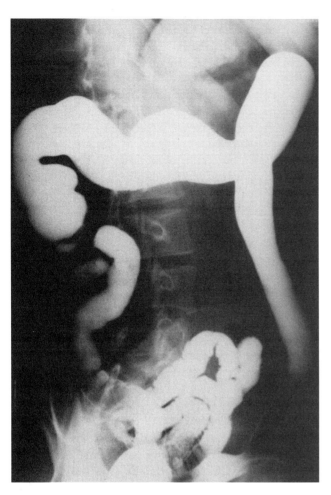

FIG. 10. "Lead-pipe colon."

tute azo-bond formulations, or delayed release preparations. These formulations bypass small bowel absorption of 5-ASA, allowing direct delivery to the colonic mucosa.

Chemotherapeutic Agents for UC

The immunomodulatory effect of corticosteroids is well known and makes it a useful agent in the treatment of UC. Steroids, however, have not been effective in preventing relapses without inducing undesirable long-term sequelae. The antimetabolite azathioprine and its hepatic conversion product 6-mercaptopurine, although controversial, have been shown to have therapeutic efficacy in a select group of patients with UC.

Surgical Therapy for UC

Drug therapy for UC is purely palliative. The only potential curative therapy rests with surgical intervention. Proctocolectomy with a Brooke ileostomy remains as the gold standard, against which all other surgical treatments for UC must be compared. It is a safe procedure with neg-

ligible mortality and a low rate of morbidity. This procedure is indicated while the surgeon is dealing with complications of a pouch operation, poor anal sphincter function, and associated severe medical problems, or when Crohn's colitis cannot be excluded.

If the rectum is spared and sphincter function is good, total abdominal colectomy with ileorectal anastomosis is a satisfactory surgical option. The procedure preserves bladder and sexual function and provides a statistically significant number of patients with adequate anorectal function. It must be recognized that inflammatory changes of the rectum may develop and the risk of cancer in the retained rectum is the same as that of the excised colon. As a consequence, regular surveillance is required.

Proctocolectomy with ileo-anal anastomosis has become an established surgical treatment of UC. It provides ideal therapy—eradication of disease, preservation of anorectal physiologic function, and return to high-quality life-style. The distal ileum is constructed into a variety of different pouches (e.g., "J," "S," "W") to provide a neorectum with reservoir capability. This pouch is then anastomosed to the anus.

Acute complications of UC that necessitate an urgent operation include (in decreasing order of frequency) toxic megacolon, perforation, and massive hemorrhage. In most emergency cases, the colon is extensively or totally involved (pancolitis). In 50% of the cases undergoing urgent surgical intervention for UC, the disease was recently diagnosed. In these emergencies, the safest operation is colectomy with ileostomy and a distal rectal mucous fistula.

Crohn's Colitis

It is accepted that Crohn's disease can affect any segment of bowel from mouth to anus. About two-thirds of patients with Crohn's disease have some involvement of the colon in addition to other segments of diseased intestine. Approximately two-thirds of patients with Crohn's colitis have a pancolitis pattern, while the remainder have a segmental distribution.

Clinical diagnosis is often difficult but is based on patient history and physical examination. The majority of Crohn's colitis patients complain of abdominal pain and rectal bleeding. Barium enema may reveal the typical segmental disease pattern but will often miss the subtle changes associated with mild and early disease. Endoscopy, particularly colonoscopy, is the only sure method of confirming inflammatory bowel disease of the colon secondary to Crohn's disease.

Principal management of Crohn's colitis consists of medical therapy, e.g., sulfasalazine, 5-ASA compounds, and corticosteroids. Most patients can maintain a stable pattern of disease with occasional exacerbations in condition with medical compliance. Infrequently, complications arise—e.g., toxic colitis, perforation, colocutaneous fistula, hemorrhage, and obstruction—that require surgical intervention. Conservative surgical resection is the current standard approach with aims of postoperative medical palliation that may obviate further colonic resection. Additionally, sphincter-saving operations involving ileum to anus anastomosis, especially in the younger individual, may prevent the psychological and social heartache that accompanies an abdominal stoma.

Diverticular Disease

Diverticular disease of the colon is a pathology endemic to Western countries. High-fat and low-fiber (low-residue) diet predispose to the development of diverticulosis. It occurs in one-third of the population over the age of 45 and in up to two-thirds of the population over 85 years of age. Of those patients with diverticulosis, 10% to 25% will progress to diverticulitis. Typically, males are affected more than females.

The vast majority of colonic diverticula are false diverticula comprised of only mucosa and submucosa. A point of weakness of the colonic wall where mesenteric blood vessels penetrate the circular muscle layer, vasa recta, allows the outpouching of mucosa and submucosa (Fig. 11). This occurs typically about the intertaenial antimesenteric colonic wall. In up to 65% of patients, diverticulosis is limited to the sigmoid colon. In ~35%, at least one other area in addition to the sigmoid colon is involved (Fig. 12).

Diverticulitis results from inflammation and subsequent perforation of a colonic diverticulum. Perforation may result in a phlegmon, abscess formation, or diffuse fecal or purulent peritonitis. The initial assessment of the patient with suspected diverticulitis is similar to that of any patient presenting with abdominal pain. A detailed history and thorough physical examination with particu-

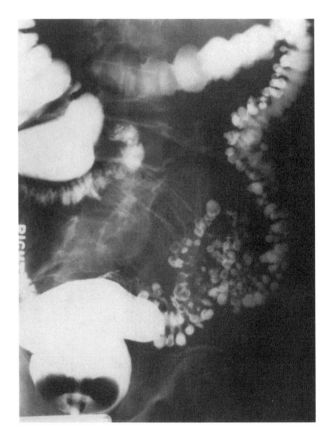

FIG. 12. Barium enema showing diverticulosis.

lar attention to the abdominal, rectal, and (in females) pelvic examinations. The majority of patients will have left lower quadrant pain (93% to 100%), fever (57% to 100%), and leukocytosis (69% to 83%). Fullness in the left lower quadrant on abdominal palpation is common and signifies an inflammatory phlegmon. Other associated symptoms may include nausea, vomiting, constipation, diarrhea, dysuria, and frequency. Other disease entities that have similar presentations include irritable bowel syndrome, colon cancer, inflammatory bowel disease, ischemic colitis, bowel obstruction, and gynecologic and urologic diseases. The diagnosis can usually be made on the basis of clinical history and examination.

In cases where the diagnosis of diverticulitis is in question, radiologic studies, such as water-soluble contrast enema, barium enema, CT scan, and ultrasound, may be performed. Barium enema should generally be avoided in patients with suspected acute diverticulitis and localized peritoneal signs because of the risk of barium extravasation and resultant barium peritonitis. Similarly, endoscopy is usually avoided in the setting of acute diverticulitis because of the risk of perforating the inflamed colon.

CT scan has become increasingly useful as the initial imaging test in patients with suspected diverticulitis. Criteria for diagnosis of diverticulitis include colonic wall thickening, pericolic fat infiltration, pericolic or distant abscesses, and extraluminal air. In the era of cost con-

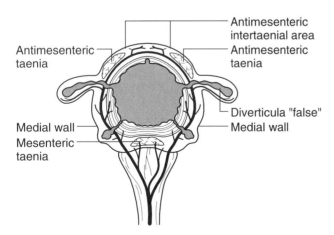

FIG. 11. Relationship of diverticula to colonic taeniae and vasculature.

tainment, a CT scan can be omitted from diagnostic studies, unless symptoms indicate the presence of a pericolonic abscess that requires percutaneous drainage.

Treatment

Conservative or medical treatment for acute uncomplicated diverticulitis entails bowel rest and intravenous antibiotics. In the majority of patients, resolution can be expected. The choice of antibiotics should be made with the knowledge that gram-negative rods and anaerobes are the usual pathogenic organisms. If the patient does not improve in several days, an abscess may be suspected and diagnostic imaging may be considered.

If the index episode of diverticulitis resolves, patients should be reevaluated preferably with colonoscopy but at least flexible sigmoidoscopy and double-contrast barium enema. Long-term fiber supplementation after the first episode of diverticulitis may prevent recurrence in >70% in the ensuing 5 years.

Complications from acute diverticulitis include abscess, fistula, obstruction, stricture, and free perforation. The Hinchey classification describes the spectrum of perforated colonic diverticulitis ranging from limited, localized inflammatory process (phlegmon) to fecal peritonitis.

Treatment of patients with diverticular abscess depends on the magnitude and location of the abscess as well as the patient's clinical condition at the time of the diagnosis. Small pericolic abscesses may resolve with antibiotic therapy and bowel rest. Large diverticular abscesses typically do not resolve with medical treatment and require either percutaneous or surgical drainage. The potential advantage of percutaneous drainage is avoidance of an operation and temporary stoma.

Abscesses that are not amenable to CT-guided percutaneous drainage or in whom clinical symptoms persist following percutaneous drainage should undergo laparotomy. Primary resection of the diseased colon segment and construction of an end proximal colostomy should be performed. The distal colon segment can be constructed to a mucus fistula or blind (Hartmann's) pouch.

Free perforation of acute diverticulitis is a surgical emergency and carries a 6% to 35% mortality rate. Emergent segmental resection with colostomy should be undertaken. Large bowel obstruction secondary to diverticulitis should be treated similarly.

Diverticular disease may also be complicated by the development of fistulas from the diseased colon to other viscera or skin. Colon to bladder (colovesical) fistulas account for about half of fistulas due to diverticulitis. Patients typically complain of urinary tract symptoms, including urgency, dysuria, pneumaturia, and fecaluria. Although rare in the past, there is an increase in the occurrence of colon to vagina (colovaginal) fistulas. The absence of a uterus predisposes female patients with diverticulitis to developing colovaginal fistulas.

Volvulus

Volvulus describes torsion of the bowel about its mesentery to cause narrowing of the bowel or strangulation of the blood vessels or both. It affects the elderly more than younger individuals especially those with a longstanding history of constipation with reliance upon laxatives or enemas and those individuals with neuropsychiatric disorders in chronic care facilities. Two major predisposing factors necessary for colonic volvulus to occur are (a) a segment of redundant mobile colon and (b) relatively fixed point or points around which the volvulus may occur. The two areas of the colon with long mesenteries that permit volvulus are the sigmoid colon (90% of cases) and the cecum (10% of cases).

Acute colonic volvulus generally presents as sudden onset of severe colicky abdominal pain, obstipation, and abdominal distention. Several radiographic findings are consistent with colonic volvulus. In many cases, distended loops of colon form a "bent inner tube" appearance. The curve loop usually points away from the obstruction, and the narrow pointed bowel points toward the obstruction. There is an air-fluid level, which tends to be single in cecal volvulus and double in transverse colon and sigmoid volvulus, owing to the "double closed loop obstruction." A "bird beak" deformity demonstrated by barium enema at the site of torsion is pathognomonic if present.

Emergent reduction of the volvulus by proctoscopy and the use of a long rectal tube passed through the sigmoidoscope is required and can be performed at the bedside provided the clinical status of the patient is stable. Upon reduction, if intraluminal sanguinous fluid is appreciated or the mucosa appears necrotic, emergent laparotomy and colonic resection must be performed. In the absence of necrotic bowel, an elective resection or rectopexy should be performed because there is an appreciable incidence of recurrence (59%) after volvulus reduction.

Ischemic Colitis

Ischemic colitis represents the most common form of gastrointestinal (GI) ischemia. It typically develops "spontaneously," in the absence of major vascular occlusion and in the presence of viable intestine elsewhere. Ischemic colitis may develop in people who are otherwise healthy, although a variety of clinical settings, such as shock, predispose to its occurrence. It usually presents as an acute abdominal illness with bloody diarrhea. Diagnosis is confirmed by colonoscopy.

Nongangrenous colonic ischemia will invariably resolve with aggressive reperfusion of the splanchnic vascular system usually and is associated with a good prognosis. Chronic colonic ischemia may lead to colonic strictures, occasionally requiring surgery.

Lower Gastrointestinal Bleed

Acute hemorrhage from the GI tract is a common clinical problem. A lower GI bleed is defined as bleeding distal to the ligament of Treitz and usually presents as the passage of maroon or bright red blood passed through the rectum. Although numerous potential causes have been identified, colonic diverticulosis and vascular ectasia (arteriovenous malformations) of the colon are the most common causes of massive lower GI hemorrhage. Bleeding from the small bowel is exceedingly rare.

Vascular ectasias typically arise in the right colon of elderly patients and present characteristically as recurring low-grade hemorrhage. Early lesions are ectatic capillaries and venules, and bleeding from these lesions usually ceases spontaneously and is rarely associated with life-threatening hemorrhage. Progression to advanced lesions (arteriovenous communications) occurs and can result in hematochezia or massive hemorrhage. Even with massive hemorrhage, however, bleeding usually ceases spontaneously in the majority of patients.

Hemorrhage from diverticular disease can be massive or occult. Because the colon can contain large volume of blood, neither the volume nor the frequency of bloody stools is a reliable guide to the rate of hemorrhage. Most patients with diverticular disease stop bleeding spontaneously; only 20% of patients suffer continued hemorrhage.

Diagnostic Evaluation of Lower GI Bleeding

Gastric aspiration is used to exclude a source proximal to the ligament of Treitz, which manifests as lower GI bleeding in 10% to 15% of cases (Fig. 13). It is the presence of bile and not the absence of blood in the gastric aspirate that excludes an upper intestinal source of lower GI bleeding. Rigid sigmoidoscopy is performed to exclude an anorectal source of hemorrhage.

In a hemodynamically stable patient who is actively passing blood per rectum, a radionuclide scan using Tc sulfur colloid or Tc-labeled autologous red blood cells is performed provided upper GI bleeding and rectal bleeding have been excluded. Sulfur colloid given intravenously is cleared rapidly by the reticuloendothelial system, but extravasation into the lumen may be detectable with bleeding rate as low as 0.1 to 0.5 ml/min. The advantage of using ^{99mm}Tc-labeled autologous red blood cells fro the index bleeding scan is that a repeat bleeding scan can be performed should recurrent bleeding occur within 24 to 48 hr of the first episode. If no active bleeding is appreciated and the patient remains clinically stable, an urgent colonoscopy can be undertaken after the large bowel is cleansed. If the bleeding scan demonstrates active bleeding, a selective mesenteric angiogram localizes bleeding as low as 0.5 to 1.0 ml/min. Intraarterial infusion of vasopressin may induce enough vasoconstriction to promote hemostasis; however, 50% of patients rebleed on cessation of therapy. Because of the extensive collateral arterial supply of the colon, selective arterial embolization is only infrequently successful.

In general, colonoscopy is a useful diagnostic procedure for determining the cause of lower GI hemorrhage in a clinically stable patient who is not bleeding profusely. The bleeding site was identified in 94% of patients using colonoscopy and upper endoscopy in a large series.

Operative intervention should be performed if other measures fail and the patient continues to bleed. If transfusion requirements exceed 4 U in the first 24 hr, there is a 50% chance that operation will be required. If there is no localization of the site of bleeding, it may be necessary to perform a total abdominal colectomy and ileorectal anastomosis in these circumstances. Preoperative localization of bleeding may help limit the amount of colon resection required.

Colorectal Polyps

Polypoid lesions of mucosa of the colon and rectum can be divided into three major classes (Table 1). Tubular adenomas consist of benign epithelium; they increase in number with age and occur about eight times more frequently than villous adenomas. About 80% are located in the rectum and sigmoid colon. The typical tubular adenoma is a pedunculated firm condensation of densely packed colonic mucosal glands that often resemble colonic epithelium. Variable amounts of nuclear atypia may be evident. The stalk typically has normal colonic mucosa. The average size is 1 to 2 cm. The bigger the size of the polyp, the greater is the probability that carcinoma exists (Table 2).

Villous adenomas typically assume a gross cauliflower like configuration. Most are confined to the sigmoid or rectum; 15% originate in the proximal colon. These lesions have a greater propensity for harboring foci of invasive carcinoma. In one large series, over half of villous adenomas of >2 cm contained histologic malignancy (Table 2).

Patients with large tumors may present with obstruction, abdominal cramps, or obstipation. Microcytic anemia from chronic occult blood loss commonly occurs. Rarely, a villous tumor may produce profuse mucous diarrhea, circulatory collapse with electrolyte and water depletion, metabolic acidosis, and prerenal azotemia.

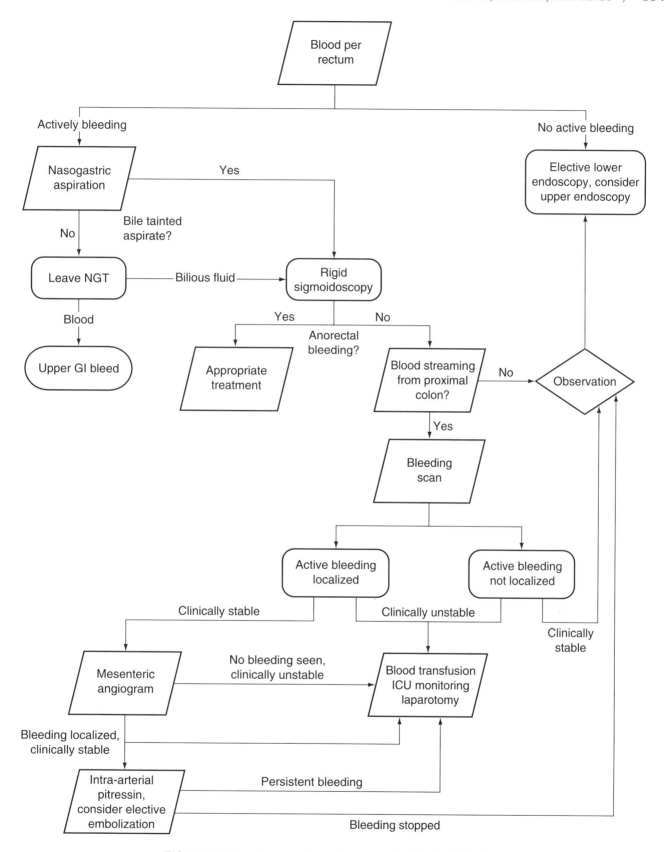

FIG. 13. Diagnostic evaluation of lower gastrointestinal bleeding.

TABLE 1. *Classification of colon polyps*

Neoplastic polyps	Nonneoplastic polyps	Unclassified polyps
Tubular	Hamartomas	Hyperplastic
Tubulovillous	Leiomyomas	Carcinoid tumors
Villous	Hemangiomas	Heterotypic
	Inflammatory	

As a general rule, all polyps of >1.0 cm in diameter should be removed for tissue diagnosis. Pedunculated polyps can contain invasive cancer, but as long as the stalk was included in the resected specimen and there is no evidence of malignancy at the margin, a curative procedure has been performed. In contradistinction, invasive cancer in sessile polyps usually necessitates colonic resection as definitive therapy.

Colorectal Cancer

Over 155,000 new cases are diagnosed each year in the United States. Adenocarcinoma of the large bowel is the second most common malignancy in the United States and the second leading cause of all cancer-related deaths. When diagnosed in its early stages, however, this malignancy is curable by surgical treatment with minimal morbidity and mortality.

Epidemiology

Dietary factors play important causative and protective roles in the development of large bowel cancers. As previously stated, the high-fat diet and low-fiber diet of Western civilization is associated with colon cancer development. Lack of antioxidant vitamins (e.g., ascorbic acid, vitamins A and E, glutathione) and minerals (e.g., selenium) in the diet are associated with a higher incidence of colon cancer.

Hereditary influences are associated with the risk of developing colon cancer. There are four genetic alterations that have been recently defined to be associated with colorectal cancer: ras gene mutations and allelic deletions of chromosomes 5q, 17p, and 18q. Several familial polyposis syndromes, characterized by numerous adenomatous polyps, are associated with a high risk for

TABLE 2. *Incidence of malignancy harbored within a colonic polyp correlated with type and size*

Type	Size	Incidence of CA
Tubular	<1 cm	<1%
	>2 cm	~35%
Tubulovillous	<1 cm	~3.5%
Villous	<1 cm	~10%
	>2 cm	~50%

the development of large bowel cancers. The most significant of these syndromes is familial polyposis coli. Innumerable adenomatous polyps develop by adolescence. This disease is inherited as an autosomal dominant trait, with 90% penetrance. Unless proctocolectomy is performed in early adulthood, virtually all affected patients develop cancer by age 55.

Gardner's syndrome is another hereditary colonic adenomatous polyp syndrome associated with osteomas of the mandible, skull, and long bones, and soft tissue tumors, including sebaceous cysts, fibromas, lipomas, and desmoid tumors. Turcot's syndrome is characterized as a familial colonic polyposis syndrome associated with malignant central nervous system tumors.

The polyp to carcinoma conversion theory is accepted as the etiology of a majority of adenocarcinomas of the colon. Clinicians need only to recognize the incidence of invasive carcinoma in villous adenomatous polyps to understand the correlation. The pathogenesis sequence of the polyp to cancer involves early metaplastic and finally dysplastic changes of the colonic mucosa. Several of the above mentioned factors and others have been implicated as causative agents.

Two types of familial colon cancer syndromes have been described that are not associated with polyposis, i.e., hereditary nonpolyposis colon cancer syndrome (HNPCC). Lynch syndrome I is an autosomal dominant trait in which patients develop multiple colon cancers much earlier than is typically seen. The cancers that develop have a predilection for the proximal colon. Lynch syndrome II, also called "cancer family syndrome," is a closely related inherited disease that includes all the features seen in Lynch syndrome I but also is characterized by the early onset of carcinoma at other sites e.g., endometrium, ovaries, and GI tract.

Pathology

The vast majority of large bowel cancers are adenocarcinomas, with the remainder histologic types being squamous cell carcinomas, adenosquamous carcinomas, lymphomas, sarcomas, and carcinoid tumors. Features associated with poor prognosis include blood vessel invasion, lymphatic vessel invasion, and absence of a lymphocytic response to the tumor, mucin production, and aneuploidy.

Diagnosis

The least expensive and potentially most informative study for colorectal tumors is the digital examination. Occult blood in the stool may be the only indication of colonic pathology. In contrast, a palpable rectal malignancy can be evaluated for circumference of rectal wall involvement, distance from anal verge and degree of fixation to sacrum. Double-contrast barium enema is sensitive in detecting small polyps or cancers. Rigid sigmoidoscopy is comparatively inexpensive but is limited to the length of bowel that can be examined and by the patient's compliance. It should be performed to exclude rectal lesions since visualization of this area is inadequate by barium enema. Colonoscopy is the most widely used diagnostic study to evaluate the colon. Polypectomies can be performed via the colonoscope. Mucosal tissue specimens can be obtained for diagnosis. The entire colon can be evaluated for synchronous lesions.

With regard to rectal cancer, endorectal ultrasound has been established as an extremely useful tool in preoperative assessment. Each of the layers of the rectum can be sonographically visualized, with a tumor usually appearing as a hypoechoic disruption of the rectal wall. The procedure may also reveal if underlying lymph nodes are affected. Most studies indicate a sensitivity and a specificity of 90%.

The impact of screening programs on reducing mortality in the general population has not yet been definitely proved. For the general population, many clinicians advocate yearly fecal occult blood tests and sigmoidoscopy every 2 to 35 years beginning at the age of 40.

Staging

The prognosis of colon cancer is not related to the size of the primary tumor but rather the degree of penetration of the tumor through the bowel wall and the presence or absence of nodal involvement. These two characteristics form the basis for all staging systems developed for this disease.

Dukes classified the depth of invasion of rectal tumors in stages from A to C. Stage A indicated penetration through the muscularis mucosa but not through the muscularis propria. Stage B represented penetration through the muscularis propria into the perirectal fat without lymph node involvement. Stage C represented metastasis to the lymph nodes regardless of the extent of bowel wall penetration. Stage D of contemporary modified Dukes classification signifies distant metastatic disease. The primary tumor/regional nodes/metastasis (TNM) classification is very similar to the Dukes classification and is the current staging system recognized by the World Health Organization (Table 3).

Surgical Therapy

The only potential curative therapy for colon cancer requires surgical extirpation of the tumor. Prior to undertaking surgical resection, a few concerns must be addressed.

The determination of metastatic disease prior to operation is not absolutely mandatory. In the presence of

TABLE 3. *Five-year survival of colon cancer related to stage of disease*

TNM	Dukes	Five-year survival
I	A	90%
II	B$_1$	75%
	B$_2$	60–70%
III	C$_1$	35%
	C$_2$	20–30%
IV	D	<5%

metastatic disease, prevention of complications of the primary tumor (e.g., intestinal obstruction, lower GI bleeding) takes clinical precedence over the metastatic foci. One must recognize that critical decisions should be individualized in patients with widespread metastasis. For rectal tumors, determination of its distance from the anal verge and its mobility are important in assessing resectability and type of operation possible. A preoperative serum carcinoembryonic antigen (CEA) level is useful in correlating the completeness of resection and in subsequent reevaluations of the patient for recurrence. CEA is a glycoprotein found in the cell membranes of many tissues including malignant neoplasms of the colon and rectum. Tissue CEA concentrations are lower in poorly differentiated colorectal cancers than in well differentiated lesions. Elevation of CEA levels is not specific for colorectal cancer and can be elevated in numerous other pathologies e.g., pancreatitis, pancreatic tumors, chronic excessive cigarette smoking, and gynecologic tumors.

Complete surgical resection of a primary colorectal cancer entails en bloc resection that encompasses an adequate amount of normal colon proximal and distal to the tumor, adequate lateral margins if the tumor is adherent to contiguous structures, and removal of the regional lymph node basin (Fig. 14). At the time of surgical resection, a thorough investigation of the abdominal viscera, particularly the liver and peritoneal surfaces, should be performed. Intraoperative ultrasound has a higher sensitivity than CT scan in detecting liver metastasis.

Adjuvant Therapy

About 25% and 50% of patients with stage II and III tumors, respectively, eventually die from growth of micrometastatic disease present at the time of primary tumor removal. Chemotherapy given after surgical resection of advanced disease (stage III and some stage II) improves disease-free and overall survival. 5-Fluorouracil combined with levamisole is standard adjuvant chemotherapy. In general, the use of radiation therapy is limited to rectal cancer. Decreased incidence of local recurrence may result by administering preoperative or postoperative pelvic radiation.

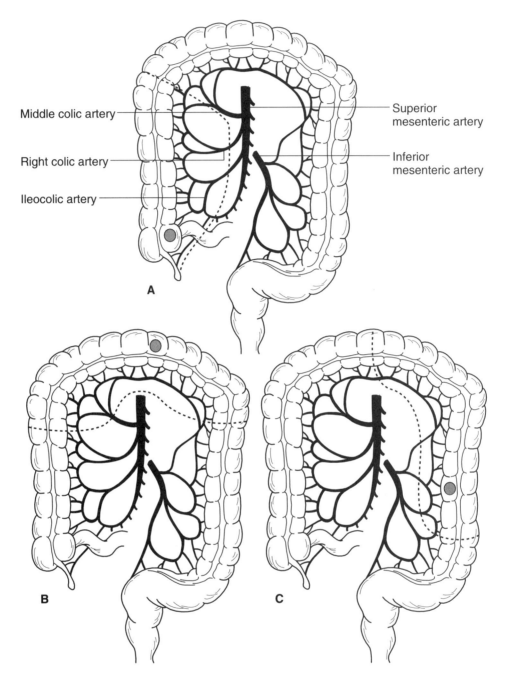

FIG. 14. Appropriate resections for colon cancer. **(A)** Right hemicolectomy for a lesion of the ascending colon. **(B)** Transverse colectomy for a lesion in the midtransverse colon. **(C)** Left hemicolectomy for lesions in the sigmoid colon.

ANORECTAL DISORDERS

Hemorrhoids

Three groups of hemorrhoidal complexes exist at the right anterior, right posterior, and left lateral areas of the anal canal. They are arterio-venous channels in the submucous space that assist in the smooth transanal passage of stool. They become symptomatic when they become engorged with blood. External hemorrhoids occur below the level of the dentate line and are easily seen on inspection of the anus. Because of its somatic innervation, thrombosis results in exquisite tenderness. Internal hemorrhoids, which occur above the level of the dentate line, are closely associated with their external components and are better appreciated by anoscopy. These typically present as painless postdefecation bleeding per anus. Thrombosis can produce a poorly localized anal discomfort.

The three cardinal symptoms of hemorrhoids are bleeding, protrusion, and pain. A burning sensation commonly accompanies engorgement of hemorrhoidal tissue. Bleeding is usually minimal, bright red, and associated with straining. Bleeding can sometimes be profuse and spontaneous.

Medical management is satisfactory in most patients except those in the acute stages of disease. A diet high in fiber together with an attempt to establish a healthy bowel habit pattern often results in temporary or permanent abatement of symptoms. The patient should be encouraged to drink at least five 8-oz glasses of water throughout the day in an attempt to maintain proper stool consistency.

Patients with external hemorrhoids that do not respond to the above measures would benefit from hemorrhoidectomy. Refractory internal hemorrhoids can be treated with sclerotherapy, infrared coagulation, or rubber banding as a more conservative approach to treatment before suggesting surgical hemorrhoidectomy. Most patients with third and fourth degree internal hemorrhoids (Table 4) would be best advised to undergo surgical hemorrhoidectomy.

Fissures

Fissure in ano is a "crack" in the epithelium of the anal canal. Ulcer in ano is a chronic fissure. The lesion is classically associated with bleeding and intense pain at the time of defecation.

A traumatic event is thought to cause fissures, such as the passage of a hard stool or severe diarrhea. In the first instance, a mechanical tear results, and in the second, a chemical burn is caused by severe alkalinity, which usually accompanies diarrhea. Many patients also present with a skin tag or a sentinel "pile" distal to the lesion, signaling the presence of a fissure just proximal to it. The most common location for fissures is in the posterior and anterior midline just below the level of the dentate line.

Most patients complain of "hemorrhoids," and only on thorough inspection of the anus is it evident that the clinical problem is due to fissure in ano. Severe undescribable pain and intense cutting, tearing, and knife-like sensations lasting many hours are classic symptoms. Bleeding is always bright red, and the pain is associated with and immediately follows a bowel movement. Lesions that are painless, especially those with extensive inflammation around the lesion, should be fully investigated. When symptoms of diarrhea and cramping abdominal pain are present, Crohn's disease should be ruled out.

Acute fissures should be treated conservatively with bulking agents to promote a softer stool. Patients should be encouraged to have a bowel movement as soon as urge comes. Lidocaine 5% applied to the anus just prior to the bowel movement is often helpful as well as nitroglycerine ointment $\frac{1}{2}$%. Oral pain medication and even a muscle relaxant such as diazepam taken for a few days may promote healing. Fissures that do not heal or those with persistent pain may benefit from surgical release of the internal sphincter/lateral subcutaneous internal anal sphincterotomy.

Perirectal Abscesses and Fistulas

The pathogenesis of perirectal abscesses and fistulas are similar and thus are discussed together. Obstruction of the submucosal glands of the anus leads to inflammation and infection. With an exception for perianal abscesses, perirectal abscesses require formal incision and drainage in the operating room.

Fistula in ano is a chronic form of perirectal abscess that is spontaneously or surgically drained, but in which the abscess cavity does not heal completely, becoming instead an inflammatory track with a primary opening (internal opening) in the anal crypt at the dentate line and a secondary opening (external opening) in the perianal skin.

There are four forms of fistula in ano based on the relation of the fistula to the sphincter muscles (Fig. 15): intersphincteric, transsphincteric, suprasphincteric, and extrasphincteric fistulae. Extrasphincteric fistulas may arise from cryptoglandular origin, trauma, foreign body, inflammatory bowel disease, or pelvic abscess.

Most patients with fistula in ano have a previous history of anorectal abscess subsequently associated with intermittent drainage. Indeed, recurrence of a perianal abscess suggests the presence of a fistula in ano. The external opening is usually visible as a red elevation of granulation tissue with purulent or serosanguineous drainage on compression.

The location of the internal opening can be predicted by Goodsall's rule (Fig. 16). Proctoscopy and flexible sigmoidoscopy is performed to rule out other lesions and inflammatory bowel disease. To adequately treat fistula in ano, surgeons must be prepared to unroof the fistula, eliminate the internal opening, and establish adequate drainage.

TABLE 4. *Internal hemorrhoids*

Type	Definition
First degree	Complex bulges and bleeds at the time of defecation
Second degree	Complex prolapses at time of defecation but spontaneously reduce
Third degree	Complex prolapses at time of defecation and requires manual reduction
Fourth degree	Complex is prolapsed and incarcerated

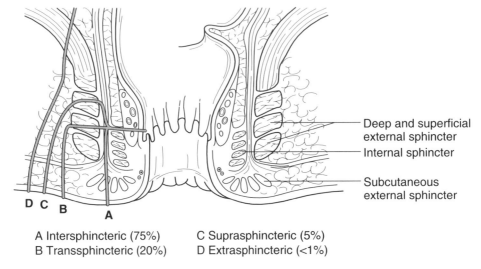

A Intersphincteric (75%)   C Suprasphincteric (5%)
B Transsphincteric (20%)   D Extrasphincteric (<1%)

FIG. 15. Incidence of fistula in ano.

Anal Condyloma

Anal condylomata acuminata are caused by a papilloma virus and are most commonly found in male homosexuals. In most patients, the warts involve the perianal skin, anal verge, and anoderm. Occasionally, the lesions also involve the mucosa of the upper anal canal and the lower rectum. The extent of the disease varies from a few small warts to an extensive mass occluding the anus. The diagnosis is usually obvious by the characteristic papillary appearance. Anoscopic examination is essential to detect intraanal involvement. Because most cases are transmitted sexually, other coexisting venereal diseases, especially gonorrhea and syphilis, should be excluded.

Small anal warts can be destroyed by applying podophyllin solution or bichloroacetic acid. Extensive warts in the perineal area or in the anal canal require electrocoagulation or excision. Recurrence is as high as 65%.

Anal Malignancy

Chronic anal wounds or irritation predisposes to an increased risk of anal malignancy. In particular, human papilloma virus, herpes simplex virus type 2, radiation exposure, and Crohn's disease have been linked to malignant development in the anogenital region. Although the exact mechanisms are yet to be defined, when risk factors are appreciated, early recognition of anal malignancy should be the goal.

Despite the knowledge that anal malignancies, when detected early, have a favorable prognosis, the vast majority of carcinomas are beyond locoregional control at the time of diagnosis and poor outcomes are common. Many patients complain of hemorrhoid pain, and often have anal bleeding and swelling. Digital anorectal examination and anoscopy are well tolerated by patients and can simply confirm or exclude the suspicion of anal malignancy. Additionally, inguinal lymph nodes require inspection should an anal neoplasm be confirmed.

Malignant melanoma of the anus carries a dismal prognosis owing to the aggressive characteristics of the disease and the propensity to disseminate in the early stages of disease. By the time symptoms of anal pressure and pain have developed, metastasis has invariably occurred. Overall 5-year survival is ~12% and correlates to the depth of penetration. Lesions with penetration of >2 mm

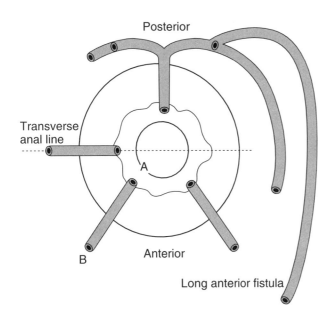

FIG. 16. Goodsall's rule.

were uniformly fatal before 5 years. Asymptomatic lesions encountered have a favorable outcome with wide local excision, provided that metastasis has not occurred. Otherwise, treatment is aimed at palliation of symptoms.

Epidermoid carcinoma of the anus (e.g., squamous cell, basaloid, mucoepidermoid) account for 1% to 2% of all large bowel malignancies. Therapy for these malignancies has evolved over the past 20 years and currently involves a multimodality approach. With an exception for the small lesion (<2 cm), which can be treated by wide local excision, larger lesions that were treated initially in the 1960s with surgery as the only therapy and then in the 1970s by radiation alone are now treated with combined neoadjuvant chemotherapy and radiation therapy (Nigro protocol). Favorable reduction in tumor burden is noted in a significant percentage of patients, some of whom will not require radical surgery for treatment (abdomino-perineal resection).

SUMMARY

Colorectal and anal disease affects a significant number of individuals every year. Clinical problem solving related to disease issues requires understanding of the principles presented here. Although many of the therapies may seem in constant evolution, it is hoped that the information will be incorporated into clinical knowledge to give confidence in fundamental treatment of patients with diseases of the colon, rectum, and anus.

STUDY QUESTIONS

1. Describe the arterial supply and venous drainage of the colon and rectum.
2. What are the embryological origins of the colon?
3. What are the predisposing risk factors for colorectal carcinoma?
4. What is appropriate treatment for patients with colorectal carcinoma?
5. Devise a screening program for colorectal cancer; devise a postoperative follow-up screening protocol for detection of recurrent/metastatic colorectal cancer.

SUGGESTED READING

Corman M.L. *Colon and rectal surgery.* 3rd ed. Philadelphia: J.B. Lippincott, 1993.

Gordon PH, Nivatvongs S. *Principles and practice of surgery for the colon, rectum and anus.* Montreal: Quality Medical Publishing, 1992.

Schwartz SI, Shires GT, Spencer FC. *Principles of surgery.* 6th ed. New York: McGraw-Hill, 1994.

CHAPTER 13

Liver, Portal Hypertension, and Spleen

Jose I. Almeida and Danny Sleeman

LIVER

Anatomy and Physiology

For centuries, the liver has been regarded as a mysterious organ with complex anatomy and physiology. The Babylonians considered the liver to be the seat of the soul. Prometheus symbolized the regenerative capability of the liver in Greek mythology. As his punishment handed down by Zeus, he was bound to a rock where a carnivorous bird preyed on his liver, which regenerated to allow the process to repeat for eternity. Hippocrates, along with many other Greek medicinal men, described the topographical and sometimes variable lobular anatomy of the liver. Galen hypothesized in the Middle Ages that the hepatic and portal vascular systems interconnected with hepatic veins within the liver. Although liver anatomy was masterfully diagrammed as early as the Renaissance period by Leonardo da Vinci, knowledge regarding hepatic anatomy remained rather rudimentary until the 19th century. In 1833, Kiernan characterized the lobule centered upon a hepatic venule as the basic unit of the liver. It was first reported in 1897 that the anatomic right and left lobes of the liver were divided not by the falciform ligament but by an anatomic line from the inferior vena cava and the gallbladder. In 1954, Couinaud described the eight lobes of the liver that are used by clinicians today to describe hepatic anatomy.

The ability to perform interventional or operative procedures on the hepatobiliary system necessitates knowledge of liver anatomy. The liver occupies most of the right upper quadrant and is protected by the right thoracic cage (ribs 5 to 10). As mentioned, the true anatomic division of the liver is drawn by a line between the gallbladder fossa and the inferior vena cava (Fig. 1). The surgical anatomy of the liver, described by Couinaud, is based on the distribution of portal veins, hepatic

veins, and intrahepatic biliary ductal systems (Fig. 2). The right lobe is subdivided into anteromedial (segments V and VIII) and posterolateral (segments VI and VII) segments. The left lobe is divided into medial (segments IV) and lateral (segments II and III segments). Segment I is comprised of the caudate lobe.

Reflections of peritoneum form ligaments that attach the liver to the abdominal wall, diaphragm, and abdominal viscera. The falciform ligament attaches the liver to the anterior abdominal wall and extends from the diaphragm superiorly to the umbilicus inferiorly. Within it runs the vestigial remnant of the left umbilical vein, which connects to the left portal vein. This umbilical vein is usually obliterated in the adult but may remain patent in patients with portal hypertension. The anterior and posterior right and left coronary ligaments connect the liver to the diaphragm. These ligaments extend laterally to form the right and left triangular ligaments.

The gastrohepatic and hepatoduodenal ligaments form the anterior layer of the lesser omentum. Within the gastrohepatic ligament courses the left gastric artery. In 15% of cases, the left hepatic artery branches off of the left gastric artery and will be found in this ligament. The hepatoduodenal ligament is the anterior boundary of the epiploic foramen of Winslow and contains the hepatic artery, portal vein, and the common bile duct. Occlusion of this ligament (the Pringle maneuver) is occasionally used to control bleeding from the liver. This interruption of blood supply is tolerated safely for up to 30 to 60 min without untoward effects after reperfusion.

The liver is afforded the luxury of a dual blood supply. The hepatic artery accounts for ~25% of hepatic blood flow. Normally, the common hepatic artery originating from the celiac trunk, gives off the right gastric and gastroduodenal arteries to become the proper hepatic artery which then bifurcates into right and left hepatic branches at the hepatic hilum (Fig. 3). However,

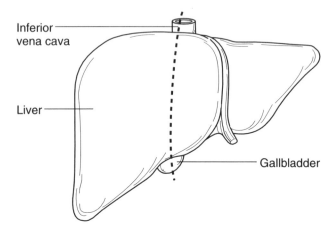

FIG. 1. *Dotted line* shows anatomic landmark dividing right and left lobes.

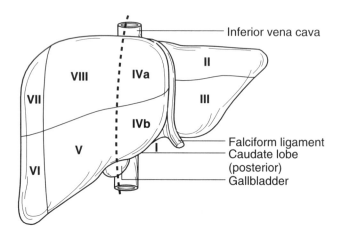

FIG. 2. Couinaud hepatic anatomy.

there is significant variability in hepatic arterial anatomy. The right hepatic artery occasionally arises from the superior mesenteric artery (17%), while the left hepatic artery sometimes arises from the left gastric artery (15%). Recognizing the existence of these variants during upper abdominal operations is crucial. The portal vein drains the splanchnic circulation and provides the liver with ~75% of its blood flow. The portal vein is formed behind the pancreas by the confluence of the superior mesenteric vein and the splenic vein. It bifurcates into right and left branches at the level of porta hepatis together with the hepatic artery (Fig. 3).

The hepatic veins begin in the liver lobules as the central veins and coalesce to form the right, left, and middle hepatic veins, which drain into the inferior vena cava. The right hepatic vein drains most of the right lobe. The left vein drains the lateral segment of the left lobe and a portion of the medial segment. The middle vein drains a portion of the anterior right lobe and medial left lobe segments. Unlike the hepatic artery, portal vein, and bile duct branches, the hepatic veins travel in planes between segments of the liver (Fig. 3).

The biliary drainage system is based upon the segmental liver anatomy. Beginning at the hepatocyte level, bile from the canaliculi drains into small intrahepatic biliary radicles that conduct the bile to segmental ducts, which ultimately terminate in the right and left hepatic ducts (Fig. 4). In up to 25% of cases, the large ducts draining segments V/VIII or segments VI/VII join aberrantly with the left ductal system (Fig. 4, inset). As with arterial anomalies, recognition of abnormal distribution of ductal drainage can prevent catastrophic complications from liver surgery.

The liver is a complex organ that performs a wide range of synthetic and metabolic functions. Some important functions of the liver include protein synthesis (e.g., albumin, coagulation factors, acute phase proteins), gluconeogenesis, glycogen synthesis, formation

of ketone bodies, cholesterol synthesis, and bile salt synthesis and metabolism. In addition, it plays a critical role in the metabolism of both water- and fat-soluble vitamins; it is the site of initial hydrolysis of vitamin D and is responsible for the metabolism of many drugs and toxins by the oxidative reactions of the cytochrome P- 450 system.

Surgical Disease of the Liver

Pyogenic and Amebic Liver Abscess

Pyogenic (bacterial) and amebic abscesses share many clinical features and are classically discussed together. The spread of bacteria or other organisms to the hepatic parenchyma may occur via (a) the portal venous system, (b) ascension from the biliary tree, (c) the hepatic artery during generalized septicemia, (d) direct extension from subhepatic or subdiaphragmatic infection, or (e) direct spread, i.e., following penetrating trauma. Intraabdominal pathology (e.g., appendicitis, diverticulitis) infrequently disseminates infection to the liver via portal venous drainage (pylephlebitis).

Both amebic and pyogenic hepatic abscesses are readily diagnosed with ultrasonography or computed tomography (CT) scan. Amebic liver abscesses follow intestinal infestation by *Entamoeba histolytica*. The most common cause of pyogenic liver abscess is biliary sepsis. These abscesses are often multiple. Treatment focuses on administration of intravenous antibiotics bacteriocidal against gram-negative rods, Enterococcus, and anaerobic bacteria. In addition to antibiotics, large pyogenic abscesses should be percutaneously drained with ultrasound or CT scan guidance. Amebic abscesses, however, have a propensity for free intraperitoneal rupture, whereas pyogenic abscesses do not. This may be related to the thin layer of granulation tissue around amebic disease compared with the more fibrous reaction

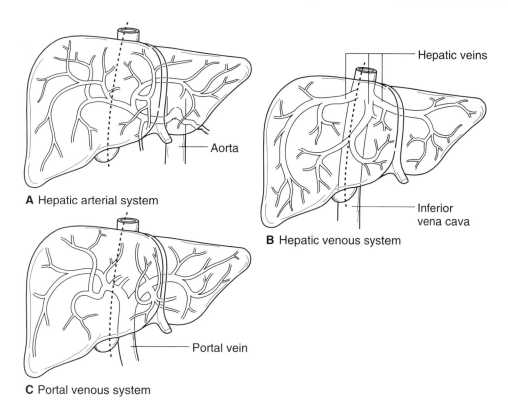

FIG. 3. **(A)** Arterial supply to the liver. **(B)** Portal vein supply to the liver. **(C)** Venous drainage from the liver.

of a pyogenic process. A positive indirect serum hemagglutination test confirms the presence of an amebic abscess. Treatment for amebic abscesses usually consists of metronidazole, although secondarily infected amebic abscesses require percutaneous drainage.

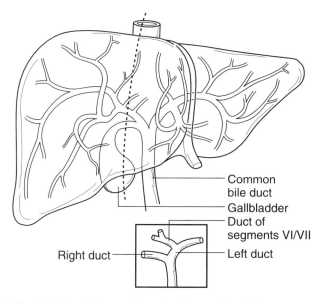

FIG. 4. Biliary drainage from the livery. *(Inset)* Segments V and VIII, or VI and VII may join aberrantly to the left.

Hepatic Cysts

Benign simple cysts are the most common cystic lesions of the liver. Virtually all are asymptomatic and are usually incidental findings on ultrasound or CT scan performed for an unrelated disorder. Benign cysts are uniform in shape, have a smooth surface, and lack septa. Operative intervention is indicated for abdominal pain secondary to cyst enlargement or when a neoplastic cyst cannot be excluded. For large simple cysts, unroofing and placement of an omental pedicle within the cavity to prevent reaccumulation of fluid is considered definitive treatment. This procedure can also be performed laparoscopically with good results. Cyst wall biopsy is mandatory to differentiate benign (cuboidal epithelium) from malignant (columnar epithelium) lesions.

Cystic neoplasms of the liver are unusual and can be diagnosed solely on the basis of CT scan or ultrasound examination. They are multilocular with irregular thick walls secondary to their columnar epithelium, which forms papillary projections. These cystic neoplasms require complete excision, whether symptomatic or not, to exclude the presence of malignancy.

Echinococcal (hydatid) cysts of the liver are the most frequent etiology of liver cysts worldwide. They are the result of the dog tapeworm *Echinococcus granulosis.* The cysts have an outer fibrous and sometimes calcific layer with an inner parasite-derived layer. The Casoni skin test has an 85% diagnostic sensitivity. The cysts are treated surgically by careful aspiration, followed by infusion of hypertonic saline. Peritoneal soiling must be avoided since the cyst fluid is highly antigenic and may result in acute anaphylactic shock.

Hepatic Neoplasms

Benign Hepatic Tumors

Cavernous hemangiomas are hamartomatous transformations of blood vessels and represent the most common benign hepatic tumors. Usually, these lesions are asymptomatic incidental findings on radiographic studies obtained for other reasons and can be observed safely. Occasionally, congestive heart failure is the result of arteriovenous malformation within the hemangioma. Platelet consumption within the hemangioma (Kasabach-Merritt syndrome) occasionally leads to thrombocytopenia. Rarely, patients have presented with hemorrhagic shock resulting from spontaneous rupture. Biopsy of a suspected hemangioma is absolutely contraindicated since the diagnosis can be made with certainty in most cases by scintigraphy, contrast-enhanced CT scans, magnetic resonance imaging (MRI), or angiography without the potential for catastrophic rupture and hemorrhage. Resection by enucleation is appropriate for symptomatic lesions, for enlarging lesions, or if the diagnosis is uncertain.

Hepatic adenoma and focal nodular hyperplasia (FNH) are benign neoplasms with both important similarities and distinguishing characteristics. Both occur commonly in women of child-bearing age. The pathogenesis of hepatic adenoma is related to the use of oral contraceptives and other exogenous steroids, and is also seen in certain glycogen storage diseases. The relationship of FNH with oral contraceptive and steroid use has been reported; however, it is not widely accepted. Hepatic adenoma may rupture and bleed in up to 50% of patients, whereas FNH rarely rupture. Malignant transformations of hepatic adenoma is well recognized, while the risk of malignancy in FNH is uncertain. Histologically, hepatic adenoma consists of hepatocytes without bile ducts or Kupffer cells and is demonstrated well by technetium-sulfur colloid scan. A central stellate scar is pathognomonic of FNH. The discontinuation of oral contraceptives is usually not associated with regression of the adenoma, and surgical resection is the therapy of choice. A clinical diagnosis of FNH, on the other hand, does not require excision, unless confusion regarding actual diagnosis exists and malignant neoplasm cannot be excluded.

Malignant Hepatic Tumors

Metastatic neoplasms are the most common malignant tumors of the liver, with the proportion of primary to secondary hepatic neoplasms estimated at 1:20. The liver is second only to regional lymph nodes as a site of metastases for tumors. Although the results are best with hepatic metastasis from colon carcinoma, liver resection has been attempted for a variety of other cancers if the disease-free interval since the primary resection is long and the liver is the only site of metastasis. Metastatic disease not amenable to surgery can be treated with intraarterial infusion of chemotherapy and cryosurgery in selected patients.

Approximately 35% of all patients with colorectal carcinoma go on to develop metastatic disease to the liver. Of these, 10% to 20% may benefit from hepatic resection. Twenty-five percent 5-year disease-free survival can be expected in patients with unilobar metastatic disease who undergo surgical resection.

Primary hepatocellular carcinoma (hepatoma) is the most common gastrointestinal malignancy worldwide. Hepatitis B infection, cirrhosis, and hemochromatosis have been associated with 80% of cases. Cirrhosis of all types is a predisposing factor in the development of hepatocellular carcinoma. Environmental toxins, i.e., aflatoxins, also play a role. Aflatoxins are the products of *Aspergillus flavus,* found in wheat, milk products, peanuts, and rice. All other primary hepatic tumors, such as primary intrahepatic cholangiocarcinoma, are not associated with cirrhosis. Angiosarcoma, the least common primary hepatic tumor, has been linked to vinyl chloride exposure. Hepatocellular carcinoma has several histologic subtypes, with the fibrolamellar variant having the best prognosis. Hepatic tumors extend by four methods: centrifugal growth, parasinusoidol extension, portal vein invasion, and lymphatic invasion.

Weight loss, weakness, and abdominal pain are frequent clinical presentations. Elevated serum alkaline phosphatase and alpha-fetoprotein (AFP) are common laboratory findings. CT scan and MRI are capable of determining the presence and extent of these tumors. CT or ultrasound-guided percutaneous needle biopsy can provide a definitive diagnosis. Ultrasound and AFP levels are recommended screening tools for all cirrhotic patients.

The staging for hepatocellular carcinoma can be summarized in Table 1.

The best treatment of hepatocellular carcinoma is surgical resection. Cirrhosis compromises the regenerative ability of the liver and is a contraindication to lobar and extended lobar resection. Segmental resections have been performed successfully. In the absence of cirrhosis, curative resection offers a 5-year survival of between 18% and 36%. Factors that predict decreased survival following resection include presence of cirrhosis, large tumor size (>4 cm), tumor multiplicity, lack of encapsulation, incomplete resection, portal or hepatic vein invasion, poor histologic differentiation, and decreased preoperative liver function. The fibrolamellar histologic variant has a better 5-year survival

TABLE 1. *TNM staging system in hepatocellular carcinoma (HCC)*

Stage	Description		
I	T_1	N_0	M_0
II	T_2	N_0	M_0
III	T_1	N_1	M_0
	T_2	N_1	M_0
	T_3	N_1, N_2	M_0
IVA	T_4	Any N	M_0
IVB	Any T	Any N	M_1

Primary tumor (T): T_1, solitary tumor of ≤ 2 cm, without vascular invasion; T_2, solitary tumor of ≤ 2 cm with vascular invasion, or multiple tumors limited to one lobe all ≤ 2 cm without vascular invasion, or solitary tumor of ≥ 2 cm without vascular invasion; T_3, solitary tumor of ≥ 2 cm with vascular invasion, or multiple tumors limited to one lobe all ≤ 2 cm with vascular invasion, or multiple tumors limited to one lobe any ≥ 2 cm with or without vascular invasion; T_4, multiple tumors in more than lobe, or tumor(s) involve(s) a major branch of the portal or hepatic vein.

Regional lymph nodes (N): N_0, no regional lymph node metastasis; N_1, regional lymph node metastasis.

Distant metastasis (M): M_0, no distant metastasis; M_1, distant metastasis.

rate. Other modalities such as direct arterial infusion of chemotherapeutic drugs have extended survival in some cases. Other therapeutic options available include liver transplantation or cryosurgery in selected cases.

CIRRHOSIS AND PORTAL HYPERTENSION

Cirrhosis

Cirrhosis is defined as a chronic disease of the liver in which diffuse destruction and regeneration of hepatic parenchymal cells occur with a diffuse increase in interlobular connective tissue, resulting in distorted lobular and vascular architecture. The mechanisms of hepatocellular injury resulting from alcohol consumption, viral hepatitis, biliary obstruction, and venous outflow obstruction (to name but a few) are well understood. The precise cause of cirrhosis and the reason why only a minority of patients develop it, however, are unknown, but it appears that multiple factors are involved.

Patient evaluation begins with a detailed history and physical examination. Stigmata of chronic liver disease include cutaneous spider angiomas, palmar erythema, gynecomastia, testicular atrophy, and encephalopathy. Splenomegaly, ascites, and visible abdominal wall veins each indicate the presence of portal hypertension. A chemistry profile, hepatitis serology, and liver biopsy may be helpful in making a specific diagnosis. Definitive diagnosis of cirrhosis is made by biopsy.

Child's classification, composed of three clinical variables (ascites, encephalopathy, and nutritional status) and two biochemical tests (serum bilirubin and albumin), is an indirect estimate of hepatic functional reserve (Table 2) and is predictive of perioperative outcome. However, the single most important parameter predictive of perioperative liver function is the prothrombin time. Of the coagulation factors produced by the liver (e.g., II, VII, IX, X) factor VII, which is the coinitiator of the extrinsic pathway, has the shortest half-life. Elevation of the prothrombin time, an in vitro measure of extrinsic pathway integrity, indicates liver insufficiency with respect to protein synthesis and metabolic function. The failure of the correction of the prothrombin time with fresh frozen plasma and vitamin K is indicative of severe liver dysfunction.

Portal Hypertension

Portal hypertension is the result of impedance to portal venous flow. In the United States, cirrhosis is the

TABLE 2. *Child's classification of liver dysfunction*

	Child's		
	A	B	C
Bilirubin	<2.0 mg/dl	2.0–3.0 mg/dl	> 3.0 mg/dl
Albumin	>3.5 mg/dl	3.0–3.5 mg/dl	<3.0 mg/dl
Ascites	None	Easily controlled	Refractory
Encephalopathy	None	Minimal	Advanced
Nutrition	Excellent	Good	Poor
Prognosis following surgery	Excellent	Fair	Poor

principal etiology of the majority of portal hypertensive patients. Schistosomiasis is the most common cause worldwide. Other etiologies of portal hypertension are listed in Table 3. If portal venous pressure is chronically elevated, spontaneous portasystemic collaterals develop in an attempt to decompress the portal system. Other complications from portal hypertension include encephalopathy, splenomegaly, ascites, and hepatorenal syndrome.

Portasystemic venous collaterals, e.g., esophagogastric varices and rectal varices, can easily rupture and result in massive gastrointestinal bleeding; these represent the most serious sequelae of portal hypertension. Up to half of patients will die from the acute bleed, reflecting not only the volume of hemorrhage but also the compromised liver function and other systemic disease. During an acute variceal bleed, the general goal of treatment is to control the bleeding as quickly as possible. Samples of patient blood should be drawn for transfusion cross-matching, hemoglobin, hematocrit, electrolytes, liver function tests, and coagulation profiles. An intravenous infusion for volume resuscitation is started. A nasogastric tube is inserted, and the stomach is lavaged with saline irrigation. Preferably, all these measures are performed in a monitored setting, i.e., intensive care unit.

Acute endoscopic sclerotherapy should be the first line of treatment. Sclerotherapy should be repeated until all esophageal varices have been eradicated. Vasopressin or propranolol may or may not be included in the initial resuscitative regimen. Vasopressin lowers portal blood flow and portal pressure by a direct constrictive action or splanchnic arterioles. Similarly, beta-receptor blockade may indirectly decrease portal venous pressure. Balloon tamponade of the esophagus with a Sengstaken-Blakemore (SB) tube was routine but is now used only when simpler methods fail. These measures are successful in stopping hemorrhage in 90% of cases, but early rebleeding rate is encountered in ~30% of cases. When bleeding is refractory to sclerotherapy or recurs, emergency portasystemic shunting is required.

If an anastomosis (shunt) between the portal and systemic venous circulations is created, the elevated portal pressure drops, and the risk of variceal bleeding is reduced. In the past, portasystemic shunting was strictly an operative procedure and when performed in an emergency setting was accompanied by an exceedingly high mortality. The advent of transjugular intrahepatic portasystemic shunting (TIPS), has established the interventional radiologist as the pivotal care-giver in this emergency setting, and surgery is withheld until all of the above measures fail.

Surgically created portasystemic shunts can be grouped into those that shunt the entire portal system (nonselective) and thus decrease the portal hypertension and those that selectively shunt blood from the gastrosplenic region while preserving the pressure-flow relationships in the rest of the portal bed (selective shunt) and thus preserve portal hypertension. Preserving portal flow to the liver is important to avoid encephalopathy. Also, liver failure is not uncommon if the portal inflow to the liver is disrupted. The distal splenorenal shunt is the first choice for elective portal decompression (Fig. 5). If ascites is present or the anatomy is unfavorable, an end-to-end portacaval shunt is preferred. Side-to-side shunts would be done for patients with severe ascites or Budd-Chiari syndrome. The mesocaval and central splenorenal shunts are reserved for special anatomic situations in which the above operations are unsuitable. The shunts are schematically illustrated in Fig. 6.

Advances in orthotopic liver transplantation have dramatically decreased morbidity and mortality. Liver transplantation is another viable option for therapy in the acute or elective setting in select patients. Some advocate transplant in young patients, since the mortality rate for all other forms of therapy within the subsequent years is high secondary to rebleeding or hepatic failure. Good transplant candidates should not be subjected to portasystemic shunts.

Ascites represents a local consequence of an imbalance of those factors that favor the exudation of fluid from the vascular compartment over those that maintain vascular volume. Starling suggested that the transudation of fluid between capillaries and tissue spaces was determined by the equilibrium of hydrostatic and osmotic forces in the two compartments. The advanced cirrhotic patient with portal hypertension has increased intravascular hydrostatic pressure (portal hypertension) and decreased vascular osmotic pressure (hypoalbuminemia), a combination of factors favoring loss of fluid into the peritoneal space. The overflow theory suggests the inappropriate sodium and water retention with expansion of plasma volume is the primary event in ascites formation. The reason for sodium retention

TABLE 3. *Portal hypertension*

Prehepatic	Portal vein thrombosis, arteriovenous malformation
Intrahepatic	
Presinusoidal	Schistosomiasis
Sinusoidal	Cirrhosis
Postsinusoidal	Central veno-occlusive disease
Posthepatic	Budd-Chiari syndrome, congestive heart failure

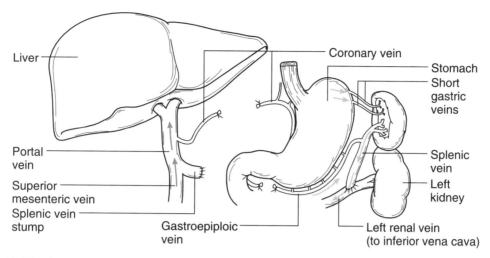

FIG. 5. Distal splenorenal shunt. Note that the portal blood supply is maintained with this selective splenorenal shunt.

remains obscure but probably involves an increased renal tubular sensitivity to aldosterone. With advancing cirrhosis and portal hypertension, the expanded extracellular and plasma compartments overflow into the peritoneal cavity.

The mainstay of therapy is sodium and fluid restriction. Diuretic therapy restricts the ability of the kidney to conserve sodium. Spironolactone, an aldosterone antagonist, favors sodium excretion and potassium absorption. Percutaneous withdrawal of ascitic fluid, paracentesis, is offered to patients with symptomatic or refractory ascites. Intravenous albumin should be administered during large-volume paracentesis to maintain circulating volume and avoid inadequate renal perfusion. Peritoneal-venous

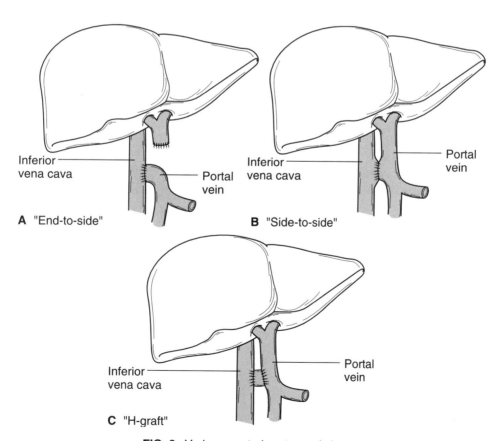

FIG. 6. Various central portacaval shunts.

shunts of the LeVeen and Denver types have effectively controlled medically intractable ascites. Improvement may be related to increased creatinine clearance and normalization of renin activity and aldosterone levels. Adverse consequences of the procedure include disseminated intravascular coagulapathy and initiation of variceal bleeding.

SPLEEN

Anatomy and Physiology

The spleen is located in the left upper quadrant along the undersurface of the left leaf of the diaphragm and protected by ribs 8 to 11. Its position is maintained by the splenophrenic, splenorenal, splenocolic and gastrosplenic ligaments. Arterial blood enters the splenic bed via the splenic artery, a branch of the celiac artery (Fig. 7). The short gastric arteries (vasa brevia) supply the spleen after traveling through the gastrosplenic ligament. The venous drainage courses through the splenic vein, which joins the superior mesenteric vein to form the portal vein.

The spleen is divided by connective tissue trabeculae. The splenic artery divides into trabecular arteries, which terminate in the white pulp, followed by the marginal zone, then the red pulp. The white pulp contains lymphatic cells, and the marginal zone contains mostly plasma, while the red pulp has cords and sinuses. The red pulp serves mainly as a filter and reservoir. It is the primary site of phagocystosis of defective red cells (requires changes in the red cell membrane). The white pulp serves mainly an immune function and is the site of IgM, lymphocytes, and plasma cell synthesis. The spleen is also a major platelet reservoir. Overactivity of splenic function leading to accelerated removal of any or all of the circulating cellular elements of the blood with resultant anemia, leukopenia, or thrombocytopenia, alone or in combination, is referred to as "hypersplenism."

Splenectomy is carried out for many reasons (Table 4). Immune thrombocytopenia purpura (ITP) is a syndrome characterized by a low platelet count caused by a circulating antiplatelet factor. The platelet count can reach dangerously low levels, predisposing patients to spontaneous and devastating bleeding. In the past, women were most commonly affected however, there has been a recent increase in ITP in homosexual males with the human immunodeficiency virus (HIV). Infusion of immunoglobulin (IgG) and corticosteroids are the first line of treatment, and an increase in the platelet count can be expected within 3 to 7 days. Splenectomy is reserved for patients who are refractory to steroid therapy or patients with recurrent ITP after discontinuation of steroids.

Thrombotic thrombocytopenia purpura (TTP) is a syndrome characterized by thrombocytopenia, microangiopathic hemolytic anemia, fluctuating neurologic abnormalities, progressive renal failure, and fever. Prognosis is poor in untreated patients. Combined therapy with antiplatelet agents, corticosteroids, and plasma is instituted at the time of diagnosis. Splenectomy is offered to those patients who do not respond favorably to medical treatment.

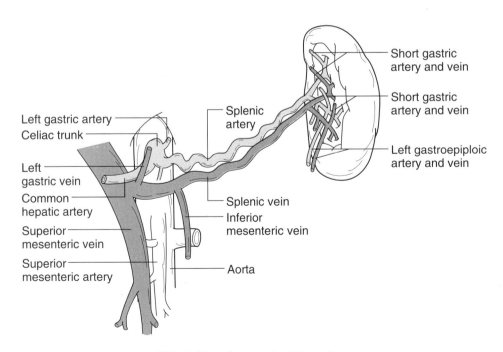

FIG. 7. Vascular supply of the spleen.

TABLE 4. *Indications for splenectomy*

Hematologic disorders	Immune thrombocytopenia purpura, congenital spherocytosis, hairy-cell leukemia
Injury	Blunt trauma, surgical trauma, splenic torsion
Part of surgical procedures	Staging of lymphomas, radical gastrectomy
Splenic lesions	Splenic tumors, cysts, and abscesses

Asplenic patients have an increased susceptibility to the development of overwhelming infection, characterized by fulminant bacteremia, meningitis, or pneumonia. Although more common in children, the postsplenectomy sepsis syndrome can occur in previously healthy adults following a mild upper respiratory infection associated with fever. Within hours, nausea, vomiting, headache, confusion, shock, and coma occur, and death ensues within 24 hr. Encapsulated organisms such as *Streptococcus pneumonia, Neisseria meningitides, Escherichia coli,* or *Haemophilus influenzae* are responsible for the majority of cases. Penicillin can be administered prophylactically or immediately with the onset of a febrile upper respiratory illness. Ideally, patients should be immunized 2 weeks prior to splenectomy with polyvalent vaccines to allow for development of protective antibodies. Thrombocytosis is another common sequelae following splenectomy when platelet count exceeds $10^6/mm^3$ blood. Most surgeons recommend an aspirin daily to prevent thrombotic complications if the platelet count reaches such a high level.

SUMMARY

Sadly, the liver's tremendous metabolic function and regenerative capabilities are taken for granted. A patient without sufficient hepatic function to manufacture energy products and proteins, combat infection, and metabolize toxins has a poor clinical prognosis. Cirrhosis and its complications are accompanied by tremendous morbidity. Likewise, complications from portal hypertension like variceal bleeding have a very high mortality rate and at times are difficult to treat effectively. Splenectomy performed infrequently for hematologic or traumatic disease is performed safely, but postsplenectomy thrombocytosis and relative immune incompetence deserve special consideration.

STUDY QUESTIONS

1. What is the blood supply of the liver?
2. What is the hepatic venous drainage of the liver?
3. What is Child's classification?
4. What is the management for variceal bleeding?
5. Describe the vascular supply of the spleen—its ligamentous attachments.

SUGGESTED READING

Cameron JL. *Current surgical therapy.* 5th ed. St. Louis: Mosby, 1995.
Economou SG, Deziel DJ, Witt TR, et al. *Rush University review of surgery.* 2nd ed. Philadelphia: Saunders, 1994.
Greenfield LJ. *Surgery: scientific principles and practice.* Philadelphia: Lippincott, 1993.
Sabiston DC Jr. *Textbook of surgery.* 14th ed. Philadelphia: Saunders, 1991.
Schwartz SI, Shires GT, Spencer FC. *Principles of surgery.* 6th ed. New York: McGraw-Hill, 1994.

CHAPTER 14

Biliary System

Dyann Yarish and Duane G. Hutson

The surgical management of biliary disease has been evolving since Carl Langenbuch performed the first cholecystectomy in 1882. Great advances in biliary surgery have been paralleled by new methods of nonsurgical management of biliary pathology. Here, we present the pathophysiologic basis of biliary disease and the currently available surgical and nonsurgical management options.

ANATOMY

The extrahepatic biliary system conducts bile produced in the liver to the duodenum, where it mixes with chyme to aid digestion (Fig. 1). The left and right hepatic ducts that drain bile from the left and right lobes of the liver merge to form the common hepatic duct that descends in the anterior portion of the hepatoduodenal ligament. The common bile duct (CBD) is formed by the confluence of the common hepatic duct and the cystic duct. The CBD passes posterior to the first portion of the duodenum, yielding the intrapancreatic segment of the CBD that enters the second portion of the duodenum at the papilla of Vater. There is tremendous variation in cystic duct anatomy as well as in the union of the biliary and pancreatic ducts (Figs. 2 and 3).

The gallbladder is a storage reservoir for bile that receives and discharges bile through the cystic duct. It has four anatomic segments—fundus, body, infundibulum, and neck (Fig. 4A). The valves of Heister that line the cystic duct are not true valves, as bile freely flows into and out of the gallbladder. Congenital absence of the gallbladder occurs in approximately three in 10,000 cases;

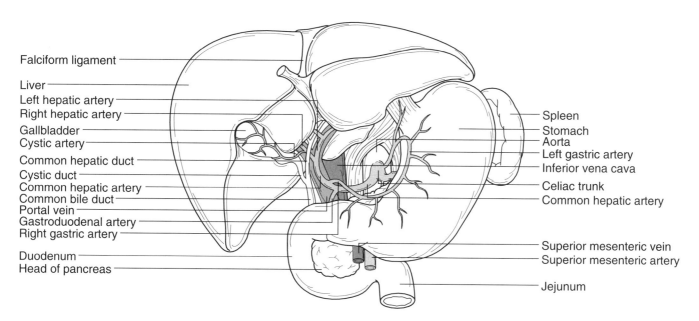

FIG. 1. Anatomic overview of biliary system (gallbladder, extrahepatic biliary system).

175

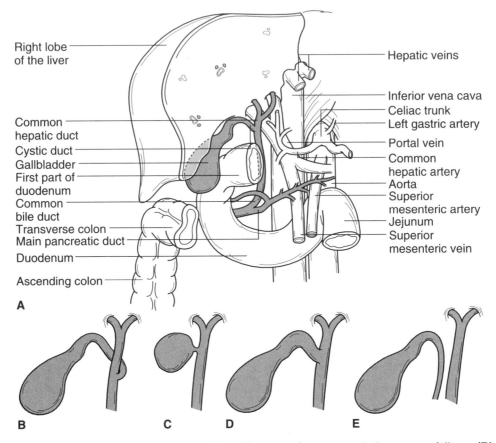

FIG. 2. (A) Complex and variable anatomy of the biliary tree. Common variations are as follows: **(B)** Cystic duct traveling posterior to common hepatic duct. **(C)** Contracted gallbladder with very short cystic duct. **(D)** Gallbladder with atypically enlarged cystic duct. **(E)** Nonunion of cystic duct and common hepatic duct. Ducts travel separately and unite within the pancreas. (Adapted from Gray JW, Skandalakis JE. *Atlas of surgical anatomy for general surgeons.* Baltimore: Williams and Wilkins, 1985.)

duplication occurs in approximately one in 4,000 cases. Intrahepatic gallbladders, partial or complete, are fairly common, however. Occasionally small bile ducts conduct bile from the liver directly to the gallbladder across the gallbladder fossa, the bile ducts of Luschka.

The blood supply to the biliary tree is derived from tributaries of the proper hepatic artery and the gastroduodenal artery. The proper hepatic artery travels medial and posterior to the biliary tree, and divides into a left and right hepatic artery in the porta hepatis. The cystic artery,

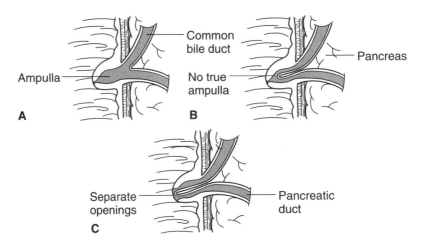

FIG. 3. Variations of the distal biliary tree.**(A)** Normal ampulla. **(B)** No true ampulla. **(C)** Separate openings. (Adapted from Gray JW, Skandalakis JE. *Atlas of surgical anatomy for general surgeons.* Baltimore: Williams and Wilkins, 1985.)

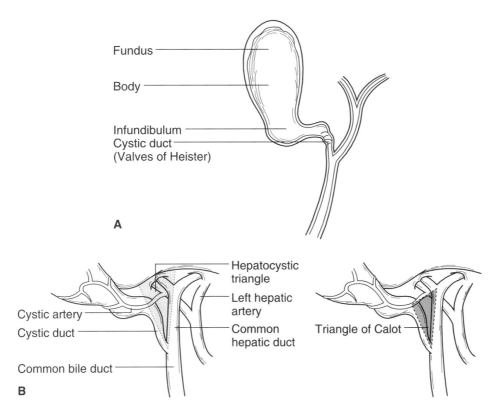

FIG. 4. (A) The anatomic segments of the gallbladder. **(B)** The hepatocystic triangle *(left)* and the triangle of Calot *(right)*.

which delivers blood to the gallbladder, is derived from the right hepatic artery and travels in the hepatocystic triangle, which is defined by the liver edge, cystic duct, and common hepatic duct. The triangle of Calot, which is contained within the hepatocystic triangle, is bounded by the cystic artery, cystic duct, and common hepatic duct (Fig. 4B). Small branches from the gastroduodenal artery

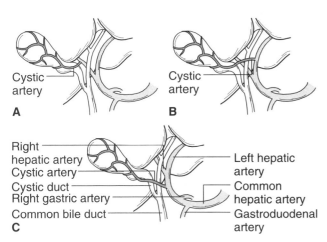

FIG. 5. Anomalous origins of the cystic artery. **(A)** Short cystic artery originating from right hepatic artery. **(B)** Cystic artery originating from the left hepatic artery. **(C)** Cystic artery originating from the common hepatic artery.

parallel the lateral surface of and supply blood to the CBD, named the 9 o'clock and 3 o'clock arteries. Similar to the biliary drainage system, there are numerous variations regarding the origin of the cystic artery as well as right and left hepatic arteries (Fig. 5). Venous drainage of the gallbladder is via a cystic vein which drains to the right portal vein. Small venules can drain directly to the liver. Lymphatic flow also drains directly to the liver.

PHYSIOLOGY

Between 500 and 1,500 cc of bile is produced and secreted by hepatocytes daily. Water, electrolytes, and organic solutes are the main components in bile. Electrolyte composition is quite similar to serum, with an exception for bicarbonate concentration. Bile contains a tremendous amount of bicarbonate, which is secreted by columnar cells of the hepatic biliary radicals under the stimulation of the hormone secretin.

The primary function of the gallbladder is to store and concentrate bile. Of the organs in the alimentary tract, the gallbladder has the greatest absorptive capacity per unit area of mucosa. The water and sodium absorption that occurs in the gallbladder can dramatically change the relative concentrations of water, electrolytes, and solutes of bile originally produced in the liver. Stimulated by the presence of lipid breakdown metabolites in the duodenum, cholecystokinin is released and acts as the most potent stimulus for gallbladder contraction. Secondarily, the hepatic branch of the vagus nerve has stimulatory effect on gallbladder contraction. Sympathetic tone opposes the parasympathetic stimulatory effect.

RADIOLOGIC EVALUATION OF THE BILIARY DUCTAL SYSTEM

An upright abdominal radiograph demonstrates gallstones in <15% of cases and is of little diagnostic value in patients with suspected biliary disease. Rarely, air in the biliary tree, pneumobilia (secondary to a biliary enteric fistula or anastomosis), or, less commonly, severe cholangitis, emphysematous cholecystitis, and biliary ascariasis is demonstrated.

In the past, oral cholecystography was commonly used in biliary and gallbladder evaluation. Oral contrast (tyropanoate or iopanoic acid) pills ingested the night prior to the examination are absorbed, taken up by hepatocytes via enterohepatic circulation and excreted into bile. About 10 hr after pill ingestion, cholecystogram demonstrates a full gallbladder. Thereafter, a fatty meal is ingested by the patient, and on sequential cholecystograms, a decrease in size of the gallbladder to >50% of baseline is considered normal. Nonvisualization of the gallbladder occurs in 15% of patients, even after a double oral dose of contrast. Persistent nonopacification of the gallbladder is 95% sensitive for gallbladder disease.

Inadequate absorption from the intestine or decreased excretion by the liver limit the usefulness of this study.

The use of ultrasound has overtaken oral cholecystogram in screening for the presence of biliary disease because it provides a quick, noninvasive, and inexpensive method of evaluation. Specifically, it offers the most sensitive detection of stones in the gallbladder (cholelithiasis) that appear as mobile, echogenic, intraluminal structures that cast acoustic shadows (Fig. 6). Intrahepatic and extrahepatic ducts as well as hepatic vasculature are demonstrated in exquisite detail. With an exception for obese patients or patients with excessive intestinal gas, distal CBD abnormalities and pathology in the head of the pancreas can be detected by ultrasound as well.

Computed tomography (CT) scan of the abdomen can complement the diagnostic accuracy of ultrasound in the area of the head of the pancreas. Distal CBD stones and periampullary neoplasia can be demonstrated with high sensitivity and specificity. CT scan is extremely useful in evaluating tumors of the gallbladder and possible involvement of the liver, but for detection of cholelithiasis, it is considered inferior to sonography.

Intravenously administered of [99m]technetium-iminodiacetic acid (IDA) compounds are extracted by hepatocytes and secreted into bile. Even with serum bilirubin of >20 mg/dl, biliary flow can be outlined by this procedure, called biliary scintigraphy. The DISIDA (or PIPIDA scan, as it is frequently termed) nonvisualization of the gallbladder confirms cystic duct obstruction that

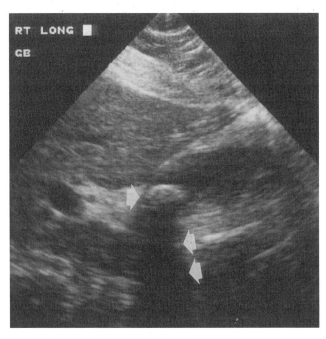

FIG. 6. Longitudinal view of the gallbladder revealing solitary stone *(arrow)* impacted at the neck of the gallbladder. Note the posterior shadowing of the stone *(double arrow)*.

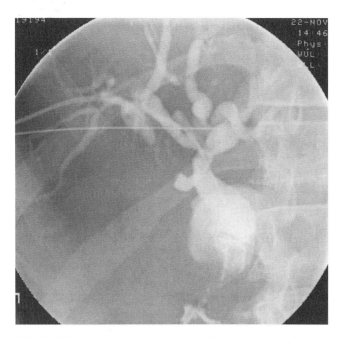

FIG. 7. This is a percutaneous transhepatic cholangiogram of a patient who has undergone pancreaticoduodenectomy. The common bile duct empties into the jejunum. Of note is moderate biliary dilatation of both left and right ductal systems suggestive of mechanical obstruction.

accompanies acute cholecystitis. In a normal study the liver, CBD, gallbladder, duodenum, and jejunum are visualized on the images obtained within 60 min.

Percutaneous transhepatic cholangiography (PTC) can be quite useful in the evaluation of patients with suspected biliary disease. PTC is performed by passing a needle through the hepatic parenchyma and into the lumen of a bile duct using fluoroscopic guidance. PTC can define the site of biliary pathology and guide placement of internal or external drainage of a biliary obstruction as well as guide balloon dilatation of ductal narrowing (Fig. 7). The procedure is much easier in the presence of intrahepatic biliary dilatation. Parenchymal bleeding and bleeding into the ductal system (hemobilia) are infrequent complications.

Since its introduction >20 years ago, endoscopic retrograde cholangiography (ERC) has assumed a principal role in the diagnosis and management of biliary tract disorders, especially obstructive jaundice. The biliary ductal system is cannulated via the ampulla of Vater under direct vision through a duodenoscope. Opacification of the biliary ducts can delineate causes of obstruction, including gallstones, malignancy, and benign strictures (Fig. 8). Nasobiliary drains can be placed endoscopically for decompression of the biliary tree, and stents can be deployed in an obstructed biliary duct.

DISEASES OF THE BILIARY SYSTEM

Cholelithiasis

In Western countries, one out of 10 individuals has gallstones, i.e., cholelithiasis. The majority of patients are females in the middle years of life. The main component of most stones is cholesterol mixed with bilirubin and calcium salts. Pigment stones, which are composed primarily of bilirubin compounds, are the source of clinical disease in a minority of patients.

The main organic solutes that contribute to biliary stone formation are bile salts, cholesterol, and phospholipids. In bile, cholesterol is maintained in solution within micelles but as the concentration of cholesterol in bile exceeds its solubility quotient cholesterol precipitates. An increase in the absolute amount of cholesterol or a decrease in the relative concentration of bile salts or phospholipids can lead to this event as depicted in Small's triangle (Fig. 9).

Many factors are associated with or contribute to the pathogenesis of cholelithiasis. There is a linear relationship between advancing age and gallstone incidence in both sexes, although there are still a greater number of women with stones. Studies demonstrate that estrogen decreases the enzymatic conversion of cholesterol to bile

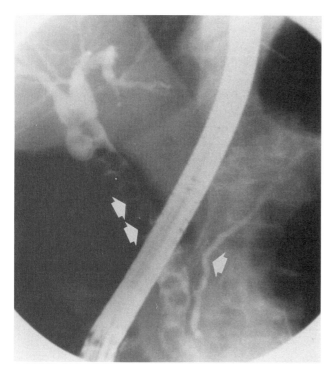

FIG. 8. Endoscopic retrograde cholangiopancreatography. The pancreatic duct *(arrow)* and the common bile duct *(double arrow)* are both opacified. Note the multiple filling defects in the common bile duct (secondary stones).

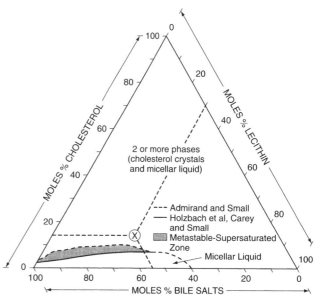

FIG. 9. Tricoordinate phase diagram for determination of cholesterol saturation index. A given single point represents the relative molar ratios of bile salts, lecithin, and cholesterol. The range of concentrations consistent with a clear, micellar solution (where cholesterol is fully solubilized) is limited to a small region in the lower left. The shaded area directly above this region corresponds to a metastable zone, in which bile initially appears clear but with time develops cholesterol crystals. All other regions (including the designated point) represent bile solutions in which the cholesterol solubilization

acids. The relative increase in cholesterol fosters precipitation out of solution. Pregnancy predisposes to gallstone formation because of high serum estrogen levels. Anyone who has interruption of the enterohepatic circulation of bile acids (e.g., short bowel syndrome) is at higher risk for gallstone formation. This is a consequence of the decreased bile acid pool, leading to a shift in the equilibrium of cholesterol solubilization.

Pigmented stones account for one-fourth to one-third of gallstones in the United States, but represent the most common type of gallstone worldwide. The formation of pigmented stones is related to supersaturation of bile by calcium hydrogen bilirubinate. Patients with chronic hemolysis may have a >10-fold increase in the bile pigment and are particularly prone to pigmented stone formation. Prevalence also increases with age, female sex, and the presence of cirrhosis. Electron microscopy reveals that 90% of pigment stones are composed of dense mixtures of bacteria and bacterial glycocalyx. Bacteria may have a role in pigment gallstone formation and may explain why patients with pigment gallstones experience sepsis more often than do those with cholesterol gallstone disease.

Cholelithiasis can intermittently obstruct the cystic duct and cause visceral pain as a result of cholecystic distention. During episodes of pain, patients typically complain of right upper quadrant or epigastric abdominal discomfort especially after the ingestion of a fatty meal due to the hormonal stimulation for gallbladder contraction. Pain may be referred also to the right scapular area and is often associated with nausea and vomiting. This constellation of symptoms is termed biliary colic. If the pain persists or progresses to local peritonitis with or without fever, acute cholecystitis has presumably developed. Jaundice, superimposed on a clinical history of biliary colic, suggests the existence of extrahepatic biliary obstruction secondary to a gallstone, i.e., choledocholithiasis.

Examination of the abdomen completes a thorough physical examination in evaluating patients with suspected biliary disease. Acute abdominal pain is discussed elsewhere in this text, but some specifics of bile duct and gallbladder pathology are presented here. Murphy's sign describes the cessation of patient's deep inspiration during palpation of the right upper abdominal quadrant. It reflects peritoneal inflammation of the gallbladder consistent with acute cholecystitis. A nontender, palpable gallbladder (Courvoisier's sign) in a jaundiced patient suggests malignant obstruction the extrahepatic biliary system anywhere along the course of the CBD.

If the patient history and physical examination is suggestive of biliary pathology, sonogram of the abdomen is utilized as the primary diagnostic test. Distal biliary obstruction and hyperbilirubinemia can be evaluated by CT scan or ERC. Each test has its risks and benefits in the evaluation of benign or malignant disease. PTC may be required if cholangiography via the ampulla cannot be accomplished.

Acute Cholecystitis

Acute inflammation of the gallbladder is exceedingly common and results from persistent obstruction of the cystic duct, usually by gallstones. Gallbladder distention leads to transmural edema that, if it is persistent, eventually results in transmural ischemia. This, combined with the bacterial overgrowth in stagnant bile, establishes an ideal scenario for inflammation and infection of the gallbladder, acute cholecystitis.

Persistent right upper quadrant abdominal pain with signs of pericholecystic peritoneal inflammation (Murphy's sign) are very suggestive of cholecystitis. Fever, nausea and vomiting are commonly associated symptoms. Leukocytosis, elevated serum liver transaminases and alkaline phosphatase can be seen in acute cholecystitis. Ultrasonography provides a quick and inexpensive method of detecting stones within the gallbladder. Classically, the visualization of a distended gallbladder with stones, a thickened gallbladder wall, and pericholecystic fluid in the presence of right upper abdominal pain is acute cholecystitis until proven otherwise. PIPIDA scan remains an excellent supplementary test should ultrasound not be available or the results of ultrasound equivocal (Fig. 10).

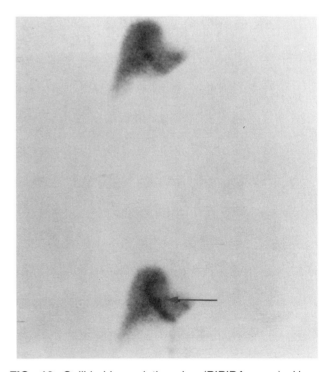

FIG. 10. Gallbladder scintigraphy (PIPIDA scan). Upper image is at 30 min; lower image is at 60 min. Both show delayed imaging of the gallbladder (arrow).

Once a diagnosis of acute cholecystitis is made, oral intake is withheld from the patient, nasogastric tube decompression is implemented if vomiting persists, and intravenous fluids are administered to correct fluid deficiencies. Empiric broad-spectrum intravenous antibiotics are administered immediately after diagnosis is made. The most common microorganisms cultured from bile in patients with acute cholecystitis in decreasing order of frequency are *Escherichia coli, Klebsiella pneumonia,* and *Streptococcus faecalis.* Other common microbes include Pseudomonas, Salmonella, and Bacterioides.

Chronic Cholecystitis

Chronic cholecystitis is due to repeated obstruction of the cystic duct that gives rise to mild cholecystitis. The chronically inflamed gallbladder becomes contracted and occasionally calcified as demonstrated by ultrasound or CT scan. The incidence of gallbladder carcinoma in calcified gallbladders (i.e., porcelain gallbladder) approaches 20%, and thus removal should be performed once diagnosis has been established.

Cholecystectomy

Surgical removal of the gallbladder, cholecystectomy, can and should be performed in many different clinical scenarios (Table 1). Patients with acute cholecystitis should be rehydrated and given intravenous antibiotics prior to urgent cholecystectomy. Emergent surgery is indicated for patients with suspected empyema or perforation of the gallbladder and for patients who deteriorate despite therapy instituted as described. Mortality from elective cholecystectomy is ~0.5%. In contrast, mortality from cholecystectomy for acute cholecystitis is ~3% in otherwise healthy individuals but approaches 7% in the elderly with comorbid medical disease.

Prior to 1990, 95% of cholecystectomy procedures were performed through a right subcostal or midline abdominal incision, the so-called open cholecystectomy. Today, 95% of cholecystectomies are performed utilizing minimally invasive surgical technology. The laparoscopic cholecystectomy, when performed by experienced and skilled surgeons, provides equivalent results when compared to the open cholecystecomy but with decreased length of hospital stay, convalescence, and postoperative

TABLE 1. *Indications for cholecystectomy*

Symptomatic biliary colic
Chronic cholecystitis
Acute cholecystitis
Sickle cell disease
Porcelain gallbladder

pain. It is widely accepted as standard treatment for patients with symptomatic gallbladder disease.

Approximately 5% of laparoscopic cholecystectomy procedures cannot be completed and must be converted to an open procedure. It should not be regarded as a complication but rather a reflection of good judgment to ensure a successful and safe removal of the gallbladder. Indications for conversion include poorly definable anatomy that precludes a safe dissection, uncontrollable bleeding, and suspected CBD injury. As experience with laparoscopy has grown, the rate of conversion has declined due in part to advancement in equipment that allows clearance of the CBD of stones laparoscopically and expanded clinical experience among surgeons.

Alternatives to Cholecystectomy

If acute cholecystitis is considered simply an infected fluid collection, removal of this fluid can relieve sequelae of this locally contained infection. Percutaneous tube cholecystostomy establishes drainage of the gallbladder. It can be performed in the operating room under local anesthesia or by interventional radiology using ultrasound or CT scan guidance. It is indicated for patients with acute cholecystitis who are otherwise too ill to tolerate an emergent cholecystectomy under general anesthesia. If the clinical condition improves, an elective cholecystectomy at a later date can be considered. In patients with a hostile abdomen secondary to previous surgery, it may be the only reasonable treatment option.

Better understanding of the pathogenesis of cholesterol gallstones has led to medical treatment for selected groups of patients. Two naturally occurring bile acids, chenodeoxycholic acid (CDCA) and ursodeoxycholic acid (UDCA) reduce cholesterol secretion in bile and are used for dissolution of cholesterol gallstones. The use of extracorporeal shockwave lithotripsy to break the stones into smaller fragments, with concurrent use of bile acids, can help speed dissolution rates. Eligible patients have small (<2 cm in diameter) radiolucent gallstones. After dissolution, disease recurrence rates approach 50% in 5 years and can have varying symptomatology.

Acalculous Cholecystitis

Acute acalculous cholecystitis occurs most commonly in patients who are critically ill from trauma, burns, or sepsis, in patients after open heart surgery, and in those patients receiving total parenteral nutrition. These patients have gallbladder stasis and biliary sludge and despite the absence of cholelithiasis are at higher risk for developing cholecystitis. Abdominal ultrasound may demonstrate gallbladder wall thickening, pericholecystic fluid, intramural gas, or a sloughed mucosal membrane. Recognizing the subpopulation of patients in which this disease entity typically occurs, cholecystectomy under general anesthesia and potential laparotomy may not be advisable. Ultrasound-guided percutaneous cholecystostomy drainage has become a favored approach in the critically ill and has led to complete resolution of symptoms often obviating the need for cholecystectomy. Infrequently, laparoscopic or open cholecystectomy may be required if resolution of symptoms does not occur. Acalculous cholecystitis is associated with a high morbidity and mortality due to the subgroup of clinical patients in which it occurs and should be remembered in critically ill patients with clinical manifestation of sepsis without a clear source of infection.

Choledocholithiasis

Approximately 10% to 15% of patients with symptomatic cholelithiasis pass stones that are formed in the gallbladder into the CBD (secondary stones). They are discovered by preoperative or intraoperative cholangiogram or in the postoperative period as a symptomatic retained common duct stone. Any stones discovered within 2 years of surgery are assumed to have been undetected at the time of first operation. Rarely, primary common duct stones, which are composed of calcium and sodium bilirubinate, develop within the intrahepatic or extrahepatic bile ducts due to bile stasis. Primary or secondary stones can cause obstructive jaundice and cholangitis in 2% of patients with biliary stone disease.

Choledocholithiasis can be diagnosed and treated via ERC. If stones are found, or if the clinical circumstances strongly suggest stones have been passed, then a papillotomy is performed. Papillotomy is rarely complicated by perforation, pancreatitis, cholangitis, and bleeding. ERC is unsuccessful in removing stones >2 cm in diameter, and for these cases, an operative CBD exploration is required.

Up to one-third of patients with acutely symptomatic gallstones can have associated CBD stones. Interestingly, however, between 3% and 5% of chronically symptomatic gallstone patients who have never experienced jaundice have stones in the CBD. Because most contemporary surgeons now perform laparoscopic cholecystectomy for symptomatic cholelithiasis, some clinical variables to select the subpopulation of patients who should undergo preoperative cholangiographic assessment or intraoperative cholangiogram have been determined (Table 2).

Absolute indications for CBD exploration are palpable calculus at the time of abdominal exploration, choledocholithiasis determined by preoperative imaging, or demonstration of a calculus on intraoperative cholangiography. Suspicion of ductal calculi, a history of obstructive jaundice, or a dilated CBD are certainly indications for an imaging study of the CBD, either in the preoperative or intraoperative period. An equivocal study is a relative indication for CBD exploration. This ductal exploration can be performed laparoscopically or via open technique.

TABLE 2. *Indicators of possible choledocholithiasis*[a]

Elevated bilirubin
Elevated alkaline phosphatase
Elevated liver transaminases (SGOT, SGPT)
Biliary pancreatitis

[a]Preoperative or intraoperative cholangiogram is indicated.

After completion of the exploration a T-tube is inserted into the common duct and retained by suture closure of the ductal opening. A completion cholangiogram is performed to ensure the duct is free of residual stones. The T-tube is then brought through the abdominal wall and placed to dependent drainage collection. If any stones are found on subsequent cholangiogram, interventional radiology-guided retrieval of the stones via the T-tube path can be performed.

Cholangitis

Cholangitis results from obstruction of bile flow and secondary bacterial colonization of stagnant bile. The most common cause in the United States is choledocholithiasis. Other causes include malignant obstruction of the bile duct, obstruction at a previous biliary anastomosis, and benign biliary strictures. Benign strictures are more common today due to the higher incidence of biliary injury from laparoscopic cholecystectomy. Cholangitis has a spectrum of clinical presentation ranging from mild forms that respond to minimal intervention to life-threatening acute suppurative cholangitis that requires decompression of the biliary system or emergent surgery.

Infection develops infrequently in a normal biliary system. Kupffer cells and tight junctions between hepatocytes help prevent bacteria and toxic metabolites from entering the hepatobiliary system from the portal circulation. The continuous flushing action of bile and the bacteriostatic effects of bile salts make the biliary tract a hostile environment for bacterial overgrowth. Secretory immunoglobulin A and mucus excreted by the biliary epithelium function as antiadherence factors that inhibits microbial colonization. In the presence of stones, strictures, or endoprosthesis, however, bacteria are not effectively cleared resulting in clinical infection. Bacteria colonize stagnant bile by ascending an obstructed CBD, bacteremia in the portal vein as a result of intestinal translocation, and, finally, from any manipulation of the biliary system (e.g., PTC, ERC). The most common microorganisms of infected bile have been elucidated earlier.

In 1877, Charcot described the classic triad of findings in acute cholangitis consisting of right upper quadrant pain, fever, and jaundice—"Charcot's triad." These signs and symptoms are manifestations of an infectious process within the biliary system. In 1955, Reynolds modified the clinical triad by adding hypotension and mental obtundation—"Reynold's pentad," signifying the profound systemic effects of widespread dissemination of biliary infection.

Leukocytosis, increased serum bilirubin, liver transaminases, and alkaline phosphatase are common in most patients with acute cholangitis. Biliary obstruction due to malignancy may have higher serum alkaline phosphatase and bilirubin levels compared with other benign causes of biliary obstruction. Ultrasound demonstrates intrahepatic and extrahepatic biliary obstruction in addition to determining the presence of stones in the gallbladder. It is limited in evaluating the intrapancreatic segment of CBD, especially in patients who are obese or those with excess intestinal gas. Again, CT scan is more useful in defining pathology in the periampullary area.

Principal care of patients with acute cholangitis begins with broad-spectrum intravenous antibiotics that have selective biliary excretion. In stable patients, semielective cholangiogram and biliary decompression is performed. Patients with toxic cholangitis require emergent biliary intervention. Subcutaneous administration of vitamin K is given to overcome deficiencies of chronic biliary obstruction.

Cholangiography and biliary drainage can be accomplished by either PTC or endoscopy (ERC). Transhepatic drainage tubes or internally placed biliary stents are successful in up to 90% of patients with a relatively low morbidity and mortality. Extraction of CBD stones is best accomplished by ERC after sphincterotomy. Biliary drainage by placement of a nasobiliary catheter or endoscopically placed biliary stents can also be performed. Overall success rates are between 90% and 98%, with a significantly lower mortality compared to surgical intervention (5% versus 21%).

However, if radiologic or endoscopic interventions are unsuccessful, surgical decompression is required. The CBD is explored to diagnose the etiology of biliary obstruction. Single choledocholithiasis and cholelithiasis is treated by cholecystectomy and T-tube drainage. Recognizing a biliary malignancy may require an extensive resection and biliary reconstruction if the patient's clinical status permits. Biliary enteric bypass is indicated in benign biliary stricture, ampullary fibrosis, or multiple choledocholithiasis.

Benign Biliary Strictures

Iatrogenic injury is the most common cause of benign biliary strictures of intra- and extrahepatic ducts. The rate of bile duct injury from laparoscopic cholecystectomy is between two to three times the rate of biliary injury from open cholecystectomy. Advocates of routine intraoperative cholangiography during laparoscopic cholecystectomy argue that injuries can be detected intraoperatively and delayed presentation can be prevented.

Although some biliary injuries are recognized at the time of operation, the majority go unnoticed and have early or late postoperative presentations. Jaundice immediately after surgery suggests complete or near complete obstruction of the common hepatic or CBD. Narrowing of biliary ducts has a variable progression often presenting with signs and symptoms of cholangitis. Unrelieved biliary obstruction can lead to biliary cirrhosis in a period of weeks to months. Cystic duct leaks commonly manifest as right upper quadrant pain and perhaps fever. A fluid collection in the subhepatic space may be demonstrated by sonogram. What must be recognized is that distal obstruction prevents transampullary flow of bile and progression to biliary cirrhosis is also likely if this is not resolved.

Suspected biliary strictures mandate immediate evaluation. Ultrasound is an excellent first test because it delineates ductal dilation and fluid collections suggestive of biloma from a presumed ductal leak. CT scan may demonstrate hepatic segmental or lobar atrophy as a result of ductal obstruction. Ultimately, cholangiography by ERC or PTC is required.

Extrahepatic biliary tract injury recognized intraoperatively can be repaired in a number of ways. Laceration, not caused by cautery, of a duct without significant tissue loss can be repaired primarily. End-to-end primary reanastomosis can be performed for complete transection of a duct if there is minimal loss of bile duct length to allow a tension free anastomosis. A T-tube is occasionally placed as an anastomotic stent . Resection of the injured segment of duct with primary reanastomosis as described can be performed provided the anastomosis is without tension. These repair techniques, especially in smaller ducts and when resection is performed, are associated with up to a 40% to 50% long-term stricture rate and should be chosen only for minimal duct injury.

Choledochoenterostomy (e.g., choledochoduodenostomy), Roux-en-Y hepatodocho- or choledochojejunostomy is performed for bile duct injuries recognized either intraoperatively or postoperatively with minimal morbidity and infrequent long-term restricture potential. For these reasons, biliary reconstruction remains the standard of care for injury to the biliary tract against which all other methods of treatment must be compared. Some surgeons fix the afferent segment of the Roux limb to the abdominal wall in a subfascial or subcutaneous position so that, should future biliary intervention be required, percutaneous access of the intestinal tract can be gained and biliary instrumentation of the anastomosis using fluoroscopic guidance can be performed with minimal patient morbidity.

Sclerosing Cholangitis

Sclerosing cholangitis is a chronic cholestatic liver disease associated with nonbacterial inflammatory narrowing of the bile ducts. The duct walls contain an increased amount of collagen and lymphoid elements that narrow the luminal diameter. Although the cause of primary sclerosing cholangitis (PSC) remains unknown, several etiologies have been proposed including bacterial and viral infection, and congenital lesions. Because approximately half of the cases are associated with inflammatory bowel disease (ulcerative colitis), autoimmune mechanisms have been implicated. Secondary sclerosing cholangitis is associated with bile duct injuries, previous common duct stones, mycotic cholangitis, viral cholangitis, cholangiocarcinoma, drug hypersensitivity, and idiopathic adult ductopenia.

PSC is seen more often in males in the mid years of life. The diagnosis is suggested by hyperbilirubinemia and elevated serum alkaline phosphatase. Cholangiogram is the gold standard diagnostic test and classically demonstrates a beaded appearance of the biliary system with sacculations. It is common to find segments of normal duct epithelium interspersed in areas of disease. There is usually a gradual appearance of mild jaundice and pruritus. An isolated diagnosis of PSC requires endoscopic evaluation of the colon for ulcerative colitis because about half of these patients will have occult inflammatory bowel disease.

The severity and progression of disease is extremely variable. The course of PSC in patients with associated ulcerative colitis is similar to those with isolated disease. In a significant number of patients, the disease is rapidly progressive, resulting in liver failure and death. Drug treatment with steroids, penicillamine, cholestyramine, and colchicine is largely ineffective. Cholestyramine will provide symptomatic relief from pruritus. Cholangiocarcinoma will develop in 10% to 15% of cases.

The use of interventional radiology is limited to percutaneous transhepatic balloon dilation of solitary dominant strictures. Because the disease is much more widespread, dilation does not inhibit progression of disease. Although symptoms may be temporarily palliated, stricture recurrence is common after balloon dilation.

Patients with isolated extrahepatic disease can be offered biliary resection and bypass with reasonable expectation of good outcome. For patients with intrahepatic PSC, repeated biliary intervention may be required to allow biliary drainage. Unfortunately, this may not prevent the development of cirrhosis. Invariably, in all patients with PSC, despite biliary reconstruction, recurrence of strictures will occur. ERC or transhepatic balloon dilatation and drainage tubes have been placed with good results. Alternatively, a defunctionalized afferent limb of the biliary enteric anastomosis placed in the subfascial or subcutaneous abdominal wall allows percutaneous access for future biliary intervention.

The incidence of cholangiocarcinoma in patients with PSC is rare but well recognized. It can emerge at any time during the course of disease and typically has an insidious progression much like that of PSC. Many feel that this malignancy represents the true end stage of PSC and the preventative clinical management often presents a dilemma that demands consideration. Orthotopic liver transplantation clearly remains the most effective therapeutic option for patients with end-stage liver disease secondary to PSC. However, advances in operative technique, intensive care postoperatively, and developments in immunosuppression have improved survival rates after transplantation including those with PSC. Some clinicians feel that preemptive transplantation, especially in young patients prior to biliary surgery, should be considered early rather than late in the course of disease. Others argue that long-term survival has been achieved with biliary reconstruction and routine regular biliary dilatation and thus the emotional and physiological demands of transplantation can be delayed or avoided. The appropriate treatment for PSC is debatable and currently evolving.

BILIARY TRACT MALIGNANCY

Gallbladder Cancer

Although carcinoma of the gallbladder is rare, it is the most common biliary tract malignancy and the fifth most common gastrointestinal tract malignancy. Approximately 5,000 new cases are diagnosed each year in the United States. Roughly 0.5% of cholecystectomy procedures reveal gallbladder cancer. Adenocarcinoma is the most common histopathology, followed by squamous, small cell, and mixed malignant tumors. The majority of patients are female and in the seventh decade of life. Gallbladder cancer incidence rates are lowest in African-Americans and highest in Southwest American Indians.

An exact etiology is unknown, but chronic irritation produced by gallstones may initiate dysplastic transformation of the gallbladder mucosa. The majority of patients with gallbladder cancer have cholelithiasis (80%), but the converse is not true. As previously mentioned, malignancy in the presence of a porcelain gallbladder is common. Gallbladder adenomas, which have been found in association with carcinoma in situ of the gallbladder, appear as pedunculated polyps either by ultrasound or on direct visual inspection of the specimen after cholecystectomy.

The pathogenesis of gallbladder cancer is insidious, and early diagnosis is rare. These early cancers are often serendipitous findings at cholecystectomy. Symptoms are localized to the right upper abdominal quadrant and usually attributed to cholelithiasis. Nausea, anorexia, and weight loss are present in two-thirds of patients. An extremely rare idiopathic dermatologic disorder, acquired hypertrichosis lanuginosa, occurs due to an overproduction of unmedullated, nonpigmented facial lanugo. This presents as part of a paraneoplastic syndrome and has been termed "malignant down."

Laboratory tests are of little value in confirming or excluding the presence of gallbladder cancer. Radiographic studies may demonstrate a calcified gallbladder in up to 25% of cases. Oral cholecystogram or PIPIDA scan demonstrates an unopacified gallbladder. Ultrasound and CT scan may show a large mass replacing the gallbladder. A mass in the region of the head of the pancreas may be seen due to lymphatic spread to nodes around the distal CBD. These modalities may also demonstrate invasion of the liver.

The management of gallbladder carcinoma varies depending on the stage at diagnosis (Table 3). After all routine as well as emergent cholecystectomy procedures, it is imperative that the gallbladder be opened. Suspicious lesions are sent to pathology for immediate microscopic analysis. If cancer is confirmed and locoregional extension of the tumor is not present, an extended resection that includes an adjacent rim of liver and hepatoduodenal lymph nodes may be performed.

Cancer of the gallbladder has an unfavorable prognosis due to late diagnosis. The vast majority of gallbladder cancers infiltrate surrounding structures such as the portal vein and hepatic artery, making a curative surgical treatment impossible. The 5-year survival in all patients is <5%. The best 5-year survival is observed in patients with T_{is} tumors diagnosed after cholecystectomy and approaches 15%. Extended cholecystectomy has been shown to improve survival for T_1 and T_2 cancers in a few retrospective studies. Five-year survival after resection for known diagnosis is <3%. There is no added survival benefit from adjuvant chemotherapy or radiation therapy, although it may offer palliative relief by reducing tumor mass, relieving pain, and alleviating jaundice.

Cholangiocarcinoma

Primary malignant tumors of the bile ducts, i.e., cholangiocarcinoma, are even less common than carcinoma of the gallbladder and in general are difficult to treat and cure. Tumor classification is according to anatomic location. Proximal tumors include the major segmental intrahepatic ducts, right and left hepatic ducts, their confluence (Klatskin tumor), and the proximal common hepatic duct. Cholangiocarcinoma of the middle biliary system involves the distal hepatic duct, cystic duct, and their confluence.

Distal cholangiocarcinoma involves the distal common duct and carcinomas of the ampulla of Vater.

Typical patients are in the sixth decade of life, and males and females are equally affected. As in gallbladder cancer, direct invasion of surrounding organs (e.g., liver, duodenum, pancreatic head) and local vascular structures (e.g., hepatic artery, portal vein) is common. The vast lymphatic network allows cancer to spread to the regional lymph nodes in the porta hepatis, celiac axis, and pancreaticoduodenal nodes. Peritoneal seeding is a late manifestation of widely disseminated carcinoma.

The etiologies behind biliary tract malignancies are many. In the Far East, chronic parasitic infestation of the bile ducts with *Clonorchis sinensis* and *Opisthorchis viverrini* predispose to the development of bile duct cancer. Exposure to carcinogens such as anabolic steroids and thorium dioxide has also been linked to cholangiocarcinoma. Congenital anomalies of the biliary tree such as choledochal cysts, microhamartomas of von Meyenburg, and congenital intrahepatic dilation of the bile ducts are associated with development of biliary cancer. As stated previously, cholangiocarcinoma can develop in the presence of PSC.

A gradual onset of jaundice is the common manifestation of biliary tract malignancy. Anorexia, pruritus, a deep discomfort in the right upper quadrant, or abdominal pain are other common signs and symptoms. Cholangitis from acute obstruction is common. With distal biliary obstruction, the gallbladder may distend and become palpable below the right costal margin (Courvoisier's sign). Patients with tumors of the hepatic or cystic duct do not develop distended palpable gallbladders.

Diagnostic studies are consistent with obstructive jaundice. Ultrasound demonstrates dilated intrahepatic and perhaps extrahepatic biliary dilatation with distal tumors. CT can reveal direct invasion of the liver and better delineation of lymphadenopathy. Magnetic resonance imaging, although not routinely used, can demonstrate displacement, or encasement of adjacent vessels, as well as distant spread (e.g., hepatic metastases, regional lymphadenopathy).

ERC and PTC are complementary in defining anatomic pathology and obtaining a bile sample for cytology analysis, which reveals malignant cells in up to 40% of cases. Often ERC is unsuccessful in opacifying the

TABLE 3. *Staging gallbladder carcinoma*

Stage	T	
I	T_{is}	Carcinoma in situ
	T_1	Intramucosal lesions
II	T_2	Involves mucosa and muscularis layer
III	T3	Penetrates to gallbladder serosa or one adjacent organ or ≤2 cm invasion of liver
IV	T4	≥2 cm invasion of liver, invasion ≥2 adjacent organs

proximal ductal system. PTC is frequently relied upon to demonstrate proximal ductal anatomy and extent of the lesion, especially with tumors involving the proximal biliary system.

Patients without evidence of metastases or locally advanced cancer are candidates for surgical intervention. At laparotomy, if the portal vein and hepatic artery are free of disease, surgery should proceed with curative intent. Tumors of the distal common duct should be treated by pancreaticoduodenectomy (Whipple procedure). Tumors of the proximal or middle duct should be resected and biliary enteric reconstruction performed. Proximal bile duct tumors may require liver resection for complete resection of disease. Extensive proximal disease may prohibit safe resection.

Curative surgery cannot be offered to patients with extensive locoregional or metastatic disease. Tube decompression of the obstructed biliary duct(s) can be accomplished surgically, percutaneously, or endoscopically, and should be considered for palliation of jaundice. Percutaneous or endoscopic deployment of stents across malignant obstruction is successful in up to 70% of patients. Uncommon complications include infection and bleeding. Stent obstruction secondary to tumor ingrowth is common.

Postoperative radiation therapy is commonly recommended to decrease local recurrence. Intraductal radiation catheters in combination with external beam irradiation can provide a wider field of coverage with enhanced locoregional control. Chemotherapy has been unsuccessful in palliating symptoms of cholangiocarcinoma.

The overall prognosis of patients with cholangiocarcinoma is dismal. A patient with adenocarcinoma of the bile duct is not expected to survive >1 year after diagnosis. The 5-year survival overall is 15%. Death ensues after progression to biliary cirrhosis, intrahepatic infection, and inanition.

SUMMARY

Biliary tract disorders are common and require practicing clinicians to understand the mechanisms behind the disease. Although gallstone disease is frequently encountered in clinical practice, it should not be disregarded as mundane. Disastrous complications can result from underestimation of clinical disease. Similarly, biliary tract injuries, when suspected, deserve immediate attention with respect to diagnosis and prevention of sequelae from untreated ductal injury. Biliary tract cancer has an overwhelmingly poor prognosis but can be effectively palliated with radiologic or endoscopic biliary intervention.

STUDY QUESTIONS

1. Define the pathogenesis of acute cholecystitis.
2. Describe the extrahepatic biliary ductal system.
3. What is the appropriate management for biliary strictures.
4. What is Charcot's triad? Reynold's pentad?
5. Describe Murphy's sign and its clinical significance.

SUGGESTED READING

Friedman G. Natural history of asymptomatic and symptomatic gallstones. *Am J Surg* 1993;165:399–404.
Pitt HA, ed. Postoperative bile duct strictures. *Surg Clin North Am* 1990;70:355–380.
Rossi R, ed. Biliary reconstruction. *Surg Clin North Am* 1994;74:825–841.
Shailesh L, Kadakia M. Biliary tract emergencies. *Med Clin North Am* 1993;77:1015–1033.

CHAPTER 15

Pancreas

David M. Levi and Joe U. Levi

Since the Middle Ages, when Galen described the function of the pancreas as merely to protect the visceral vessels, a tremendous understanding of the pancreas has evolved. In the late 1800s, the research of many scientists elucidated the fundamentals of pancreatic exocrine function. At about the same time, Fitz characterized the inflammatory process of pancreatitis. Banting and Best in 1921 described the endocrine functions of the pancreas. Clinicians today use management principles that have emerged from knowledge regarding the pathogenesis and pathophysiology of pancreatic disease.

ANATOMY

The pancreas is an elongated, yellow-tan, lobulated, solid organ located in the retroperitoneum intimately associated with the duodenum, stomach, and spleen (Figs. 1 and 2). The anatomical, segments of the pancreas are the head, uncinate process, neck, body, and tail (Fig. 3). The head is encompassed by the duodenum and

surrounds the distal common bile duct. The uncinate process extends from the head posteriorly to lie behind the superior mesenteric vein near its union with the portal vein. The neck, the narrowest portion of the gland, extends anterior to the superior mesenteric vessels and is posterior to the pylorus and first portion of the duodenum. The body continues from the neck obliquely across the retroperitoneum anterior to the first lumbar vertebrae. The body merges into the tail, which ends near the hilum of the spleen. On average, the pancreas weighs 80 to 90 g and measures 15 to 20 cm in length.

Embryologically, the pancreas develops from two endodermal outpouchings of the foregut at ~4 weeks of gestation (Fig. 4). The dorsal portion arises from the duodenum and makes up the bulk of the gland. The ventral portion, which is a part of the hepatic diverticulum, makes up part of the head of the pancreas and the uncinate process. At ~6 weeks of gestation, the duodenum rotates and folds and the ventral pancreas rotates posteriorly behind the duodenum to fuse with the dorsal pancreas. Abnormal rotation or fusion of the ventral portion

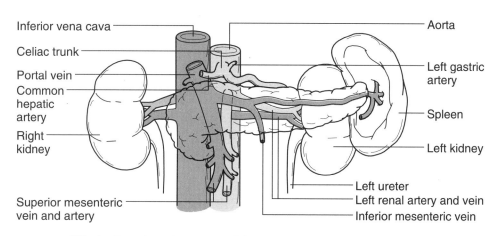

FIG. 1. Overview of anatomy of the pancreas, including blood supply.

187

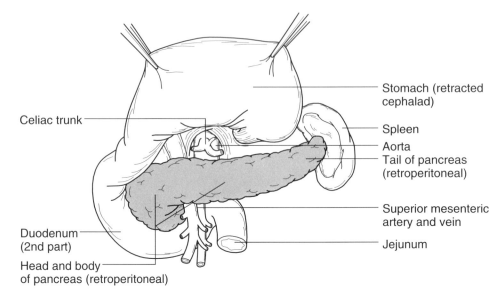

FIG. 2. Location of pancreas in relation to stomach.

with respect to the dorsal portion can result in annular pancreas (Fig. 5). Annular pancreas is a rare anomaly in which a strip of pancreatic tissue encircles the duodenum and usually manifests in children as partial or complete intestinal obstruction.

The arterial supply to the pancreas is derived from the splenic and pancreaticoduodenal arteries (Fig. 6). Multiple branches from the splenic artery, which travel along the superior border of the gland, supply the neck, body, and tail of the pancreas. The superior and inferior pancreatic arteries course transversely through the pancreas with many connections to branches of the celiac trunk and superior mesenteric arteries. The head and uncinate are supplied by the superior and inferior pancreaticoduodenal arteries. The former is a branch of the gastroduodenal artery, and the latter originates from the superior

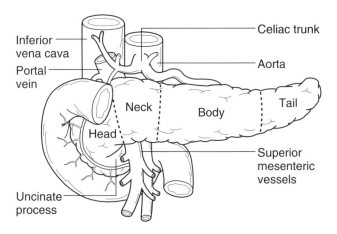

FIG. 3. Anatomical segments of the pancreas are the head, uncinate process, neck, body, and tail.

mesenteric artery. The superior and inferior pancreaticoduodenal arteries each have anterior and posterior branches that interconnect, providing a rich blood supply for the head of the pancreas and duodenum. Because of this shared blood supply, resection of the entire pancreatic head requires resection of the duodenum as well.

The venous drainage of the pancreas parallels the arterial supply (Fig. 7). Similarly named veins empty into the portal venous system. Along the length of the pancreas, multiple small veins empty into the splenic vein. In the head portion, pancreaticoduodenal veins empty into the portal and superior mesenteric veins. Often, the anterior branch of the superior pancreaticoduodenal vein joins the gastrocolic trunk at the inferior border of the neck on its way to the superior mesenteric vein. Numerous small veins from the uncinate empty directly into the superior mesenteric vein. The pancreas has a rich lymphatic network that drains into regional lymph nodes.

The main pancreatic duct (duct of Wirsung) represents a fusion between the ducts of the embryological ventral and dorsal pancreas. From the tail of the gland, it traverses the length of the pancreas slanting downward in the head to enter the duodenum with the common bile duct via the ampulla of Vater. The accessory duct (duct of Santorini) is derived from the dorsal portion of the gland and drains the superior aspect of the pancreatic head. It enters the duodenum proximal to the ampulla of Vater via an accessory ampulla. In pancreatic divisum, the ventral and dorsal ducts fail to fuse and the duct of Santorini acts as the primary ductal drainage for the pancreas. Pancreatic divisum has been implicated as an infrequent cause of pancreatitis and will be discussed later.

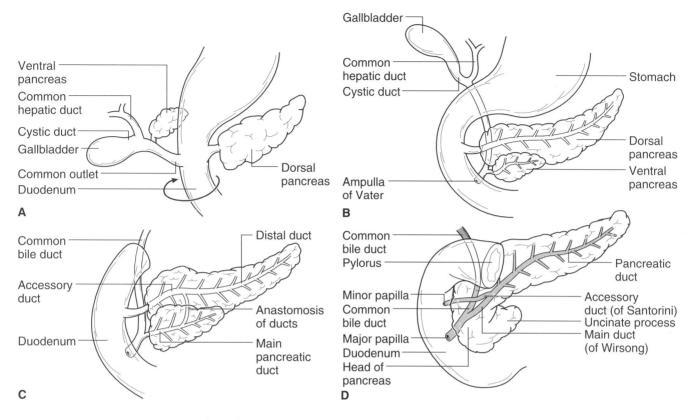

FIG. 4. (A–D) Embryological development of the pancreas.

PHYSIOLOGY

The pancreas has both endocrine and exocrine functions. The endocrine pancreas consists of clusters of cells, the islets of Langerhans, that are scattered throughout the pancreas comprising 2% of the total weight of the gland. Glucose homeostasis is the primary role of the endocrine pancreas, but the pancreas also contributes to the regulation of exocrine function. Important products of the islet cells that are released into the portal circulation include insulin, glucagon, somatostatin, and pancreatic polypeptide. The functional unit of the exocrine pancreas is composed of a cluster of acinar cells joined with centroacinar cells that lead into small ductules. The acinar cells produce an array of enzymes essential in the breakdown of proteins, carbohydrates, lipids, and nucleic acids. Centroacinar cells are rich in carbonic anhydrase and generate a tremendous amount of bicarbonate ion. Collectively, acinar and centroacinar cells secrete between 2 and 3 L of fluid rich in proenzymes and bicarbonate, which is conducted to tributaries of the main duct to ultimately reach the duodenum. It is there where these digestive enzymes are converted to the active form and mix with chyme for digestion.

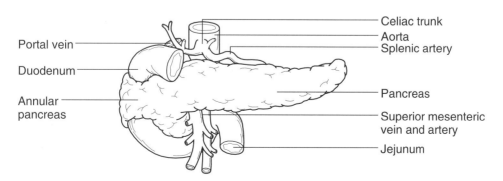

FIG. 5. Annular pancreas.

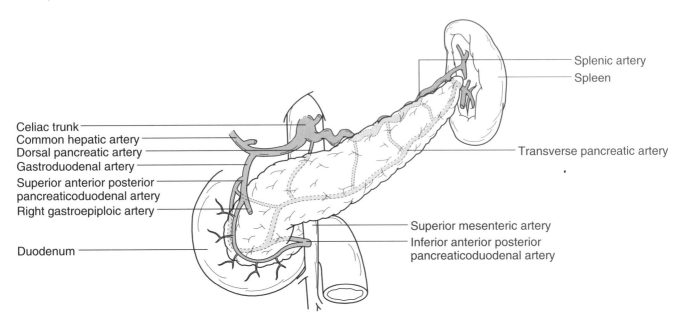

FIG. 6. Arterial supply to the pancreas is derived from the splenic and pancreaticoduodenal artery.

Endocrine Pancreas

Insulin is produced by the islet β-cell, the predominant cell in the pancreatic islet. Insulin production and release are stimulated by hyperglycemia. To a lesser degree, insulin is regulated by vagal control and various inhibitory peptides. Insulin facilitates the uptake of circulating glucose by a number of tissues and cell types.

Glucagon is produced and released from islet α-cells and functions as a counterregulatory hormone to insulin. In the liver, it promotes gluconeogenesis, glycogenolysis, and ketogenesis. In adipose tissue, it stimulates lipolysis.

Additionally, glucagon acts as an inhibitor of intestinal peristalsis, an inhibitor of gastric acid production, and an inhibitor of pancreatic exocrine secretion.

Somatostatin, from islet δ-cells, and pancreatic polypeptide have a modulatory role in gastrointestinal function and metabolism. Somatostatin has an inhibitory effect on bowel motility, gastric acid and pancreatic exocrine secretion, and islet cell function. In addition, it acts as a splanchnic vasoconstrictor and reduces intestinal blood flow. Of note, somatostatin is produced in other areas of the body, including the small intestine and the brain. The function of pancreatic polypeptide is less well

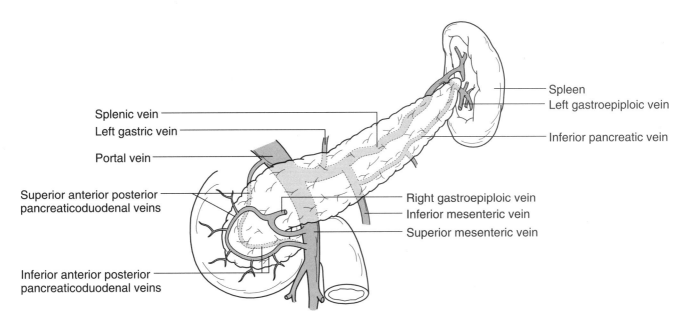

FIG. 7. Venous drainage of the duodenum and pancreas

defined. When released in response to a meal, it alters biliary motility and pancreatic exocrine function, and it probably has a role in glucose metabolism.

Exocrine Pancreas

The acinar cells package their products as zymogen granules that are released into the ductules by exocytosis. The specific endopeptidases produced include trypsin, chymotrypsin, elastase, and kallekrein. The exopeptidases include carboxypeptidase A and B. The peptidases are secreted in an inactive form to prevent autodigestion of the gland and are activated upon entering the duodenum. Duodenal mucosal enterokinase converts inactive trypsinogen to trypsin, which in turn activates the other peptidases. Other enzymes produced by the acinar cells include amylase, lipase, colipase, phospholipase, and nucleases. Acinar cell stimulation and zymogen granule release is promoted primarily by cholecystokinin and acetylcholine. Cholecystokinin is produced by the duodenum in response to luminal protein and fat.

The primary stimulus for electrolyte and water secretion by the pancreas is secretin. Secretin is produced by the proximal small intestine in response to luminal acid and bile. Normally, pancreatic fluid is isotonic, with a pH of 8, and sodium and potassium concentrations similar to plasma. As the rate of pancreatic fluid secretion increases, so does the bicarbonate ion concentration. In contrast, the chloride ion concentration decreases, but isotonicity is maintained. Bicarbonate and chloride ion concentrations are controlled by active transport mechanisms.

Neurohormonal mechanisms regulate pancreatic exocrine function during different phases of digestion. During the cephalic phase, direct parasympathetic stimulation of acinar cells through efferent vagal pathways promotes exocrine secretion. In addition, the site and smell of food stimulate gastric acid and bile production, which, when recognized in the duodenum, promotes pancreatic exocrine secretion. During the gastric phase, antral distention and protein content promote G-cell secretion of gastrin, which increases gastric acid production. Duodenal acidification, in turn, further stimulates pancreatic bicarbonate secretion. The intestinal phase starts after recognition of amino acids, fatty acids, and bile in the proximal small bowel and is mediated by direct vagal stimulation and cholecystokinin and secretin effect upon the exocrine pancreas.

DISEASES OF THE PANCREAS

Acute Pancreatitis

The term "acute pancreatitis" encompasses a broad spectrum of pancreatic inflammation. The clinical presentation and associated pathology range considerably. In addition, the complications of acute pancreatitis are diverse and present difficult challenges to the clinician. Only a minority of patients with pancreatitis will need surgical intervention. The astute clinician must be able to diagnosis and treat pancreatitis effectively, recognize severe cases, and decide when and for whom surgery is indicated.

Many etiologies of acute pancreatitis are recognized, including alcohol abuse, gallstones, hyperlipidemia, hypercalcemia, trauma, pancreatic divisum, and drugs. Worldwide, >90% of cases of acute pancreatitis are due to alcohol or gallstones. Common to all etiologies of pancreatitis appears to be the extravasation of activated pancreatic enzymes from the ductal system into the surrounding parenchyma. This initiates autodigestion of the gland with leakage of enzyme-rich fluid into parapancreatic tissues and potential spaces in the retroperitoneum and lesser sac. A systemic inflammatory response ensues that produces the clinical manifestation of acute pancreatitis.

Alcohol abuse has long been associated with acute pancreatitis. The disease usually ensues within 48 hr following excessive alcohol ingestion. Although the pathogenesis is not completely clear, alcohol is known to increase gastric acid production, which leads to duodenal acidification and increased pancreatic secretion. Simultaneously, alcohol increases the sphincter tone at the ampulla. The resultant pancreatic hypersecretion coupled with increased resistance at the ampulla leads to intraductal hypertension and extravasation of pancreatic enzymes that become activated and begin autodigestion of the parenchyma. Additionally, alcohol metabolites that directly cause pancreatic injury in experimental models and transient hyperlipidemia secondary to alcohol ingestion have been implicated as causes of acute pancreatitis.

Biliary pancreatitis was first recognized by Opie in 1901. According to his common channel theory, gallstone impaction at the ampulla results in bile reflux into the pancreatic duct via a shared segment of duct just proximal to the ampulla. Bile was thought to irritate the gland and cause acute pancreatitis. While most patients with biliary pancreatitis do have a common channel between the pancreatic and common bile ducts, it has since been learned that gallstone impaction is not required to initiate pancreatitis. Rather, the passage of a stone through the ampulla and the ensuing ampullary edema may be all that is necessary to facilitate bile reflux into the pancreatic duct. Regardless of the exact mechanism, gallstones clearly can cause acute pancreatitis. Perhaps the best evidence is provided by the fact that cholecystectomy and clearance of stones from the biliary tree prevents future attacks of the disease.

Less is known about the other etiologies for acute pancreatitis, but their recognition is important because management of the underlying etiology may protect against recurrent episodes of pancreatitis. Hypercalcemia-related acute pancreatitis is usually due to hyperparathyroidism, which often can be effectively treated. Blunt abdominal trauma may fracture the pancreas at the neck of the pancreas, where it overlies the spine and can cause pancreatitis. Pancreatic divisum results when the ductal systems from the dorsal and ventral portions of the gland fail to join and, thus, drain separately into the duodenum. This variation in ductal anatomy affects nearly 10% of the population and has been cited as a cause of pancreatitis. Acute pancreatitis secondary to pancreatic divisum or blunt abdominal trauma may dictate specific treatments that may be curative. In a minority of patients, the cause is never found.

The clinical presentation of acute pancreatitis can range from a stable patient with mild abdominal pain to an obtunded patient with sepsis, hemodynamic instability, and multiple organ system failure. A careful history may reveal recent alcohol abuse or biliary stone disease. Classically, the patient presents with epigastric pain that radiates through to the back with associated nausea and vomiting. Right or left upper quadrant pain may predominate. Fever, tachycardia, abdominal tenderness, and distention may be noted on physical examination. Abdominal tenderness is due to retroperitoneal irritation and distention is a sign of paralytic ileus. In severe cases, the patient may present in hypovolemic shock due to massive retroperitoneal fluid sequestration or hemorrhage. In this subgroup of patients, aggressive resuscitation and intensive care monitoring are required.

The diagnosis of acute pancreatitis rests on accurate assessment of clinical presentation and results of specific laboratory tests and radiologic studies. An elevation in the serum amylase is the most common laboratory abnormality seen in acute pancreatitis. It is, however, neither sensitive nor specific. A normal amylase level does not eliminate the possibility of acute pancreatitis. Additionally, an elevated serum amylase is associated with a broad range of disorders, including intestinal obstruction and infarction, peptic ulcer disease, peritonitis, salpingitis, ruptured ectopic pregnancy, salivary gland disease, severe burns, pneumonia, and head trauma. Measurement of amylase isoenzymes and urinary amylase levels can improve the utility of amylase as a diagnostic marker. Elevation of serum lipase level serves as a more accurate indicator of acute pancreatitis because lipase originates solely from the pancreas.

Other laboratory abnormalities reflect the pathophysiology of acute pancreatitis. An elevated hematocrit results from hemoconcentration. Calcium deposition in the retroperitoneum results in hypocalcemia. Transaminase, alkaline phosphatase, and bilirubin elevation are associated with biliary pancreatitis. Pancreatic endocrine insufficiency may result in hyperglycemia. Leukocytosis, hypoxemia, and metabolic acidosis are all nonspecific findings but are important predictors of disease severity.

A variety of radiologic studies are used to evaluate patients suspected or known to have acute pancreatitis. Abdominal ultrasound may reveal signs of pancreatic inflammation including gland enlargement, edema, and fluid collections. Ultrasound is excellent for detecting cholelithiasis and biliary tract pathology, thereby revealing the etiology of the disease in a large number of cases. Endoscopic retrograde cholangiopancreatography (ERCP) is sometimes used after resolution of the acute disease to reveal a ductal stenosis or pancreatic divisum. It may also be used to detect and treat choledocholithiasis. Dynamic computerized tomography (CT) scanning of the abdomen is the best radiographic study for visualizing the pancreas. It illustrates findings indicative of acute pancreatitis including pancreatic enlargement, edema, fat stranding, necrosis, and fluid collections including abscesses and pseudocysts. Additionally, CT-guided needle aspiration of pancreatic fluid collections may reveal evidence of infection, or it can direct catheter placement for drainage of pseudocysts. In rare cases of acute pancreatitis, the inflammatory process erodes branches of the splenic artery or pancreaticoduodenal arcade, resulting in massive hemorrhage. Selective angiography and embolization of a bleeding vessel may be life saving. Angiography, however, has no role in the diagnosis of acute pancreatitis.

In most patients, acute pancreatitis is self-limiting and requires only supportive care. However, in a minority of patients, the disease is severe, necessitating intensive care monitoring and support. Predicting which patients need this increased support is problematic, but a number of scoring systems have been devised to predict morbidity and mortality associated with acute pancreatitis. The ability to recognize the critically ill patients early and treat them aggressively may decrease the mortality and morbidity from acute disease.

The most well known of these scoring systems was established by Ranson in 1974. He described 11 variables (Table 1) consisting of five measured on admission and six within 48 hr of admission. Prognosis in patients suffering from acute pancreatitis can be determined on the basis of these criteria (Table 2). This system is useful in predicting disease severity and may aid selection of patients that would benefit from intensive monitoring and more aggressive intervention.

The management of acute pancreatitis is predominantly nonoperative in nature and begins with pancreatic exocrine suppression. By decreasing pancreatic exocrine function, the severity of acute pancreatitis is lessened, and episodic exacerbation of disease symptoms due to gland stimulation can be prevented. Modalities used to suppress the exocrine pancreas include withholding oral intake, nasogastric suction as needed for persistent vomiting, and antacids and H_2 receptor antagonists. These measures suppress the gland by inhibiting gastric distention and acid production. If the patient is malnourished or is not expected to resume oral intake soon, then hyperal-

TABLE 1. *Ranson criteria of acute pancreatitis*

At admission	Within 48 hr of admission
Age of >55	HCT decrease of >10 points
WBC of >16,000 cells/mm^3	BUN elevation of >5 mg/dl
Serum glucose of >200 mg/dl	Serum Ca^{2+} decrease of <8 mg/dl
Lactate dehydrogenase of >350 IU/L	Arterial pO_2 of <60 mm Hg
GOT of >250 U/dl	Base deficit of >4 meq/L
	Fluid requirement of >6 L

imentation is indicated. Narcotic agents are given for pain control. Meperidine is favored over morphine because it has less spasmodic effect on the ampullary sphincter.

The intense inflammatory response seen in acute pancreatitis has a wide range of effects. Significant retroperitoneal fluid sequestration can result in critical intravascular volume depletion and hemodynamic instability if untreated. Thus, fluid and electrolyte replacement and volume status should be closely monitored. Severe pancreatitis can result in a variety of pulmonary problems ranging from atelectasis to respiratory failure. Some patients may require endotracheal intubation and positive pressure ventilation. The use of antibiotics in acute pancreatitis is somewhat controversial, but most agree that broad spectrum agents are indicated in severe cases to decrease the incidence of infectious complications. Specific treatment for acute pancreatitis geared toward halting the sequence of events that cause gland destruction and necrosis is an active area of research.

Although the majority of patients who develop acute pancreatitis will recover without operative intervention, there are specific cases in which surgery is indicated. These include infection of the pancreas and deteriorating clinical status despite optimal support and treatment of the underlying cause. Rarely, diagnostic uncertainty occasionally warrants exploratory laparotomy because there exists no definitive test to exclude or confirm acute pancreatitis.

Infection of the pancreas encompasses pancreatic abscess and infected necrosis and should be considered in those patients that do not respond to supportive measures, especially in those patients with signs of ongoing sepsis. Differentiating between sterile necrosis of the gland and secondary infection can be difficult. Dynamic CT scan may reveal air bubbles in the retroperitoneum from gas-forming organisms. In difficult cases CT scan–guided

needle aspiration of peripancreatic collections with Gram stain and culture may be the key to confirming the diagnosis of pancreatic abscess or infected necrosis. Enteric organisms are the most common pathogens.

The surgical management involves debridement of the retroperitoneum, and wide drainage and often multiple reexplorations are required. Some surgeons prefer closing the abdomen after placing large peripancreatic catheters for continuous postoperative irrigating and drainage. Others debride the lesser sac and leave it open packed with moist gauze dressing, termed "marsupialization." The dressing is removed daily either in the intensive care unit or operating room so the pancreatic bed can be irrigated and repacked. A high incidence of morbidity and mortality that accompanies the above procedures has brought forth an evolution in alternative methods of therapy for infected pancreatic necrosis. In this particular subgroup of patients who otherwise have minimal symptoms, repetitive interventional radiology-guided percutaneous irrigation and drainage has achieved similar results to operative intervention with avoidance of increased morbidity and mortality. As yet, though, it is not widely recognized as standard of care because it is less effective at draining the thick and viscous necrotic tissue. Those patients that decompensate or have incomplete resolution of infected pancreatic collections require operative drainage.

The clinical management of biliary pancreatitis deserves special consideration. Gallstone-induced pancreatitis is encountered frequently in clinical practice; however, fundamental management principles are often overlooked because of failure to understand the natural history of this particular disease. Similar to other types of pancreatitis, pancreatic injury ranges from minimal peripancreatic inflammation to frank necrosis. However, unique to biliary pancreatitis is the short duration of serum hyperamylasemia that usually resolves within a 48-hr period. The clinical condition of the patient corresponds to the extent of destruction of pancreatic parenchyma. Biliary pancreatitis has an extremely high short-term recurrence rate. Therefore, despite complete resolution of clinical symptoms, patients suffering from an episode of biliary pancreatitis should not be discharged prior to cholecystectomy and cholangiographic exclusion of residual common bile duct stones.

TABLE 2. *Mortality predicted from Ranson criteria*

# Ransom criteria	Mortality
<3	0%
3 or 4	15–40%
5 or 6	near 50%
7 or more	approaching 100%

Pancreatic Pseudocyst

Pseudocysts are the most common complication of acute pancreatitis. A pseudocyst, as the name implies, is not a true cyst because it lacks an epithelial lining. Pancreatic ductal disruption due to inflammation or trauma permits exocrine secretions to leak around the gland. This invokes an inflammatory response that walls off the fluid forming a cystic collection. This fibrous wall may be adherent to adjacent organs. The communication between the pancreatic duct and a pseudocyst may persist or be obliterated. Pseudocyst fluid has a high amylase content and can be mixed with blood and debris.

The presence of a pseudocyst should be considered in the patient who has persistent pain, hyperamylasemia, or an ileus at >2 weeks after a bout of acute pancreatitis. A palpable mass or fullness is often detected on abdominal examination. The pain is usually localized to the epigastric region or left upper quadrant and can be associated with fever, nausea, and malaise.

To study a suspected pseudocyst, a CT scan should be chosen because it accurately characterizes size and relationship to the pancreas and adjacent viscera. Ultrasound is also useful, especially when serial exams over time are needed for longitudinal follow-up. ERCP is sometimes helpful in demonstrating a communication between the pseudocyst and pancreatic duct but is not used routinely.

Many pseudocysts will resolve spontaneously. Some, however, persist and cause a number of problems. A pseudocyst can become secondarily infected, and when this occurs, it should be treated like a pancreatic abscess. Other complications seen with pseudocysts include rupture into the peritoneal cavity, intestinal or biliary obstruction due to extrinsic compression, and bleeding from erosion into nearby vessels. Complications are more often seen with large pseudocysts.

The preferred treatment of pseudocysts depends on a number of variables, including size, location, duration, associated symptoms, and the manifestation of complications. Most agree that small diameter (<6 cm) asymptomatic lesions require no specific treatment. Previously, it was believed that larger pseudocysts should be treated even if asymptomatic, due to the risk of serious complications. Several recent studies suggest that large, asymptomatic pseudocysts can be managed expectantly. Symptomatic or complicated pseudocysts require treatment in the form of percutaneous drainage, surgical drainage, or surgical excision.

Percutaneous catheter drainage of pseudocysts performed with ultrasound or CT guidance has gained popularity in recent years. This technique requires meticulous patient compliance with regard to long-term outpatient care. Some clinicians advocate ERCP prior to percutaneous drainage to exclude a communication between pseudocyst and pancreatic duct that would pre-

dispose to treatment failure. In these cases, surgical drainage may be a better alternative.

The surgical options for the management of pseudocysts include internal drainage, external drainage, and excision. Internal drainage via surgical anastomosis of the pseudocyst and hollow viscera is the preferred method of treatment for most pseudocysts. The stomach (cystogastrostomy) is chosen when the pseudocyst is adherent to the posterior gastric wall. A jejunal limb (cystojejunostomy) is the most versatile option and is commonly used. The duodenum is acceptable for internal drainage (cystoduodenostomy) when the pseudocyst is in the head of the pancreas. External drainage is reserved for grossly infected pseudocysts that have a thin wall. Pseudocysts are rarely excised due to extraordinary inflammatory reaction encountered. Occasionally, a pseudocyst in the head of the pancreas causing biliary and duodenal obstruction can be excised by performing a pancreaticoduodenectomy (Whipple procedure).

Chronic Pancreatitis

Chronic pancreatitis is the end result of long-term inflammatory injury to the pancreas. It is an entity that can be thought of as pancreatic failure in much the same way one considers cardiac or hepatic failure. It is characterized by exocrine insufficiency, endocrine insufficiency, and chronic pain. The majority of patients with chronic pancreatitis have alcohol-induced disease. Years of injury to the gland results in atrophy and fibrosis. Calcification of the pancreas is a classic finding often detectable radiographically. The pancreatic duct often has strictures with interposed segments of dilatation, i.e., "chain of lakes."

The patient with chronic pancreatitis usually has had several bouts of acute pancreatitis over several years. Unfortunately, the disease may progress even if the patient abstains from alcohol ingestion. Eventually, intermittent epigastric pain slowly becomes constant and unrelenting, and most patients become dependent upon narcotic medications. Anorexia and weight loss are common. Exocrine insufficiency results in steatorrhea, and endocrine dysfunction manifests as diabetes mellitus. Occasionally, a scarred, fibrotic head of the pancreas may impinge on the distal common bile duct resulting in biliary obstruction. Similarly, these lesions may cause duodenal obstruction. Pseudocysts are common in the presence of chronic pancreatitis also. Chronic inflammation may cause splenic vein thrombosis with resultant segmental portal hypertension. Finally, pancreatic carcinoma may develop in the presence of chronic pancreatitis.

The diagnosis of chronic pancreatitis is suspected based on the patient's history and presentation. There are no laboratory studies specific for chronic pancreatitis.

Diffuse pancreatic calcifications is invariably diagnostic of chronic pancreatitis.

The primary indication for surgery in chronic pancreatitis is unrelenting pain. Typically, pain is severe, exceedingly intractable, and refractory to medical management. Prior to operative intervention, investigation should be undertaken to exclude biliary or duodenal obstruction. If found, the procedure should be designed to relieve these processes. Pseudocysts are managed similar to those encountered with acute pancreatitis. Resection of suspected pancreatic malignancy should always be offered. Finally, if the patient is not yet a diabetic, endocrine function should be preserved.

The cause of pain in chronic pancreatitis is not completely understood but relative pancreatic ductal obstruction and hypertension are thought to be contributory. Several drainage procedures have been devised to relieve this obstruction. A side-to-side pancreaticojejunostomy (Puestow procedure) is a favored procedure of contemporary pancreatic surgeons. In this operation, a defunctionalized limb of jejunum is opened longitudinally and sewn to the side of the pancreas after opening the duct along its length. This procedure is most effective when most or all of the pancreatic duct is dilated. Total pancreatectomy is another surgical option, but should be done only if the patient is an insulin dependent diabetic. Removing 95% of the pancreas while preserving the common bile duct and blood supply to the duodenum is yet another option. Biliary and duodenal obstruction is treated either by bypass of the lesion or resection. Chronic pancreatitis in the head of the pancreas with associated distal common bile duct obstruction is often indistinguishable from pancreatic cancer and should be treated as such by performing a pancreaticoduodenectomy if there is no evidence of metastatic disease. A final measure for pain control is celiac nerve block with alcohol. This can be done intraoperatively or percutaneously.

Pancreatic Neoplasms

Benign neoplasms of the pancreas are exceedingly rare and will not be discussed here. Our focus is on primary malignancies of the pancreas, of which there are three types. The first arises from the ductal epithelium, namely, adenocarcinoma. The second consists of endocrine tumors of the pancreas. The third involves cystic pancreatic neoplasms.

Pancreatic Carcinoma

The incidence of pancreatic cancer has increased threefold in the past 40 years. There are ~28,000 new cases diagnosed each year. It is the second most common gastrointestinal tract malignancy and the fourth most common cause of death from cancer. The incidence of pancreatic cancer increases with age and peaks in the eighth decade of life. Men are affected twice as frequently as women. Over half of the lesions are localized to the head, one-fifth are located in the body, <5% are located in the tail, and 20% are multicentric throughout the entire gland.

Cancer of the head of the pancreas comprises the vast majority of periampullary malignancies, including duodenal/ampullary cancer and distal common bile duct cholangiocarcinoma. Periampullary malignancies present with similar findings, but for the context of this text, all references will be made to cancer of the head of the pancreas. Findings typically noted on physical examination include jaundice and, infrequently, a palpable nontender gallbladder (Courvoisier's sign). Palpation of an abdominal mass or supraclavicular node is suggestive of distant metastasis. Laboratory studies are nonspecific but often support the diagnosis of obstructive jaundice. Abdominal ultrasound will reveal biliary dilatation and, less often, a mass at the head of the pancreas. CT scan of the abdomen is helpful in confirming the presence of a mass in the head of the pancreas, though dramatic pancreatic and biliary ductal dilatation may be present even before the tumor is large enough to be detected by CT scan. Encroachment or encasement of the portal vein and superior mesenteric vessels demonstrated by CT predicts against resectability. Likewise, visualization of metastatic disease to the liver and other organs is another unfavorable predictor of resectability.

ERCP may reveal a duodenal or ampullary lesion, and a pancreatogram may provide more data regarding ductal anatomy. Irregular narrowing of both the intrapancreatic common bile duct and the pancreatic duct ("double duct sign") is pancreatic cancer until proven otherwise. However, if the pancreatic duct and biliary tree are dilated and well visualized by CT, then ERCP may not be necessary. Some surgeons prefer transhepatic cholangiography to evaluate the nature of the obstruction and to decompress the biliary tree in preparation for surgery. Previously, operating on a patient with obstructive jaundice was thought to be dangerous. Clinical experience has not proven this to be true, and routine preoperative biliary decompression is not absolutely necessary. A biopsy of the pancreatic lesion is also not necessary unless the patient is not a candidate for surgery and a tissue diagnosis is needed. Frequently, the best pancreatic biopsy is the surgical specimen. Laparoscopy can be used preoperatively to look for metastatic disease too small to be seen by CT scan.

The goal of surgery for pancreatic cancer is cure. The procedure of choice for resectable tumors in the head of the pancreas is pancreaticoduodenectomy (Whipple procedure). Biliary-enteric, gastroenteric, and pancreaticoenteric anastamoses reestablish alimentary tract continuity.

Tumor diameter of >3.0 cm, lymph node involvement, and perineural invasion are poor prognostic indicators. Perioperative mortality which previously was as high as 20% has dramatically declined to <5% with experienced surgical teams. Furthermore, the morbidity after pancreaticoduodenectomy has also declined in recent years. Gastric atony and pancreaticoenteric anastomotic leak remain the most common postoperative complications. Unfortunately, less than one-fourth of these malignancies prove to be resectable at the time of operation. For patients with unresectable disease, relief of biliary obstruction and relief or prevention of duodenal obstruction are goals of palliation. Intraoperatively, biliary diversion is accomplished by choledochoenteric or cholecystoenteric anastamoses, while doudenal obstruction is relieved by gastrojejunostomy. Alternatively, stents placed percutaneously or endoscopically can decompress biliary obstruction.

Five-year survival after curative resection approaches only 20% in all patients. However, a significant minority of pancreatic head tumors are not pancreatic adenocarcinoma and carry a much better prognosis. Despite the generalized pessimism regarding the clinical management of pancreatic cancer, postoperative chemotherapy and radiation therapy has value. Adjuvant multimodality therapy involving radiation sensitization followed by intensive chemotherapy appears to improve short-term survival; however, no improvement in long-term survival has been appreciated. Palliative chemoradiation therapy for patients with distant metastasis without evidence of biliary or duodenal obstruction has been disappointing with only a negligible increase in short-term survival reported.

Pancreatic cancer of the body and tail has a silent insidious growth pattern. Weight loss (up to 20% of total body weight), pain, and metastatic disease (e.g., Blumer's shelf, Virchow's node, etc.) are the predominant signs and symptoms. CT scan of the pancreas may demonstrate a lesion in the distal pancreas. Surgical excision of this tumor involves distal pancreatectomy, splenic hilar node dissection, and splenectomy. Unfortunately, <10% of patients have resectable lesions at laparotomy, and long-term survival in patients with this type of pancreatic cancer is rare.

Endocrine Tumors

Endocrine tumors of the pancreas originate from islet cells. They can present as functional tumors, secreting an array of neurohormonal products, or they can exist as nonfunctional tumors. They are classified as neoplasms that possess amine precursor uptake and decarboxylation properties (APUDomas). These relatively rare tumors are associated with specific syndromes, and their study has allowed much insight regarding gastrointestinal endocrine physiology. The endocrine tumors include the insulinoma, gastrinoma, and glucagonoma. Each can pre-

sent with local symptoms but usually are suspected by the manifestation of endocrine imbalances.

An insulinoma is islet β-cells that produce insulin without regulation. Classically, patients are overweight or obese from the continual necessity to eat to prevent hypoglycemic episodes. Patients present with profound hypoglycemia usually preceded by weakness, confusion, hunger, and convulsions. These symptoms resolve immediately with glucose administration. The diagnosis is confirmed during a 72-hr fast during which time the patient is given nothing to eat. As glucose levels drop, the patient becomes symptomatic. Immediately insulin, c-peptide, and serum glucose levels are drawn followed by the administration of glucose. Whipple's triad describes findings during the 72-hr fast, including (a) fasting-induced hypoglycemia, (b) associated symptoms, and (c) complete resolution of the symptoms with glucose ingestion. Approximately 10% of insulinomas are malignant, and half of these are metastatic. There is no effective medical treatment for insulinoma. Surgical extirpation of the tumor is required. The best preoperative localization study is a CT scan, but if the lesion cannot be found intraoperative ultrasound and palpation of the gland localize the lesion in the vast majority of cases. Enucleation of the tumor followed by a thorough exam of the remaining gland to exclude residual disease is the surgical management principle. If intraoperative localization studies have failed to find the lesion, blind pancreatic resection, albeit controversial, is done in some instances.

In 1955, Zollinger and Ellison characterized hypergastrinemia that manifested as refractory peptic ulcer disease. The gastrinoma, as they found, is an ulcerogenic tumor of pancreatic islet cells responsible for what is now termed "Zollinger-Ellison (ZE) syndrome." The majority of these tumors are located in the gastrinoma triangle defined by three landmarks: the confluence of the cystic and hepatic duct, the junction of the second and third portions of the duodenum, and the neck of the pancreas. Sixty percent of these tumors are frankly malignant. One third are associated with multiple endocrine neoplasia (MEN I), whereas the remainder are sporadic. The pattern of peptic ulcer disease is complicated in that distribution of ulcers can extend into the distal duodenum and jejunum in a significant percentage of cases and that many patients have multiple ulcer sites. Frequently, patients have been treated for ulcer disease and have had persistence or recurrence despite maximal therapy, including definitive surgical therapy.

The current therapy for ZE syndrome has evolved from the previous standards. ZE syndrome in association with MEN I is invariably multifocal disease and surgically unresectable. Administration of H^+ proton pump blockade, however, is quite successful in medical control of this disease. Highly selective vagotomy is reserved for patients that fail medical management. Patients with nonfamilial gastrinoma should be offered surgical therapy for disease. Preoperative localization is ideal and can be obtained frequently by endoscopy or with CT scan or somatostatin scintigraphy scan. Unfortunately, however, attempts at preoperative localization are frequently unsuccessful, but this should not preclude the attempt at surgical resection of tumor. Upon laparotomy, thorough search for primary disease as well as metastatic disease should be sought. Occasionally, intraoperative ultrasound and endoscopy can assist in localization. Disease localized to the pancreas is excised with a rim of normal pancreas. Large lesions in the head of the pancreas may require pancreaticoduodenectomy. Failure to localize the lesion is an indication for highly selective vagotomy. Patients with isolated locoregional metastasis should be resected for palliation of ulcer symptoms. Total gastrectomy and blind pancreatectomy are no longer favored as treatment of ZE because of the tremendous associated morbidity. The success from chemotherapeutic agents (e.g., streptozocin, 5-FU) has been disappointing.

Cystic Pancreatic Neoplasms

Cystic tumors of the pancreas make up <5% of pancreatic neoplasms and include cystadenoma and cystadenocarcinoma. They are much more prevalent in women than men. Epigastric pain and back pain are the usual complaint. A palpable mass is often present. These lesions are typically found in the body and tail of the pancreas, and abdominal ultrasound or CT scan are the best imaging studies for this disease. Serous cystadenomas are typically small, multiple lesions and are benign. Mucinous cystadenomas are often large, solitary perhaps septated lesions and invariably harbor malignancy.

It is sometimes quite difficult to distinguish between a cystic neoplasm and a pseudocyst of the pancreas; however, if the patient has no history of pancreatitis, one must be suspicious of a cystic neoplasm. Unlike pseudocysts, cystic tumors are not adherent to adjacent organs. Also, amylase in the cyst fluid can be low or high, whereas the amylase in pseudocysts is usually quite high. Finally, biopsy of the cyst wall or cytology of the fluid may reveal epithelial cells indicative of a cystic neoplasm. These tumors are considered low-grade malignancies and

should be surgically excised. For lesions in the distal pancreas, distal pancreatectomy with splenectomy completely removes the lesion. Cystic neoplasms at the head of the pancreas require pancreaticoduodenectomy. Five-year survival in large series approaches 50% in all patients with resectable lesions.

SUMMARY

Disease of the pancreas is quite common and requires an understanding of the anatomy, physiology, and pathophysiology of pancreatic diseases. The pancreas occupies a central anatomical position and is in close proximity to vascular structures as well as other abdominal organs. It has both endocrine and exocrine function, and the degree of dysfunction is vital to clinical decision making. Most diseases of the pancreas that concern the surgeon can be classified as inflammatory or neoplastic. Despite this simple classification and the rather unassuming appearance of the pancreas on visual inspection, it is only too clear to general surgeons that the pancreas can pose a formidable array of clinical problems unmatched in the alimentary tract with respect to severity, complexity, and treatment.

STUDY QUESTIONS

1. Describe the arterial supply and venous drainage of the pancreas.
2. Embryologically, where does the pancreas arise from?
3. When is surgery indicated for the treatment of pancreatitis?
4. What is the proposed mechanism behind the pathogenesis of chronic pancreatitis?
5. Describe the typical presentation of a patient with a periampullary carcinoma.

SUGGESTED READING

Cameron J, ed. Pancreatic neoplasms. *Surg Clin North Am* 1995;75.
Ranson JH, Rifkind KM, Roses DF, et al.: Prognostic signs and the role of operative management in acute pancreatitis. *Surg Gyn Obstet.* 1974;139, 69–81.
Reber H, ed. The pancreas. *Surg Clin North Am* 1989;69.

CHAPTER 16

Acute Abdomen and Appendicitis

Enrique Ginzburg and Jorge de la Pedraja

An acute abdomen is defined as severe abdominal pain that is often sudden in onset or can be an exacerbation of chronic abdominal disease. The pain and associated symptoms may be manifestations of either surgical or nonsurgical abdominal illness. Obtaining a thorough patient history and performing a complete physical examination is fundamental in evaluating abdominal pain. Selective laboratory and radiologic studies should be obtained based on specific data from the history and physical examination.

The abdominal cavity is commonly divided into four quadrants by imaginary lines that cross vertically and horizontally at the umbilicus (Fig. 1). Alternatively, the abdomen is divided into nine areas by vertical mid-clavicular lines and transverse lines across the costal angles and anterior superior iliac spines (Fig. 2). Accurate clinical assessment requires recognition of intraabdominal

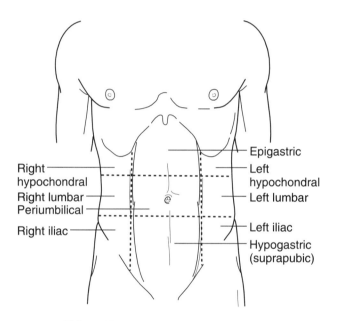

FIG. 2. The nine areas of the abdomen.

anatomy and related disease patterns within each respective area (Table 1).

HISTORY OF PRESENT ILLNESS

Perhaps the most important step in clinical assessment is obtaining a detailed patient history. Onset of pain (e.g., spontaneous, chronic, episodic), location (e.g., right upper quadrant [RUQ], flank, back), and severity (e.g., intense, moderate discomfort) should be determined. Equally as important are the quality of the pain (e.g., cramps, burning, intermittent, steady) as well as referred or associated pain (e.g., epigastric pain with radiation to the mid-back, RUQ pain with reference to the ipsilateral scapula). Clinicians must inquire whether the patient has ever experienced this type of pain in the past, what meth-

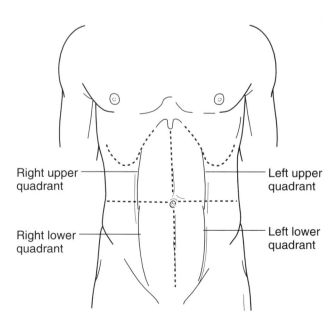

FIG. 1. The four quadrants of the abdominal cavity.

TABLE 1. *Abdominal contents divided into quadrants and areas*

RUQ
  Gallbladder
  Pancrease
  Stomach
  Liver
  Duodenum
  Right adrenal
  Right kidney
  Hepatic flexure
RLQ
  Appendix
  Cecum
  Ascending colon
  Right ureter
  Right ovary
Epigastric
  Stomach
  Pancreas
  Transverse colon
Umbilical
  Small bowel
Suprapubic
  Urinary bladder
  Uterus
LUQ
  Spleen
  Pancreas
  Stomach
  Left adrenal
  Left kidney
  Splenic flexure
LLQ
  Sigmoid colon
  Descending colon
  Left ureter
  Left ovary
  Left fallopian tube

RUQ, right upper quadrant; RLQ, right lower quadrant; LUQ, left upper quadrant; LLQ, left lower quadrant.

ods of pain relief the patient has attempted, and if any relief was experienced with these interventions.

Gastrointestinal dysfunction is frequently associated with abdominal pain. Nausea and vomiting are often primary presenting symptoms. Occasionally, nausea and vomiting may precede the onset of pain. The onset of pain may become evident only after meals. Conversely, eating may be the sole event that relieves abdominal pain. A change in bowel habits is an important detail in patient history that may suggest an etiology of abdominal pain. Bloody, mucus-laden diarrhea is associated with inflammatory, infectious, or ischemic bowel disease. Profuse watery diarrhea may be associated with gastroenteritis. Gross blood per rectum, hematochezia, implies colonic pathology, whereas black tarry stools, melena, suggests upper intestinal disease. Evaluation of patients with alternating bouts of constipation and diarrhea or change in

stool caliber may reveal an obstructing distal colon lesion.

Accurate diagnosis remains a challenge in female patients in whom clinical disease that can manifest as acute abdominal pain is diverse. Questions about the patient's last menstrual period, regularity of her menstrual cycle, and past or present pregnancies are essential. Inquiries regarding sexual activity and promiscuity, presence of an intrauterine device (IUD), as well as a history of pelvic inflammatory disease (PID) are important data that can improve diagnostic accuracy.

Finally, a patient history is incomplete without investigation into coexisting medical diseases, previous surgical procedures, and review of systems. Exacerbations of chronic medical conditions such as sickle-cell anemia and systemic lupus erythematosus can manifest as acute abdominal pain. Chronic disease may also be a marker for associated pathology that can present clinically as acute abdominal pain, i.e., peripheral vascular disease as a marker for mesenteric ischemia. Previous surgical procedures (e.g., appendectomy, cholecystectomy, colectomy) will eliminate those specific possibilities from the differential diagnosis. A patient who has undergone previous abdominal surgery and who claims progressive nausea and vomiting in the presence of abdominal distention certainly deserves evaluation for bowel obstruction. A complete review of systems may detect other sources of nonsurgical abdominal pain such as myocardial ischemia, rare systemic illnesses (systemic lupus erythematosus, porphyria), or common regional disease such as urinary tract infections. Race and ethnic heritage are clinically important, as demonstrated by increased incidence of sickle-cell disease in African-Americans and familial Mediterranean fever seen in Sephardic Jews and Armenians.

PHYSICAL EXAMINATION

A complete physical examination is essential to the assessment of patients with abdominal pain. However, to exhaustively review every detail of patient examination is beyond the scope of this discussion. A directed approach to abdominal examination will be presented.

Observation is a subjective but quick method of assessing the intensity and nature of a patient's abdominal pain. Facial expressions or body position often relate the severity of pain. Scleral jaundice suggests hepatobiliary pathology. Cutaneous manifestations of abdominal pathology (e.g., spider angiomata, pyoderma gangrenosum) may be present. The presence of surgical scars on the chest, abdomen, and back consistent with previous surgery should be noted; if these were not described by the patient in the history taking, thorough inquiry should be made into these issues. Ecchymosis about the periumbilical area, "Cullen's sign," or about the flanks, "Grey Turner's sign," indicates extraperitoneal or retroperitoneal hemorrhage, respectively. Any abdominal wall hernias or masses must be evaluated.

Auscultation of abnormal abdominal sounds suggests intraabdominal pathology. Normally, bowel sounds can be heard every 5 to 10 sec. "Absent bowel sounds" describes the lack of bowel sounds during 2 min of continuous auscultation. Intestinal ileus, intestinal ischemia, or diffuse peritonitis are typical clinical situations in which bowel sounds are absent. Hyperactive bowel sounds with high-pitched rushes, borborygmi, are heard in bowel obstruction. The presence of an abdominal bruit may correlate with renal, mesenteric or suprainguinal vascular disease.

Percussion of the abdomen can determine abnormal dullness, tympany, or presence of fluid that is suggestive of intrabdominal pathology. A normal liver span is ~9 to 10 cm. A spleen that is detected by percussion is enlarged and considered abnormal. Significant tympanitic sounds are often elicited with dilated small bowel, large bowel, or stomach. The presence of shifting dullness or a fluid wave implies ascites. Also, abdominal tenderness to percussion is very suggestive of peritonitis.

Palpation completes the abdominal examination and may yield the most important clinical information with regard to the location of pain, quality of pain, and presence of an abnormal mass. Initially, ask the patient to indicate where maximal pain is felt in the abdomen. Begin palpating in another remote area directing toward this region of maximal pain. Light palpation followed by deep palpation may elicit different responses or may detect tender masses or enlarged organs. While palpating, note if voluntary or involuntary contraction of the abdominal muscles (guarding) is present on palpation. Rebound tenderness describes pain elicited upon quick release of a deeply palpating hand and is suggestive of peritonitis. Recall that percussion of the abdomen may elicit signs of peritonitis as well. Table 2 lists eponyms of abdominal pain and abdominal pathology.

A rectal exam must always be performed in evaluating a patient with acute abdominal pain. Occult or gross blood in the stool can be caused by hemorrhoids, malignancy, colitis, or peptic ulcer disease. Localized tenderness with fluctuance is suggestive of infectious pathology. Abnormal masses may be primary rectal neoplastic

TABLE 2. *Peritoneal signs*

Sign	Description	Interpretation
Rovsing's sign	Abdominal tenderness felt in the right lower quadrant during palpation of the left lower quadrant	Right lower quadrant peritonitis consistent with acute appendicitis
Obturator sign	Abdominal tenderness felt in the right lower quadrant upon flexion of the right thigh at the hip and either medial or lateral rotation	Right lower quadrant peritonitis in the pelvic retroperitoneal area consistent with acute appendicitis located in the pelvis
Psoas sign	Abdominal tenderness felt in the right lower quadrant upon extension of the thigh at the hip or, alternatively, raising the thigh in the supine position	Right lower quadrant peritonitis in the retroperitoneal area consistent with acute appendicitis located in a retrocecal position
Chandelier's sign	Exquisite cervical motion tenderness on bimanual gynecologic examination	Pelvic peritonitis consistent with pelvic inflammatory disease
Kehr's sign	Pain referred to the left shoulder secondary to left hemidiaphragm irritation	Commonly caused by localized hemoperitoneum from splenic laceration
Murphy's sign	When asked to inspire deeply while the examiner is palpating the right upper quadrant where the gallbladder is located, the patient hesitates in mid-breath secondary to cholecystic peritoneal inflammation	Acute cholecystitis
Charcot's triad	Clinical symptoms of jaundice, fever, and right upper quadrant abdominal pain	Acute suppurative ascending choloangitis, nonseptic
Reynolds-Dargan pentad	Charcot's triad in addition to altered mental status and hypotension	Acute suppurative ascending cholangitis, septicemic shock
Valentino's sign	Right lower quadrant peritonitis	Perforated peptic ulcer with translocation of purulence to the right lower quadrant
Dance's sign	Absence of bowel sounds in the right lower quadrant	Ileocolic intussusception
Ballance's sign	"Shifting dullness" with percussion of the right flank, lack of "shifting dullness" on the left flank	Ruptured spleen
Chaussier's sign	Epigastric pain in a pregnant female	Eclampsia
Fothergill's sign	Abdominal wall mass that does not cross the midline, remains palpable when muscle contracted	Rectus muscle hematoma
Küstner's sign	Palpable mass anterior to ovary	Dermoid cyst

disease or metastatic disease. Blumer's shelf masses describe metastatic tumors that have seeded the peritoneal reflection at mid-rectum. These masses are typically palpable at the distal tip of the examining digit on the anterior rectal wall. In males, the prostate must be examined for nodules, enlargement or tenderness.

A bimanual gynecologic exam must be performed on all females with abdominal pain. The adnexa, uterus, and ovaries are palpated to exclude a gynecologic source of abdominal pain. Cervical motion tenderness suggests PID. An adnexal mass may represent an ectopic pregnancy, tuboovarian abscess or malignancy.

LABORATORY TESTS

After patient history is obtained and physical examination performed, directed laboratory tests are an essential component in determining the etiology of abdominal pain. An elevated white blood cell count with increased number of primitive leukocytes (left shift) is consistent with an acute infection. Recognize that elderly or immunocompromised patients may not manifest a leukocytosis in response to acute infection. The hemoglobin or hematocrit can indicate acute or chronic anemia or imply hemoconcentration from dehydration. Blood in the urine may be a manifestation of urologic disease ranging from nephrolithiasis to malignancy. White blood cells in the urine (pyuria) is consistent with a urinary tract infection. A urine pregnancy test must be obtained in all females of child-bearing age. Hepatic transaminases and alkaline phosphatase in the serum, as well as a serum bilirubin profile should be obtained if evaluation suggests hepatobiliary pathology. Similarly, serum amylase and lipase levels should be checked to confirm suspicion of pancreatitis. An arterial blood gas may reveal metabolic acidosis compatible with septic shock or mesenteric ischemia. Serum electrolytes may be required to guide fluid management in the presence of excessive fluid loss associated with acute abdominal pain, e.g., intractable vomiting, voluminous diarrhea.

RADIOLOGIC STUDIES

Appropriate radiologic studies are also important in the accurate diagnosis of acute abdominal pain. Flat and upright radiographs of the abdomen detect calcific masses and abnormal bowel gas patterns. For example, renal stones are visualized in up to 90% of cases. In contrast, biliary stones are radiopaque in only <20% of cases. Although infrequently seen, a fecalith (appendicolith) may be seen in the right lower quadrant (RLQ). In the patient with intestinal ileus, gas is present in both the large and small bowels with moderate distention and air-fluid levels throughout. Intestinal obstruction may present with similar radiographic findings, especially in the

situation of a distal obstruction. The absence of bowel gas in the large bowel should raise suspicion for small bowel obstruction. Pneumoperitoneum is detected best by an upright chest radiograph. However, if the patient cannot voluntarily undergo multiple views of the chest, a left lateral decubitus film should be obtained to evaluate for abnormal air-fluid levels or the presence of pneumoperitoneum demonstrated as air between the liver and abdominal wall. Air in the biliary tree seen in a radiograph may be due to a biliary-enteric anastomosis (i.e., choledochojejunostomy) or a gas-forming infection causing cholangitis. Pneumobilia in combination with small bowel obstruction is the "sine qua non" of gallstone ileus. Ultrasonography of the abdomen is a popular diagnostic test to correlate physical examination with the presence of intraabdominal pathology. Sonogram is quite sensitive in detecting minimal amounts of free fluid and evaluating the gallbladder and biliary system. Pelvic ultrasonography can distinguish between gynecologic and abdominal pathology when the clinical diagnosis is unclear. It is particularly useful in differentiating cystic from solid structures as well as locating fluid collections, especially in women of child-bearing age. Computed tomography (CT) scanning of the abdomen and pelvis, when indicated, defines anatomy, inflammation, abnormal masses, and abscesses within the abdomen. CT scan is the test of choice to evaluate the soft tissue structures of the retroperitoneum. The enormous diagnostic value of CT scanning must be balanced against radiation exposure and use of intravenous contrast, which may cause systemic allergic reactions.

APPENDICITIS

Originally called "perityphlitis," appendicitis was recognized ~500 years ago. Milier, in 1827, described appendicitis as an "iliac tumor." In 1886, Reginald Fitz characterized the pathology and symptoms of appendicitis and recommended appendectomy. Senn, in 1889, was the first to successfully diagnose appendicitis and remove it prior to rupture. In the same year, McBurney described the symptoms of appendicitis, including the region of maximal pain (McBurney's point). Today, appendicitis is the most common etiology of an acute surgical abdomen and affects ~6% of the population, predominantly between ages 5 and 35. Accurate diagnosis can be difficult in the very old or very young patient. Delay in treatment may result in perforation.

Anatomy and Pathophysiology

In adolescence, the appendix is predominantly a lymphoid organ with high concentrations of Peyer's patches in the submucosa. Progressively with age, these lymphoid patches become more diffuse and are sparse in maturity.

Normally, the appendix is 8 to 13 cm in length, and its base is located at the posteromedial cecum intimately related to the anterior taenia coli. Blood supply to the appendix comes from the appendiceal artery, a terminal branch of the ileocolic artery that originates as a branch of the superior mesenteric artery. Venous drainage is similarly named and follows splanchnic venous drainage to the superior mesenteric vein and ultimately the portal vein.

The pathogenesis behind acute appendicitis begins with obstruction of the appendiceal lumen. The most common cause of luminal obstruction in the young is lymphoid hyperplasia, while in adults fecaliths obstruct the appendiceal lumen. Rare causes of appendicitis are inspissated barium, parasitic worms (e.g., pinworm), cancer of the cecum, and carcinoid tumors. Obstruction of the lumen in the presence of continued mucosal secretions results in appendiceal distention. At this point, irritation is limited to visceral peritoneum of the appendix and thus vague abdominal pain is referred to the periumbilical area. Bacterial colonization of stagnant luminal fluid occurs. Subsequently, decreased venous outflow and eventually decreased arterial blood supply develops secondary to prolonged luminal distention. The ensuing ischemia allows bacterial colonization to progress to frank infection. Parietal peritoneum of the RLQ abdominal wall becomes irritated, and somatic innervation localizes pain in the RLQ. Perforation occurs because of transmural gangrene.

Evaluation

Diagnosis of appendicitis is based mostly on the patient history and physical examination. Classically, abdominal pain is initally vague and poorly localized at the periumbilical area. Nausea, vomiting, and anorexia ensue. After a period of time, the patient begins to localize pain in the RLQ and on palpation commonly exhibits rebound tenderness. Recognize that an atypically located appendix (e.g., retrocecal appendix) that is acutely inflamed may not manifest exquisite abdominal pain on examination. Digital rectal examination may demonstrate tenderness to palpation in the right lateral rectum. In cases of nonperforated appendicitis, patients may be afebrile or have a low-grade temperature on presentation.

Plain abdominal radiographs are not usually helpful unless an appendicolith is seen. A "sentinel" loop in the RLQ may represent an area of localized ileus secondary to the local inflammatory process. Often seen on plain film is the disappearance of the right psoas shadow that indicates retroperitoneal inflammation. In patients with an unclear presentation, ultrasonography of the RLQ may demonstrate a distended noncompressible appendix with surrounding free fluid. In a significant percentage of cases of patients with acute appendicitis cases, a CT scan will reveal right lower abdominal inflammation or phleg-

mon. The leukocyte count is usually elevated (12,000 to 20,000/mm^3) with a "left shift." Interestingly, urinalysis may reveal pyuria that is a result of retroperitoneal irritation of the ureter.

Appendiceal rupture increases patient morbidity and mortality dramatically, and should be suspected in patients that present with prolonged symptoms of >36 hr, leukocyte count of >20,000, or temperature of >101.5°F. The mortality from a nonruptured appendix is <1% but increases to 3% to 4% in perforated cases. Mortality in elderly patients, especially those with preexisting medical disease, can approach 15%. The incidence of wound infection and postoperative intraabdominal abscess is increased after perforated appendicitis. Distant spread of infection can occur with appendicitis, especially in the presence of appendiceal rupture via suppurative thrombophlebitis of the portal vein (pylephlebitis). Hepatic abscess formation as a result of this condition is common and has a staggering mortality rate. In women, perforated appendicitis increases the rate of infertility by threefold. During pregnancy, perforated appendicitis increases the rate of spontaneous abortion.

Treatment

With exception for periappendiceal abscesses, which will be discussed later, surgical removal of the appendix is the only acceptable treatment for acute appendicitis. Traditional appendectomy is performed via a RLQ incision centered about McBurney's point (two-thirds the distance from the umbilicus to the right anterior superior iliac spine). A McBurney incision is a predominantly oblique incision (Fig. 2), whereas a Rocky-Davis incision is predominantly a transverse incision. Perioperative antibiotics are indicated to reduce rates of wound infection. If perforated appendicitis is evident, an extended course of intravenous antibiotics is recommended. Occasionally, drains are placed in the presence of residual purulence and allowed to drain externally. The surgical wound is left open and allowed to heal by secondary intention. Laparoscopic appendectomy has been popularized, but cost-benefit ratio of patient care appears inferior to traditional appendectomy. It remains, however, a viable option to fulfill patients personal desires.

If clinical assessment is based on a thorough patient history and physical examination, then diagnosis of acute appendicitis is frequently straightforward. However, atypical abdominal pain, especially right-sided abdominal pain, often requires attention to subtle details of patient history. Additionally, sequential physical examinations may indeed prove more helpful than sheer knowledge of clinical facts. The evaluating physician must focus on the clinical objective, which is to confidently exclude acute appendicitis. Certainly, there are circumstances in which this goal cannot be met, and the only treatment option is to exclude appendicitis by surgical removal.

If symptoms have been present for >7 days but have resolved, a periappendiceal abscess may exist. Abdominal examination may reveal a nontender RLQ mass or fullness. CT scan of the abdomen and pelvis may demonstrate a fluid collection in the corresponding area. Percutaneous drainage and interval appendectomy (10 to 12 weeks later) is the recommended treatment of choice.

"SPECIAL SITUATIONS"

No Appendiceal Pathology

When an operation is performed based on signs and symptoms and a physical examination consistent with appendicitis, ~20% of cases will reveal no appendiceal pathology. In this scenario, the appendix is removed to exclude it from future pathogenesis, and the search begins for the actual source of the RLQ pain. Initially, a peritoneal fluid culture is obtained. Subsequently, all potential organ systems that can produce pain that mimics appendicitis must be evaluated. Locally, the terminal ileum is palpated and visually evaluated to exclude inflammatory bowel disease or intraluminal pathology. Acute inflammation of a Meckel's diverticulum, which are found ~70 to 90 cm from the ileocecal valve, can mimic acute appendicitis. Bacterial, viral, or granulomatous ascending colitis and right colon diverticulitis can also produce appendicitis-like pain. Regionally, the kidney and ureter should be palpated to appreciate any abnormalities. In the female, the uterus, along with each fallopian tube and each ovary, must be visualized to exclude pelvic disease. Distant organs such as the gallbladder, liver, and duodenum require palpation to appreciate pathology that may have resulted in RLQ symptoms.

Malignancy

Rarely, appendiceal malignancy or cancer involving another abdominal organ is the etiology behind the appendicitis-like pain. Mid-gut carcinoid tumors arise most commonly in the terminal ileum and appendix. Carcinoids of the appendix are rarely malignant. Routine appendectomy for a tumor of <2 cm in diameter is curative. Tumors of >2 cm in diameter require a right hemicoloectomy. With liver metastasis, the 5-year survival rate drops significantly to between 20% and 40%.

A mucocele resulting from a benign mucinous cystadenoma of the appendix may present as appendicitis-like pain. The appropriate treatment is simply appendectomy. A mucocele resulting from a malignant mucinous cystadenocarcinoma can also mimic acute appendicitis. Interestingly, it frequently ruptures producing pseudomyxoma peritonei. Adenocarcinoma of the appendix is rare, but resembles adenocarcinoma of the colon. Intraluminal or intramural neoplasms within the cecum or ascending colon can also produce symptoms that mimic appendicitis. Malignant lesions of the appendix, cecum, or ascending colon generally require a right colectomy for proper treatment.

Crohn's Disease of the Appendix

When Crohn's disease involves the appendix, a clinical dilemna is placed before the operating surgeon. Crohn's disease limited to the distal appendix can be treated by a standard appendectomy. However, involvement of the base of the appendix and cecum would prohibit appendectomy, as the incidence of postoperative colocutaneous fistula is unacceptably high. In this case, it is recommended that the appendix be left in situ and the patient be informed in detail of the fact that the appendix remains within the abdomen.

Appendicitis During Pregnancy

Appendicitis is the most common etiology of acute abdominal pain requiring surgery during pregnancy. It is well known that, as the uterus enlarges during pregnancy, the cecum and appendix are superiorly and laterally displaced. Thus, because of atypical symptoms and abdominal examination, the diagnosis of acute appendicitis is too often ignored or overlooked. Clinicians must be persistent in their quest to exclude appendicitis in pregnant females with persistent abdominal pain in order to prevent increased fetal and maternal mortality. The incidence of perioperative mortality of pregnant females with nonperforated appendicitis is identical to nonpregnant females with acute nonperforated appendicitis. Similarly, the incidence of fetal mortality from spontaneous abortion is significantly lower in nonperforated as compared to perforated appendicitis. In a pregnant female with persistent abdominal pain but atypical symptoms and physical examination, thorough evaluation of appendicitis is mandatory.

ACUTE ABDOMEN

It cannot be overemphasized that a complete history and physical examination should direct the clinician's thought process regarding abdominal pain. As well, one should recognize that age, gender, history of comorbid disease, and social history are important details that clinicians should remember when formulating a reasonable differential diagnosis. Details of this segment of discussion are limited to essentials of common intraabdominal pathology.

Virtually any organ or structure within the abdomen can become pathologic and cause exquisite abdominal pain. To accurately diagnose intraabdominal pathology, an understanding of anatomical and physiologic relationships, rather than recall of memorized lists, is required. Reconsider specific abdominal regions and structures within those areas that commonly cause abdominal pain (Table 1).

Right Upper Quadrant and Epigastric Pain

Often, RUQ and epigastric pain have the same etiology. The majority of pathologies in these regions consist of biliary, hepatic, gastroduodenal, and pancreatic disease. Infrequently, disease in the right adrenal gland, the upper pole of the right kidney and the lower lobe of the right lung can produce abdominal pain in the RUQ and epigastrium. Patient history can frequently distinguish these processes.

Biliary pathologies that can present clinically with acute abdominal pain include biliary colic and acute or chronic cholecystitis. Typical patients are middle aged, obese females with a history of recurrent episodes of RUQ and sometimes epigastric pain after consumption of fat-rich meals. The pain is described as colicky or crampy often associated with nausea and vomiting. Pain may radiate to the right scapula and shoulder, due to shared afferent/efferent innervation between the gallbladder and diaphragm. Episodic pain that resolves in combination with normal laboratory and diagnostic tests describes biliary colic. Conversely, persistent pain especially with abnormal laboratory tests and fever suggests cholecystitis. Physical examination of the abdomen in these cases usually demonstrates localized pain to the RUQ (diffuse peritonitis implies perforated cholecystitis or other abdominal pathology). Specifically, palpation of the right subcostal area during patient respiration may elicit a Murphy's sign, which refers to hesitation during deep inspiration when simultaneously palpating the gallbladder. This implies pericholecystic peritoneal inflammation and correlates in the majority of cases with acute cholecystitis. Ultrasonography is the diagnostic modality of choice for biliary tract disease. The classic sonographic findings in acute cholecystitis include cholelithiasis, gallbladder wall thickening with luminal distention, and pericholecystic fluid.

Frequently, an episode of pain may be extremely severe with protracted nausea and vomiting. If cholelithiasis is noted by ultrasound and an elevated serum amylase is found, appropriate treatement for biliary pancreatitis should be started. Jaundice may be a manifestation of impaired biliary flow and suggests choledocholithiasis. Jaundice in association with RUQ pain and fever (Charcot's triad) implies ascending suppurative cholangitis and requires emergent endoscopic extraction of the common bile duct stone and decompression of the biliary tree. Infrequently, biliary or periampullary malignancy may be the cause of jaundice, and appropriate diagnostic studies should be employed.

Patients with peptic ulcer disease complain primarily of constant burning pain, occasionally associated with meals located predominantly in the epigastric area. Patients with sudden onset severe abdominal pain and a history of peptic ulcer disease must be evaluated for acute perforation. Physical examination in these patients reveals abdominal distention, involuntary guarding, and signs of acute peritonitis. Upright plain radiograph of the chest demonstrates pneumonperitoneum in 75% of cases. Surgical treatment is mandatory and primarily involves covering the transmural perforation with a tongue of omentum, the Graham patch procedure. A definitive antiulcer operation can also be performed in selected patients.

Pancreatitis not associated with biliary calculi is another cause of acute abdominal pain. A history of alcohol abuse or recurrent episodes of pancreatitic pain secondary to metabolic abnormalities suggests the diagnosis of pancreatitis. Patients typically describe mid-epigastric stabbing pain that radiates directly posterior due to the central retroperitoneal location of the pancreas. Protracted nausea and vomiting are common complaints. An elevated serum amylase is noted with acute pancreatitis. In chronic pancreatitis, however, because of diffuse parenchymal destruction, serum amylase levels often do not correlate with the level of disease. Dynamic CT scan of the abdomen and pelvis is required to document pancreatitis complicated by parenchymal hemorrhage, pseudocyst, or peripancreatic infection.

RUQ pain from pulmonary, renal, and adrenal structures rarely manifest an abdominal examination consistent with peritonitis. Right lower lobe pneumonia with pleuritis can refer pain to the upper abdomen. Pathology involving the kidney typically causes a chronic boring pain radiating to the flank or back. Hematuria without clots is also indicative of renal pathology. Endocrine abnormalities or external stigmata may suggest adrenal pathology.

Left Upper Quadrant Pain

Most pathologic processes that manifest as left upper quadrant (LUQ) abdominal pain originate from the stomach, spleen, splenic flexure of the colon, and tail of pancreas. Other infrequently involved organs include the left adrenal gland and upper pole of the left kidney.

Gastritis is mucosal ulceration of the stomach resulting from a variety of etiologies. Chronic alcohol abuse, nonsteroidal antiinflammatory drugs, aspirin, corticosteroids, and postoperative stress are some common causes. Clinical manifestations of gastritis are similar to other etiologies of upper gastrointestinal bleeding including nausea, hematemesis, and melena. Pain is felt mainly in the epigastric and LUQ area. Persistent upper intestinal bleeding with hemodynamic stability requires emergent upper endoscopy for diagnostic and therapeutic purposes. Gastric neoplasms can also produce abdominal pain and may be associated with either hematemesis or melena. Often, however, a change in eating habits over a period of time, e.g., progressive early satiety to frank gastric outlet obstruction, is noted by the patient. An upper endoscopy should be performed to biopsy tissue for diagnosis in cases of a intramural or intraluminal lesion.

Distal pancreatic lesions (e.g., pseudocysts, neoplasms) can produce symptoms of left upper abdominal pain. Dynamic CT scan is the preferred diagnostic test of choice. Splenic lesions can present with abdominal pain located predominantly in the LUQ and with radiation or referral of pain to the left shoulder, left back, or left chest. Left lower lobe pneumonia with pleuritis can refer pain to the LUQ. Lesions in the splenic flexure of the colon infrequently may present as localized left abdominal discomfort or pain. Clinical presentation of renal and adrenal pathology are comparable in both the left and right upper quadrants.

Right Lower Quadrant Pain

Any suggestion of right lower abdominal pain mandates an evaluation of and perhaps operation for appendicitis. In addition to appendicitis and the clinical scenarios discussed above, still other etiologies should be evaluated. Pain along the lower abdomen or flank with radiation of pain to the testicles suggests either a renal or ureteral irritation. The triad of flank pain, hematuria, and a palpable abdominal mass implies renal cell carcinoma. Malignancies in regionally located organs can manifest as lower abdominal pain. Microperforation of gastroduodenal peptic ulcer disease with translocation of purulence to the RLQ can present as acute abdominal pain with signs of peritonitis, Valentino's sign.

Left Lower Quadrant Pain

Diverticular disease can affect any region of the colon but has predilection for the descending and sigmoid colon. Diverticulosis is a disease of Western civilization affecting patients predominantly over the age of 50 and is associated with sedentary life and consumption of low-residue diet. Uncomplicated diverticulitis presents clinically with fever, pain on palpation of the left lower quadrant (LLQ) perhaps with localized peritonitis. A mass or fullness may be appreciated. Endoscopic procedures and contrast enema radiography are contraindicated in the presence of colonic inflammation. CT scan of the abdomen and pelvis is quite sensitive in detecting diverticulitis. Typical findings include diverticulosis with inflammatory thickening of the colonic wall. A high-grade fever and localized tenderness is suggestive of pericolonic abscess and requires CT scanning for

accurate diagnosis. CT-guided percutaneous drainage of localized abscesses is the preferred treatment modality. If percutaneous drainage is not possible or successful, surgical drainage with diverting colostomy may be required. Colonic perforation with fecal peritonitis requires abdominal exploration and, typically, proximal fecal diversion (colostomy) and drainage of inflammatory area.

Pelvic and Suprapubic Pain

In females, gynecologic processes are the predominant source for pelvic and suprapubic pain. In males, prostate disease presents with midline lower abdominal pain. In both sexes, bladder and rectal pathology have similar presentation in the pelvis and suprapubic area.

Salpingitis, otherwise known as PID, affects females, particularly sexually active individuals between ages of 15 and 35 years. Salpingitis in virgin patients usually occurs at the end of a patient's menses. Pain is localized to the suprapubic area and lower quadrants. The patient may report vaginal discharge. Physical examination typically demonstrates fever in the presence of bilateral lower quadrant pain on palpation perhaps with signs of peritonitis. An appropriate bimanual gynecologic exam should be performed, and may reveal cervical purulence and severe cervical motion tenderness. A smear and culture of any drainage will assist in treatment that involves high-dose intravenous antibiotics. If serial abdominal examinations or fever do not show improvement, a missed diagnosis should be considered and evaluated.

An ectopic pregnancy can also present with severe abdominal pain. The exact date of the patient's last menses is paramount, and all women of child-bearing age must submit a urine pregnancy test as part of their evaluation for acute abdominal pain. On pelvic examination, blood in the vagina, cervical motion tenderness, and a palpable adnexal mass may be appreciated. Culdocentesis demonstrates blood in the case of ruptured ectopic pregnancy. If the diagnosis remains uncertain, ultrasound may be helpful in differentiating between gynecologic and gastrointestinal causes of acute abdomen. Ultimately, laparoscopy may be required to exclude gynecologic pathology.

Ovarian cysts grow and decrease in size depending on the menstrual cycle and are common causes of acute abdominal pain in women. If the cyst ruptures, peritonitis may be present. Likewise, torsion of the ovary will cause excruciating ipsilateral pain in the lower quadrant and may be associated with nausea and vomiting.

Diffuse Abdominal Pain

There are many disease processes that manifest as diffuse abdominal pain. Gastroenteritis, pneumonia, myocardial infarction, sickle-cell crisis, collagen vascular disorders, and uremia are but a few examples of chronic medical conditions that can present with diffuse abdominal pain.

Mesenteric ischemia requires brief discussion because of its disastrous complications if the diagnosis is not suspected. Inadequate oxygen supply to intestines is the fundamental pathogenesis behind mesenteric ischemia. Typical patients have preexisting central and peripheral vascular disease, and complain of vague postprandial abdominal pain, i.e., abdominal angina. Alternatively, acute or chronic cardiac arrhythmias, e.g., atrial fibrillation, may be a source of arterial emboli that can occlude mesenteric vascular supply to the intestines. Accurate diagnosis requires a high degree of suspicion based on the history of acute and chronic disease. Classic physical examination demonstrates pain out of proportion to the physical exam. Virtually all diagnostic tests, including base deficit, multiple view abdominal radiographs, and CT scan, are not consistently sensitive or specific to completely exclude ischemic bowel. Lateral view mesenteric angiogram remains the gold standard diagnostic modality for mesenteric ischemia. Early diagnosis and revascularization of the bowel is imperative to prevent massive bowel resection for intestinal gangrene.

Intestinal obstruction is another abdominal process that presents as diffuse abdominal pain and requires brief discussion. Etiologies of obstruction in decreasing order of frequency are postoperative adhesions, hernias, and intraabdominal malignancy. Other causes include intestinal volvulus, intussusception, diverticulitis, inflammatory bowel disease, and extrinsic compression from large abdominal tumors. Typical patient history reveals crampy abdominal discomfort with intermittent flares of pain. Patients often describe progressive intolerance to oral intake and nausea with voluminous vomiting. Clear fluid suggests an obstruction proximal to the ampulla of Vater while green, bilious fluid suggests a more distal obstruction. Copious, foul-smelling brown fluid suggests an obstruction involving the distal small bowel or colon.

Physical examination in patients with suspected intestinal obstruction begins with notation of previous surgical scars or obvious abdominal wall hernias. With exception of a proximal small bowel obstruction, a distended tympanic abdomen with hyperactive bowel sounds and intermittent rushes, especially during a flare of pain is typical. Although presentation of bowel obstruction and intestinal ileus is similar, bowel sounds are typically absent in an paralytic ileus. Multiple view radiographs of the abdomen show multiple air- and fluid-filled loops of bowel proximal to the obstruction. If the plain films are inconclusive, a CT scan may show the cause of obstruction.

Intestinal obstruction in the absence of previous abdominal surgery (especially if no abdominal hernias are appreciated) mandates urgent abdominal exploration after cardiovascular stability and adequate urine output have been achieved. In elderly patients, acute appendicitis and malignancy are common etiologies of bowel obstruction in these situations. The most serious complication of an unrelieved obstruction is bowel wall ischemia from strangulation and resultant perforation. Peritonitis and sepsis soon follow. According to LaPlace's law, increased luminal diameter results in increased intestinal wall tension. The thin cecal wall, for example, cannot withstand acute distention and is at high risk for perforation. Cecal diameter of >10 cm may require urgent endoscopic decompression.

In postoperative bowel obstruction, a conservative approach, involving nasogastric decompression and intravenous fluid replacement to allow satisfactory urine output, is undertaken. Clinical impatience and early surgical lysis of adhesions will only serve to induce redevelopment of intraabdominal adhesions and a more severe bowel obstruction in the future. If, however, resolution of symptoms is not perceived within 24 to 48 hr, surgical exploration for release of adhesive bands should be considered. Additional indications to abort the conservative treatment approach in a postoperative intestinal obstruction include, progressive acidosis, persistent leukocytosis, tachycardia, tachypnea, and progressive fever.

SUMMARY

Proper evaluation of acute abdominal pain is a skill that must be learned early in one's medical career. Patient evaluation is based on precise knowledge of the anatomy and pathophysiology of intraabdominal and retroperitoneal disease. Accurate diagnosis is based on a detailed patient history and thorough physical examination and correct interpretation of radiologic and laboratory data. The ability to distinguish a surgical from a nonsurgical acute abdomen requires insight and a logical thought process, and remains a challenge to all practitioners of medicine. Finally, it is acceptable to observe patients with abdominal pain without a provisional diagnosis provided that early surgical consultation is obtained and sequential physical examinations are performed (preferably by the same clinician) in an effort to define the true source of abdominal symptoms. In this manner, missed diagnosis and potential disasters can be avoided.

STUDY QUESTIONS

1. Describe the pathogenesis of acute appendicitis.
2. Explain the different clinical presentations of acute appendicitis in pregnancy, in childhood, and in elderly and immunocompromised patients.

3. Name 20 different differential diagnoses for right lower quadrant pain.
4. What are the most common causes of small bowel obstruction?
5. Define the importance of laparoscopy in the evaluation of the acute abdomen.

SUGGESTED READING

Cameron JL. *Current surgical therapy.* 5th ed. St. Louis: Mosby, 1995.

Sabiston DC. *Textbook of surgery.* 14th ed. Philadelphia: Saunders, 1991.

Schwartz SI. *Principles of surgery.* 6th ed. New York: McGraw-Hill, 1994.

Silen US. *Cope's early diagnosis of the acute abdomen.* 18th ed. New York: Oxford University Press, 1991.

Swartz MH. *Textbook of physical diagnosis.* Philadelphia: Saunders, 1989.

CHAPTER 17

Endocrine Surgery

Patrick C. Mangonon, Jodeen E. Boggs, and Alan S. Livingstone

THYROID GLAND

Surgical Anatomy

The thyroid is the first endocrine gland to appear in the fetus. During the third week of fetal life, epithelial tissue arising from the foramen cecum evaginates at the base of the tongue, and during its descent anterior to the pharyngeal gut, this primordial tissue incorporates parafollicular cells (C cells) derived from mesoderm. At the third month of gestation, the thyroid gland comes to final rest as a bilobed organ draped anterior to the trachea below the cricoid cartilage. Anterior to the thyroid lie the strap muscles. Posterior and lateral to the gland are the carotid sheath vessels and vagus nerve. The adult gland weighs ~20 g and typically features a thyroid isthmus that bridges the two lateral lobes. Occasionally, a pyramidal lobe extends superiorly from the isthmus, representing a trail of thyroid tissue left from its developmental descent (Fig. 1).

The vascular system of the thyroid gland is complex (Fig. 2). The arterial blood supply to the thyroid gland is derived from paired superior and inferior thyroid arteries. The superior thyroid artery is often the first branch of the external carotid artery, whereas the inferior thyroid artery arises from the thyrocervical trunk of the subclavian artery. The venous drainage of the thyroid gland consists of superior, middle, and inferior thyroid veins. The superior thyroid vein parallels the superior thyroid artery and empties into the internal jugular vein. The middle thyroid vein does not have a corresponding artery and empties into the internal jugular vein, whereas the inferior thyroid vein conducts blood to the innominate vein. Lymphatic drainage of the thyroid gland includes the prelaryngeal delphian node and digastric nodal group which drain the superior lobes. The inferior thyroid lobes drain to the pretracheal and innominate nodes and the lateral lobes drain to the jugular and paratracheal nodes.

The recurrent laryngeal nerve, a branch of the vagus nerve, innervates the true vocal cords and is anatomically related to the inferior thyroid artery. If the recurrent laryngeal nerve is inadvertently injured during thyroid surgery, temporary or permanent hoarseness of voice may result from ipsilateral vocal cord paresis. Bilateral nerve injury often results in permanently closed vocal cords requiring tracheostomy to maintain airway patency. The cricothyroid muscle is supplied by the external branch of the superior laryngeal nerve and if accidentally damaged, may result in loss of high pitch tone of voice.

Physiology

The thyroid gland produces thyroid hormones, T_4 and T_3, that modulate human basal metabolic rate. Thyroid hormone synthesis is dependent upon the body iodine content. Dietary iodide taken up by the thyroid and stored in the follicular cell is chemically bound to a tyrosine residue on thyroglobulin. This monoiodotyrosine (MIT) binds with another MIT to yield diiodotyrosine (DIT). Subsequently, DIT combines with another DIT or MIT to yield thyroid hormones, T4 and T_3, respectively.

$$MIT + MIT = DIT$$

$$DIT + DIT = T_4$$

$$DIT + MIT = T_3$$

Broadly, however, thyroid hormone synthesis is regulated by the hypothalamic-pituitary-thyroid endocrine axis as depicted in Fig. 3. Synthetic T_4 was discovered in the early 1920s and has significantly impacted the treatment of many thyroid disorders.

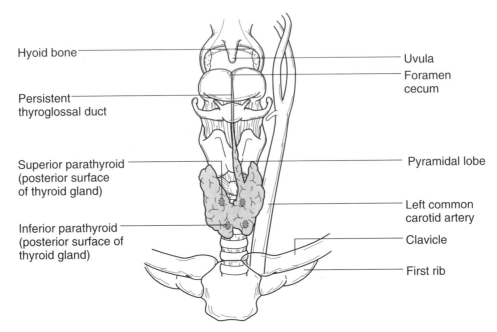

FIG. 1. Thyroid gland. (Adapted from Gray JW, Skandalakis JE. *Atlas of surgical anatomy for general surgeons.* Baltimore: Williams and Wilkins, 1985.)

Physical Examination of the Thyroid

Complete examination of the thyroid should be a routine part of patient examination. Visual inspection of the neck from anterior and lateral views helps appreciate thyroid enlargement or asymmetry. Following visual survey, palpation of the thyroid gland is performed by standing behind a sitting patient. Manual palpation of each lobe of the thyroid allows detection of small nodules that are characterized as firm or hard and fixed or mobile in relation to overlying strap muscles. The act of swallowing moves the patient's thyroid under the clinician's palpating hands, confirms appropriate examination of the thyroid, and accentuates palpation of thyroid masses. Performing

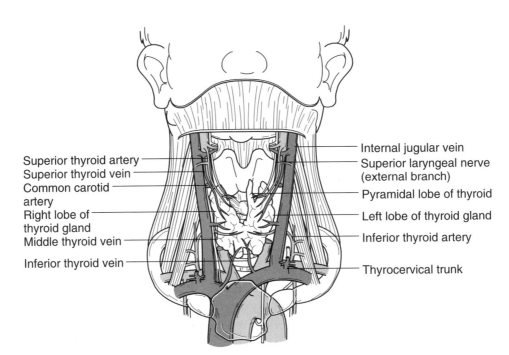

FIG. 2. Vascular supply of thyroid gland. (Adapted from Gray JW, Skandalakis JE. *Atlas of surgical anatomy for general surgeons.* Baltimore: Williams and Wilkins, 1985.)

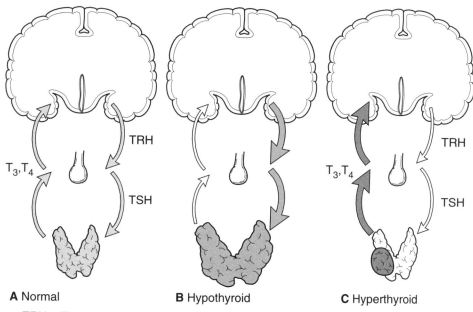

FIG. 3. Thyroid hormone synthesis is controlled by both hypothalamic RTH and pituitary TSH secretion in a classic negative feedback loop. Low levels of T_3 and T_4 stimulate the release of TSH and RTH. **(A)** Normal. **(B)** Hypothyroid. In individuals with biosynthetic defects in T_3 and T_4 synthesis, TRH and TSH are increased. The persistent stimulation of the thyroid by TSH results in the development of the thyroid enlargement (goiter). **(C)** Similarly in patients with elevated levels of T_3 and T_4 (toxic adenoma), release of TRH and TSH are suppressed. (Adapted from Gray JW, Skandalakis JE. *Atlas of surgical anatomy for general surgeons.* Baltimore: Williams and Wilkins, 1985.)

similar maneuvers while the patient's head is turned to either side may allow discovery of subtle thyroid masses.

Diseases of the Thyroid

Thyroglossal Duct

The development of the thyroid evolves from evagination of epidermal tissue from the foramen cecum and its descent anterior to the trachea. Persistent patency of this evagination, a thyroglossal duct, is infrequently found but can occur anywhere along the pathway of the thyroidal descent. A thyroglossal duct cyst describes fluid trapped in the duct lumen but generally causes no symptoms in the absence of infection. An enlarging midline anterior neck structure commonly near the hyoid bone are common findings. A cyst that communicates with skin or oropharynx is known as a thyroglossal fistula. Complete excision of the tract of thyroid descent as well as the hyoid bone is usually required for definitive therapy.

Thyroid Goiter

Enlargement of the thyroid gland, a goiter, has been recognized for >4,000 years. In 1958, the World Health Organization recorded >200 million people (roughly 7%

of the world population) with goiter disease. In the United States, the incidence has decreased dramatically ever since dietary iodide was made widely available in commonly consumed products. There remain, however, endemic areas in the United States as well as worldwide. Outside endemic areas, sporadic and compensatory goiters are commonly discovered during routine physical examination of the neck. Familial or iatrogenic goiter disease is uncommon.

A nontoxic thyroid goiter is defined arbitrarily as diffuse or nodular enlargement of the gland as compensation for insufficient thyroid hormone production. Elevated serum levels of thyroid stimulating hormone (TSH) and other growth factors, secondary to hypothyroidism, stimulate varying rates of thyroid growth. The thyroid gland can reach 20 times normal with multiple nodules. Nodular goiters are the most common form of thyroid enlargement and are usually due to iodine deficiency. Congenital goiter of infancy is due to either a maternal iodine deficiency during pregnancy or autosomal recessive transmission of thyroxine synthesis deficiency. A diffuse colloid goiter is seen primarily in adolescent females, and spontaneous regression is common. Substernal goiter describes an enlarged thyroid that has grown into the mediastinum through the thoracic inlet.

The incidence of thyroid enlargement is more common in females and increases markedly in patients over the

212 / GENERAL SURGERY

age of 50. The majority of cases are asymptomatic and found incidentally on routine physical examination. Symptoms relate to mass size and compression of the esophagus and trachea. Hemorrhage within the goiter may cause pain. Excessive thyroid hormone levels with symptoms (thyrotoxicosis) is an infrequent presentation. Recurrent laryngeal nerve entrapment is unusual in benign disease, and voice hoarseness should raise suspicion of malignancy.

The diagnosis of goiter disease is usually made by patient history and physical examination. A nodular goiter is usually easily palpable. A fine needle aspiration (FNA) of a solitary nodule should be performed to confirm thyroid goiter disease or identify a suspected malignancy. Thyroid chemistry profiles in compensatory goiters depict an elevated TSH level in the presence of euthyroid state. Thyroid hormone elevation is not frequently encountered. If mass size and clinical history suggest respiratory or alimentary tract compression, a chest radiograph should be obtained. A computed tomography (CT) scan of the neck and upper chest should be obtained if the chest radiograph demonstrates thoracic extension.

Administration of supplemental iodine and T_4 suppresses TSH levels and causes regression in the majority of asymptomatic patients with nontoxic goiter. However, surgical resection of thyroid goiters must be considered in certain clinical situations. Substernal thyroid goiters grow within a confined space and can cause trachea compression with only mild enlargement. These goiters rarely involute despite adequate medical suppression and should be resected. Similarly, underlying malignancy should be suspected, especially in individuals with recent hoarseness, an equivocal FNA, or a rapidly enlarging goiter despite administration of T_4. Large cervical goiters may cause esophageal or airway obstructive symptoms from progressive growth and should be removed. Finally, patients with cosmetically disfiguring goiters that have failed to regress with thyroid hormone supplementation are candidates for surgical resection.

Historically, thyroid surgery was fraught with complications until Theodore Kocher, a physiologist and surgeon practicing in an endemic goiter belt in Switzerland, recognized the importance of hemostasis and preservation of the parathyroid glands and the recurrent laryngeal nerves. Through his experience of >5,000 thyroid resections, he reduced the perioperative mortality rate from 13% to 0.5%. Also because of his recognition of postthyroidectomy hypothyroidism, for which he won the Nobel prize in 1909, contemporary surgeons administer thyroid hormone to suppress TSH levels and prevent disease recurrence. Similarly, thyroid hormone supplementation should be administered prior to thyroid resection to ensure a euthyroid state and avoid anesthetic risk from hypothyroidism.

In contrast to previous experience, the well-recognized complications after thyroidectomy, when performed by an experienced surgeon are rare. Because of the extremely confined space within the fascial planes of the neck, small hematomas can have catastrophic consequences. Suspicion of airway compromise from a postoperative hematoma mandates emergent wound exploration and hematoma evacuation (occasionally at the bedside). Signs of recurrent laryngeal nerve injury are immediately apparent and manifest as respiratory distress or inability to spontaneously ventilate after endotracheal extubation. Parathyroid injury is rare if all parathyroid glands are visualized and are left undisturbed. Characteristic clinical features of hypocalcemia from parathyroid damage include circumoral numbness, distal extremity paresthesia, twitching of the facial muscles upon tapping of the facial nerve area (Chvostek's sign), and forearm carpopedal spasm upon application of sphygmomanometric pressure to the upper extremity (Trousseau's sign).

Hyperthyroidism

Hyperthyroidism is defined as an abnormally increased level of thyroid hormone in the absence of normal hormonal feedback mechanisms. The most common cause of hyperthyroidism in the United States is diffuse toxic goiter (Grave's disease) secondary to the endogenous production of antibodies directed at the TSH receptor. Other causes include toxic nodular goiter (Plummer's disease), thyroiditis, drug induced hyperthyroidism (iodine, thyroxine, amiodarone), ectopic hyperthyroidism (struma ovarii), trophoblastic tumors such as hydatidiform moles, and metastatic thyroid cancer.

Clinical signs and symptoms reflect the increase in basal metabolic rate and include weight loss, cardiac arrhythmias, anxiety, and heat intolerance. Older patients may complain only of muscle weakness or present with new onset atrial fibrillation. Classic ophthalmopathy (exophthalmos) is distinctive to hyperthyroidism, particularly in Grave's disease; however, the etiology remains unclear. Thyrotoxicosis ("thyroid storm") is rarely seen today but typically occurs in undiagnosed hyperthyroid patients who are undergoing emergency surgery or have an underlying exacerbation of systemic disease. Hyperthermia, vomiting and diarrhea may progress to hemodynamic instability and coma. Thyrotoxicosis secondary to a toxic adenoma possesses striking similarities to Grave's disease with an exception for the absence of exophthalmos. Generally, this process more commonly affects older individuals and presents with more cardiac symptoms.

The fundamental objective in treating patients with hyperthyroidism is establishing a clinically euthyroid state. Antithyroidal medications (e.g., propylthiouracil, methimazole) and β-adrenergic receptor blockade reduce the quantity and effect of thyroid hormone and should be utilized as primary therapy. Administration of ^{131}I is effective in ablating thyroid tissue but is complicated by postablation hypothyroidism and an unacceptable percentage of patients require long-term thyroid supplementation. This modality is contraindicated in pregnancy and in pediatric patients because of radiation exposure.

Appropriate treatment for thyroid storm includes rehydration, application of a cooling blanket, and administration of supplemental oxygen, glucose, and medications to ablate hyperthyroid symptoms (e.g., reserpine, β-adrenergic receptor blockade). Exophthalmos will invariably regress after thyrotoxicosis has resolved, and no surgical therapy directed at oculoplasty is required.

Surgical intervention is indicated for failure of medical management and usually involves subtotal thyroid resection to render the patient euthyroid. For patients with toxic adenoma, medical therapy is largely ineffective in treating hyperthyroidism and radioablative therapy has an unacceptable rate of hypothyroidism. Surgical resection is safe and considered a much better alternative to radioablative therapy.

Thyroiditis

Thyroiditis is characterized by an acute, progressive, or chronic inflammation of thyroid tissue. Hashimoto's thyroiditis is a result of autoimmune destruction of the thyroid and represents the most common cause of hypothyroidism in areas outside endemic goiter regions. Early in the course of disease, diffuse lymphocytic infiltration causes gradual painless enlargement of the thyroid but levels of free T_4 remain normal. Many patients are found with a positive serum microsomal antibody test and elevated erythrocyte sedimentation rate (ESR). Eventually, hypothyroidism and an elevated serum TSH level predominate. Initial treatment for Hashimoto's thyroiditis is thyroid hormone supplementation. Dyspnea or dysphagia as a result of thyroid compression of the trachea or esophagus is an indication for thyroidectomy.

Subacute granulomatous (DeQuervain's) thyroiditis is rare but is thought to follow an upper respiratory tract infection. Occurring primarily in middle aged women, clinical symptoms include a suddenly enlarged and painful thyroid with pain radiating to the jaw and ears. Thyroid function is normal during the initial phase of disease but thyrotoxicosis from release of thyroid hormone followed by hypothyroidism from parenchymal destruction may occur. Eventually, however, resolution and euthyroidism prevail. Microscopic analysis of subacute granulomatous thyroiditis reveals granulomas surrounding thyroid follicles, with invasion of thyroid parenchyma by granulocytes and inflammatory cells. Nonsteroidal antiinflammatory medications and supportive care are successful in treating this disease.

Reidel's thyroiditis is another rare thyroid inflammatory process but is associated with other similar disorders like sclerosing cholangitis and mediastinal fibrosis.

The patients are usually euthyroid and present with a hard but nonpainful enlargement of the thyroid gland. Occasionally, on palpation, the thyroid gland seems to be fixed to the strap muscles and trachea. Again, surgery is reserved for symptoms of tracheal or esophageal compression.

Acute suppurative thyroiditis is a bacterial infection of the gland commonly the result of contiguous spread from adjacent structures, e.g., pharynx and lymph nodes. Less commonly, hematogenous spread of bacteria secondarily infects the thyroid. Patients present with fevers, chills, and a painful, swollen thyroid gland. Thyroid function is usually normal, except when extensive parenchymal destruction results in release of thyroid hormone into the systemic circulation. Abscesses require surgical drainage, and bacteria cultured should be treated with appropriate systemic antibiotics. The most common organisms isolated are Streptococcus and Staphylococcus, although fungal and parasitic infections may occur as well.

Thyroid Nodule

Thyroid nodules are very common and are found in ~4% of the population. Understanding the common disease entities that result in development of thyroid nodules (Table 1) as well as appropriate work up of thyroid nodules must be embraced by all clinicians. Details of patient history, including radiation exposure during infancy or adolescence, family history of papillary or medullary carcinoma, and nodule characteristics, (e.g. rate of onset and growth) are essential aspects of patient evaluation. Thorough examination of the thyroid as previously outlined should be practiced routinely to detect the asymptomatic thyroid nodule.

A thyroid adenoma is the most common benign thyroid nodule. These are solid encapsulated nodules that often contain colloid. Rapid painful enlargement of a nodule suggests hemorrhage within a benign nodule; however, rapid painless growth suggests malignancy, especially if the nodule was not present on a previous examination. Children and adolescents as well as elderly patients are at higher risk of malignancy within a thyroid nodule. Symptoms of vocal cord paralysis are suggestive of thyroid cancer. Physical examination revealing solitary nodules fixed to surrounding muscles suggests thyroid carci-

TABLE 1. *Differential diagnosis of thyroid nodules*

Thyroid adenoma
Cyst
Colloid nodule
Thyroiditis
Abscess
Malignancy

noma. On the other hand, tracheal or esophageal compression is not a good indicator of malignancy.

Laboratory tests are not particularly sensitive nor specific in the evaluation of a thyroid nodule. Clinical thyrotoxicosis seen in toxic adenomas may be confirmed with a thyroid chemistry profile. Medullary thyroid carcinoma (MTC) may be confirmed with a calcitonin level. Radionuclide scanning with ^{131}I depicts the endocrine function of thyroid nodules as nonfunctioning ("cold"), normal ("warm"), or hyperfunctioning ("hot"). Radionuclide scanning, unfortunately, does not clearly or consistently distinguish between benign or malignant nodules. Although malignant cells do not trap iodine and show as a cold nodule, the vast majority of cold nodules are benign. Additionally, a small minority of warm and hot nodules have been found to harbor thyroid cancer also.

FNA biopsy is safe, inexpensive, and accurate—and, with few exceptions, is viewed as the most important diagnostic test in evaluating a thyroid nodule. Palpable lesions are easily biopsied by FNA. Nonpalpable lesions detected by scintigraphy study of other means may be biopsied with the assistance of ultrasonography to guide needle aspiration biopsy of these lesions. A benign nodule may be observed or treated with thyroid hormone supplementation to suppress TSH stimulation. Regardless of which modality is chosen, however, careful periodic reexamination is mandatory to evaluate for dysplastic changes within the nodule. Follicular adenomas and the histologic variant, Hürthle cell adenoma, vary according to the degree of differentiation, but often benign tumors cannot be distinguished from carcinoma; thus, these results are indications for thyroidectomy for diagnosis. Similarly, benign papillary adenomas rarely occur, and papillary carcinoma must be presumed, which should be resected. Unsatisfactory results indicate the need for repeat biopsy, but, ultimately, surgical excision of suspicious masses may be the only definitive diagnostic test.

Thyroid Cancer

Although thyroid nodules are very common, thyroid malignancy is extremely rare, affecting <0.004% of the population. Despite this fact, though, thyroid carcinoma is the most common endocrine carcinoma. Approximately 11,000 patients per year are treated for this disease, and ~1,000 patients per year die from this disease in the United States. Past radiation exposure is a known etiology of thyroid carcinoma. Goiterogenic drugs or iodide deficiency have been implicated in the development of thyroid cancer. Likewise, rapid growth of a thyroid nodule with or without symptoms of hoarseness, dysphagia or dyspnea suggests malignancy until proven otherwise.

Thyroid carcinoma can range from slow-growing lesions to rapidly advancing tumors. The most common subtype of thyroid cancer is papillary thyroid carcinoma, which is considered a well-differentiated cancer with an excellent long-term prognosis. Follicular thyroid carcinoma is considered a well-differentiated thyroid cancer subtype with an overall favorable long-term prognosis dependent on specific subclassification. In contrast, anaplastic thyroid cancer is the most aggressive and has an extremely poor prognosis. MTC is a malignancy of the parafollicular C cells throughout the entire gland. Medullary, papillary, and anaplastic carcinoma are diagnosed with >90% accuracy with FNA biopsy. Follicular carcinoma is less accurately diagnosed (40%) because of the similarities between adenoma and carcinoma morphology. Thyroid lymphoma may arise spontaneously or may be seen in a patient with a long history of thyroiditis. Although this tumor may be diagnosed by FNA, a biopsy is usually required to correctly classify the type of lymphoma.

Well-differentiated thyroid cancers include papillary and follicular thyroid carcinoma. Papillary carcinoma tends to be multifocal and bilateral with dissemination occurring through the lymphatic system. Histologically psammoma bodies or layered calcification are seen within the papillary carcinoma. Follicular carcinoma typically presents as a solitary enlarged mass of the thyroid. Despite the fact that the nodule is encapsulated, irregular edges and microscopic invasion of the capsule are indicative of malignancy. Tumor invasion is subclassified into minimally invasive and extensively invasive lesions.

Although specific differences in prognosis exist between papillary and follicular thyroid cancer, certain generalities are common knowledge. In 1987, the Mayo Clinic published data from a retrospective review of patients with well-differentiated thyroid cancer. Prognosis regarding local recurrence rates, distant metastasis rates, and mortality was found to be related to patient *a*ge, histologic *g*rade of tumor, *e*xtracapsular spread of tumor, and *s*ize of lesion (AGES). Women over the age of 50 and men over the age of 40 have higher recurrence rates and distant metastasis rates. Local recurrences were higher in cases of extracapsular spread of disease. A poorer prognosis is noted in patients that present with larger tumors (>2 cm in diameter). With regard to specific differences, it appears that the mortality from follicular carcinoma is twice that of papillary carcinoma and is related to certain indicators. Poorly differentiated and extensively invasive follicular carcinomas, as expected, have a worse prognosis. Hürthle cell carcinoma is a histologic variant of follicular carcinoma that mimics extensively invasive follicular carcinoma in character, and invades locally or metastasizes in the blood or lymphatic system. Thyroid cancer staging is defined in Table 2.

MTC arises from parafollicular cells, also known as C cells. Because the parafollicular cells are predominantly located in the superior and middle aspects of the thyroid gland, it is in these areas where medullary thyroid cancer prevails. These tumors are typically multifocal and not

TABLE 2. *Staging thyroid cancer*

Stage	Description
I	Intrathyroid foci
II	Cervical lymph node metastasis, lymph nodes are not fixed
III	Cervical lymph node metastasis, lymph nodes are fixed to surrounding structures
IV	Metastasis beyond confines of the neck

encapsulated. Metastasis occurs via either the lymphatic or hematogenous systems. These tumors are commonly associated with multiple endocrine neoplasia (MEN) syndromes.

Anaplastic (undifferentiated large cell) thyroid carcinoma is one of the most aggressive malignancies known in medicine and fortunately comprises only 10% of all thyroid cancers. This malignancy typically occurs in older individuals with a long-standing history of goiter or nodular thyroid. Aggressive local invasion compressing the trachea is the usual course of this tumor. Patient survival beyond 3 to 6 months after diagnosis is exceedingly rare.

Treatment

Clearly, surgical resection of well-differentiated thyroid cancer remains the primary focus of curative therapy. However, the extent of resection and need for cervical lymphadenectomy are heavily debated. Patients who are at low risk for recurrence, such as a man younger than 40 and a woman younger than 50, and who have a small tumor (<2 cm in diameter) may be candidates for limited resection. Patients with high risk of local recurrence or distant metastasis (e.g., adolescents, elderly, patients with large tumors) are candidates for a total thyroidectomy. Although no clear survival benefit has been shown with total thyroidectomy, proponents argue that adjuvant radioablative ^{131}I therapy is more effective in treating residual local disease or metastatic foci, the utilization of nuclear scintigraphy is more reliable in detecting recurrent disease, and that in expert hands, morbidity is no different than that after conservative resection. Dissenters point to the fact that residual thyroid often remains after complete resection, incidence of parathyroid damage and recurrent laryngeal nerve damage are higher, and although these well-differentiated cancers have a tendency to be located in bilateral thyroid lobes, these foci are easily controlled with thyroid hormone supplementation for TSH suppression and the clinical importance of these lesions is negligible. The benefits of thyroid lobectomy versus total thyroidectomy must be weighed against the operative risk to the patient.

Thyroid suppression after a subtotal thyroidectomy may be considered but is not required. The follow-up in patients with well-differentiated thyroid carcinoma should include a physical examination, thyroglobulin levels, and ^{131}I radionuclide scans. Adjuvant radiation is reserved for lesions that do not take up iodine. Response to multiagent chemotherapy in those patients is reserved for patients with metastatic disease; multiagent chemotherapy may increase survival, but prospective randomized studies are yet to be completed.

Total thyroidectomy with removal of affected cervical lymph nodes is recommended in patients with medullary carcinoma due to the fact that C cells are located throughout the gland. Patients with medullary carcinoma should be followed with calcitonin levels. An elevated calcitonin level postoperatively indicates recurrent metastatic disease. Patients with anaplastic thyroid cancer are rarely cured with surgery. Multimodality therapy consisting of surgery, radiation, and chemotherapy is the only chance of survival in these patients.

Prognosis

Still, the prognosis for patients with thyroid cancer is quite favorable overall and is dependent on the histologic subtype, size, and stage of disease as well as age and sex of the patient. The most important factors in thyroid carcinoma include the grade, the extent, and the size of the tumor. Women fare better than men, and furthermore, women younger than 50 years of age survive longer than similarly aged men.

PARATHYROID GLANDS

Surgical Anatomy

Parathyroid glands are intimately associated with the thyroid gland. There are usually four glands, two superior and two inferior parathyroid glands, but there may be anywhere from two to five. Grossly, they appear as small, yellowish glands sometimes resembling fat. The superior and inferior parathyroid glands arise from the fourth and third pharyngeal pouches respectively during the fifth week of embryological development. The superior parathyroid glands usually descend with the developing thyroid gland, whereas the inferior parathyroid glands migrate with the thymus. The distance of superior gland migration is shorter, and variations in their location are few. In contrast, the location of the inferior glands (ranging from the pharynx to the mediastinum) is due to the greater distance of migration. Blood is supplied to the parathyroid glands typically by the inferior thyroid artery and less commonly by the superior thyroid artery. The superior, middle, and inferior thyroid veins drain the parathyroid glands.

Physiology

Parathyroid hormone (PTH) is produced by the parathyroid gland and acts as the principal regulator of calcium and phosphate homeostasis. PTH has two main target organs, bone and kidney. In bone, PTH stimulates demineralization by osteoclasts. At the renal tubule, calcium reabsorption and phosphate excretion are affected by PTH, whereas in the renal parenchyma, production of $1,25(OH)_2$ vitamin D_3 is stimulated. Figure 4 depicts the normal regulatory hormonal feedback mechanisms of PTH secretion.

The most common cause of hypercalcemia (Fig. 5) of the general population is primary hyperparathyroidism. In hospitalized patients, however, malignancy (e.g., hematologic malignancies, solid tumors with bony metastasis, solid tumors without bony metastasis) is the most common cause of hypercalcemia. Hematologic malignancies, such as multiple myeloma, lymphoma, and leukemia, produce hypercalcemia from direct bone involvement. Metastatic breast, lung, and prostate carcinoma produce hypercalcemia as a result of direct destruction of bone or stimulation of osteoclast demineralization of bone. Solid tumors without bony metastasis that produce a hyperparathyroid state secondary to paraneoplastic secretion of parathyroid or parathyroid-like hormone include squamous cell carcinoma of the lung and esophagus, renal cell carcinoma, and ovarian cancer. Hypercalcemia is infrequently associated with sarcoidosis, although the exact mechanism is unknown. Patients with vitamin D intoxication, long-term use of lithium and thiazides, prolonged immobilization, and peptic ulcer disease treated with oral antacids and milk (milk-alkali syndrome) are clinically prone to developing hypercalcemia. Other diseases associated with hypercalcemia include familial hypocalcemia hypercalcemia, thyrotoxicosis, and chronic renal failure (secondary hyperparathyroidism).

Disease of the Parathyroid Glands

Primary Hyperparathyroidism

Nonfamilial primary hyperparathyroidism is defined as excessive production of PTH from a solitary adenoma (80%) or multiglandular hyperplasia (20%). Parathyroid carcinoma is found in <1% of all patients with primary hyperparathyroidism. Patients with hyperparathyroidism associated with MEN typically have multiglandular hyperplasia. There are ~100,000 new cases of primary hyperparathyroidism per year diagnosed in the United States. The etiology is largely unknown, but radiation exposure has been implicated. Statistically, the disease occurs in approximately one in 500 women and in one in 1,000 men over the age of 60.

The clinical presentation of primary hyperparathyroidism was first characterized by von Recklinghausen in 1891 and until recently was referred to as the disease of "bones, stones, abdominal groans and psychological moans." The constellation of symptoms that this phrase refers to reflects the increased PTH levels and their effect at the target organs (e.g., painful bone disease, renal calculi, abdominal discomfort) as well as neuropsychiatric symptoms. Because of an increased awareness of hyperparathyroidism, hypercalcemia detected on routine serum calcium levels has detected more patients early in the course of disease, and thus an increasing percentage of patients today are asymptomatic at the time of diagnosis. It should be emphasized, however, that hypercalcemia does not always equate with hyperparathyroidism.

Renal consequences of primary hyperparathyroidism range from renal calculi to renal dysfunction. Renal calculi develop from hypercalcemia and the tubular precipitation of calcium despite the effect of increased PTH. Once considered the hallmark of primary hyperparathyroidism, the incidence of renal calculi has decreased because of earlier diagnosis. Direct tubular damage from calcium or intravascular hypovolemia may be contributory to decreased renal function. Lytic bone lesions are the result of PTH action on bone osteoclasts. Bony changes range between subperiosteal resorption of the phalanxes to osteitis fibrosis cystica. The latter patients have an increased incidence of pathological fractures. The pathogenesis of abdominal pain with associated nausea, anorexia, and vomiting secondary to hypercalcemia is less clear but may rest with the related gastric hyperacidity in these patients. Similarly, psychological changes ranging from mild depression or inability to concentrate to lethargy, confusion, and coma due to hypercalcemia are known but not well understood. Hypercal-

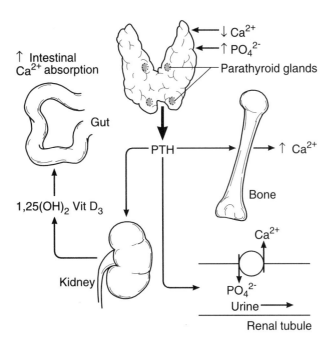

FIG. 4. Calcium homeostasis.

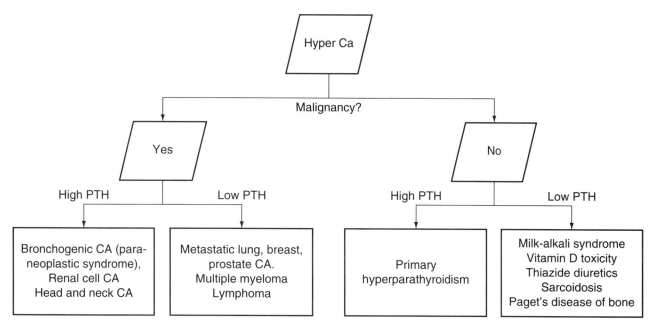

FIG. 5. Differential diagnosis of hypercalcemia.

cemic crisis is arbitrarily defined as a serum calcium of >15 mg/dl associated with clinical symptoms of nausea, vomiting, lethargy, and even coma. Aggressive intravenous rehydration, administration of intravenous diphosphonates, and loop diuretics are the primary therapies instituted in the midst of prompt evaluation for the cause of hypercalcemia.

A careful history and physical examination to exclude other causes of hypercalcemia are critical in diagnosing primary hyperparathyroidism. Although there is no single test that confirms primary hyperparathyroidism, an elevated serum calcium, an elevated intact PTH level, and normal renal function are extremely sensitive markers of disease.

The diagnosis of primary hyperparathyroidism is an indication for parathyroidectomy. Prior to operation, imaging studies (e.g., ^{99m}technetium sestamibi scan, ultrasonography, MRI) localize hyperfunctioning glands in up to 80% of cases, but false-positive and false-negative results taint the utilization of these tests. Many contemporary endocrine surgeons do not rely upon preoperative localization in the patient who has not had previous neck surgery. The standard surgical approach to a patient with primary hyperparathyroidism who has not undergone previous neck surgery is four-gland exploration with histologic confirmation of normal parathyroid glands. Enlarged glands are removed and normal appearing glands are carefully biopsied.

Hypercalcemia within 6 months of a neck exploration is characterized as persistent hyperparathyroidism, whereas hypercalcemia developing 6 months after parathyroidectomy defines recurrent hyperparathyroidism. Re-exploration is mandated in either case, but preoperative use of

parathyroid localization studies are recommended. Patients undergoing re-exploration are at higher risk for developing the operative complications of hypocalcemia and injury to the recurrent laryngeal nerve.

Secondary Hyperparathyroidism

In contradistinction to hyperparathyroidism where hypercalcemia predominates, secondary hyperparathyroidism is generally the result of physiologic compensation of hypocalcemia from chronic renal failure. Phosphate retention, decreased 1,25(OH)$_2$ vitamin D$_3$ production, and the resultant decreased serum calcium level lead to increased synthesis of PTH and parathyroid gland hyperplasia. This clinical scenario is distinguished from tertiary hyperparathyroidism in which parathyroid adenomas develop in patients with chronic secondary hyperparathyroidism.

Management of the primary disease process, renal failure, is required to manage secondary hyperparathyroidism, and surgery is rarely necessary. In cases refractory to medical management, standard surgical practice involves total parathyroidectomy with autotransplantation of one-half of one gland either in the forearm of the strap muscles of the neck. This allows easy access to glands in the rare event of recurrent hyperplasia that would require further resection.

Hypoparathyroidism

Hypoparathyroidism is most commonly caused by injury to the parathyroid glands during total thyroidectomy. In patients with hyperparathyroidism and bone disease, calcium deposition into bone can occur following resection of parathyroid, and clinical symptoms can mimic hypoparathyroidism.

Clinical signs and symptoms correlate directly with decreased serum ionized Ca^{2+}, leading to circumoral and digital numbness and tingling. Mental symptoms include confusion and anxiety. Tetany, carpopedal spasm, tonic-clonic convulsions, and laryngeal stridor may also occur. Acute treatment requires intravenous calcium chloride or calcium gluconate. Long-term medications require vitamin D and oral calcium supplementation.

Parathyroid Carcinoma

Because carcinoma of the parathyroid gland is rare, there are few large series reported, but some general concepts are known. First, most parathyroid carcinomas secrete PTH, and although some nonfunctioning parathyroid cancers exist, diagnosis of parathyroid carcinoma is usually linked to a preoperative diagnosis of hyperparathyroidism. Intraoperative appreciation of a hard parathyroid gland adherent or fixed to adjacent tissues and the strap muscles is suggestive of parathyroid cancer. Additionally, diagnosis of parathyroid carcinoma is based on certain histologic features including capsular and vascular invasion, mitotic figures, and lymph node metastasis. If associated hyperparathyroidism is promptly diagnosed and surgical excision of the carcinoma not delayed, long-term postoperative survival is the rule. There appears to be no benefit from adjuvant radiation or chemotherapy for metastatic or recurrent disease.

ADRENAL GLAND

Anatomy and Physiology

Bilateral adrenal glands form between the fourth and sixth weeks of fetal life. The adrenal cortex develops during the fourth week of embryogenesis from mesodermal tissue and evolves into steroid secreting cells. During the seventh week, ectodermal cells (pheochromoblasts) migrate from the neural crest into the adrenal mass to become the adrenal medulla. The cortex and medulla function as discrete endocrine units housed within a common capsule. Normal sized glands are ~4 to 5 g, but this varies widely with states of critical disease or exogenous corticosteroid administration.

The adrenal cortex is composed of three functional layers. The zona glomerulosa makes up the outer cortical layer and synthesizes mineralocorticoids, the most important of which is aldosterone. Elevated serum levels of angiotensin II and potassium increase secretion of aldosterone from the adrenal cortex to act at primarily the distal tubule of the nephron to cause increased absorption of sodium and increased excretion of potassium and hydrogen ion. The zona fasciculata occupies the mid-cortex region and blends with the zona reticularis, the innermost region of the adrenal cortex. These two zones are important in the production of glucocorticoids (cortisol) and androgens (testosterone). The production of glucocorticoids is regulated by the hypothalamus-pituitary-adrenal axis (Fig. 6). Cortisol is influential in carbohydrate metabolism by promoting gluconeogenesis. Additionally, it inhibits mast cell histamine release, inhibits osteoblasts, and stimulates osteoclasts. As an immunosuppressant, cortisol blunts hyperthermia in response to infection, suppresses lymphocyte proliferation, and promotes cytolysis of T-lymphocytes. By inhibiting the aggregation of inflammatory cells in an area of inflammation, corticosteroids retard wound healing and promote bacterial infection. Androgens are important in anabolic protein synthesis and maturation of sexual organs.

The adrenal medulla is composed of cells that produce biologically active amine compounds called "catecholamines" (dopamine, epinephrine, and norepinephrine). Neural crest cells migrate to the adrenal medulla and other nonadrenal tissues during embryonic life. Normally, these nonadrenal tissue areas regress; however, abnormal persistence of these neural crest cell clusters into adult life may produce symptoms secondary to elevated catecholamine levels.

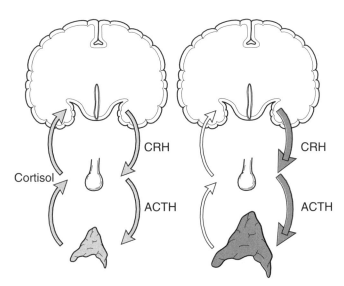

CRH = Corticoptropic releasing hormone
ACTH = Adreno corticotropic hormone

FIG. 6. Adrenal cortisol synthesis is controlled by both hypothalamic CRH and pituitary ACTH in a classic negative feedback loop. In individuals with defects in cortisol biosynthesis, CRH and ACTH are increased. The persistent stimulation of the adrenal by ACTH results in adrenal cortical hyperplasis. (Adapted from Gray JW, Skandalakis JE. *Atlas of surgical anatomy for general surgeons.* Baltimore: Williams and Wilkins, 1985.)

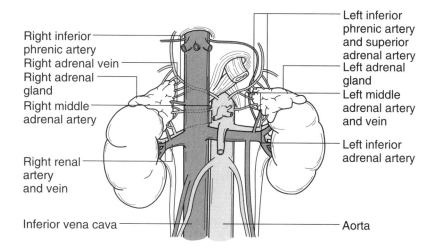

Right inferior phrenic artery
Right adrenal vein
Right adrenal gland
Right middle adrenal artery
Right renal artery and vein
Inferior vena cava

Left inferior phrenic artery and superior adrenal artery
Left adrenal gland
Left middle adrenal artery and vein
Left inferior adrenal artery
Aorta

FIG. 7. Vascular supply of adrenal gland. (Adapted from Gray JW, Skandalakis JE. *Atlas of surgical anatomy for general surgeons.* Baltimore: Williams and Wilkins, 1985.)

The vascular system of the adrenal gland is quite complex (Fig. 7) and is separated into superior, middle and inferior vessels. The right superior gland receives blood from the inferior phrenic artery. The right middle and inferior gland receive blood from the aorta and right renal artery. The left adrenal gland is supplied by the aorta to its superior and middle regions, and by the left renal artery to its inferior pole. The venous drainage of the superior lobe of the right adrenal gland conducts blood directly to the inferior vena cava, whereas that of the inferior right adrenal gland is brought to the right renal vein. In contrast, virtually all the venous blood of the left adrenal gland is delivered to the left renal vein.

Diseases of the Adrenal Gland

Cushing's Syndrome

In 1912, Harvey Cushing first described a pattern of symptoms that reflects chronic exposure to inappropriately elevated levels of cortisol. Cushing's syndrome is due to excessive corticotropin-releasing hormone/adrenocorticotropic hormone (ACTH) production (more appropriately termed "Cushing's disease"), autonomous adrenocortical hyperfunction, and ectopic ACTH production or exogenous ingestion of corticosteroids. Pituitary adenoma (usually microadenoma), adrenal adenoma, adrenal carcinoma, and ectopic ACTH production are the disease processes in decreasing order of frequency, resulting in primary hypercortisolism. In this review, attention is focused on pituitary and adrenal disease.

The disease is more common in females, with the peak age of clinical presentation between 35 and 50 years of age. "Pseudocushing" syndromes can be seen in alcoholism and in patients with primary obesity. Common clinical signs and symptoms are listed in Table 3.

Establishing the diagnosis of Cushing's syndrome is challenging; however, by recognizing the endocrine negative feedback axis of the adrenal gland with respect to glucocorticoid production, localizing the pathology is straightforward. Persistently elevated serum cortisol levels after administration of low-dose dexamethasone (2 mg/day for 2 days) distinguish patients with true hypercortisolism from normal individuals, whose cortisol levels will be suppressed. In patients with true hypercortisolism, serum ACTH levels are normal or elevated from a pituitary adenoma or ectopic ACTH production. In contrast, with autonomous adrenal hyperfunction, ACTH levels are low. In patients with elevated serum ACTH, suppression of serum cortisol levels after administration of high-dose dexamethasone (8 mg/day for 2 days) identifies a pituitary adenoma, whereas persistently elevated serum glucocorticoid levels indicates ectopic ACTH production. Low serum ACTH in the presence of elevated serum cortisol suggests an adrenal adenoma or adrenal carcinoma, and CT of the abdomen will demonstrate disease with high sensitivity (Fig. 8).

Isolated primary adrenal adenomas require unilateral adrenalectomy through either a flank or transabdominal approach. A recent advance has been a laparoscopic approach to remove adrenal adenomas. Pituitary disease was formerly treated with bilateral adrenalectomy. Currently, trans-sphenoidal excision of anterior neurohypophyseal adenomas has been proven safe and effective and is considered the standard treatment for Cushing's

TABLE 3. *Signs and symptoms of Cushing's disease*

Weight gain
Oligomenorrhea
Hirsutism
Glucose intolerance
Depression
Obesity
"Moon facies"
Hypertension
Striae
"Buffalo hump"

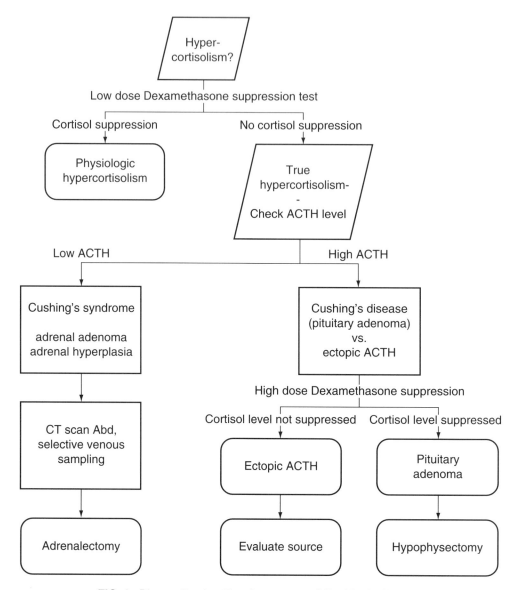

FIG. 8. Diagnostic algorithm for suspected Cushing's disease.

disease. Refractory cases, disease recurrence, or the inability to safely remove the entire adenoma are indications for pituitary irradiation or bilateral adrenalectomy. If primary adrenal hyperplasia is the pathologic process, bilateral adrenalectomy is indicated. The removal of *both* adrenal glands necessitates postoperative administration of low-dose oral corticosteroids and mineralocorticoids. Infrequently, a pituitary tumor develops ≥3 years after bilateral adrenalectomy, and is manifested by progressively increasing skin pigmentation, amenorrhea, and visual field disturbances (Nelson's syndrome).

Hyperaldosteronism (Conn's syndrome)

In 1955, Conn described the case of a patient with weakness, hypertension, and polyuria, with serum chem-istry revealing hypernatremia, hypokalemia, and metabolic alkalosis. Surgical removal of the adrenal gland, which was found to harbor an aldosterone-producing tumor, resulted in resolution of metabolic abnormalities in the postoperative period. The most common pathologic processes responsible for hypermineralocorticoidism include adrenocortical adenoma followed by bilateral adrenocortical hyperplasia. Rare etiologies include glucocorticoid suppressible hypercortisolism, adrenocortical carcinoma, and ovarian neoplasms producing excess aldosterone.

Clinical suspicion is raised when initial evaluation of a patient who is not on diuretics has hypertension and a decreased serum potassium (<3.5 meq/L). Elevated urinary K^+ and HCO_3^- levels in the presence of high serum aldosterone and low serum renin all but confirm the existence of primary hyperaldosteronism. CT scan of the abdomen should be obtained to detect adrenal disease. Failure to clearly localize adrenal pathology in patients with confirmed hyperaldosteronism may require performance of posture studies to identify which patients are best treated by medical or surgical therapy (Fig. 9). Early in the morning, after the patient has been in a recumbent position overnight, a serum aldosterone level is obtained. A second serum aldosterone level is drawn 4 hr later, after the patient has been standing for some time. Normally, serum aldosterone levels rise slightly after standing, but in idiopathic adrenal hyperplasia, a greater rise from baseline level is noted. The presence of an adrenocortical adenoma is suggested by a paradoxical fall in serum aldosterone. Sometimes a

presumed adenoma will be missed on a routine screening CT scan. However, localization can usually be accomplished with thin-slice CT scanning of the abdomen, nuclear scintigraphy, or selective renal vein sampling.

Surgical removal of a unilateral adrenocortical adenoma is performed safely via flank or abdominal incision and successfully resolves metabolic abnormalities in >90% of cases. Adrenal hyperplasia is managed with spironolactone and routine follow-up evaluation. Long-term spironolactone may disrupt the menstrual cycle and cause breast pain in the female and gynecomastia in males. This may result in termination of medical therapy and consideration of surgical therapy.

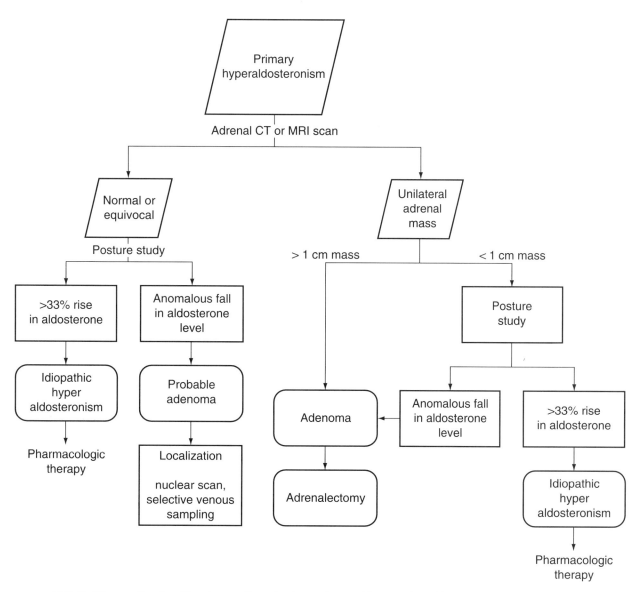

FIG. 9. Diagnostic algorithm for confirmed primary hyperaldosteronism. (Adapted from Young WF Jr., Hogan MJ, Klee GG, et al.: Primary hyperaldosteronism: dignosis and treatment. *Mayo Clin Proc* 1990;65:96–110.)

Addison's disease (Hypoadrenalism)

In 1855, Addison described tuberculous destruction of the adrenal gland which even today is still prevalent in medically and disease acquired immunocompromised patients. Hypoadrenalism is succinctly defined as adrenocortical insufficiency with hypoaldosteronism. Idiopathic adrenal insufficiency is the most common variety. Abrupt cessation of exogenous corticosteroid therapy and stress (trauma) are infrequent but well-recognized etiologies. Autoimmune destruction of the adrenal gland has been implicated. Females outnumber males, and a higher incidence of associated diseases like hypothyroidism, diabetes mellitus, gonadal dysfunction, hypoparathyroidism, and pernicious anemia is seen.

Symptoms are related to deficiencies of glucocorticoid and mineralocorticoid hormones. Fatigue, weight loss, and hyperpigmentation of skin (especially palmar creases) and buccal and tongue mucus membranes are common findings. Laboratory values of significance include hyponatremia, hyperkalemia, and fasting or reactive hypoglycemia. Elevated ACTH levels in combination with low serum cortisol levels are diagnostic. Treatment for both acute and chronic disease involves supportive care and replacement of cortisol and mineralocorticoid hormones. In evaluating these patients, it is imperative to differentiate primary from secondary hypoadrenalism. If the patient has panhypopituitarism, hypothyroidism must also be treated.

Adrenocortical Carcinoma

Adrenocortical carcinoma is a rare and extremely aggressive malignancy that is diagnosed at an advanced stage in the majority of cases. The etiology of this cancer remains to be elucidated, but chromosomal alterations have been implicated. Between one-third to one-half of patients with adrenocortical cancer produce some adrenal hormone (cortisol, aldosterone, or androgens). Nonfunctioning tumors present clinically with weight loss, abdominal pain, increased abdominal girth, and nausea.

Adrenocortical carcinoma should be suspected in rapidly progressive adrenal hormonal syndromes (e.g., Cushing's and Conn's syndromes) or when large adrenal masses appear by CT scan to invade adjacent structures. Percutaneous biopsy of large lesions of the adrenal gland (>6 cm) should be avoided unless curative surgical excision of the adrenal mass will not be offered to the patient secondary to prohibitive operative risk. Total en bloc resection of the adrenal gland and adjacent involved structures is definitive therapy. Unfortunately, most cases are diagnosed late, and long-term survival is poor. Chemotherapy protocols using mitotane have had partial, unsustained responses in a small minority of patients and have been disappointing with regard to improved survival.

Pheochromocytoma

Catecholamines are normally retained within postganglionic neurons and sympathetic nerves, taken up and degraded in nonspecific fashion in peripheral tissues, or excreted in urine as measurable degradation products including normetanephrine, metanephrine, and vanillyl mandelic acid (VMA). A pheochromocytoma is autonomous tissue producing excess levels of catecholamines and usually arises from the adrenal medulla. Occasionally, other tissues that had incorporated neural crest cells become autonomous secretors of catecholamines. An example is the Organ of Zuckerkandl, which represents tissue at the origin of the inferior mesenteric artery or near the aortic bifurcation.

Patients with pheochromocytomas commonly present dramatically in hypertensive crisis with diaphoresis, headache and palpitations. An evolving stroke or myocardial infarction is not infrequently seen. Myocarditis secondary to increased catecholamines has been reported. Associated diseases are listed in Table 4. Although hypertension is the most consistent clinical sign, persistent hypertension occurs in less than one-half of the patients. Paroxysmal hypertension can be induced by physical exercise, sexual intercourse, labor and delivery, and even laughing or coughing. In nonfamilial cases of pheochromocytoma, 10% are considered malignant, 10% are extraadrenal in location, and 10% are harbored in both adrenal glands ("rule of tens"). This contrasts sharply with familial cases, in which the majority are likely to be multiple, bilateral, extraadrenal, and malignant.

Clinical suspicion is based on the classic patient history of hypertension and the triad of headache, palpitations, and diaphoresis. Biochemical confirmation is easily accomplished by demonstrating increased urinary levels of VMA, metanephrine, and catecholamine. CT scanning of the abdomen usually localizes lesions of >1 cm. Nuclear scintigraphy utilizing ^{131}I-metaiodobenzylguanidine (MIBG scan) is an alternative diagnostic test and is particularly helpful in localizing extraadrenal tumors.

Surgical excision of the tumor has the greatest potential for cure. A well-timed operation in a well-prepared patient is of paramount importance. Preoperative α-adrenergic receptor blockade is commonly administered over a 2-week period utilizing phenoxybenzamine. If tachycardia persists after adequate α-blockade, β-adrenergic receptor blockade is started. Initial blood pressure control and

TABLE 4. *Diseases associated with pheochromocytoma*

Multiple endocrine neoplasia IIa
Multiple endocrine neoplasia IIb
Neuroectodermal dysplasias, e.g., neurofibromatosis
Tuberous sclerosis
Sturge-Weber syndrome
von Hippel-Lindau disease

reduction to the point of moderate hypotension allows intravascular volume reexpansion. These patients have contracted blood volumes secondary to physiologic compensation for chronic hypertension. Foods high in tyramine (beer, wine, cheese) can increase the frequency of paroxysmal events and should be avoided. Intraoperative anesthetic management must be undertaken by an experienced team. Sodium nitroprusside, a potent vasodilator, must be ready for immediate infusion to combat potential episodic hypertensive surges with tumor manipulation. Finally, blood pressure monitoring during the postoperative period is important as profound hypotension from relative hypovolemia may manifest.

Incidental Adrenal Mass

The wide utilization of CT scanning of the abdomen and pelvis has led to increasing discovery of asymptomatic adrenal masses. Despite the fact that the overwhelming majority of these masses are benign nonfunctional adenomas, the concern obviously is the possibility of malignancy. Review of large series has stratified these masses according to size. Virtually all nonfunctioning masses of <3.0 cm in diameter are benign, and should be treated expectantly and followed with serial CT scans. The majority of tumors of >6.0 cm in diameter are still benign, but a significant minority harbor malignancy and should be excised for diagnostic reasons. Lesions between 3.0 and 6.0 cm in diameter that are nonfunctional fall into intermediate risk, and their treatment should be individualized.

MULTIPLE ENDOCRINE NEOPLASIAS

The syndrome of MEN is a familial disease in which endocrine neoplasms, both benign and malignant, develop in synchronous or metachronous fashion in various sites. The types of MEN are distinguished by the organs involved and the differences in clinical presentation (Table 5).

Patients with MEN I classically have involvement of the parathyroid glands, pancreas, and pituitary gland. The most common presentation is hypercalcemia, reflecting parathyroid hyperplasia. Gastrinoma is the most common islet cell pancreatic tumor, followed by insulinoma. Prolactinoma of the anterior hypophyseal gland is the most common pituitary neoplasm. Occasionally, tumors will grow large enough to produce visual dysfunction due to compression of the optic nerves.

MEN II syndromes are expressions of abnormalities of organs and tissues derived from neural crest cells and the classic presentation is the association of medullary thyroid cancer and pheochromocytoma. MTC is usually the first abnormality detected, and calcitonin, the product of C cells, serves as a tumor marker for MTC. The majority

TABLE 5. *Multiple endocrine neoplasia (MEN) classification*

	Site	Pathology
MEN I	Parathyroid	Hyperplasia
	Pancreas	Gastrinoma, insulinoma
	Pituitary	Prolactinoma
MEN IIa	Thyroid	Medullary thyroid carcinoma
	Adrenal	Pheochromocytoma
	Parathyroid	Hyperplasia
MEN IIb (III)	Thyroid	Medullary thyroid carcinoma
	Adrenal	Pheochromocytoma
	Soft tissue	Mucosal neuroma, ganglioneuroma of GI tract, skeletal abnormalities, marfanoid appearance

of pheochromocytoma lesions that develop are bilateral in distribution but are invariably limited to the adrenal medulla. Virtually all lesions are benign. In MEN IIa, parathyroid hyperplasia is the common metabolic abnormality, whereas in MEN IIb, soft tissue conditions predominate.

Accurate diagnosis is based on clinical suspicion from patient history, family history, and physical examination. Serum chemistry and urine markers serve as excellent, cost-effective screening tests. The appropriate diagnostic tests for the respective endocrine neoplasm have been outlined here.

The algorithm for treating these patients follows the logic of addressing the most serious condition first. Pheochromocytoma and insulinoma are considered serious processes that demand priority treatment and urgent surgical resection. MTC tends to be multifocal and is best treated by total thyroidectomy; lymph node dissection may be necessary. Recently, genetic research has identified a mutation in the RET proto-oncogene associated with MEN IIa, MEN IIb, and familial non-MEN medullary thyroid cancer. The presence of this genetic mutation in patients at risk distinguishes individuals in which it is hoped that preventative thyroidectomy will eliminate the emergence of MTC. Long-term studies are required to demonstrate that the operative morbidity is low and that the operation effectively cures or prevent medullary thyroid cancer. Gastrinoma in patients with MEN I tends to be multicentric in distribution, and although complicated peptic ulcer disease is frequent, antacid therapy utilizing the H^+ proton pump inhibitors is quite effective and is the initial treatment of choice. Refractory cases may benefit from highly selective vagotomy to modulate acid secretion. Trans-sphenoidal hypophysectomy is standard treatment for prolactinoma. In patients with hyperparathyroidism associated with MEN, total parathyroidectomy and autotransplantation of one-half of one gland into the sternocleidomastoid muscle or into the forearm is standard treatment. This ectopic tissue becomes revascularized and functional, which prevents permanent hypocalcemia, seen after a total parathyroidectomy.

STUDY QUESTIONS

1. What is the blood supply to the thyroid and parathyroid glands?
2. Describe the different types of thyroid cancer and factors related to prognosis.
3. What are the symptoms of hypercalcemia? What is the differential diagnosis of hypercalcemia?
4. What are the potential complications from thyroidectomy and from parathyroidectomy?
5. What are the clinical signs of hypocalcemia?
6. Describe the embryological development of the adrenal gland.
7. Characterize the vascular system of the adrenal gland.
8. Describe appropriate evaluation of a patient with suspected Cushing's disease.
9. What are typical signs and symptoms of Conn's syndrome? How do clinicians properly evaluate patients with suspected hyperaldosteronism?
10. Characterize the different syndromes of MEN.

SUGGESTED READING

Cady B, Rossi R. *Surgery of the thyroid and parathyroid glands.* Philadelphia: Saunders, 1991.

Jossart G, Clark O. Well-differentiated thyroid cancer. *Curr Probl Surg* 1994;31:933–1012.

Lyerly HK, Leight G, Wells SA, Lairmore TC. The thyroid gland. In: Sabiston D, ed. *Textbook of surgery: the biological basis of modern surgical practice.* Philadelphia: Saunders, 1991.

Mazzaaferi E. Management of a solitary thyroid nodule. *N Engl J Med* 1993;328:553–559.

Wells SA, Ashley SW. The parathyroid glands. In: Sabiston D, ed. *Textbook of surgery: the biological basis of modern surgical practice.* Philadelphia: Saunders, 1991.

Wells SA, Soybel DI. The pituitary and adrenal glands. In: Sabiston D, ed. *Textbook of surgery: the biological basis of modern surgical practice.* Philadelphia: Saunders, 1991.

CHAPTER 18

Vascular Surgery

Utpal S. Desai and Anselmo Nunez

Peripheral and central vascular disease is a major cause of disability and death worldwide. In the United States, the increasing life expectancy of males and females directly correlates with an increasing prevalence of vascular disease as well as associated comorbid diseases. The cost of health care for acute vascular disease is tremendous. Similarly, financial expenses required for rehabilitation and chronic care of patients suffering from complications of vascular disease are staggering.

Vascular disease can be divided into arterial, venous, and lymphatic disease. Although considered a systemic disease, arterial vascular disease is described in four vascular regions of the body: the coronary arteries (see Chapter 20), the arteries of the cervicothoracic great vessels and upper extremities, the visceral arteries, and infrarenal aorta and arteries of the lower extremities. Arterial disease can be further subcategorized into aneurysmal, occlusive, and inflammatory disease. Venous and lymphatic disease is present predominantly in the lower extremities.

This chapter is by no means an exhaustive dissertation on the recognition and treatment of vascular disease; however, it is hoped that it will impart some basic principles of clinical management. Accurate clinical assessment of vascular disease is based upon understanding of vascular pathophysiology, which will be discussed in detail. Additionally, an explanation of proper examination skills that correlate to the pathophysiology of vascular disease as well as the basic principles of management of occlusive and aneurysmal disease will be discussed. Finally, diagnostic tests currently in use to confirm the presence of vascular disease will be reviewed.

ARTERIAL DISEASE

Histology

Intima is the innermost layer of the arterial wall and extends from the luminal surface to the inner elastic lamina (Fig. 1). The intima is lined by endothelium with few scattered leukocytes, smooth muscle cells, and connective tissue. The endothelium provides a pliable surface that permits nutrient diffusion and compliance, and a smooth surface for the red blood cell to travel through the artery. The media extends from the internal elastic lamina to the adventitia and contains elastic fibers combined with smooth muscle in varying ratios. For example, in larger arteries that function merely as conduits, elasticity is an important quality, and hence these vessels, e.g., aorta and large branches, contain high concentrations of elastic fibers in the media. In contrast, small arteries and arterioles contain high concentration of smooth muscle to act as the resistor component of arterial system. According to LaPlace's law,

$$T \sim P \times R$$

(which T is arterial wall tension, P is arterial pressure, and R is luminal radius) with increased pressure in the arterial system, smooth muscle contraction can decrease the luminal radius to maintain constant wall tension. The external elastic lamina, although not always present, separates the media and adventitia. The adventitia is composed primarily of fibrocellular tissue, making it the strongest component of the arterial wall. Vasa vasorum are neurovascular bundles that penetrate the adventitia and outer portion of the media of larger arteries. Within

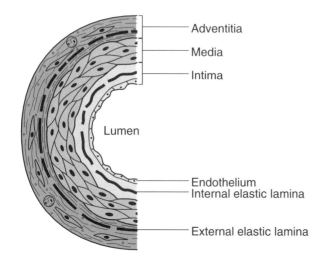

FIG. 1. Diagrammatic representation of the main components of a vascular wall.

the vasa vasorum, small arteries deliver nutrients to arterial tissue, whereas nerves within the bundle mediate smooth muscle tone and contraction.

Arterial Occlusive Disease

Atherosclerosis is the principal disease process affecting arteries. It is characterized by accumulation of cell matrix fibers, lipids, and tissue debris in the subintimal layer, which may result in narrowing of the lumen and obstruction of blood flow. Atherosclerotic lesions may also lead to ulceration, embolization, and thrombosis. Associated risk factors for atherogenesis include hyperlipidemia (cholesterolemia), cigarette smoking, hypertension, diabetes mellitus, obesity, and family history.

The pathogenesis of atherosclerosis is complex and probably multifactorial. The endothelial injury hypothesis postulates that mechanical forces (increased arterial wall stress from hypertension), metabolic intermediates (hyperlipidemia, nicotine) or immunologic reactions cause endothelial injury and desquamation. Exposed subendothelial tissue promotes platelet aggregate accumulation, cellular proliferation, and eventual plaque formation. Additionally, humoral mediators, growth factors, and cytokines from altered endothelial cells and from inflammatory cells interacting with other arterial cells are important mediators of macrophage infiltration, smooth muscle proliferation, and lipid deposition. Although injury may not initiate atherosclerosis, biologic reactions of the endothelium and arterial wall during injury and repair may play an important role in plaque formation. Recent reports have uncovered some new information which suggests that atherosclerotic plaque localizes preferentially to regions of low shear stress. In susceptible areas of low-flow velocity, atherogenic substances are cleared slowly, increasing residence time and favoring atheroma formation (Fig. 2). Arterial

wall thickening also occurs in response to increases in tangential tension, but this thickening occurs not by increases in media thickness but by intimal thickening. For example, in patients with hypertension, arterial-arteriolar intimal thickening occurs as a response to increased arterial wall tension.

The fibrous plaque is the characteristic lesion of atherosclerosis (Fig. 3). The fibrous cap is a subendothelial well-organized layer of smooth muscle and connective tissue. A necrotic core occupies the deep central regions containing amorphous and crystalline droplets of lipids. Over time, the media layer thins and allows outward bulging of atheroma. Atheroma calcification is a feature of advanced plaques, distinguishing it from newer lesions, which are soft and friable in character.

As intimal plaques enlarge, a closely associated enlargement of the affected artery tends to limit the stenosing effect of enlarging intimal plaque. Arterial enlargement keeps pace with rate of luminal narrowing, until ~40% stenosis (Fig. 4), but progression of disease beyond this degree of narrowing cannot be overcome by arterial enlargement, and eventually blood flow across the

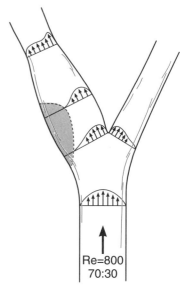

FIG. 2. Axial velocity profiles measured with laser Doppler anemometry in a glass model carotid bifurcation under conditions of steady flow (Reynolds number, 800; flow division ratio of internal carotid to external carotid, 70:30). The velocity profile is skewed toward the inner wall of the carotid bifurcasion, resulting in a steep velocity gradient and high wall shear stress. Along the outer wall of the internal carotid sinus, the velocity profile is flat and there is an area of flow separation with very low flow velocities (dotted line) and very low wall shear stress. It is in this region of the human carotid bifurcation that intimal plaques form. (Adapted from Zarins CK, Giddens DP, Bharadvaj BK, et al. Carotid bifurcation atherosclerosis: quantitative correlation of plaque localization with flow velocity profiles and wall shear stress. Circ Res 1983;53:502.)

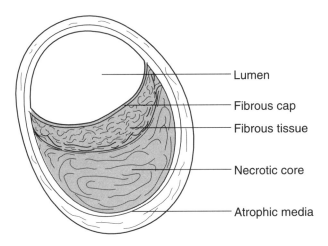

FIG. 3. Cross-section of a human artery with an advanced atherosclerotic plaque. The fibrous cap is a well-organized layer of smooth muscle cells and fibrous tissue that separates the necrotic core of the plaque from the lumen. The media beneath the plaque may become thin and atrophic. The lumen contains a gelatin cast used to redistend and maintain lumen contour.

stenosis is compromised. Hypertension contributes to and modulates the development of atherogenesis but, despite exhaustive research, has not been shown to be a principal etiology of atherosclerosis. Similarly, turbulence, contrary to clinical intuition, has not been shown to be atherogenic. Poststenotic dilation, however, may play a role in atheroma complication (e.g., plaque disruption, thrombogenesis).

Arterial Aneurysmal Disease

An arterial aneurysm can be defined as >50% increase in luminal diameter compared to the diameter of an unaffected artery. Structural weakness, overcome by mechanical and hemodynamic forces, leads to aneurysm formation. Analysis reveals a substantial loss of elastin in the media as well as a similar degree of loss of collagen in the

adventitia layer. An increased concentration of inflammatory cells in the latter may be contributory in aneurysmal disease. Although the majority of arterial aneurysms were once thought to be secondary to atherosclerotic disease, this theory has come under heavy scrutiny. The exact mechanism of progression of disease has not been clearly identified, it is apparent that many factors play key roles in the development of arterial aneurysms.

The association between atherosclerosis and arterial aneurysms had been recognized for decades. As mentioned earlier, compensatory arterial enlargement up to a certain point keeps pace with atheroma luminal narrowing but at the expense of media layer atrophy. Reduction of plaque volume by plaque regression and absorption combined with the thinned media layer exposes an abnormal artery to increased wall tension resulting in progressive arterial dilation and aneurysm formation. Current literature proposes, however, that atheroma may be a secondary occurrence rather than a initiating factor. What has been brought to the forefront of recent clinical research in aneurysm development is genetic susceptibility. Multiple studies have reported hereditary or familial aneurysmal disease. The most recent large-scale report suggests autosomal recessive transmission of aneurysmal susceptibility. It is now theorized that those who have risk factors for atherosclerotic disease (e.g., cigarette smoking, diabetes mellitus, hypertension) combined with genetic susceptibility traits are at highest risk for aortic aneurysm development.

Beyond atherosclerosis and degenerative theories, a host of other etiologies are common and deserve consideration (Table 1). Syphilis at one time was a frequent cause of aortic aneurysms, but now, after the near eradication of tertiary syphilis, it rarely causes aneurysmal disease. Subacute bacterial endocarditis is a common source of embolomycotic aneurysms. Today, in the age of medical and disease-induced immunosuppression, opportunistic organisms like anaerobic and fungal microbes are frequently encountered. The etiology behind inflammatory aneurysms is unclear. A dense fibrotic wall adherent

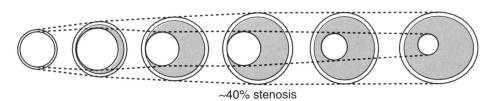

~40% stenosis

FIG. 4. Possible sequence of changes in atherosclerotic arteries in response to enlarging atherosclerotic plaques. In the early stages of intimal plaque deposition, the lumen remains normal or enlarges slightly (left). When intimal plaque enlarges to involve the entire circumference of the vessel and produces >40% stenosis, the artery is no longer able to enlarge at a rate sufficient to prevent narrowing of the lumen. (Adapted from Zarins CK, Giddens DP, Bharadvaj BK, et al. Carotid bifurcation atherosclerosis: quantitative correlation of plaque localization with flow velocity profiles and wall shear stress. *Circ Res* 1983;53:502.)

TABLE 1. *Other etiologies behind arterial aneurysmal disease*

Connective tissue disorders, e.g., Ehlers-Danlos syndrome
Pregnancy-associated splenic artery aneurysms
Infectious (syphilis)
Embolomycotic
Inflammatory

to surrounding structures (e.g., duodenum, ureters, inferior vena cava) with increased concentration of inflammatory cells is the typical histopathology. The explanation behind the heightened inflammatory reaction is yet to be elucidated.

Evaluating a Patient With Arterial Vascular Disease

Despite its locoregional manifestations, vascular disease is invariably a systemic process. A detailed history is unequaled in the evaluation of patients with suspected vascular disease. The mere presence of vascular pathology or a history consistent with poor blood flow mandates clinical consideration of the probable coexistence of chronic cardiac disease. Furthermore, a majority of patients reveal long-time tobacco use or a history of diabetes mellitus. Likewise, a thorough physical examination is mandatory in evaluating patients with vascular disease. A comprehensive review of the complete physical examination is not presented, but considerations toward special aspects of examination of a patient with vascular disease are presented. Blood pressure in each upper extremity should be obtained to determine the existence of upper extremity arterial occlusive disease and to calculate the ankle-brachial index (ABI), which is discussed below. Ophthalmoscopic examination may demonstrate evidence of chronic hypertension. Auscultation of the carotid and precordial areas may reveal bruits or murmurs consistent with extracranial vascular disease or cardiac valvular disease. Bruits heard on auscultation of the abdomen suggest vasculo-occlusive disease in the visceral, renal, or iliac arteries. A pulsatile midline abdominal mass palpable on examination is suggestive of an abdominal aortic aneurysm. Finally, documentation of pulses in all normally palpable areas is mandatory to discern asymmetry implying unilateral vascular disease or monitor unexpected postoperative vascular insufficiency. A stick figure is a practical way of documenting peripheral pulses (Fig. 5).

Noninvasive Studies of the Vascular System

The use of tests that do not require venous or arterial access or expose patients to radiation are collectively referred to as noninvasive testing and are an essential part of evaluating suspected vascular disease. Segmental limb

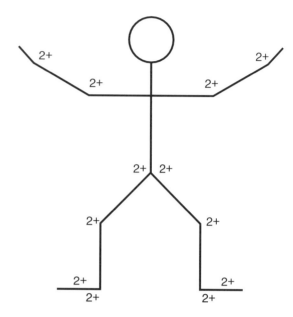

FIG. 5. Stick figure that can be drawn for easy documentation of peripheral pulses. Scale of 1 to 4, with 2 being normal.

pressure is widely accepted because of its simplicity, reproducibility, low cost, and availability. Systolic occlusion pressure is determined by elevating pressure in a cuff placed at different limb segments (e.g., thigh, calf, and foot) until the pulse becomes absent. A systolic blood pressure gradient of ≥20 mm Hg between contiguous segments usually is indicative of a hemodynamically significant lesion. Because atherosclerotic occlusive disease infrequently affects the upper extremity, segmental pressure measurements of the arm often truly reflect the central aortic systolic pressure. The occlusion pressure measured at the ankle divided by the measurement in the arm defines the ABI, which is an accurate indicator of arterial occlusive disease in the lower extremity. Normal ABI is essentially 1.0; values of <0.8 signify vascular occlusive disease. The ankle segmental pressure, though, reflects a summation of all arterial stenotic lesions proximal to the ankle. Stiff arteries typical of chronic diabetes and renal failure falsely elevate segmental pressure measurements leading to erroneous ABI measurements.

Pulse volume recording (PVR) measures the pulsatile increase in volume in an extremity and localizes hemodynamically significant lesions accurately (Table 2 and Fig. 6). Volumetric measurements, also termed "plethysmography," does not require complete occlusion of arterial flow as is necessary with PVR. A blood pressure cuff placed at the thigh, calf, ankle, and mid toe records waveforms as normal (with a dicrotic notch), moderate stenosis (no notch, with a flatter waveform), and severe stenosis (flattened waveform with a more gradual upstroke and downstroke). Abnormalities in waveforms imply only segmental arterial disease and can make no inference to which individual artery is diseased.

TABLE 2. *Sample of a patient with intermittent claudication of the right leg*

	Systolic Doppler pressures at rest	
	Right	Left
Brachial	140	140
Thigh	Not done	Not done
Calf	Not done	Not done
Ankle	84	140
Metatarsal	Not done	Not done
Toe	Not done	Not done
ABI	0.6	1

ABI, ankle brachial index (ratio of ankle to highest brachial).

(waveform). The spectrum of waveforms are triphasic (normal), minimized with loss of reverse flow velocity (moderate stenosis), and blunted with gradual upstroke and a prolonged downstroke (severe stenosis). Color duplex, also known as color sonoangiography, characterizes arterial flow velocity by assigning color to specific Doppler frequencies. Venous flow can be distinguished from arterial flow by color; similarly, antegrade versus retrograde flow within an arterial segment can be depicted. In well-trained hands, arterial anatomy and pathology is exquisitely demonstrated by duplex study, and advocates predict that its use will at least supplement invasive arteriography if not supersede it in the near future.

Ultrasound gives accurate two-dimensional analysis of arterial wall and lumen with respect to the presence of aneurysm disease, plaque character, lumen diameter, and the presence and quality of luminal thrombus. It is unable, however, to characterize blood flow. Doppler-ultrasound (Duplex) utilizes the imaging quality of ultrasound and quantitates the flow velocity in an artery by recognition of Doppler signal and reproduction into graphic display

Computed Tomography Scan

Computed tomography (CT) scan of the abdomen and pelvis accurately demonstrates the presence and extent of aneurysmal disease. Axial-spiral CT scanning capability may provide equivalent visualization results regarding mesenteric vessels. Radiation exposure and rare intravenous contrast nephropathy are disadvantages to its use.

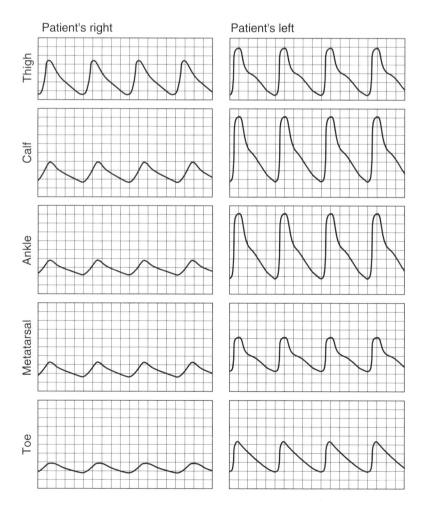

FIG. 6. Pulse volume recording (PVR) and ankle brachial index (ABI) of the lower extremity in a patient with intermittent claudication.

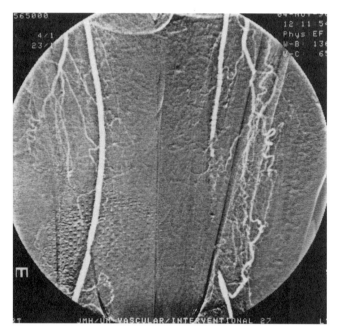

FIG. 7. Angiography of the right and left superficial femoral arteries (SFA). Note the segmental occlusion of the left SFA with reconstitution of flow at the above knee segment of popliteal artery.

Angiography

An arteriogram accurately demonstrates vascular anatomy in exquisite detail and localizes multiple segments of luminal stenosis that correlate with clinical presentation (Fig. 7). It is considered the diagnostic gold standard but is reserved for preoperative evaluation. Disadvantages are few and infrequent but well-recognized. Postprocedure groin hematoma is the most common complication resulting from inadequate hemostasis. Similarly, inadequate hemostasis can result in pseudoaneurysm formation. Occasionally, arteriovenous fistula complicate percutaneous arterial access. Infrequently, renal failure or systemic anaphylaxis occurs as a result of contrast administration. Rarely, acute limb ischemia from arterial thrombosis may supervene.

Preoperative Evaluation

For surgical intervention to be warranted, the risk of loss of life or limb from existing vascular disease and the patient's perioperative risk from coexisting medical conditions must be outweighed by the relative benefit to be derived from the procedure. Recognizing that patients with vascular pathology invariably have serious comorbid disease necessitates well-planned preoperative evaluation. A thorough patient history, with particular attention to review of cardiac reserve and systemic disease, can identify patients that might benefit from advanced diagnostic studies. Control of diabetes mellitus, hypertension, and optimization of respiratory status further decrease perioperative morbidity.

VASCULAR DISEASE OF THE INFRARENAL AORTA AND LOWER EXTREMITY ARTERIAL SYSTEM

Occlusive Disease

Occlusive arterial disease in the infrarenal aorta and lower extremity system can result in diminished oxygen delivery to the lower extremity that manifests as chronic or acute limb ischemia. At the cellular level, a decreased oxygen delivery to peripheral muscle is compensated by the increased oxygen extraction and increased aerobic metabolic capability of the muscle. When the critical threshold is crossed, beyond which compensatory mechanisms can no longer keep pace with oxygen demand, ischemia results and manifests as muscular pain. Pain in the muscles of the affected extremity produced by exercise and relieved by rest is termed "claudication" (Latin *claudio*, to limp). Symptoms usually occur in the muscle region(s) distal to the arterial occlusion. Specifically, pain is experienced in the thigh, buttocks, or calf muscles while walking variable distances and is relieved with cessation of exercise. Claudicants typically have an ABI of 0.5 to 0.8. The length of time or distance before the onset of muscle pain is directionally proportional to the compensatory reserve and conditioning of the muscles of the affected limb. The reported prevalence of claudication in the general population is between 1.0% and 2.0%.

The prognosis for limb salvage in patients with intermittent claudication is good, provided certain preventative measures are followed and that compensatory physiology remains undisturbed. Although strict control of atherosclerotic risk factors (e.g., hypercholesterolemia, diabetes mellitus, and hypertension) may lower complications rates in patients with claudication, absolute cessation of smoking has been shown in a number of studies to diminish progression of disease. Furthermore, in those patients that in spite of the cessation of smoking still require surgery, adverse cardiovascular outcomes in the postoperative period are decreased and limb salvage rates after revascularization are improved. Beyond stopping cigarette use, routine exercise programs to augment compensatory physiology improve or eliminate symptoms in a large percentage of patients. Rheologic agents, like pentoxifylline, increase red blood cell membrane deformability and decrease blood viscosity and are thought to increase blood flow through stenotic vessels in the distal extremity. The efficacy of this drug is controversial. Because the prognosis of intermittent lower extremity claudication is favorable, operative intervention is generally chosen only for patients with life-style–disabling symptoms.

Severe narrowing of the main arterial conduits and collateral circulation necessitates establishment of alternative circulation pathways in the face of chronic limb ischemia. Increased blood delivery to the distal lower extremity is partially accomplished, utilizing gravity as hydrostatic pressure source to push red blood cells through dilated cutaneous capillaries, dependent rubror. With progression of disease, however, a critical level of unpaid oxygen debt at the muscle cell level reaches a critical level and manifests as persistent pain despite the lack of muscle activity, i.e., rest pain. Classically, the distribution of pain in the lower extremity is in the forefoot and toes, particularly worse at night in a recumbent position. Not surprisingly, pain improves if the patient dangles the feet at the bedside or walks. The ankle brachial index is usually <0.5. Up to half of these patients will require some form of revascularization in the near future for limb preservation. The presence tissue loss or gangrene constitutes a relative surgical emergency, and evaluation for revascularization should proceed.

Cutaneous ulcers and other evidence of tissue loss are ischemic ulcers from underlying vascular insufficiency. Usually found on the lower third of the leg on the dorsal aspect of the foot, they are painful and deep with a necrotic base. Although diabetic foot ulcers are the result of an autonomic neuropathy and tissue trauma, the coexistence of vascular disease is common and may prevent successful wound healing.

Gangrene is either the result of either thrombosis superimposed on a preexisting arterial stenosis or thromboembolic phenomenon. Dry gangrene refers to the mummified appearance of the gangrenous tissue and is typically uninfected. Wet gangrene refers to the purulent discharge and surrounding inflammatory reaction around the gangrenous tissue. Associated hemodynamic instability secondary to sepsis is an indication for emergent surgical debridement.

Aortoiliac Occlusive Disease

For the most part, atherosclerotic disease of the abdominal aorta and iliac arteries represents but an involved segment of diffuse vascular disease (Fig. 8). Infrequently, however, it occurs as an isolated disease process with specific clinical manifestations. Although patients chief complaints center around thigh and buttock claudication worsened by exercise, a thorough clinical assessment may reveal much more information relevant to arterio-occlusive disease in this region. Leriche syndrome are classic clinical symptoms of aortoiliac occlusive disease characterized by thigh and buttock claudication, impotence in men, and absent femoral pulses.

Clinical diagnosis can be made after thorough patient history and physical examination. Frequently, the lower extremities in patients with isolated aortoiliac disease are well perfused by established collateral blood flow. Segmental pressure measurements reveal an abnormal thigh values and an abnormal thigh-brachial index. PVR are often helpful after exercise, when resting segmental pressures are normal but patient history is strongly suggestive of aortoiliac occlusive disease. In isolated aortoiliac disease, there is no progressive decrease in the thigh and ankle pressure tracings.

Nonoperative therapy as outlined has favorable results. Indications for surgery include disabling claudication, rest pain, ischemic ulceration, pregangrenous skin changes. Aortobifemoral bypass (ABF) grafting is the most frequently chosen operation to reestablish arterial blood flow to the femoral arteries (Fig. 9). Perioperative mortality is <2%, and 5-year graft patency approaches 90%. For patients in whom aortic cross-clamping presents prohibitive perioperative risk, axillobifemoral bypass may be used (Fig. 10). For patients with unilateral disease, a femorofemoral bypass may be used provided the contralateral iliac artery has no evidence of atherosclerotic disease that may compromise blood flow through the bypass conduit (Fig. 11). Primary patency rates (which refer to primary "assisted" patency in which secondary interventions may have been performed to salvage a narrowed but not occluded graft) after femorofemoral bypass is ~80% at 5 years; after axillobifemoral bypass, 5-year patency approaches 75%. Early complications include graft thrombosis, infection, lymphocele formation, or distal emboli. Late occurring morbidity include thrombosis, infection, pseudoaneurysms, or graft-enteric fistula.

Femoropopliteal Occlusive Disease

Compared to aortoiliac occlusive disease, isolated femoropopliteal occlusive disease is not uncommon. Solitary segmental atherosclerotic narrowing about the adductor canal (Hunter's canal) is the most frequent lesion causing femoropopliteal arterial symptoms. Diffuse narrowing throughout the superficial femoral artery (SFA) produces similar symptoms. Patients complain chiefly of calf rather than thigh and buttock claudication. Physical examination of the distal extremity may reveal signs of chronic ischemia (e.g., thin brittle skin with lack of hair, hypertrophic toenails). Segmental pressure measurements between thigh and calf demonstrate a gradient of ≥20 mm Hg.

Claudication from femoropopliteal artery occlusive disease is treated by smoking cessation, exercise program, and rheologic agents with favorable results. Evidence of rest pain, gangrene, or nonhealing ulcers indicate critical ischemia that requires urgent revascularization. Patients with life-style–limiting claudication that have failed medical management are also candidates for revascularization. For isolated femoropopliteal arterial narrowing, bypass from the common femoral artery to

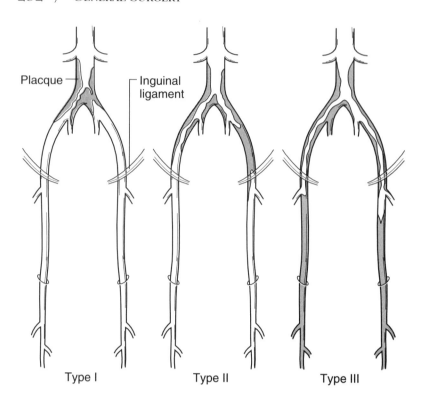

FIG. 8. Anatomic variants of aortoiliac disease. (Adapted from Braunwald E, ed. *Atlas of heart diseases. Vol. VII. Vascular disease.* St. Louis: Mosby–Year Book, 1996.)

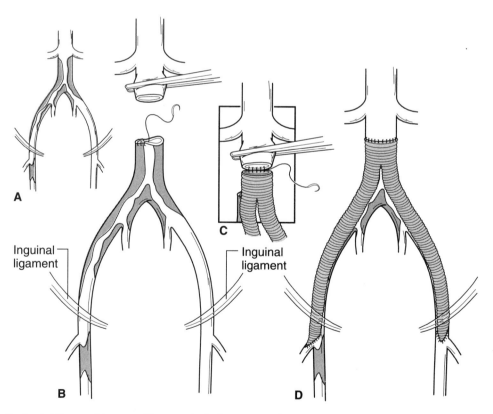

FIG. 9. Aortobifemoral bypass. The surgical placement of a prosthetic aorto-bi-iliac bypass graft from the infrarenal aorta to the femoral arteries is the most frequently employed surgical approach for aortoiliac disease. **(A)** Schematic preoperative angiogram. **(B)** Resection of the diseased aorta with oversewing of the distal aortic stump. **(C)** End-to-end anastomosis of the aorta to the proximal bypass graft. **(D)** The entire aorto-bifemoral graft in place. (Adapted from Braunwald E, ed. *Atlas of heart diseases. Vol. VII. Vascular disease.* St. Louis: Mosby–Year Book, 1996.)

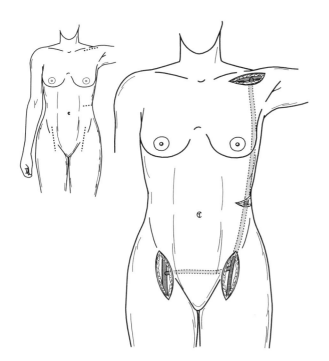

FIG. 10. Axillobifemoral bypass. (Adapted from Braunwald E, ed. *Atlas of heart diseases. Vol. VII. Vascular disease.* St. Louis: Mosby–Year Book, 1996.)

popliteal artery is performed. Although the routine use of a synthetic material is proven for ABF, the success of autogenous saphenous vein versus polytetrafluoroethylene (PTFE) for femoropopliteal artery bypass depends on location of distal anastomosis. When the anastomosis is created to the above-knee segment of the popliteal

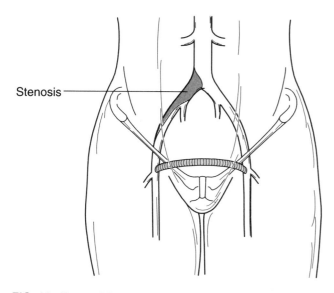

FIG. 11. Femoral-femoral bypass, which is used to treat unilateral iliac occlusive disease. (Adapted from Braunwald E, ed. *Atlas of heart diseases. Vol. VII. Vascular disease.* St. Louis: Mosby–Year Book, 1996.)

Stenosis

artery, 5-year patency rates for saphenous vein and PTFE are comparable (~70%). With anastomosis below the knee, autologous vein and PTFE have similar patency rates at 2 years postprocedure. Subsequently, however, 5-year patency rates favor use of vein (70%) rather than PTFE (15%).

Two techniques are employed when performing infrainguinal arterial bypass with autogenous vein: in situ bypass grafting or reversed saphenous vein grafting. When using the saphenous vein in situ, a valvulotome is passed within the lumen of the vein to make the valves incompetent and allow antegrade arterial flow. Reversed saphenous vein grafting refers to the placement of the vein within the bypass field in reverse direction and does not require use of the valvulotome. Despite theoretical advantages of each method, both techniques show equivalent patency rates at 5 years.

Nonatherosclerotic Vasculo-Occlusive Disease of the Lower Extremity

Vasculitides are collectively other pathologic processes that narrow arterial luminal diameter resulting in occlusive disease. Examples include polyarteritis nodosa (PAN), Kawasaki's disease, hypersensitivity angiitis, Wegener's granulomatosis, temporal arteritis, Takayasu's arteritis, and Buerger's disease. An extensive discussion regarding these entities is beyond the scope of this chapter; however, some important examples are considered briefly. Buerger's disease affects both the lower extremity arterial system and is included here. Takayasu's arteritis and temporal arteritis have important clinical symptoms in the cervicothoracic great vessel artery region and are presented in a subsequent section of this chapter.

Buerger's disease (thromboangiitis obliterans) is an occlusive vasculitis of medium sized and smaller arteries of both the lower and upper extremity typically in middle aged men. It is prevalent in the Far and Middle East populations. Although an exact etiology remains unknown, a clear relationship between tobacco use and occurrence and recurrence of disease is recognized. Once thought a disease found almost exclusively in men, unfortunately, because of increased tobacco consumption among women, the incidence of Buerger's disease has increased in females. The natural history of Buerger's disease in patients who have abandoned smoking is generally uneventful. In those with trophic gangrenous lesions, limb salvage can often be accomplished by absolute tobacco restriction and supportive care without necessitating surgery. Characteristic pathology demonstrates a fresh thrombus with characteristic microabscesses consisting of multinucleated giant cells, epithelioid cells and leukocytes. The vasculitis is nonspecific, affecting the distal aspects of the upper and lower extremities. Angiography shows segmental lesions, often resulting in corkscrew-shaped collaterals. Therapy is directed toward smoking cessation and is otherwise supportive. Arterial bypasses, however, can be performed successfully.

Acute Lower Limb Ischemia

Acute ischemia of the lower extremity occurs abruptly from either emboli or in situ thrombosis of existing arterio-occlusive disease. Clinical presentation of acute arterial occlusion can be characterized by the five "p's": **p**ain, **p**aresthesia, **p**allor, **p**ulselessness, and **p**aralysis. Lack of well-developed collateral circulation can result in irreversible tissue ischemia in 4 to 6 hr. On the other hand, in limbs with chronic vascular insufficiency but developed collateral flow, successful revascularization and reperfusion may be possible after up to 12 hr of ischemia. Limb salvage rates are inversely proportional to the tolerance of tissue within the circulatory bed to ischemia and duration of inadequate blood flow. Thus, recognition of acute limb ischemia demands emergent revascularization.

Many etiologies behind acute arterial occlusion are known (Table 3), and the majority are related to cardiovascular disease. Patient history and physical examination are crucial in determining the etiology of acute vascular insufficiency. Simultaneously, protection of the circulatory bed distal to occlusion from thrombosis is achieved with systemic heparinization. Evidence of isolated embolism to an arterial branch of the lower extremity requires emergent operative thromboembolectomy. Should revascularization after embolectomy be inadequate, arterial bypass with the assistance of intraoperative angiography is required. History of preexisting vascular disease or clinical evidence of other vascular pathology, on the other hand, generally requires preoperative arteriography to delineate all contributory vascular disease and provide a roadmap for optimal revascularization. In certain selected circumstances, thrombolytic therapy directed by angiographic catheter placement may dissolve obstructing thrombus and successfully revascularize an ischemic limb without requiring

surgery. Best outcomes are seen in thrombosis treated within 4 hr of occlusion.

ANEURYSMAL DISEASE

Abdominal Aortic Aneurysm

The incidence of true aneurysms of the abdominal aorta is ~40 per 100,000 population. Because of increasing prevalence with increasing age, aneurysmal disease of the abdominal aorta, the classic example being the common infrarenal abdominal aortic aneurysm, was categorized as degenerative in nature. A causal relationship between atherosclerotic disease and degenerative aneurysms developed from the coexistence of both processes in a majority of cases. It has recently come to light that the two entities may in fact not be related and traditional thoughts regarding risk factors for abdominal aneurysmal disease have been subjected to reinterpretation. Although it is true that hypertension and smoking are risk factors for atherosclerosis and that atheroma lesions are common in infrarenal aortic aneurysms, a large minority of patients with disease did not give a clinical history of the accepted risk factors for atherosclerosis. Furthermore, in postmortem studies of several patients with infrarenal aortic aneurysms, atheroma were either absent or soft in quality relating to the subacute rather than chronic nature of the lesion. In light of recent research into hereditary aneurysm disease of the abdominal aorta, it has been proposed that patients with risk factors for atherosclerotic disease (e.g., cigarette smoking, diabetes mellitus, hypertension) in combination with genetic susceptibility are at highest risk for aortic aneurysm development. What has been known for some time is the absence of vasa vasorum in the infrarenal aorta compared to the suprarenal aorta which may enhance progression of media layer atrophy during arterial dilation. Other, less common causes of aneurysmal transformation of the aorta are syphilis, mycotic infection, and Marfan's syndrome.

Diagnosis

The vast majority of patients with aortic aneurysms are asymptomatic. Clinical appreciation of peripheral vascular disease should raise suspicion for aneurysmal disease, especially in the elderly patient. Peripheral artery aneurysms, particularly in the popliteal region, frequently coexist with abdominal aortic aneurysms, and should one be found, diagnostic evaluation of the abdominal aorta should be pursued. Family history of abdominal aortic aneurysms should raise suspicion of disease. Symptoms of aortic aneurysms are vague and nonspecific but usually center around abdominal pain or back pain. Rarely, massive gastrointestinal hemorrhage is the clinical pre-

---

TABLE 3. *Etiologies of acute arterial occlusion*

Emboli
    Atrial fibrillation
    Rheumatic heart disease or other valvular source
    Central or peripheral vascular aneurysm with mural
        thrombus
In situ thrombosis
    Superimposed upon native vessel stenosis
    Graft thrombosis
    "Low-flow" states, e.g., severe congestive heart failure,
        acute myocardial infarction
Other
    Vascular inflammatory disease
    Severe venous disease (phlegmasia cerulea dolens)
    Hypercoagulable states
    Intravenous drug abuse

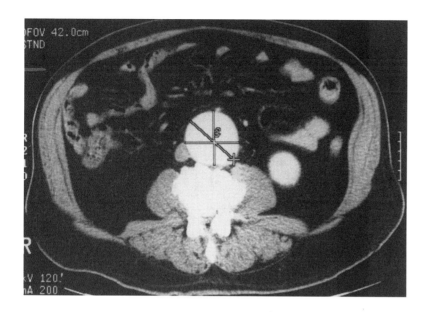

FIG. 12. Axial-spiral computed tomography of the abdomen demonstrating an abdominal aortic aneurysm. Note that the contrast administered opacifies the entire lumen of the aneurysm, which lacks mural clot.

sentation of an aortoenteric fistula secondary to aneurysmal disease.

Ultrasonography offers noninvasive detection of aneurysms of the abdominal aorta with high sensitivity and specificity. Accurate determination of size is consistent, although adequate determination of proximal and distal extent of the aneurysm is difficult. CT scanning is a very sensitive and specific imaging tool that provides not only accurate size determination but also information regarding proximal and distal extent of disease (Fig. 12). It is, however, significantly more expensive than ultrasound and exposes the patient to radiation. Aortography, previously performed routinely in all patients with aneurysmal disease, is being utilized selectively now by contemporary vascular surgeons. By virtue of the fact that mural clot develops about the circumference of the aneurysm from decreased blood flow velocity in that region, angiographic contrast administered directly within the arterial system opacifies only the true lumen that is either narrowed or normal in appearance. Angiography is not considered helpful in evaluating aortic aneurysmal disease but in select patients with a clinical history of splanchnic artery or renal artery stenosis or in patients with evidence of lower extremity occlusive disease, angiography may provide information to guide clinical management. Axial-spiral CT, in addition to demonstrating anatomic details, may provide equivalent evaluation of mesenteric arterial branches compared with aortography.

Treatment

The clinical management of abdominal aortic aneurysms has evolved from previous reports of untreated aneurysms. A report from the Mayo Clinic in 1950 showed that, among patients who died with known aortic aneurysms, well over half were a result of aneurysm rupture. Subsequent to that report, studies of patients with symptomatic aneurysms reported 75% mortality within 6 months and 80% mortality within 1 year of symptom onset. Although in retrospect, the high prevalence of large and symptomatic aneurysms probably resulted in clinical bias of data, it was nonetheless important in revealing the risk of aneurysm rupture. Numerous studies have followed reporting on either patients with abdominal aortic aneurysms examined at autopsy or patients followed with known aneurysms but considered unfit for surgery. From these analyses, the risk of rupture has been stratified based on size of the aneurysm. For aneurysms of >7.0 cm in maximum diameter, the risk of rupture over a 5-year period exceeds 75%, whereas for aneurysms between 5.0 and 5.9 cm in diameter, rupture rate is ~25% over the same time period. Recent literature suggests the risk of rupture for aneurysms 4.0 to 5.5 cm in diameter approaches 4% per year, which extrapolates to 20% rupture rate over 5 years.

Surgical repair of abdominal aortic aneurysms should be performed when relative patient benefit (prevent risk of rupture) far outweighs patient operative risk. When performed by experienced surgeons, mortality rates in all comers is <5%. Surgical repair of asymptomatic aneurysms of >5 cm in diameter is considered standard of care for eligible patients. Certainly symptomatic aneurysms, including those of <5 cm in diameter, should be repaired. Because asymptomatic aneurysms between 4.0 to 5.0 cm rupture, albeit infrequently, repair can be justified provided patient age, physiologic reserve, and coexisting medical disease that additively contribute to operative risk is considered on a case by case basis. Occasionally, operations related to systemic vascular disease (e.g., carotid endarterectomy, coronary artery bypass) are performed before elective aneurysm repair to prevent potential perioperative complications.

The first resection and repair of an abdominal aortic aneurysm was performed by Dubost in 1951. Since then, tremendous surgical advancements have been made with a dramatic decrease in morbidity and mortality. Aneurysm excision and replacement with a prosthetic graft, aneurysmorrhaphy, can be done via the transabdominal or retroperitoneal approach (Fig. 13). By far, the majority of early perioperative complications are cardiac in nature including myocardial infarction, arrhythmia, and congestive heart failure. Other early morbidity include respiratory insufficiency, stroke, renal insufficiency, gastrointestinal complications, and distal arterial embolization. Because the inferior mesenteric artery is routinely ligated and blood supply to the colon is dependent on collateral

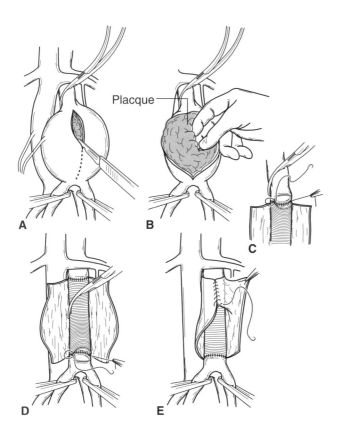

FIG. 13. Surgical technique for repair of infrarenal abdominal aortic aneurysm. **(A)** Following retroperitoneal exposure, the aneurysm is isolated between occluding cross-clamps and the sac is excised longintudinally. **(B)** Intraluminal thrombus is evacuated by backbleeding lumbar vessels are oversewn. **(C)** The proximal anastomosis is formed by continuously suturing the graft end-to-end to the neck of the aneurysm. **(D)** The distal anastomosis is completed at the aortic bifurcation, also using monofilament suture. **(E)** After flow is restored, the wall of the aneurysm is reapproximated over the graft to protect adjacent viscera. (Adapted from Braunwald E, ed. *Atlas of heart diseases. Vol. VII. Vascular disease.* St. Louis: Mosby–Year Book, 1996.)

blood flow, colonic ischemia must be considered in the postoperative period in the presence of bloody diarrhea or intraabdominal sepsis. Late complications include graft infection, aortoenteric fistula, anastomotic aneurysms, and graft occlusion.

Special Concerns

A patient with known abdominal aortic aneurysm who presents with (a) back pain, (b) hypotension, and (c) a pulsatile abdominal mass is exhibiting symptoms of aneurysm rupture until proven otherwise. This clinical scenario constitutes a surgical emergency and requires emergent operative intervention. Treatment of infectious aortitis complicated by rupture usually requires complete aneurysmectomy and extra-anatomic bypass (axillobifemoral) for definitive therapy. Infrequently, in situ interposition grafting is performed necessitating chronic antibiotic administration.

Patients with thoracoabdominal aneurysms (Fig. 14), if not repaired, have a 2-year survival of 24%. Successful repair of the thoracoabdominal aneurysms requires experienced surgical and anesthesiology teams. Important aspects of intraoperative management include control of blood pressure and myocardial function during thoracic or supraceliac cross-clamping. Unfortunately, paraplegia is a disastrous complication of aneurysmorrhaphy occurring in ~16% of thoracoabdominal aneurysm repairs (compared with <1% of infrarenal aortic repairs). Blood supply to the spinal cord is provided via the anterior spinal artery, the artery of Adamkowicz, arising between T_8 and L_1. Infrequently, however, the anterior spinal artery is discontinuous making the distal spinal cord dependent on the internal iliac arteries for its blood supply. Disruption or temporary occlusion of this collateral blood supply results in spinal cord ischemia and paraplegia. Methods that have been suggested to reduce the incidence of paraplegia include selective reimplantation of the intercostal arteries, partial cardiopulmonary bypass, and cerebrospinal fluid pressure monitoring and decompression.

Peripheral Arterial Aneurysms

Ninety percent of peripheral artery aneurysms involve the popliteal and femoral arteries. Popliteal artery aneurysms are the most common and are true aneurysms. In contrast, false aneurysms (pseudoaneurysms) are common in the femoral artery region as a result of incomplete hemostasis following percutaneous arterial access. True aneurysms are infrequently found in the femoral artery area. Peripheral artery aneurysms are complicated by distal embolization or thrombosis. Pseudoaneurysms commonly produce pain from local compression of nerves but may also rupture or become infected.

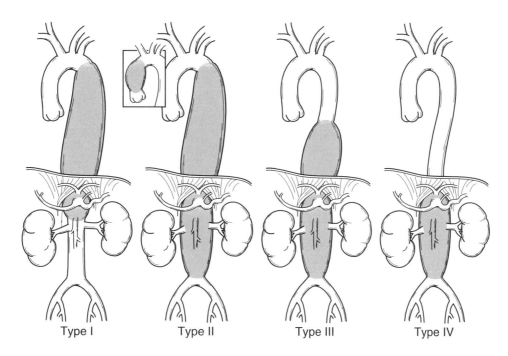

FIG. 14. DeBakey's classification of thoracoabdominal aortic aneurysms. (Adapted from Braunwald E, ed. *Atlas of heart diseases. Vol. VII. Vascular disease.* St. Louis: Mosby–Year Book, 1996.)

Type I   Type II   Type III   Type IV

Popliteal artery aneurysms are frequently associated with aneurysms other arterial and occur almost exclusively in men. The incidence of bilateral popliteal artery aneurysms is ~50%. Of greatest importance, however, is the fact that abdominal aortic aneurysms are found associated with popliteal artery aneurysms in 25% of cases. Coexisting femoral and iliac artery aneurysms are found less frequently. A prominent or widened popliteal pulse is suggestive of aneurysmal transformation. The most common symptoms include distal embolization, thrombosis, and venous compression producing leg edema. Suspicion mandates evaluation with ultrasound of the popliteal fossa and if aneurysm disease is found, study of the contralateral popliteal fossa and abdominal aorta should be performed. Recommended therapy is repair of all popliteal artery aneurysms, symptomatic and asymptomatic, using autogenous vein conduit.

The most common etiology of femoral artery aneurysms is atherosclerosis. Pseudoaneurysms of the femoral artery are infrequently the complication of percutaneous transluminal angioplasty for peripheral or coronary artery disease. The incidence of disease appears to be increasing because of the increased utilization of this procedure. Ultrasound guided compression of pseudoaneurysm is used to induce thrombosis of the false cavity while preserving the patency of the true lumen. If this procedure is unsuccessful, surgical closure of the defect in the arterial wall is performed. Approximately 50% of true femoral artery aneurysms are associated with abdominal aortic aneurysms and occur almost exclusively in men. Half are associated with popliteal aneurysms and about half are bilateral in location. Pain from local compression of the femoral nerve is the most common symptom of femoral artery aneurysms. Limb-threatening thrombosis or embolization often occurs after the onset of symptoms. Therefore, symptomatic aneurysms of the femoral artery are best treated by urgent repair. In contrast, asymptomatic femoral artery aneurysms, unlike their popliteal artery counterpart, rarely cause symptoms and are observed after diagnosis.

VASCULAR DISEASE OF THE VISCERAL ARTERIAL SYSTEM

Occlusive Disease

Renovascular Hypertension

In 1934, Goldblatt's landmark experiment showed that renal artery constriction produced renal atrophy and hypertension in dogs. By far, the most common causes of renal artery stenosis are atherosclerosis and fibromuscular hyperplasia. Figure 15 depicts the pathophysiology of renal artery stenosis in which decreased renal blood flow leads to renin release and ultimately significantly increased levels of angiotensin II. Angiotensin II, beyond being a potent vasoconstrictor, stimulates the production

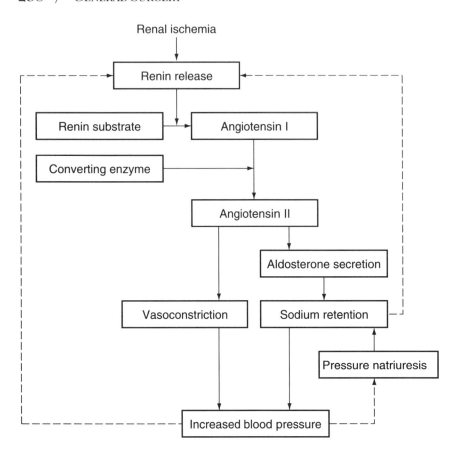

Renal ischemia

Renin release

Renin substrate → Angiotensin I

Converting enzyme →

Angiotensin II

Aldosterone secretion

Vasoconstriction   Sodium retention

Pressure natriuresis

Increased blood pressure

FIG. 15. The effect of renal ischemia on the renin-angiotensin-aldosterone system in renovascular hypertension. (Adapted from Braunwald E, ed. *Atlas of heart diseases. Vol. VII. Vascular disease.* St. Louis: Mosby–Year Book, 1996.)

of aldosterone by the adrenal glands. Thus, intravascular hypervolemia because of secondary hyperaldosteronemia and vasoconstriction as a result of increased angiotensin II levels elevate systemic blood pressure in renovascular hypertension.

Although 95% of hypertension is idiopathic or essential, 5% is secondary and potentially curable. Renovascular hypertension is thought to affect 5% to 10% of the hypertensive population and represents the most common form of secondary hypertension. Infrequently, a bruit auscultated on abdominal examination is suggestive of renal artery disease. Patients with suspected renal artery stenosis should undergo duplex study to determine flow velocity across the renal artery. Selective renal vein sampling for renin may supplement ultrasound localization of disease. Renal arteriography remains the gold standard diagnostic test for renal artery stenosis, although no cause-effect relationship with clinical hypertension can be inferred solely with this finding.

The advances in interventional radiology have been applied to renal artery occlusive disease also. In select cases (e.g., nonostial short-segment lesions limited to the main renal artery), results compare equally to operative techniques. However, for all other cases especially ostial stenosis or distal renal artery involvement, aortorenal bypass remains the standard therapy.

Mesenteric Ischemia

Chronic mesenteric ischemia commonly affects individuals between the fifth and seventh decade of life. Females with disease outnumber males. The vast majority of cases are caused by ostial narrowing secondary to atherosclerosis. Other causes include but are not limited to radiation injury, systemic lupus erythematosus, and cocaine abuse. The clinical presentation of chronic mesenteric ischemia results from oxygen demand that exceeds oxygen supply and is analogous to claudication. Specifically, visceral discomfort follows inadequate postprandial hyperemic intestinal arterial flow. Symptoms are not usually present until at least two out of three splanchnic arteries are highly stenosed or occluded (Fig. 16). Occasionally, isolated superior mesenteric artery occlusion results in intestinal ischemia. In contrast, isolated occlusion of the celiac or inferior mesenteric artery is well tolerated.

Pain described as colicky or vague discomfort located predominantly in the midabdominal region and occasionally radiating to the back is the typical symptom. Patients frequently have had several evaluations for abdominal disease. Pain usually begins 15 to 30 minutes after eating and can last for up to 3 hrs. Although early in the course of disease food is consumed without pain, with progres-

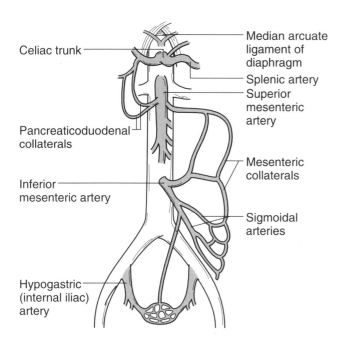

FIG. 16. Diagrammatic representation of the mesenteric arterial anatomy showing the rich collateral network, interconnecting celiac, superior mesenteric, inferior mesenteric, and internal iliac vascular beds. (Adapted from Braunwald E, ed. *Atlas of heart diseases. Vol. VII. Vascular disease.* St. Louis: Mosby–Year Book, 1996.)

sion of disease patients associate eating with abdominal pain. This food fear may result in tremendous weight loss, which is occasionally mistaken for incurable malignancy.

Mesenteric arteriography remains the gold standard diagnostic test but is not without risks. Noninvasive Doppler ultrasound provides high sensitivity and specificity for disease, but testing accuracy is limited by many patient-related factors. Aortomesenteric bypass is performed in patients with disabling symptoms.

Acute intestinal ischemia is characterized as the acute reduction in intestinal blood flow of sufficient magnitude to potentially result in infarction. The abrupt occlusion occurs in a proximal portion of a major splanchnic arterial trunk (usually the superior mesenteric artery) and is the result of either thromboembolism or thrombotic occlusion superimposed on untreated chronic mesenteric arterial occlusive disease. The majority of cases are in females in the seventh and eighth decade of life. Typical clinical history is sudden onset and unrelenting abdominal pain without evidence of peritoneal irritation on physical examination—pain out of proportion to physical findings.

Mesenteric ischemia is a diagnosis made with difficulty. Laboratory studies are generally not helpful in confirming or excluding disease. Duplex ultrasound is extremely limited in the setting of acute disease. The use of angiography in the presence of acute ischemia is controversial. Advocates claim that early diagnosis improves patient outcome,

and confirmation of a nonocclusive etiology (e.g., low-flow state) may obviate the need for operation. Opponents argue that the procedure unnecessarily delays potential life-saving operation in patients with overwhelming evidence of acute intestinal ischemia. For thrombosis of mesenteric arterial occlusive disease, aortomesenteric bypass is performed. In cases of thromboembolic phenomenon, embolectomy to reestablish arterial inflow to the gut is attempted. If unsuccessful, aortomesenteric bypass is performed. Prior to the development of intestinal necrosis, mortality rates approach 10%. In contrast, after bowel infarction has set in, mortality exceeds 70% in most large series.

Splanchnic Arterial Aneurysmal Disease

Although splanchnic artery aneurysms are uncommon, up to one-fourth of cases unfortunately present as surgical emergencies with a large minority resulting in death. In general, morbidity and mortality is associated with rupture, either into peritoneal cavity or into the intestines. In contrast to abdominal and lower extremity aneurysms, females outnumber males by a ratio 4:1. Loss of elastin fibers and decreased smooth muscle concentration is proposed as the mechanism of medial degeneration. The overwhelming majority of splanchnic artery aneurysms are located in the splenic artery followed by, in decreasing order of frequency, hepatic, superior mesenteric, and celiac arteries. With exception for splenic artery aneurysms, aneurysm repair with interposition bypass is generally required if collateral blood supply is insufficient.

Splenic artery aneurysms are associated with portal hypertension and chronic pancreatitis. There is also a strong association with multiparity. The majority of lesions are asymptomatic. Occasionally, vague left upper abdominal pain or epigastric discomfort that radiates to the back are frequent symptoms. Free rupture into the peritoneal cavity and rupture into intestinal tract occur with equal frequency. Acute rupture is the leading cause of death from splenic artery aneurysms. Should diagnosis be made, urgent ligation and exclusion of the aneurysm is definitive therapy. No arterial bypass is required.

ARTERIAL DISEASE OF THE CERVICOTHORACIC GREAT VESSELS AND UPPER EXTREMITIES

Carotid Artery Stenosis

Cerebrovascular accident (CVA), or as it is commonly termed, "stroke," is the third leading cause of death and the second leading cause of cardiovascular death in the United States. The incidence of stroke in the general population is ~200 per 100,000 (0.2%), although in the elderly stroke rates are about seven times higher (1.4%). Beyond the crippling disability to patients sustaining major strokes is the socioeconomic burden to patient, family, and society. The cost of health care provided to patients who have suffered a stroke exceeds $16 billion per year.

Atheromatous plaque at the carotid bifurcation causing stenosis or ulcerations within the internal carotid arteries is the principal etiology behind cerebrovascular ischemic disease. Less than 10% of cases combined are due to fibromuscular dysplasia, arterial kinking, traumatic occlusion, and arterial dissection. Atherosclerotic disease of the carotid artery can cause transient ischemic attacks (TIAs) and stroke as a result of thrombosis, low-flow states, and thromboembolism from the plaque (most common). TIAs are neurologic deficits caused by insufficient hemispheric cerebral blood flow including contralateral weakness, ipsilateral cranial nerve deficit, or monocular blindness (amaurosis fugax). Patients describe the latter classically as a curtain drawn over visual field. TIAs in the left hemisphere may present with speech impairment. Neurologic deficits, however, resolve within 24 hr. Reversible ischemic neurologic deficits (RIND) have similar presentation but last up to 72 hr.

Stroke represents irreversible neurologic deficits from cerebral ischemia. Contralateral upper and lower extremity weakness or paralysis, decreased intellectual function and difficulty speaking are crippling complications of CVA. Unfortunately, the majority of patients sustaining CVA do not have antecedent transient ischemic symptoms. Furthermore, it appears that in excess of 25% of patients with resolved transient ischemic symptoms will have suffered occult cerebral infarction demonstrated by CT scan.

Based on the randomized prospective North American Symptomatic Carotid Endarterectomy Trial (NASCET) comparing medical and surgical treatment, carotid endarterectomy offers the best definitive therapy for prevention of stroke secondary to symptomatic high grade (70% to 99%) atherosclerotic stenosis of the extracranial internal carotid artery. Treated patients with symptomatic carotid artery stenosis (i.e., TIA, nondisabling stroke) had a 17% decrease in the absolute risk of stroke. Another randomized prospective trial compared medical and surgical therapy for asymptomatic carotid artery stenosis (ACAS). The study demonstrated the incidence of stroke in untreated patients was 3% to 5% per year, the majority without warning symptoms, and that endarterectomy performed for severe stenosis (>75% diameter narrowing) was of significant clinical benefit without increased morbidity. The risk of stroke in patients treated medically was 10.6% compared to 4.8% of patients treated surgically. In general, patients with risk factors for vascular disease and with neurologic symptoms should undergo carotid duplex screening to look for critical carotid artery stenosis. Contemporary vascular surgeons now agree that, provided surgical complications rates are low, carotid endarterec-

tomy is indicated for all critical carotid stenosis with exception for patients with shortened life expectancy secondary to systemic disease and patients recently sustaining major ischemic stroke.

Ultrasound and duplex study of the carotid artery accurately demonstrates plaque characteristics (e.g., ulceration) and increased flow velocity consistent with critical stenosis. The gold standard continues to be arteriography. As the accuracy of ultrasound and duplex have continued to improve in the examination of the extracranial carotid circulation, controversy has arisen about the use of routine diagnostic arteriography. Today, many surgeons obtain preoperative aortic arch and great vessel arteriography, although some vascular surgeons with dedicated and experienced vascular laboratory technicians comfortably embark on endarterectomy based solely on data obtained from duplex and ultrasound with excellent results and decreased health care costs.

Perioperative complications include stroke (<1%) caused by cerebral hypoperfusion or by plaque embolization. Cranial nerve injury may occur from extended proximal dissection, although the injury is usually transient and self-limiting. Late complications are limited to carotid artery restenosis, which can occur in up to 15% of patients on routine postoperative carotid duplex study. Fortunately, only ~1% of patients will experience symptoms of cerebral ischemia requiring reoperation. Restenosis is more frequently seen in women and patients who continue to smoke after the operation.

Aneurysms of the extracranial carotid artery, in contrast to intracerebral artery aneurysms are rare. These lesions are most frequently found in the common carotid followed by internal and external carotid artery. The natural history of carotid aneurysmal disease is unknown because of the small number of reported cases, however, review of autopsy data suggests unfavorable outcomes from untreated disease. Stroke rates exceeding 50% in untreated cases have been reported. Therefore, diagnosis usually mandates surgical repair in eligible patients.

Takayasu's arteritis is an arteriopathy of unknown etiology affecting the aorta and its major branches. Although once thought to occur only in Asians, women typically in the second to third decade of life of all races and nationalities have been diagnosed with the disease. Accurate diagnosis is difficult partly due to the nonspecific clinical symptoms early in the course of disease, i.e., fever, myalgia, headache. Heavy inflammatory cell concentration in the arterial wall and giant cells in the media layer have implicated an autoimmune etiology. Because of occlusive disease of the thoracic great vessels and aortic arch, cerebral ischemia is the most important late clinical presentation. Renovascular hypertension (also known as middle aortic syndrome) from renal artery stenosis is an infrequent complication. Medical management with corticosteroids is controversial. Surgical revascularization is required for many patients with symptoms.

Temporal arteritis is similar to Takayasu's arteritis regarding clinical presentation early in the course of disease, i.e., flu-like symptoms. However, jaw claudication and a tender, erythematous temporal artery region are distinguishing features. Ocular complications (e.g., amaurosis fugax, monocular blindness or bilateral blindness) are the dreaded manifestations of disease and occur in up to 60% of patients. Diagnosis is made by temporal artery biopsy. Steroids are the treatment of choice especially in the presence of ocular symptoms.

Vertebrobasilar Disease and Subclavian Steal

Cerebellar ischemia from vertebrobasilar arterial insufficiency is due to critical stenosis of the vertebral artery at the origin of the subclavian artery or thromboembolic phenomenon. Symptoms include bilateral circumoral sensory deficits, peripheral motor weakness or ataxia, postural disturbances, vertigo, diplopia, and drop attacks. Endarterectomy and bypass have been used in the treatment of vertebrobasilar disease.

The subclavian steal syndrome occurs as a result of ostial occlusive disease of the subclavian or innominate artery from the takeoff of the aorta. With occlusive disease proximal to the origin of the vertebral artery, retrograde flow through the vertebrobasilar circulation provides blood flow to the upper extremity circulation via the subclavian artery. This stealing of circulatory flow is marked during increased demand for blood flow in the upper extremity, as during exercise. Upper extremity effort claudication, dizziness, syncope, or nausea are common symptoms. Therapy for symptomatic subclavian steal syndrome involves a subclavian artery revascularization via carotid-subclavian bypass, axilloaxillary bypass, or aortosubclavian bypass.

Thoracic Outlet Syndrome

Thoracic outlet syndrome is a constellation of neurologic and vascular symptoms caused by compression of the brachial plexus or the subclavian vessels by bony or soft tissue abnormalities. Neurogenic thoracic outlet syndrome is the most common form (95%) and results from soft tissue or bony compression of the trunks or roots of the brachial plexus. Characteristic symptoms are pain, as well as paresthesia and weakness. The arterial and venous forms of the syndrome are uncommon. The arterial variety is the result of compression of the subclavian artery at the thoracic outlet with poststenotic dilatation and is detected clinically by the presence of a palpable supraclavicular pulsatile mass. Aneurysm formation, distal extremity thromboembolism, and subclavian artery occlusion are clinical complications. The venous form of the syndrome results from axillary vein thrombosis most

often after upper extremity exercise, also known as effort thrombosis.

Neurogenic thoracic outlet syndrome responds favorably to exercise, physical therapy, analgesics, and muscle relaxants. Surgical therapy in the form of scalenectomy, scalenotomy, or first rib resection may be necessary to relieve irritation of the brachial plexus in refractory cases. The arterial form of the disease is invariably associated with a cervical rib and requires surgical therapy. Resection of the first rib and cervical rib (if present) and subclavian artery bypass with resection of aneurysm or poststenotic arterial dilation is standard therapy. Venous effort thrombosis occurs typically in young otherwise healthy individuals. Arm heaviness and extremity discomfort exacerbated by activity and relieved by rest are the usual symptoms. A multidisciplinary approach utilizing thrombolysis, long-term anticoagulation, and surgical decompression of the thoracic outlet appears to offer the best patient outcome.

VENOUS DISEASE

Venous disease of the lower extremity has plagued the human race for centuries. Superficial varicose veins are in the least unsightly and at most painful and the cause of cutaneous ulcers and venous inflammatory reactions, phlebitis. Deep venous thrombosis (DVT) is a source of morbidity from pulmonary embolus and required long-term anticoagulation therapy.

The superficial venous system, greater and lesser saphenous veins, the deep venous system, common iliac, superficial and deep femoral veins, and the perforating veins comprise the venous system of the lower extremity. Unlike the arterial system, dynamic venous pressure is low, ~15 to 20 mm Hg. Hydrostatic venous pressure, defined as pressure within the venous channels in a standing position, often greatly exceeds the dynamic pressure. Tremendous venous capacitance allows ~250 cc of circulating blood to accumulate in each leg in the standing position. Muscle pump action of the lower extremity assures adequate venous return to the heart and protects against orthostatic blood pressure changes on standing. Perhaps the most important anatomic feature of the venous system is the presence of valves. Delicate bicuspid structures facilitate forward flow of venous blood en route to the heart. Perforating veins (communicating veins) bridge the superficial and deep system at several locations in the lower extremity. Normally, valves within these communicating veins remain competent and separate the superficial from the deep systems.

Ambulatory venous hypertension initiates progressive valvular incompetence of the iliofemoral deep venous system allowing increased hydrostatic pressure to be transmitted to valves in the lower venous system which then become incompetent and so on. When communicat-

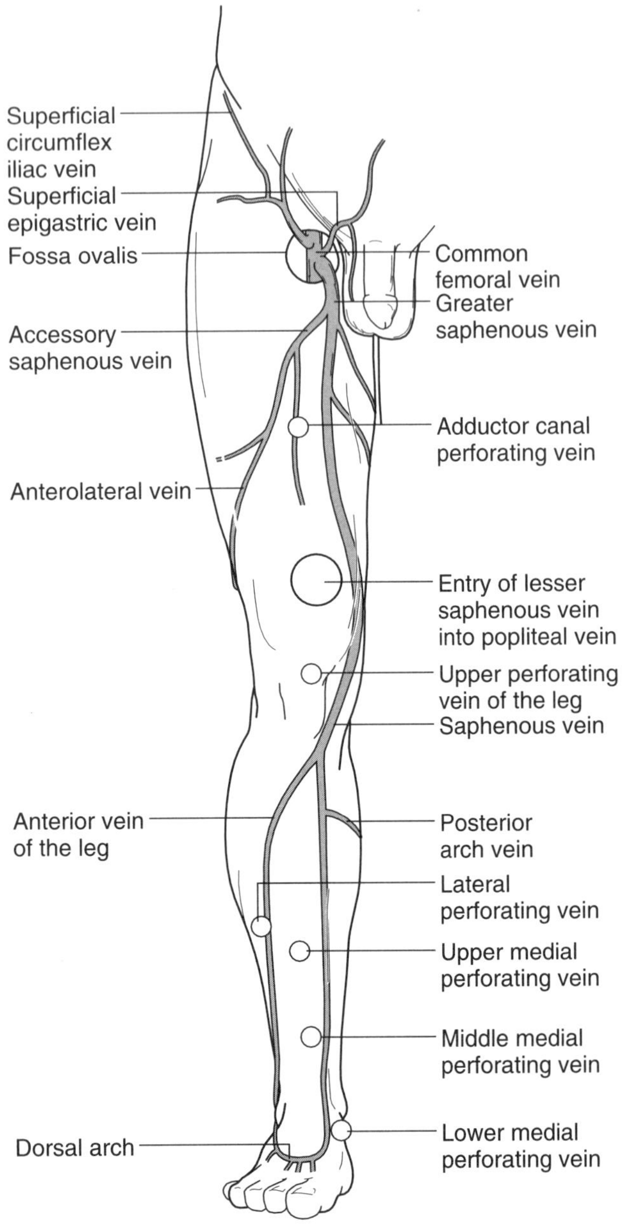
Superficial circumflex iliac vein
Superficial epigastric vein
Fossa ovalis
Accessory saphenous vein
Anterolateral vein
Anterior vein of the leg
Dorsal arch
Common femoral vein
Greater saphenous vein
Adductor canal perforating vein
Entry of lesser saphenous vein into popliteal vein
Upper perforating vein of the leg
Saphenous vein
Posterior arch vein
Lateral perforating vein
Upper medial perforating vein
Middle medial perforating vein
Lower medial perforating vein

FIG. 17. The superficial venous drainage system of the lower extremity.

ing veins become incompetent, venous reflux occurs from the deep to the superficial system (Figs. 17 and 18). Varicose veins are distended superficial veins with poor blood flow. Thrombophlebitis is common and presents as pain, tenderness, and erythema about a thrombosed varix. Symptoms arise from a local inflammatory reaction and a common misconception among clinicians is that this process is infectious in nature. Intravenous antibiotics are unnecessary in sterile thrombophlebitis. In contrast, suppurative thrombophlebitis, caused by infection of chronic indwelling venous catheters, requires vein excision inclusive of all affected vein. Although an extraordinarily high mortality accompanies untreated disease, fortunately, it is an infrequent complication among hospitalized patients.

The vast majority (95%) of venous thrombosis occurs in the deep venous system of the lower extremity. DVT develops due to venous stasis, systemic hypercoagulability, or venous endothelial injury—Virchow's triad. Venous stasis is particularly common in surgical patients during procedures under general anesthesia. Hypercoagulability is prevalent in patients with cancer.

Calf swelling, tenderness, and calf pain on dorsiflexion of the foot, Homans' sign, are some symptoms suggestive of DVT. Phlegmasia alba dolens, phlegmasia cerulea dolens, and venous gangrene represent different phases along a spectrum of massive DVT and fortunately are rare occurrences (Fig. 19). Unfortunately, physical examination is notoriously unreliable as evidenced by numerous reports in which a significant majority of patients with DVT (some found at autopsy) were without clinical signs of venous thrombosis. Venous plethysmography indirectly detects venous obstruction by measuring the filling and emptying of leg veins after inflation of a thigh pressure cuff but cannot exclude the presence of a venous thrombus. Currently, detection of DVT is more reliable (95%) with the use of duplex venous ultrasound. Noncompressible veins, venous distention, a lack of flow, or direct visualization of clot are demonstrated by duplex in patients with DVT. Recent advances in ultrasound technology have decreased the reliance upon indirect tests and venography. Although still considered the gold standard study for detection of DVT, venography is an expensive, invasive test not without risk from use of intravenous dye or percutaneous access of the venous system.

In 1986, the NIH consensus reported that 50,000 deaths and 300,000 hospitalizations in the United States were due to DVT. Sadly, inadequate prophylaxis and wide variations in prophylaxis methods contribute to its prevalence in hospitalized patients. Prevention is the best form of therapy against DVT. Ambulation, particularly after a surgical procedure if possible, and intermittent pneumatic venous compression devices, *or* subcutaneous low-dose heparin are the cornerstones of preventative therapy. Once a DVT has been diagnosed, prevention of thrombus progression by anticoagulation with continuous intravenous heparin to elevate the partial thromboplastin time to two times normal is standard. Breakdown of the clot is achieved by the patient's endogenous fibrinolytic system. Long-term anticoagulation is achieved with oral warfarin compounds to maintain the prothrombin time at 1.5 to 2.0 times normal. Contraindications to anticoagulation include recent stroke, intracerebral arteriovenous malformation, recent surgery, and hematologic disorders.

Pulmonary embolism (PE) is a common and frequently fatal problem, with an incidence of 630,000 cases per year and a mortality rate of 30%. Virchow first promoted the idea that PE is embolic in origin. The majority of PE originate from the proximal deep veins in the pelvis and

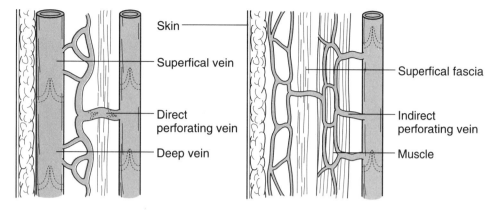

FIG. 18. Incompetent valves between the superficial and deep venous systems.

thigh. Three variations in clinical presentation of PE are recognized. Rapid onset dyspnea, cyanosis, right heart failure, and systemic hypotension is the result of a massive pulmonary embolus causing pulmonary artery obstruction. Pulmonary infarction usually occurs in the presence of recent PE that was not diagnostically pursued and presents clinically with pleuritic pain, dyspnea, and hemoptysis. Symptoms of acute pulmonary embolus include sudden dyspnea, vague complaints of malaise, mild tachycardia, and tachypnea.

PE can occur in any patient predisposed to DVT formation, not just surgical patients. Of 200,000 patients who died from a PE, 10% died within 1 hr, and among patients diagnosed incorrectly (70%), 30% died. Conversely, of patients correctly diagnosed, the mortality rate was 8%. Accurate diagnosis and prompt treatment is predicated upon a high index of suspicion (Fig. 20). Clinical suspicion of PE mandates obtaining a chest radi-

ograph, electrocardiogram, and arterial blood gas. Typical chest radiographs of patients sustaining PE demonstrate decreased vascular markings in the affected lung (Westermark sign). Electrocardiogram may show right heart dilatation. Venous thrombus in lower extremity or pelvic veins by duplex in the face of acute respiratory symptoms implies PE. Pulmonary angiography remains the definitive diagnostic test.

Treatment of PE begins with prevention of further emboli by systemic heparinization. With persistent elevation of right heart pressures, fibrinolytic therapy has been shown to be successful in improving pulmonary blood flow by angiogram, although a significant survival benefit has not been shown. Patients with persistent hemodynamic instability and hypoxemia should be taken to the operating room without delay for pulmonary artery embolectomy. Survival is best in patients who have not suffered preoperative cardiac arrest. In all cases com-

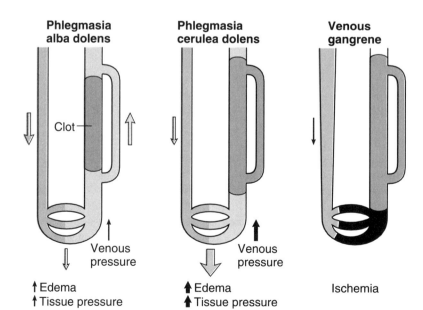

FIG. 19. Pathophysiology of increasing severity of venous obstruction. (Adapted from Rutherford RB, ed. *Vascular surgery.* 4th ed. Philadelphia: Saunders, 1995.)

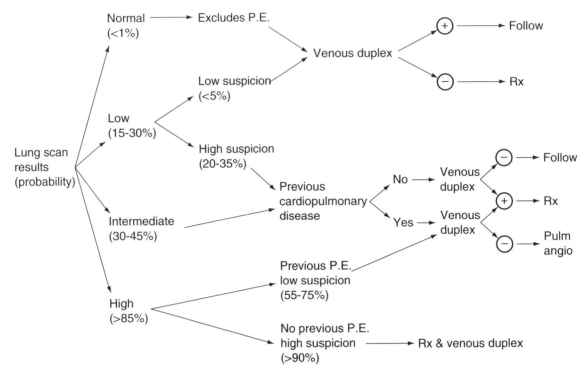

FIG. 20. Diagnostic algorithm for pulmonary embolism (PE) based on lung scanning results. Numbers in parentheses indicate the likelihood of PE. (From Comerota AJ, Rao AK. Pulmonary thromboembolism. In: Cameron JL, ed. *Current surgical therapy.* 4th ed. Philadelphia: BC Decker, 1992.)

bined, however, pulmonary artery embolectomy is accompanied by an 80% mortality.

LYMPHATIC VESSEL DISEASE

The lymphatic system transports protein rich interstitial fluid and immune cells to the central venous circulation in the cervicothoracic veins. Lymph vessel obstruction results in lymphedema which leads to cosmetic deformity, chronic physical disability, and may be complicated by bacterial infection, immunodeficiency and occasionally malignancy. Primary lymphedema is rare, typically occurring in females with an incidence of less than one per 100,000 population. Primary lymphedema is classified as congenital, praecox, and familial. Secondary lymphedema is caused by well-defined disease processes that obstruct the lymph vessel system. Worldwide, filariasis infestation is the most common etiology. In North America and Europe, surgical ligation or irradiation of lymph vessels (e.g., after modified radical mastectomy) is the most common cause. Lymphedema may be the first presentation of malignancy. Lymphangitis, commonly caused by β-hemolytic Streptococcus, can cause lymphedema as well. Diagnosis is made by lymphoscintigraphy, CT scan, and

magnetic resonance imaging (MRI). Conservative, nonoperative management is the mainstay of treatment. Specifically, regular use of high-compression elastic stockings and intermittent pneumatic compression pump devices offer long-term control of lymphedema. Occasionally, in patients with refractory disease or extensive lymphedema with skin changes, affected skin and soft tissue can be resected followed by cosmetic reconstruction.

SUMMARY

Complete care of patients with acute and chronic vascular disease requires careful consideration of all disease processes and management implications. A thorough patient history and physical examination are requisite to diagnostic accuracy. Indications for operative intervention for arterial occlusive disease are simply categorized as life-style–disabling claudication and limb-threatening ischemia. Aneurysmal disease of the arterial system, with few exceptions, requires resection and repair. Venous and lymphatic diseases of the lower extremities are both physically disfiguring and the source of many complications. Treatment is essentially nonoperative, with surgical therapy reserved for refractory cases.

STUDY QUESTIONS

1. Describe the normal anatomy of the arterial wall. What are some proposed mechanisms of atherosclerosis?
2. Describe an adequate assessment of a patient with arterial vascular disease.
3. Name some etiologies of arterial aneurysmal disease.
4. What is Virchow's triad? Describe an adequate regiment of DVT prohylaxis.
5. How is PE embolism diagnosed and treated?

SUGGESTED READING

Braunwald E, ed. *Atlas of heart disease. Vol. VII. Vascular disease.* St. Louis: Mosby–Year Book, 1996.

Gewertz B, ed. Lower extremity arterial vascular disease. *Surg Clin North Am* 1995;75:545–805.

Pearce W, Yao J, eds. Noninvasive diagnosis of vascular disease. *Surg Clin North Am* 1990;70:1–249.

Rutherford RB, ed. *Vascular surgery.* 4th ed. Philadelphia: Saunders, 1995.

Surgical Specialties

CHAPTER 19

Thoracic Surgery

Patrick C. Mangonon and Richard J. Thurer

Chest surgery progressed slowly, until advances in anesthesia and knowledge of cardiopulmonary physiology allowed procedures to be performed safely. In 1869, Trendelenberg used a percutaneous "tracheal tube" to administer chloroform in a patient breathing spontaneously. Fell and O'Dwyer in the 1890s used bellows to insufflate the lungs via transoral endotracheal intubation. Later, pioneers Meltzer (1905), Eggers (1910), and Peck (1912) refined methods of administration of anesthesia, which allowed surgeons to perform difficult procedures on the lung and esophagus, though not without risk. Negative pressure operating rooms were popularized by Sauerbruch in the early 1900s as a method of preventing the postthoracotomy pneumothorax, a major concern of the time. Understanding of pleural physiology led to thoracostomy (chest) tube drainage, which obviated the need for these special operating rooms. With increasing confidence, thoracic surgeons began performing more complex procedures. In 1933, Evarts Graham performed the first successful one-stage pneumonectomy. Shortly thereafter, Churchill and Belsey described limited pulmonary resection as a less morbid alternative for surgically treated lung disease.

Thoracoscopy originated in 1910, when Jacobaeus placed a cystoscope into the pleural space to divide adhesions and collapse the lung as treatment for pulmonary tuberculosis. Although formal thoracotomy with resection became the definitive therapy of tuberculosis of that era, thoracoscopy remained useful for evaluating pleural effusions, obtaining tissue from pleural, or mediastinal masses, and draining empyema. The primitive light source in early equipment, however, restricted visualization and limited the applicability of thoracoscopy. Fiberoptic light and microcamera technology of today's modern thoracoscope (Fig. 1) has repopularized its use in the aforementioned procedures as well as in complex procedures, including limited pulmonary resection, pericardiotomy, and evaluation of thoracic injury.

The field of thoracic surgery has also attained its current status thanks to advances in specific equipment such as the fiberoptic bronchoscope. Computerized tomography (CT) scanning, magnetic resonance imaging (MRI), and quantitative nuclear lung scans have supplemented and, in some cases, replaced outdated diagnostic tests. Modern thoracoscopy and new stapling devices have made minimally invasive chest surgery a viable alternative in treating certain thoracic disease.

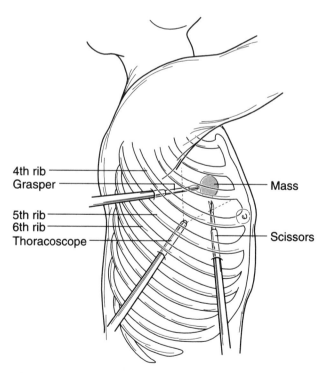

FIG. 1. Removal of anterior mediastinal mass. The thoracoscope is introduced through the sixth intercostal space in the posterior axillary line. Graspers and scissors positioned in the fourth intercostal space posteriorly and the fifth intercostal space anteriorly allow dissection of the mass from surrounding tissues.

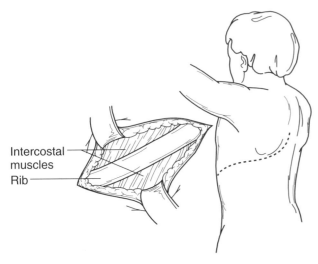

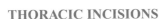

FIG. 2. Incision location and muscular anatomy encountered in a posterolateral thoracotomy.

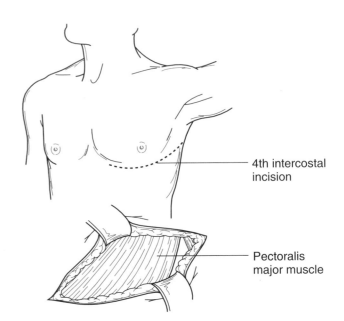

FIG. 3. Anterolateral thoracotomy.

THORACIC INCISIONS

Lateral thoracotomy, anterior thoracotomy, and median sternotomy are the principal incisions used in chest surgery. The posterolateral thoracotomy is performed with the patient in the lateral decubitus position (Fig. 2). A curvilinear incision is made beginning at the anterior axillary line at about the fourth rib and ending medial to the ipsilateral scapula. This approach offers generous exposure for most lung resections and operations in the hemithorax. With the patient supine, an anterior thoracotomy incision extends from the sternum at the fourth rib in an oblique direction, finishing in the posterior axillary line (Fig. 3). It provides excellent

emergent access to the thoracic cavity and pericardium. Median sternotomy is the standard approach for operations on the heart, great vessels, and superior mediastinum and is performed by splitting the sternum vertically with an electric saw.

Mediastinoscopy is performed through a small suprasternal incision and involves placing an endoscope in the pretracheal space within the superior mediastinum for visualization and biopsy of tissue, usually lymph nodes (Fig. 4). Anterior mediastinotomy is an alternative proce-

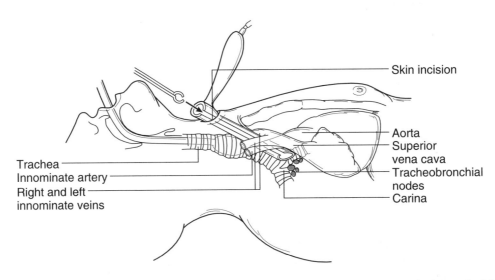

FIG. 4. Lateral view of mediastinoscopy performed through a small transverse cervical scan incision to view the superior mediastinum between the great vessels and trachea. Suspicious lymph nodes can be biopsied using this technique.

dure to access the mediastinum and is performed through a small transverse parasternal incision.

CHEST WALL AND PLEURA

Anatomy and Physiology

The chest wall is a musculoskeletal "cage" that gives the thorax a conical shape with a broad base and narrow apex. The sternum is comprised of the manubrium, body, and xiphoid process. The superior seven ribs, "true ribs," articulate independently with the sternum, whereas the five inferior ribs have either shared articulation with the sternum or, as in the case of the 11th and 12th ribs, are "floating." Muscles covering the chest include the pectoralis group anteriorly, the latissimus dorsi posteriorly, and the serratus group laterally. The diaphragm, innervated by the phrenic nerve, in combination with intercostal muscles function as the primary muscles of respiration. Scalene and "strap" muscles of the neck along with pectoralis and serratus groups comprise accessory muscles that may provide the increased respiratory effort required to overcome decreased pulmonary compliance in clinical disease states. The neurovascular bundle consisting of the intercostal nerve, artery, and vein course beneath the intercostal muscles along the inferior aspect of each rib.

Parietal pleura is the mesothelial lining on the inner surface of each hemithorax. It invaginates at the pulmonary hilum to become the visceral pleura and cover each lung. The parietal and visceral pleura enclose a "potential" space lubricated by serous fluid. Protein-free fluid travels from parietal to visceral pleura, driven primarily by a gradient between the high-pressure systemic capillaries and low-pressure pulmonary capillaries. Additionally, a higher net oncotic pressure at the visceral pleura combined with the extensive pulmonary lymphatic system augments the absorption of fluid from the pleural space to the pulmonary circulation (Fig. 5).

Pleural Space Disease

Pneumothorax/Hemothorax

"Pneumothorax" is defined as air within the pleural space, whereas blood in the pleural space is termed a "hemothorax." Hemothoraces are almost always caused by trauma and will be discussed elsewhere in this book. Spontaneous pneumothoraces occur secondary to rupture of pleural blebs ("air cysts") that typically occur in young athletic men and in patients with chronic obstructive pulmonary disease (COPD). Obviously, penetrating chest trauma can cause both a pneumothorax and hemothorax separately or in combination. In the setting of blunt chest trauma, pneumo- and hemothoraces can occur in the pres-

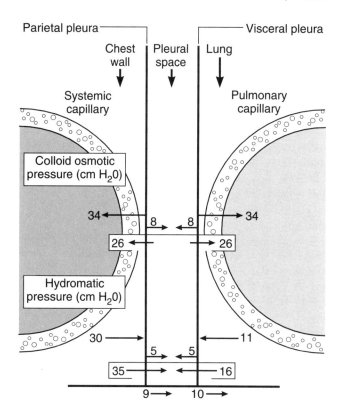

FIG. 5. Schematic representation of pleural fluid pressures. (Adapted from Fraser RG, Pare JAP. *Organ physiology: the structure and function of the lungs.* 2nd ed. Philadelphia: Saunders, 1977.)

ence or absence of rib fractures. Pain and respiratory distress are common but not always present. In pneumothorax, physical examination typically reveals decreased breath sounds along with hyperresonance to percussion in the hemithorax in question. If the patient's clinical status allows, an upright chest radiograph should be obtained to confirm the diagnosis.

Thoracostomy (Chest) Tube Placement

Pneumothorax, in the presence or absence of a hemothorax, usually requires placement of a chest tube. The posterior axillary line and a transverse line at the xiphoid process defines a "box" wherein chest tubes can be safely inserted through the fourth or fifth intercostal space. After skin preparation at the proposed insertion site, local anesthesia is infused into subcutaneous tissue, through the intercostal space, and when possible, the pleura, remembering the intercostal vessels located on the inferior aspect of the rib. The needle may be passed into the pleural space. The aspiration of air or fluid not only confirms the diagnosis but indicates a trajectory and distance to pleural entry. An incision made in the anesthetized area is carried down to fascia and with blunt finger dissection a tract above the rib is created. A large clamp is then carefully but

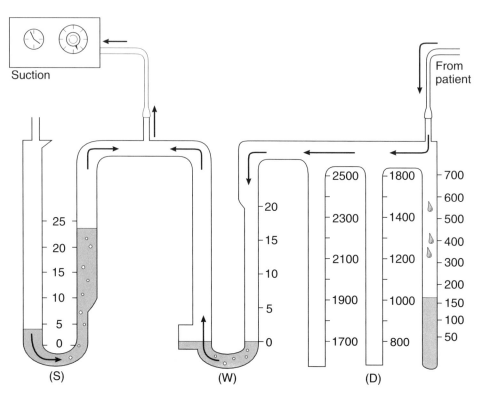

FIG. 6. Pleur-evac collection system, analogous to a three-bottle collection system. The area labeled *D* is the drainage collected from the patient; *W* is the water-seal chamber; *S* is the suction-control chamber. *Arrows* demonstrate the direction of airflow. (Adapted from Light R. *Pleural Disease.* Philadelphia: Lea & Febiger, 1983.)

forcefully guided *over* the rib to enter the pleural space. A "rush of air" or outpouring of fluid confirms entry. The clamp is held in position, opened widely, and withdrawn. Quickly, a finger is placed into the thoracic cavity and swept along the parietal pleura in all directions to lyse local adhesions or dislodge debris. The tube is then placed into the pleural space and directed toward the apex of the thoracic cavity. Ideally, chest tubes are positioned posteriorly for fluid drainage or anteriorly for aspiration of pneumothorax. A chest radiograph is obtained to confirm appropriate placement of the tube. The tube is secured to the skin with suture and connected to a suction system.

The "Pleur-evac" system (Fig. 6) is a commercially available chest tube collection apparatus that houses the classic "three-bottle" collection system. Fluid from the patient drains to the collection chamber (first bottle) that is connected to the water-seal chamber (second bottle) by a connecting tube submerged underwater to "seal" against air movement into the thorax. The suction control chamber (third bottle) has a "vent" submerged under variable water level equal to the intensity of suction.

Special Situations

Observation of a small nontraumatic pneumothorax is a valid treatment option in select patients if they have adequate respiratory reserve and minimal symptoms. Extreme caution should be employed in placement of a chest tube for traumatic pneumo/hemothoraces as fractured ribs may be encountered that are sharp and potentially injurious to the operator. When a visceral pleural flap acts as a "one-way" valve and traps increasing volumes of air in the pleural space, a "tension" pneumothorax exists that ultimately compresses the mediastinum. A clinical diagnosis is made by appreciating tracheal deviation, absent breath sounds in the hemithorax and hemodynamic compromise. Emergent decompression must be performed by placing a large gauge needle in the second intercostal space at the midclavicular line or by performing a "mini-thoracotomy" to release the air. Definitive therapy involves placement of a thoracostomy tube.

Pleural Effusion

Despite the extraordinary fluid resorptive capabilities of the lung, fluid may collect within the pleural space, i.e., a pleural effusion. Various causes of pleural effusions are listed in Table 1. A transudate is low protein fluid resulting from an imbalance in the pleural absorption equilibrium while an exudate is protein rich fluid caused by changes in capillary permeability.

TABLE 1. *Etiology of pleural effusions*

Transudate
  CHF
  Cirrhosis
  Peritoneal dialysis
  Other
    Nephrotic syndrome
    Myxedema
    Meigs' syndrome
Exudate
  Malignancy
  Thoracic infection
  Intraabdominal disorders, eg., pancreatitis
  Autoimmune disorders, e.g., rheumatoid arthritis

Pleural effusion may be symptomatic or asymptomatic, depending on its size and rapidity of development. Physical examination reveals decreased breath sounds and a level of dullness to percussion in the hemithorax containing the effusion. Various radiographic techniques can visualize effusions well, but the true diagnostic test remains thoracentesis. This is done best with the patient in a sitting position bent forward (Fig. 7) remembering that the posterior costophrenic sulcus is located at the 12th rib, and attempts at thoracentesis must be well above this level. Using principles of chest tube placement, the needle is always passed above a rib until fluid is aspirated which confirms entry into the pleural space. A postprocedure chest radiograph is obtained to exclude a pneumothorax.

Fluid obtained is sent for analysis (Table 2). Transudative effusions, with an exception for those causing dyspnea, are generally not drained completely until the primary cause is treated. Conversely, exudative effusions are aggressively drained as most causes can be treated.

Rapid reexpansion of chronically compressed pulmonary parenchyma can result in pulmonary edema.

Chylothorax describes accumulation of chyle in the pleural space. Chyle is composed primarily of chylomicrons, lymphocytes, electrolytes, and other ingested nutrients and is transported from the abdomen to the systemic venous circulation by the thoracic duct. A chylothorax can be produced by tumor, trauma and miscellaneous causes. It may be idiopathic as well. Malignancy is responsible for 50% of cases, the majority of which are lymphoma. Trauma to the thoracic duct during surgical procedures (aortic repair, esophageal resection, etc.) and penetrating injuries account for 25% of cases. Idiopathic and miscellaneous causes make up the remainder. Symptoms, physical examination, and radiographic findings are identical to those encountered in patients with pleural effusions. Nutrient and lymphocyte depletion is proportional to the duration and volume of lymph drainage. A 2-week trial of fluid and electrolyte replacement, medium chain triglyceride diet, and immune monitoring can be attempted, though it must be recognized that malnutrition and immunodeficiency can rapidly develop. If the latter occurs or if no improvement is noted, surgical treatment should be undertaken without delay. Ligation of the thoracic duct at the esophageal hiatus via right thoracotomy should resolve the persistent leak.

Malignant Effusion

Malignancy within the thoracic cavity can invade venous and lymphatic vessels and increase capillary permeability, resulting in effusion. Thoracentesis yields cytology diagnostic of malignancy in 80% of patients with malignant effusions. Thoracostomy tube drainage

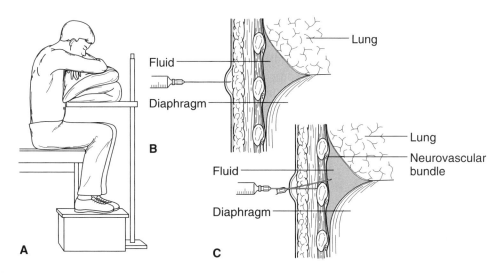

FIG. 7. (A) Recommended position of the patient for diagnostic or therapeutic thoracentesis. **(B)** Local anesthetic is administered to perform the procedure. **(C)** Needle is inserted through the subcutaneous tissue against the rib and advanced over the superior aspect of the rib to avoid the neurovascular bundle. (Adapted from Light R. *Pleural Disease.* Philadelphia: Lea & Febiger, 1983.)

TABLE 2. *Differentiating transudative versus exudative pleural effusions*

Character	Transudate	Exudate
Color	Clear, yellow	Cloudy, tan, "milky" (chylothorax)
White blood cells	<1,000/mm^3	>1,000/mm^3
Red blood cells	<10,000/mm^3	>10,000–100,000/mm^3
Glucose	NL	Low
Protein	<3.0 g/dl	>3.0 g/dl
Ratio (pleura/serum)		<0.5 >0.5
Specific gravity	<1.016	>1.016
LDH	NL	>67% of upper normal
Ratio (pleura/serum)		<0.6 >0.6
pH	Arterial	<7.2 (empyema); if <6.8, consider esophageal perforation
Amylase	Negative	Positive in esophageal perforation and pancreatitis
Culture	Negative	Positive (empyema)
Cytology	Negative	Positive, often bloody (malignancy)

Adapted from King T, Smith C. Chest wall, pleura, lung, and mediastinum. In: Schwartz S, ed. *Principles of surgery.* 6th ed. New York: McGraw-Hill, 1994:693.

treats the effusion by evacuation of fluid to relieve symptoms. By instilling agents such as talc, bleomycin, or tetracycline derivatives into the pleural space, an induced inflammatory reaction fuses the parietal and visceral pleura and prevents reaccumulation.

Malignant Mesothelioma

Malignant pleural mesothelioma is a rare malignancy with a poor prognosis. The association of mesothelioma with asbestos exposure is well understood, with known high-risk groups identified, including pipe fitters, construction workers, railroad workers, boilermakers, and shipbuilders. Sporadic cases of mesothelioma have been reported in which irradiation and exposure to minerals such as nickel have been implicated.

Malignant mesothelioma is predominantly a diffuse process that rarely invades the lung. Pleural involvement, however, may be so extensive that distinguishing normal lung from pleura may be impossible. A typical patient is middle-aged and has had exposure to asbestos in the distant past (20 to 30 years). Progression can be insidious, with as many as 25% of patients exhibiting symptoms for >6 months before seeking medical attention. Nonpleuritic chest pain with associated dyspnea, presumably from lung compression, is seen in most patients. Dyspnea may be alleviated by thoracentesis, although failure to do so is common and suggests "entrapped" lung. Chest radiograph classically demonstrates a pleural effusion with diffuse pleural nodularity and thickening. Interestingly, thrombocytosis (>400,000 platelets/mm3) is present in 60% to 90% of cases. Diagnosis requires pleural biopsy by thoracoscopy or thoracotomy.

Although distant metastases to the contralateral lung, liver, adrenal gland, and kidney occurs quite frequently, most patients with mesothelioma die from local complications of the disease. Progressive respiratory compro-

mise results from sheer tumor bulk or malignant effusion. Unless limited disease is found incidentally, the role of surgical therapy is rarely curative. Extrapleural pneumonectomy is a radical operation with a high morbidity and mortality and generally poor clinical results. Though there is no apparent improvement in long-term survival, limited resection (pleurectomy) seems to have a better palliative effect with lower patient morbidity and may be combined with brachytherapy (operative placement of radiation emitting "seeds"), external beam radiation, and chemotherapy for local control of disease.

MEDIASTINUM

Anatomy

The mediastinum is bounded by the pleura (laterally), diaphragm (inferiorly), and thoracic inlet (superiorly). Three compartments (Fig. 8) comprise the mediastinum: (a) the anterior-superior that contains the thymus and lymphatic tissue; (b) the middle that contains the heart, pericardium, aortic arch, trachea, and lymph nodes; and (c) the posterior that contains the descending aorta, esophagus, autonomic nerve roots, and the thoracic duct.

Diseases of the Mediastinum

Mediastinitis

Suppurative mediastinitis describes a fulminant infectious process that has a very high mortality rate. Cardiac surgery and esophageal perforation are the most common etiologies. Certain factors predispose to mediastinitis, which develops in 1% to 2% of all median sternotomies. Preoperative patient factors include malnutrition, poor clinical condition and diabetes. Intraoperative factors recognized include reoperation, use of bilateral internal

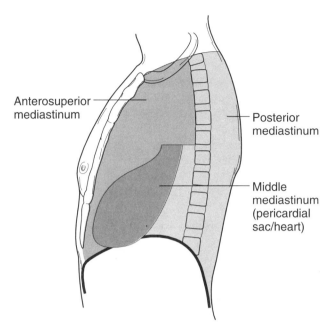

FIG. 8. A commonly used schema of the subdivision of the mediastinum. (Adapted from Hardy JD, Ewing HP. The mediastinum. In: Glenn WWL, ed. *Thoracic and cardiovascular surgery.* 4th ed. Norwalk, CT: Appleton-Century Crofts, 1983: 182.)

TABLE 3. *Distribution of mediastinal masses*

Anterior-superior
  Thymoma
  Lymphoma
  Teratoma
  Other
    Parathyroid adenoma
    Goiter
    Lymphadenopathy
    Seminoma
    Thymic cyst
Middle
  Teratoma
  Lymphoma
  Lymphadenopathy
  Other
    Bronchogenic cysts
    Pericardial cysts
Posterior
  Neurogenic tumors
  Other
    Goiter
    Spinal lesions
    Lymphadenopathy
    Aortic aneurysms
    Bronchogenic cysts
    Enteric cysts

mammary arteries for coronary bypass, extended cardiopulmonary bypass time (>3 hr), valve replacement procedures and lack of adequate hemostasis. Rarely, distant infection can contribute to the development of mediastinitis. Patients are ill-appearing, often complaining of chest pain well beyond the usual period of incisional pain. Dysphagia or dyspnea are common complaints. Wounds exhibit the hallmarks of inflammation: erythema, heat, induration, and pain. The sternum may be unstable or draining frank pus. Extreme cases present with high fever, septic shock, and cervical or upper thoracic crepitus from the rapid spread of infection through connective tissue planes. Chest radiograph occasionally is normal but may reveal pleural effusion, air in the neck, and subcutaneous tissue, or frank air-fluid levels within the mediastinal silhouette. CT scan will show the anatomic location of fluid collections. Intravenous antibiotics and surgical debridement and drainage are standard treatment. Wound closure may be difficult in the face of widespread infection. Soft tissue coverage using omentum or muscle flaps of rectus or pectoralis groups has been employed with good success.

Mediastinal Tumors

Up to one-half of mediastinal tumors (Table 3) are either asymptomatic or the source of nonspecific complaints (i.e., chronic cough or chest pain). Dyspnea or dysphagia can be caused by mass effect of the tumor while direct involvement of the recurrent laryngeal nerve results in dysphonia (hoarseness). Invasion of the superior cervical sympathetic ganglia can result in ipsilateral ptosis, meiosis and anhidrosis (Horner's syndrome). The presence of symptoms mandates evaluation for malignancy, which is present in a significant percentage of cases. In contrast, most asymptomatic mediastinal masses are benign. Beyond the standard chest radiograph, CT scan discerns cystic from solid masses, and MRI has value in evaluating vascularity of the tumor.

Neurogenic Tumors

Neurogenic tumors are the most common benign or malignant posterior compartment tumor in the adult and child. Peak incidence is in young adulthood, and 10% to 20% of cases are malignant. Masses detected at an earlier age have a higher incidence of malignancy. In children, 20% to 40% of cases are malignant. Neurilemomas and schwannomas are benign tumors found frequently. Neurofibromas, seen with von Recklinghausen's disease, are malignant in about one-fourth of cases. Paraganglionic tumors, such as pheochromocytomas, can invade vertebral bodies and the spinal canal. In such cases, MRI is essential in evaluation, particularly with regard to depth of extension and involvement of the spinal canal. Operation is indicated for all posterior mediastinal masses, and complete excision is the goal in both benign and malignant processes.

Thymomas

Thymomas are the most common anterior compartment tumor and second most common in overall frequency. One-third are found incidentally, whereas the remainder have nonspecific symptoms or are associated with paraneoplastic syndromes or myasthenia gravis. Over half are benign. Wide resection, approached via median sternotomy, is indicated in virtually all cases.

Lymphomas

Lymphomas are the most frequent malignant tumors of the anterior mediastinum. Children and adults have similar incidences of malignant lymphomas. The majority of cases have spread beyond the mediastinum at time of diagnosis. Standard treatment includes radiation and chemotherapy. Surgery is reserved for diagnosis, complicated or large tumors that bleed during chemotherapy treatment, and residual disease after chemotherapy.

Teratomas

Teratomas account for <10% of mediastinal masses and are found predominantly in the anterior compartment. Many evolve from congenital branchial cleft/pouch anomalies. Chest radiograph may reveal a large well-circumscribed anterior mediastinal mass with calcifications in about one-third of cases. CT scan is frequently performed to assess involvement of adjacent structures that makes surgical excision difficult. The majority of teratomas are benign. Elevated serum alpha-fetoprotein or carcinoembryonic antigen levels, however, suggests malignancy. Wide excision via median sternotomy is the treatment of choice.

Special Cases

Granulomatous diseases, tuberculosis, and histoplasmosis of the hilar lymph nodes can cause traction diverticula in the middle third of the esophagus. Systemic sarcoidosis manifests as bilateral hilar lymphadenopathy and can be associated with hypercalcemia in a significant number of cases. Corticosteroid treatment is usually successful in ameliorating symptoms of sarcoidosis. Aberrantly located inferior parathyroid glands are infrequently found within the superior mediastinum. Likewise, an enlarged thyroid goiter may descend into the superior mediastinum and may require median sternotomy for surgical excision. Although not malignant, these pathological entities have clinical importance and should be recognized.

LUNG

Embryology

The primitive airway develops from an out-pouching of the foregut in the fourth week of embryonic life. The lateral tracheo-esophageal grooves grow toward the midline and unite to divide the trachea from the esophagus. Sequential branching of the primitive trachea and arborization of the bronchiolar tree gives rise to the respiratory system.

Anatomy and Physiology

The trachea bifurcates to mainstem bronchi that yield increasing numbers of lobar, then segmental, and finally terminal bronchi, a total of 16 generations of airways (Fig. 9). The epithelium of tracheal and bronchial passages is composed of ciliated columnar cells interspersed with goblet cells. Because there is no respiratory epithelium in these airways, this volume of ~150 cc is considered "dead space." Each terminal bronchiole gives rise to seven generations of respiratory airways consisting of smooth muscle–lined respiratory bronchioles, which then yield alveolar ducts and sacs that comprise the basic respiratory unit where gas exchange occurs.

Deoxygenated systemic venous blood is pumped by the right heart through the pulmonary artery to segmental arterioles and ultimately to the pulmonary capillaries that engulf alveolar sacs. Oxygen from inspired air and carbon dioxide from the blood diffuse across a thin barrier, 0.5 μm, the alveolar-capillary interface. The amount of gas exchanged is proportional to the area of diffusion, which in a normal patient is ~70 m^2, the size of a tennis court. Oxygenated blood returns via the pulmonary veins to the left heart for systemic delivery.

Minute ventilation, defined as respiratory rate multiplied by tidal volume, can increase with minimal increase in energy expenditure because of the high compliance characteristic of the pulmonary parenchyma. Similarly, the pulmonary circulation can accept eight- to 10-fold increases in blood flow without significant change in pulmonary arterial pressure because of the high capacitance quality of the pulmonary vasculature. Consider how these physiologic properties of the lung compensate for increased oxygen demand.

Because of gravity, a greater proportion of blood perfuses the dependent regions of the lung at rest. Ventilation is slightly decreased in these same regions because of lower compliance though to a lesser degree than the difference in blood flow. During states of increased physiologic work, increased blood flow and ventilation recruits vasculature and alveoli of nondependent lung regions. Thus, increased alveolar ventilation (V) is "matched" to increased perfusion (Q) to increase oxygenation capa-

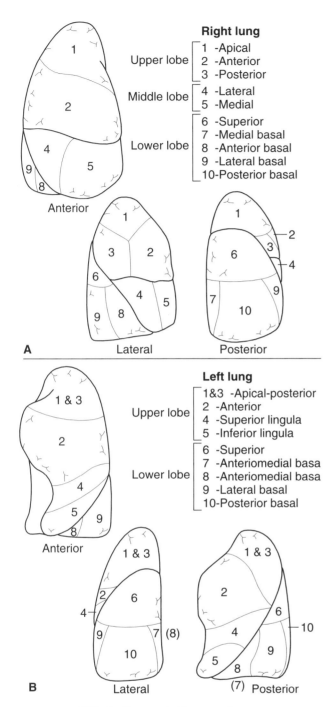

Right lung

Upper lobe
1 -Apical
2 -Anterior
3 -Posterior

Middle lobe
4 -Lateral
5 -Medial

Lower lobe
6 -Superior
7 -Medial basal
8 -Anterior basal
9 -Lateral basal
10-Posterior basal

Anterior

Lateral Posterior

A

Left lung

Upper lobe
1&3 -Apical-posterior
2 -Anterior
4 -Superior lingula
5 -Inferior lingula

Lower lobe
6 -Superior
7 -Anteriomedial basa
8 -Anteriomedial basa
9 -Lateral basal
10-Posterior basal

Anterior

Lateral (7) Posterior

B

FIG. 9. Segmental lung anatomy.

bility at the alveolar level and meet systemic oxygen demand. During periods of pulmonary disease, high or low V/Q ratios correspond to dead space ventilation and pulmonary shunting respectively.

Other important functions occur in the lung. Type II alveolar cells synthesize new alveolar cells as well as surfactant. Angiotensin I is converted to angiotensin II by an angiotensin-converting enzyme in the pulmonary vascular system. The mucociliary defense transports inhaled debris cephalad for expectoration. "Filtering" of thrombi and other blood debris occur within the capillary system.

Solitary Nodule

A solitary pulmonary nodule is typically detected incidentally on a standard chest radiograph and describes a "coin" lesion of <3 cm in diameter. Approximately one-half of all solitary nodules are malignant. Patient age correlates with the incidence of malignancy. Virtually all nodules noted in patients over 80 years of age are malignant, whereas nodules detected in those younger than 35 years of age are usually benign. Benign nodules are predominantly infectious granulomas but may also be hamartomas or noninfectious granulomas.

When discovered incidentally, the clinical objective must be to exclude cancer within the solitary nodule. Previous radiographs are extremely helpful and may indicate that the nodule has been stable over time or is the end stage of a benign process. High-resolution CT scan can often distinguish lesions with smooth well-demarcated edges and density consistent with fat or calcifications (benign) from lesions with lobulated blurred margins associated with internal spiculation (malignant). Tissue biopsy from large central lesions can be obtained by bronchoscopy. For peripheral lesions, transthoracic needle aspiration biopsy is performed with the assistance of fluoroscopy or CT scan. With history of a concurrent extrapulmonary tumor, tissue biopsy of the nodule is mandatory to diagnose a metastatic lesion that would necessitate a thorough search for other metastasis before resection is undertaken. Despite the fact that up to 30% of biopsies yield indeterminate results and ~15% of biopsies yield false-negative results, cautious observation of a small "benign" mass can be performed. Serial radiographs and CT scans are required to follow the mass in question recognizing that detecting an occult malignant lesion must be the purpose of this period of observation.

Clearly, when diagnostic evaluation has revealed malignancy, management protocols are followed to achieve maximum survival (discussed in later section). However, if all diagnostic methods have yielded equivocal results or the mass enlarges on follow-up examination, the solitary nodule should be resected. Thoracoscopic excision is a popular method of diagnosis especially in patients with poor operative risk. Formal wedge resection or lobectomy via a thoracotomy are the standard methods of excision. Metastatic spread of a primary lung cancer or widespread metastasis of an extrapulmonary primary tumor must be excluded prior to operation. Although resection of a benign lung nodule exposes the patient to an "unnecessary" thoracotomy or thoracoscopy, the benefit of excluding a malignancy in most cases outweighs the risk of surgery. Clinicians who discover solitary nodules are continually challenged to diagnose malignancy and define its extent or exclude malignancy and prevent unnecessary surgery.

Cancer of the Lung

Epidemiology

In the United States in 1994, nearly 170,000 new cases of lung cancer were recorded. In the same year, >153,000 deaths were due to lung cancer. It is the leading cause of death from cancer in men and has surpassed breast cancer as the leading cause of cancer death among women. In the Surgeon General's Report of 1989, C. Everett Koop contended that 90% of all lung cancers are caused by tobacco smoke. Since 1973, the consumption of tobacco products in the United States was on a steady annual decline. In the 1990s, however, the decreased use of tobacco among white males, resulting in a modest decrease in the incidence of lung cancer in this group, has been supplanted by an increased use of cigarettes by women and minorities which has led to an increased rate of deaths from lung cancer in those groups. Thus, the consumption of tobacco products in the United States since Koop's report has not decreased appreciably. Unfortunately, effective methods of early detection resulting in increased survival have not been found.

Pathogenesis

In the early part of this century, Evarts Graham was among the first to recognize the association between tobacco smoke and the development of lung cancer. It has been shown that DNA of replicating bronchial epithelial cells undergoes mutations after chronic exposure to carcinogens contained in cigarette smoke. Epithelial metaplasia progresses to irreversible dysplasia and carcinoma in situ. Other inhaled carcinogens, such as asbestos, act synergistically with tobacco smoke and potentiate its carcinogenic effect.

Pathology

The majority of bronchogenic carcinomas arise from pulmonary epithelium and mucus glands. The four types and their relative frequencies of occurrence are as follows: squamous cell (epidermoid) carcinoma, 30%; adenocarcinoma, 25%; small-cell (oat-cell) carcinoma, 20%; and large cell carcinoma, 15%. Other types accounting for <10% of cases include carcinoid, undifferentiated, adenosquamous, anaplastic, and miscellaneous tumors. Adenocarcinoma has become more prevalent, particularly in females, and is the most frequent lung cancer found in nonsmokers.

TABLE 4. *Symptoms of carcinoma of the lung*

Cough
Hemoptysis
Dyspnea
Pneumonia
Chest, shoulder, or arm pain
Weight loss
Bone pain
Hoarseness
Headaches or seizures
Swelling of the face or neck

Evaluation

New respiratory complaints such as cough and hemoptysis often cause previously healthy patients to seek medical attention. In patients with chronic pulmonary disease, in whom it may be difficult to appreciate new respiratory problems, evidence of unresolving atelectasis or pneumonia should raise the suspicion of cancer (Table 4). In both groups, a screening chest radiograph should be obtained to exclude the presence of a mass or nodule in the lung. If a mass is detected, noninvasive and invasive staging procedures should be performed to evaluate the primary tumor and the extent of regional nodal and metastatic involvement. Tissue diagnosis by bronchoscopy or transthoracic needle aspiration biopsy is imperative as the respective treatments for small-cell and non–small-cell lung carcinoma are significantly different.

Contemporary thoracic surgeons utilize selective mediastinoscopy in the evaluation of locoregional metastasis of non–small-cell bronchogenic carcinoma. It is clear that mediastinal lymphadenopathy detected by high-resolution CT scan mandates mediastinoscopy and biopsy. In the absence of mediastinal lymphadenopathy, it is generally accepted that mediastinoscopy will not detect a significant percentage of occult nodal disease and is not compulsory in every patient with non–small-cell lung cancer. The perseverance in evaluation should be individualized to match the clinical suspicion with attendant risks of invasive procedures.

Distant metastatic sites include liver, adrenal glands, brain, and bone. Obtaining a CT scan of the upper abdomen to exclude hepatic or adrenal nodules is standard. A CT scan of the brain, however, should be obtained only in patients with specific complaints or symptoms (i.e., headache or neurologic symptoms). Likewise, selective bone scanning should be performed for bone pain.

Special Situations

Shoulder and arm pain is commonly attributed to cervical musculoskeletal pathology, when in fact a superior sulcus carcinoma of the lung may be the cause of these symptoms. As the tumor enlarges, it can invade the brachial

TABLE 5. *Reasons for inoperability in patients with lung cancer*

Distant metastasis
Involvement of trachea or contralateral main bronchus with
  carcinoma
Mediastinal lymph node metastasis (contralateral)
Superior vena cava obstruction
Malignant cells in pleural effusion
Recurrent laryngeal nerve paralysis from carcinoma
Histologic diagnosis of small-cell carcinoma

TABLE 6. *Mean survival from small-cell carcinoma*

Stage	Treated	Untreated
Limited	14 months[a]	9 months
Extensive	9 months[b]	6 months

[a]Surgery and postoperative radiation/chemotherapy.
[b]Chemotherapy alone.

plexus, C7 and T1, first and second thoracic vertebra or the stellate ganglion. Pancoast's tumor describes the superior sulcus tumor with shoulder and arm pain in the presence of Horner's syndrome. Hoarseness can result from invasion of the recurrent laryngeal nerve, while edema of the head and upper extremities can be a manifestation of encasement and obstruction of the superior vena cava. Paraneoplastic syndromes (e.g., syndrome of inappropriate secretion of antidiuretic hormone, hyperparathyroidism) occur frequently with bronchogenic carcinoma.

As will be discussed shortly, surgery is the primary treatment in patients with non–small-cell lung cancer. Oncologists and surgeons must select patients who not only will tolerate the physiologic stress of the operation but will also withstand the physiologic demands of the postoperative period. Inoperability (Table 5) stems from disease or patient factors. Malignant effusion, superior vena cava syndrome, and extension to contralateral hilar lymph nodes are examples of incurable disease. Patient-related factors such as severe comorbid systemic disease and predicted inadequate pulmonary function after resection increase perioperative morbidity and should preclude patients from surgical resection. Poor outcomes after pneumonectomy are more frequently seen in patients with a preoperative arterial blood gas pCO_2 of >50 mm Hg or absolute predicted postoperative FEV_1 of <0.8 L/sec or FVC of <2.0 L. Nuclear medicine "split-function" studies quantify patients functional lung volume that will be removed by surgery. Consider a quantitative lung scan in a patient scheduled for right pneumonectomy with an FEV_1 of 1.5 L/sec that reveals 40% of ventilation occurs in the left lung. An FEV_1 of 0.6 L/sec postpneumonectomy is predicted, and such a patient is not a suitable candidate for resection.

Staging and Treatment

Small-Cell Carcinoma

Because of the aggressive nature of small-cell carcinoma, staging has been simplified to describe extent of disease: limited disease, confined to one hemithorax and ipsilateral lymph nodes, or extensive disease. An overwhelming majority of patients have extensive disease at the time of diagnosis, and are not candidates for surgical resection. For these patients, multidrug chemotherapy protocols have surprisingly good early results with up to 2 to 3 years of tumor "regression" though not without significant toxicity. Recently, a retrospective review of past experience with limited disease suggests that surgical resection combined with aggressive postoperative (adjuvant) chemotherapy may improve survival compared to nonoperative therapy. The addition of radiation in this group of patients resulted in only a modest increase in survival but a significant rate of complications. Radiation therapy for extensive disease is limited to palliation for site specific metastasis (e.g., brain, bone, superior vena cava, etc.) (Table 6).

Non–small-cell carcinoma

Surgical extirpation remains the primary treatment of choice (Table 7 and Figs. 10–13). Overall, 50% of patients with a solitary nodule on chest radiograph are suitable for exploratory thoracotomy, and of these patients potentially half will be cured by resection. In stage I disease, lobectomy is definitive resectional therapy with excellent long-term prognosis, whereas pneumonectomy is reserved for tumors that invade the mainstem bronchi or hilum or involve multiple lobes. In certain cases, wedge or segmental resection can be performed for peripheral lesions especially in those patients who will not tolerate a more extensive resection. Adjuvant (postoperative) radiotherapy has not been beneficial in improving survival after resection of stage I non–small-cell lung cancer. In patients who cannot undergo thoracotomy, radiation as the sole modality of treatment gives moderate cure rates, particularly if the tumor is small.

With extension of disease to lymph nodes, the cure rate after resection drops significantly. The use of radiation and chemotherapy has been studied for potential benefits, particularly in stage II and IIIA patients. Adjuvant radiation therapy after resection in stage IIIA disease is recommended but to date has shown no consistent improvement in long-term survival. Control of local disease recurrence appears to be improved. Neoadjuvant (preoperative) chemotherapy with or without radiation in controlled trials suggested "downstaging" effect on the tumor but as yet is not accepted as standard therapy. Palliative radiation is particularly useful in resolving supe-

TABLE 7. *TNM staging for lung carcinoma*

Stage	Characteristics		
Occult	T_x	N_0	M_0
Stage 0	T_{is}	N_0	M_0
Stage I	T_1	N_0	M_0
	T_2	N_0	M_0
Stage II	T_1	N_1	M_0
	T_2	N_1	M_0
Stage IIIA	T_1	N_2	M_0
	T_2	N_2	M_0
	T_3	N_0	M_0
	T_3	N_1	M_0
	T_3	N_2	M_0
Stage IIIB	Any T	N_3	M_0
	T_4	Any N	M_0
Stage IV	Any T	Any N	M_1

Primary tumor (T): T_x, primary tumor cannot be assessed, or tumor proven by the presence of malignant cells in sputum or bronchial washings but not visualized by imaging or bronchoscopy; T_0, no evidence of primary tumor; T_{is}, carcinoma in situ; T_1, tumor of ≤3 cm in greatest dimension, surrounded by lung or visceral pleura, without bronchoscopic evidence of invasion more proximal than the lobar bronchus (i.e., not in main bronchus) (note that the uncommon superficial tumor of any size with its invasive component limited to the bronchial wall, which may extend proximal to the main bronchus, is also classified as T_1); T_2, tumor with any of the following features of size or extent: >3 cm in greatest dimension, involving main bronchus ≥2 cm distal to the carina, invading the visceral pleura, or associated with atelectasis or obstructive pneumonitis that extends to the hilar region but does not involve the entire lung; T_3, tumor of any size that directly invades any of the following: chest wall (including superior sulcus tumors), diaphragm, mediastinal pleura, or parietal pericardium, or tumor in the main branchus <2 cm distal to the carina but without involvement of the carina, or associated atelectasis or obstructive pneumonitis of the entire lung; T_4, tumor of any size that invades any of the following: mediastinum, heart, great vessels, trachea, esophagus, vertebral body, carina; or a tumor with a malignant pleural effusion. Note that most pleural effusions associated with lung cancer are due to tumor; however, there are a few patients in whom multiple cytopathologic examinations of a pleural fluid are negative for tumor; in these cases, fluid is nonbloody and is not an exudate; when these elements and clinical judgment dictate that the effusion is not related to the tumor, the effusion should be excluded as a staging element and the patient should be staged T_1, T_2, or T_3.

Regional lymph nodes (N): The regional lymph nodes are the intrathoracic, scalene, and supraclavicular nodes; N_x, Regional lymph nodes cannot be assessed; N_0, no regional lymph node metastasis; N_1, metastasis in ipsilateral peribronchial and/or ipsilateral hilar lymph nodes, including direct extension; N_2, metastasis in ipsilateral mediastinal and/or subcarinal lymph node(s); N_3, metastasis in contralateral mediastinal, contralateral hilar, ipsilateral, or contralateral scalene or supraclavicular lymph node(s).

Distant metastases (M): M_x, presence of distant metastasis cannot be assessed; M_0, no distant metastasis; M_1, distant metastasis.

Adapted from Beahrs OH, Henson DE, Hutter RVP, Kennedy BJ, eds. *American Joint Committee on Cancer manual for staging of cancer.* 4th ed. Philadelphia: Lippincott, 1992.

rior vena cava syndrome or in relieving persistent cough or hemoptysis from tumor mass at the hilum. Although chemotherapy has been disappointingly unsuccessful in the past, a recent trial (Rosell, et al.) suggests that patients with advanced non–small-cell lung cancer given preoperative chemotherapy may experience extended overall and disease-free survival. Other data suggest that neoadjuvant chemotherapy may be effective in downstaging tumor with minimal toxicity and no increase in surgical complications. The use of adjuvant chemotherapy and radiotherapy for stage IIIA disease may improve local control, but as yet no long-term survival benefit has been appreciated.

Prognosis

Prognosis is related to the stage at presentation and type of bronchogenic carcinoma (non–small-cell vs. small-cell). Five-year survival from non–small-cell lung cancer correlates inversely with the size of tumor and lymph node involvement at time of resection. For example, for nodules ≤3 cm in size without lymph node involvement (stage I) a 5-year survival of 70% has been reported, whereas primary lesions of >3 cm or extension to N1 nodes carries a 5-year survival of 40% to 60% (Table 8).

Thoracic Infections

Surgical therapy for lung abscess, bronchiectasis, and chronic granulomatous disease was common as recently as 30 years ago. Antibiotics, greater diagnostic capabilities, and improved public health measures predicted that complicated pulmonary infection would be relegated to areas of the world without these advances. However, because of induced or acquired states of immunosuppression (e.g., transplant medications, chemotherapy for malignancy, or AIDS), the prevalence of serious pulmonary infection appears to be increasing. The following is a brief discussion regarding the diagnosis and management of empyema, bronchiectasis, lung abscess, empyema, fungal infections, and pulmonary tuberculosis.

Empyema thoracis is defined as a suppurative infection within the pleural space. When caused by trauma, penetrating chest injury and retained hemothorax appear to be the major predisposing factors. In the majority of nontraumatic cases, empyema occurs after pneumonia, a parapneumonic infection. Infrequently, secondary infection of a hemothorax, pulmonary infarction, lung or esophageal resection, and intraabdominal abscess can result in empyema. The diagnosis must be considered in all patients with an unresolving febrile illness and pleural effusion on chest radiograph. CT scan may demonstrate a loculated heterogeneous effusion surrounding pulmonary

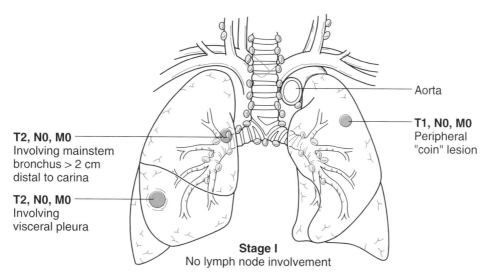

FIG. 10. Stage I disease. (Adapted from Mountain CF. A new international system for staging lung cancer. *Chest* 1986:89[suppl]:2255–2335.)

consolidation. A thoracentesis should be performed and will reveal an exudative effusion with a high leukocyte count (Table 2). Without aggressive treatment immediately after diagnosis, the initial "exudative" stage can progress over time to become "fibrinopurulent" and finally "organized" in character. Empyema due to staphylococcal pneumonia in children responds well to antibiotics alone, and invasive therapy is rarely required. Conversely, in the adult, aggressive treatment is mandatory and consists of thoracostomy tube drainage, obliteration of the empyema cavity, and intravenous antibiotics

directed at cultured bacteria especially in the initial exudative stage. In chronic fibrinopurulent or organized empyema, fibrous adhesions compartmentalize or even "entrap" the lung within the thoracic cavity. Open or, in select cases, thoracoscopy-assisted decortication is performed to relieve respiratory embarrassment and control infection. In difficult cases, thoracoplasty or muscle flap or omental transposition can be performed to obliterate the chronic empyema space.

Bronchiectasis is a chronic suppurative infection that results in pathologic dilation of segmental bronchi. Most

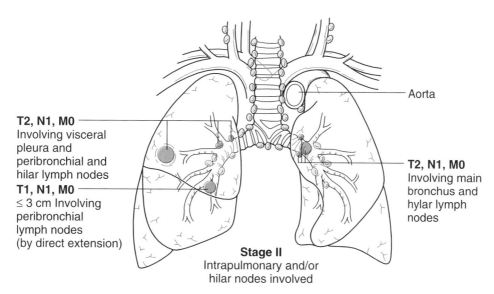

FIG. 11. Stage II disease. (Adapted from Mountain CF. A new international system for staging lung cancer. *Chest* 1986:89[suppl]:2255–2335.)

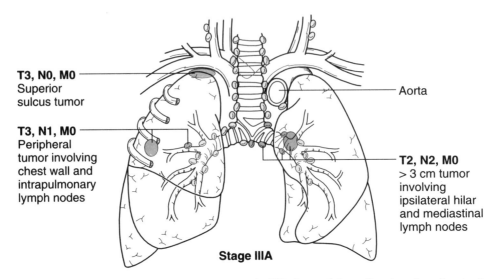

T3, N0, M0
Superior
sulcus tumor

T3, N1, M0
Peripheral
tumor involving
chest wall and
intrapulmonary
lymph nodes

Aorta

T2, N2, M0
> 3 cm tumor
involving
ipsilateral hilar
and mediastinal
lymph nodes

Stage IIIA

FIG. 12. Stage IIIA disease. (Adapted from Mountain CF. A new international system for staging lung cancer. *Chest* 1986:89[suppl]:2255–2335.)

cases are caused by chronic bronchial obstruction (e.g., tumor, foreign body) or chronic pulmonary infections such as cystic fibrosis or Kartagener's syndrome (situs inversus, pansinusitis, and bronchiectasis). Grossly dilated bronchi are filled with mucus and pus and occasionally an obstructing broncholith. Microscopically, the columnar epithelium of bronchial mucosa become pseudostratified. Patients manifest recurrent pulmonary infection with chronic cough, copious mucopurulent sputum, and infrequently hemoptysis. High-resolution CT scan has replaced the bronchogram as the diagnostic standard. In the majority of patients, conservative treatment involving postural drainage and intravenous antibiotics is success-

ful. Surgery is indicated in cases of conservative management failure, resectable limited disease, recurrent hemoptysis, or pediatric patients who fail to thrive.

Lung abscess is an infrequent complication of community-acquired or hospital-acquired pneumonia. Rarely, colonization of devitalized pulmonary tissue from infarction or an obstructing carcinoma can progress to abscess. Patients are typically edentulous with poor oral hygiene or have a history of alcoholism. Clinically they are ill-appearing, febrile, and producing foul-smelling purulent sputum. The pattern of sputum production is usually acute and episodic as the abscess intermittently "drains" into the airways. Surprisingly, dyspnea is not a common

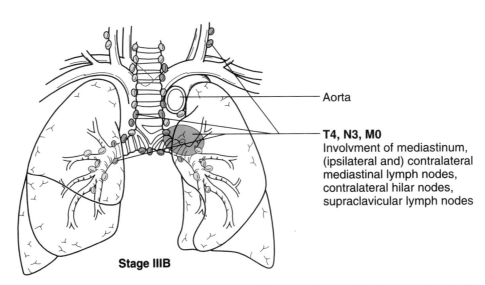

Aorta

T4, N3, M0
Involvment of mediastinum,
(ipsilateral and) contralateral
mediastinal lymph nodes,
contralateral hilar nodes,
supraclavicular lymph nodes

Stage IIIB

FIG. 13. Stage IIIB disease. (Adapted from Mountain CF. A new international system for staging lung cancer. *Chest* 1986:89[suppl]:2255–2335.)

TABLE 8. *Mean survival from non–small-cell carcinoma*

Stage	Incidence	Five-year survival
I	10%	50–70%
II	20%	30–40%
IIIA	15%	15%
IIIB	40%	5%
IV		1%

symptom. Hemoptysis can occur and may be massive. Chest radiograph reveals cavitary lesions with air-fluid levels amidst pulmonary consolidation. With spontaneous drainage, the vast majority of pulmonary abscesses are effectively treated by a 6- to 10-week course of intravenous antibiotics. For undrained abscesses, bronchoscopy is excellent in aspirating cavities and creating internal drainage pathways. Pneumonostomy tube drainage can also be used in very ill patients with poor cavity drainage via the bronchial tree. Surgical drainage is required in <10% of cases and can only be performed if pleural symphysis is present. "Marsupialization" of the abscess cavity is performed to drain the pus externally. It must be recognized that premature unroofing of an immature collection can allow dissemination throughout the pleural cavity and convert a localized collection into an empyema. Resection may be performed in cases of inability to exclude cancer or in patients with serious hemorrhage that usually originates from the pulmonary arterial system.

Fungal infections and "fungal-like" bacterial infections typically occur in immunocompromised hosts. Conservative treatment involving intravenous antibiotics, amphotericin B, or newer antifungal agents is generally successful. Surgical resection is reserved for medical failure or the inability to exclude carcinoma.

Actinomycetes is an anaerobic bacillus with hyphae and spores that is a normal inhabitant of the oral cavity. Clinical features of thoracic infection due to Actinomycetes include suppuration, abscess, sinus tracts and rib and mediastinal involvement. Microscopically, sulfur granules are present that help in diagnosis but do not distinguish it from Nocardia, Staphylococcus, or fungi. Fortunately, these organisms are sensitive to penicillin and sulfonamides, and successful treatment is expected.

Nocardia is an aerobic, weakly acid-fast bacillus with hyphae that inhabits the soil, and is carried by domestic animals. As with Actinomycetes, infection can lead to sinus tract formation and chest wall involvement, but infected patients generally exhibit a much more aggressive clinical course, commonly developing extensive pulmonary necrosis and abscesses. "Metastatic" dissemination to the central nervous system and elsewhere is a distinctive pathologic feature. Despite the invasive nature of Nocardia, it is surprisingly susceptible to penicillin and sulfonamides, and conservative treatment is usually successful.

Histoplasma capsulatum is a dimorphic fungus that is endemic to the great river valleys of the midwest and currently is the most common fungal infection in the United States. Pulmonary infection is initially seen on chest radiograph as interstitial infiltrates that can quickly progress to "patchy" alveolar consolidation. Cavitation and hemoptysis accompanies end stage disease. Fibrosing mediastinitis and mid-esophageal traction diverticula are distinctive of chronic histoplasma mediastinal disease. Blastomycetes dermatitidis is a single round budding yeast commonly inhabiting the soil of the southeastern United States. Although aspiration is the only route of transmission, cutaneous dissemination is unique to blastomycosis. Typically, erythematous crusted lesions are found on the face and abdomen. Coccidioides immitis is another dimorphic fungi that is endemic in the American southwest and is the second most common fungal infection. Acute valley fever is a syndrome of pneumonitis, erythema nodosum, and arthralgia resulting from disseminated coccidioidomycosis. Occasionally, cavitary lesions rupture into the pleural space resulting in pneumothorax and empyema. Aspergillus is an invasive fungus that, in immunocompromised hosts, manifests as three distinct clinical patterns: (a) "asthma" symptoms secondary to allergic bronchitis, (b) cavitation with development of a "fungus ball," or (c) invasive necrotizing bronchopneumonia. In 50% of patients with a "fungus ball," hemoptysis is present; in 20% of these patients, it is severe and may require emergent surgical resection. In blastomycetes, coccidioides, and disseminated aspergillus, amphotericin B is employed for serious infection, and successful resolution is expected.

As early as 6000 B.C., tuberculosis was well known as the "King of diseases." Though treatment has progressed significantly since the turn of the century when it was the leading cause of death, tuberculosis remains an important world health problem with >8 million new cases and >3 million deaths recorded each year. It is estimated that in the year 2005, the number of new cases per year will rise to nearly 12 million. There are ~1 billion infected persons worldwide, making tuberculosis one of the most prevalent infections of this era. Indeed, it is the leading cause of death worldwide from a single infectious agent. Presently, in the United States, >30,000 new cases and 1,700 recorded deaths occur every year secondary to tuberculosis.

Mycobacterium tuberculosis (MTB) is a common opportunistic pathogen in patients with AIDS, but also in the elderly, individuals with diabetes, pulmonary silicosis, or reticuloendothelial malignancies. Apical and posterior segments of the upper lobe or superior segments of the lower lobe are the usual sites of infection. Clinical presentation includes chronic productive cough with hemoptysis, weight loss, chest pain, fever, and night sweats. Once the diagnosis is made, multiple-drug therapy is mandatory to combat the emergence of drug-resistant strains. Surgery is required in <2% of all treated patients. Indications for surgical resection include extensive pulmonary destruction with bronchopleural fistula or empyema, inability to exclude bronchogenic carcinoma, massive hemoptysis, or persistently positive sputum cultures with cavitation. In rare cases, thoracoplasty to collapse the tuberculous cavity or pleural space may be indicated.

SUMMARY

Historically, the field of thoracic surgery made significant progress thanks in large part to advances in airway and anesthesia management. Also with better diagnostic methods, both invasive and noninvasive, detection and at times observation of certain thoracic disorders have become easier. Modern thoracoscopy allows lung resections to be completed with decreased incisional pain and minimal morbidity. Perhaps because of technological and medical advances, the incidence of lung infections and the detection of solitary pulmonary nodules are on the rise. Sadly, effective screening for the leading cancer death among both men and women in the United States is not yet available, but new ideas in multimodality therapy for lung cancers may improve overall and disease-free survival in patients with advanced disease.

STUDY QUESTIONS

1. Describe the pathophysiology of a tension pneumothorax.
2. List differences between a transudative and exudative pleural effusion.
3. Be able to explain the "three-bottle" chest tube collection system.
4. Describe the segmental anatomy of the left and right lung.
5. Describe the pathogenesis of empyema thoracis.

SUGGESTED READING

Light R. *Pleural disease.* Philadelphia: Lea and Febiger, 1983.
Matthay RA, ed. Lung cancer. *Clin Chest Med* 1993;1:1–201.
Ravitch M, Steichen F. *Atlas of general thoracic surgery.* Philadelphia: Saunders, 1988.
Rosell R, Gomez-Codina J, Camps C, et al. A randomized trial comparing preoperative chemotherapy plus surgery with surgery alone in patients with non-small-cell lung cancer. *N Engl J Med* 1994;330: 153–158.
Sabiston D, Spencer F, eds. *Surgery of the chest.* 5th ed. Philadelphia: Saunders, 1990.
Schwartz S, ed. *Principles of surgery.* 6th ed. New York: McGraw Hill, 1994.

CHAPTER 20

Cardiac Surgery

Patrick C. Mangonon and Richard A. Perryman

Cardiac surgery has progressed at an unprecedented rate over the past 30 years, perhaps more so than any other surgical subspecialty. Advances in cardiology, pediatrics, and neonatology have decreased perioperative morbidity of cardiac procedures for patients with previously inoperable or early fatal disease. Perhaps the largest contributions to cardiac surgery, however, have been the development in cardiopulmonary bypass and improved knowledge in intraoperative myocardial protection.

Cardiopulmonary bypass describes diversion of deoxygenated venous blood to an extracorporeal "oxygenator," where it becomes reoxygenated and returned, via pump, to the patient's arterial system. Research by Gibbon in the 1930s culminated in 1953 when he used the pump successfully during surgical repair of an atrial septal defect (ASD). Kirklin and Lillehei furthered Gibbon's work in the early 1950s at the Mayo Clinic and successfully used a pump oxygenator during repair of a ventricular septal defect (VSD). Arguably, however, it is improved understanding of myocardial preservation techniques that has allowed cardiac procedures to be performed with minimal morbidity. In critically ill patients, myocardial protection starts preoperatively by augmenting coronary perfusion and decreasing oxygen demand, i.e., beta-blockade, calcium channel blockers, and vasodilators. Intraoperative use of pulmonary artery catheters, invasive peripheral arterial monitoring, and electrocardiographic ST segment monitoring reduces periods of hypoperfusion and undetected myocardial ischemia. Contemporary cardioplegia solution originated from the early work of Melrose, which was further developed by pioneers Buckberg (United States), Gay and Ebert (United States), and Hearse and Baimbridge (Britain). Infusion of cardioplegia into the coronary system of a patient on cardiopulmonary bypass induces immediate cardiac arrest but permits continued myocardial cell energy production that protects myocytes against ischemia. The combination of cardioplegia and cardiopulmonary bypass provides the ideal motionless and bloodless field for open heart surgery.

CONGENITAL HEART DISEASE

Pursuant to discussing congenital heart disease (CHD), it is important to understand normal fetal circulation and transition to postbirth circulation. In the fetus (Fig. 1), two umbilical arteries bring deoxygenated blood to the placenta for gas exchange. Reoxygenated blood is carried away via two umbilical veins. Half of this reoxygenated blood is conducted to the ductus venosus and then empties into the inferior vena cava (IVC), while the remainder travels through the hepatic circulation and then to the IVC. Desaturated blood from the lower body joins oxygenated blood above the liver in the IVC, but a "streaming effect" segregates oxygenated blood to the left and deoxygenated blood to the right within the IVC. Upon its return to the heart, virtually all the oxygenated blood of the IVC is shunted across the foramen ovale into the left atrium and then to the left ventricle. Most of this volume is pumped into the great vessels of the aortic arch proximal to the ductus arteriosus. The remaining venous return to the heart contributed by the IVC and the superior vena cava (SVC) empties into the right ventricle. Because of increased pulmonary vascular resistance in utero, this relatively deoxygenated blood is conducted through the pulmonary outflow tract but is then shunted through the ductus arteriosus and into the distal systemic circulation.

Consider the following adaptations of fetal circulation and the changes that occur after birth. In the fetus, the pulmonary and systemic vascular systems are "parallel circuit" (Fig. 2) in which the right ventricle pumps deoxygenated blood ultimately to the placenta for reoxygenation, while the left ventricle pumps oxygenated blood to the heart and brain. Although the average arterial satura-

265

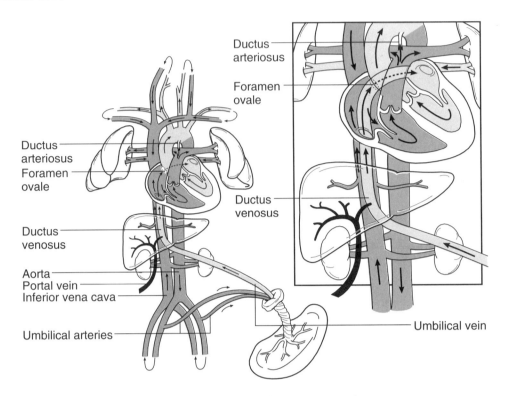

FIG. 1. Fetal circulation. Circulation in series.

tion of fetal hemoglobin is only 65%, corresponding to O2 partial pressure of 35 mm Hg, the compensatory P50 is 18 mm Hg, which facilitates both oxygen "unloading" at the peripheral tissues and oxygen absorption at the placenta. A normally high resting heart rate further increases cardiac output. These physiological changes in utero maximize oxygen delivery in a hypoxic environment. Within minutes after birth, expansion of the lungs decreases pulmonary vascular resistance and increases pulmonary blood flow eight- to 10-fold. Because of increased pulmonary blood flow, increased left atrial pressure facilitates closure of the foramen ovale. Increased O2 content in the systemic circulation combined with a decreased serum prostaglandin level causes contraction of smooth muscle in the ductus arteriosus and closure occurs within hours to days after birth. The ductus venosus closes spontaneously and becomes the ligamentum teres. Disconnection from the placenta increases systemic vascular resistance. After birth, the pulmonary and systemic circulations are placed in series so that oxygenated blood is carried to the lungs for reoxygenation and presented to the left heart for systemic distribution.

Abnormal Postbirth Circulation

Left to right shunting describes systemic blood flow abnormally diverted back to the pulmonary circulation. With large shunts, increased cardiac workload from

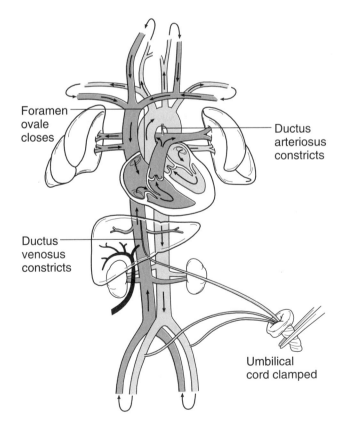

FIG. 2. Postbirth circulation. Parallel circuits.

increased blood flow results in both left and right ventricular hypertrophy. Decreased compliance of the left ventricle raises pulmonary interstitial pressure and can lead to pulmonary edema. Increased pulmonary artery blood flow can cause pulmonary hypertension and can result in irreversible histologic changes in the endothelium and smooth muscle of the pulmonary vascular system. If large shunts progress untreated, an equilibration between pulmonary and systemic vascular resistance occurs resulting in bidirectional shunting, called Eisenmenger physiology. This leads to decreased pulmonary blood flow and pulmonary edema and infections abate. However, clinical improvement is short-lived as progressive cyanosis develops from right to left shunting.

Cyanosis in infants born at term results from right to left shunting in which deoxygenated blood bypasses the lungs and is redistributed systemically or when insufficient pulmonary blood flow exists. A complete right to left shunt is incompatible with life so that, in these situations, some degree of left to right shunting must be present for survival.

Acyanotic Lesions

VSD is the most common form of CHD (Fig. 3), accounting for up to 25% of cases. VSD can occur as an isolated lesion or in association with other heart defects. It is accepted that small VSD, when diagnosed early in infancy, will progressively diminish or close completely. In contrast, large defects invariably lead to delayed growth from failure to thrive, cardiac failure, and pulmonary edema. The amount of flow across a VSD is proportional to the pressure gradient across the defect, the size of the defect, and the difference between systemic and pulmonary vascular resistance. Because systemic vascular resistance is significantly higher than pulmonary vascular resistance, shunt flow is usually directed from left to right ventricle. In patients with large shunts, physical examination typically reveals a diaphoretic, underdeveloped child in respiratory distress. A systolic thrill is palpable on a pigeon breast chest wall deformity that develops because an enlarged right ventricle pushes against a growing sternum. A holosystolic murmur is heard best at the left lower sternal border. Echocardiogram is an excellent method of evaluating left ventricular function and determining location, size, and hemodynamic flow gradients across the defect. Primary or patch closure must be performed to prevent sequelae of irreversible pulmonary hypertension.

ASDs account for up to 15% of all CHD and are caused predominantly by incomplete development of the ostium secundum (Fig. 4). Less commonly, an underdeveloped ostium primum can yield an ASD and is frequently associated with a cleft mitral valve leaflet. A sinus venosus defect near the entrance of the SVC may function as an

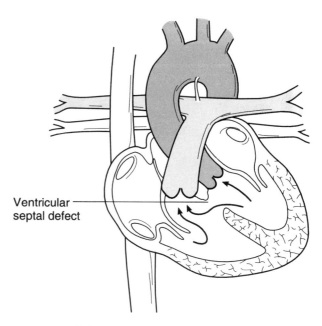

FIG. 3. Ventricular septal defect.

ASD with partial anomalous venous return. The amount of flow across an ASD is proportional to the difference in compliance between the left and right ventricle. Normally, the left ventricle is less compliant, favoring flow from left to right atrium. Despite the increased pulmonary blood flow, the majority of lesions are asymptomatic. Occasionally, children can mature to adulthood undiagnosed. A systolic ejection murmur heard at the upper left sternal border occurs because of increased blood flow across the pulmonary valve along with a fixed splitting of the second heart sound. When a pulmonary to systemic blood flow ratio of 1.5:1 or greater is present, progressive pulmonary hypertension can develop. Atrial arrhythmias are common, particularly in adulthood. If spontaneous closure does not occur in 1 year, surgical closure is required. Primary repair or patch closure is performed with low morbidity and mortality. Percutaneous interventional device closure has become an alternative in selected patients.

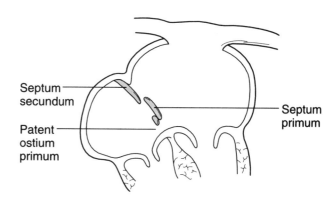

FIG. 4. Atrial septal defect.

Patent ductus arteriosus (PDA) accounts for up to 10% of all CHD (excluding premature infants). Shunt flow is dependent on size of the PDA and difference between pulmonary and systemic vascular resistance. Small PDAs are usually asymptomatic, whereas large PDAs present with symptoms of left to right shunts as previously described. Physical examination typically reveals a machine-like continuous murmur heard best at the upper left sternal border. Echocardiogram is performed to differentiate from other causes of continuous murmurs. In premature babies, closure of the PDA can be accomplished by infusing the prostaglandin inhibitor, indomethacin. Persistence of the PDA can result in prolonged mechanical ventilation secondary to pulmonary congestion and associated complications, e.g., necrotizing enterocolitis or intraventricular cerebral hemorrhage. A large PDA found in the asymptomatic infant will remain patent without surgical closure. Though successful use of interventional catheter closure has been reported in children, surgical closure of the patent ductus through a left mini-thoracotomy remains the standard of care.

Cyanotic Lesions

The pathology of tetralogy of Fallot (TOF) (Fig. 5) was originally described in 1672 but was made widely known in 1888 by Fallot. It accounts for 9% of all CHD. Classic anatomic pathology consists of pulmonary stenosis, a VSD with an overriding aorta, and right ventricular hypertrophy. Cyanosis and polycythemia vary with the degree of right to left shunt. Severe pulmonary stenosis or atresia causes intense cyanosis upon closure of the ductus arteriosus. With moderate pulmonary stenosis,

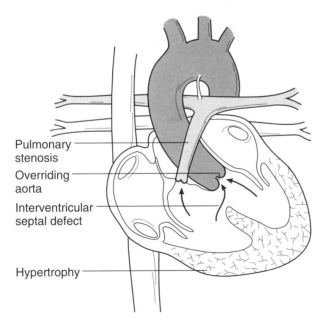

Pulmonary stenosis

Overriding aorta

Interventricular septal defect

Hypertrophy

FIG. 5. Tetralogy of Fallot.

deoxygenated blood enters the pulmonary circulation, and minimal cyanosis can be present at rest. However, with increased activity or pulmonary outflow tract dynamic obstruction, acute decompensation and hypoxia from increased shunt flow may occur, a so-called "tet spell." In cases of minimal pulmonary stenosis, a net left to right shunt may exist with only a minor degree of arterial desaturation, "pink tetralogy." Physical examination typically reveals a cyanotic infant with a palpable thrill about the precordium and an audible murmur along the left sternal border. Echocardiogram is an excellent noninvasive method of diagnosis, but cardiac catheterization may be required to determine the size of the pulmonary vasculature and coronary anatomy, and evaluate coexistent anomalies that could complicate surgical treatment. As expected, the natural history of TOF is not favorable. Only 50% of untreated cases survive beyond 2 years of age, with only an occasional patient maturing to adolescence. Immediate surgical correction, however, is not required, thanks in large part to intravenous prostaglandin analogs that maintain patency of the ductus arteriosus to maintain pulmonary blood flow during acute cyanosis. A palliative subclavian artery to pulmonary artery bypass to increase pulmonary blood flow in preparation for the definitive surgical therapy was originally described by Blalock and Taussig (the "Blalock-Taussig shunt") in 1945 and has since been modified with the use of an artificial conduit bypass. Much experience indicates that the corrective procedure can be performed with minimal morbidity at 3 months to 1 year of age. Permanent closure requires reconstruction of the pulmonary outflow tract and closure of the VSD to separate pulmonary and systemic circulation.

Transposition of the great vessels (TGV) is the most common cyanotic heart defect (Fig. 6), accounting for ~10% of all CHD. Inappropriate septation and migration of the truncus arteriosus in utero causes the aorta to originate from the right ventricle and the pulmonary trunk to arise from the left ventricle. Commonly associated cardiac anomalies include ASD, VSD, PDA, right-sided aortic arch, and subvalvular left ventricular outflow tract obstruction. Coexistent abnormal coronary artery anatomy is common as well. Cyanosis manifests early in the newborn and the degree of arterial oxygen desaturation is inversely related to the amount of mixing between systemic and pulmonary venous blood through bidirectional shunts. Fortunately, echocardiogram easily delineates the coronary anatomy and cardiac catheterization is rarely necessary. In 1966, Rashkind extended the use of catheterization by performing balloon atrial septostomy to increase "crossover" flow. This maneuver may stabilize intensely cyanotic infants and obviate emergent surgical intervention so that a thorough cardiac evaluation may be undertaken. In untreated cases, a 50% mortality within 2 months and 100% mortality at 1 year is commonly observed.

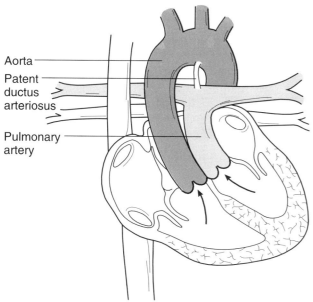

Aorta
Patent ductus arteriosus
Pulmonary artery

FIG. 6. Transposition of great vessels.

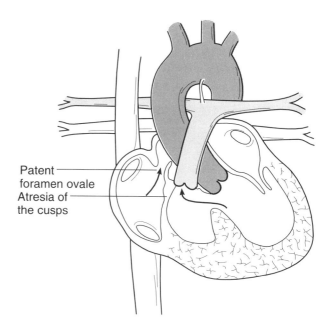

Patent foramen ovale
Atresia of the cusps

FIG. 7. Tricuspid atresia.

Surgical correction should be attempted as early as possible. Senning in 1959 ingeniously utilized atrial wall to construct autogenous "baffles" that directed reoxygenated blood to the right ventricle which pumped blood systemically. In 1963, Mustard constructed a similar baffle using pericardium. Studies comparing both procedures have shown similar results and short-term mortality rates; however, postoperative atrial arrhythmias and poor long-term hemodynamics of a right ventricular-driven arterial system were found unacceptable. The physiologically appropriate procedure involves reconnection of the pulmonary and aortic outflow tracts to the right and left ventricles, respectively. Mustard performed the so-called arterial switch operation in 1954. However, the procedure was temporarily abandoned due to disastrous results until 1975, when Jatene successfully performed an arterial switch with coronary artery reimplantation for TGV. The tremendous benefit of restoring left ventricular anatomy and avoidance of postoperative arrhythmias or right ventricular failure overshadows the slightly increased morbidity and mortality of the Jatene procedure when compared to the Mustard or Senning procedure. Currently, the Jatene procedure is the primary operation for simple transposition or transposition of the great arteries with a VSD and is usually performed within the first 2 weeks of life.

Tricuspid atresia (TA) (Fig. 7) is the third most common cyanotic CHD behind TOF and TGV. Absence of direct communication between the right atrium and right ventricle shunts all venous return through the atrial septum. The ASD is usually very wide with minimal resistance to flow. Clinical symptoms vary depending on the level of pulmonary blood flow. Congestive heart failure from volume overload on the left ventricle can occur. Echocardiography is an excellent noninvasive method of diagnosis. Early death is common, with only one out of three untreated cases surviving to 1 year of age. Because immediate corrective surgery for TA is not safe, a Blalock-Taussig shunt is performed to reverse cyanosis from decreased pulmonary blood flow. If pulmonary blood flow is excessive, pulmonary artery banding is performed. When a definitive procedure is finally considered, the presence of a hypoplastic right ventricle makes complete surgical reconstruction impossible. In 1971, Fontan concluded that a right ventricle is not necessary for pulmonary circulation and published results of a series of patients who underwent a procedure of diverting venous blood directly to the pulmonary artery bypassing the right ventricle. This procedure that bears his name has subsequently undergone multiple variations. A detailed discussion of each procedure is well beyond the scope of this review.

ACQUIRED CARDIAC DISEASE

Ischemic Heart Disease

Coronary artery disease (CAD) is the leading cause of death and disability in all industrialized nations. In the United States, it is estimated that 750,000 deaths attributed to ischemic heart disease occur annually. The economic burden of coronary disease exceeds $100 million per year. Although age-related mortality has declined over the past decade, the absolute incidence of ischemic heart disease has increased because of the increased population within the age group susceptible to CAD.

Anatomy

Left and right coronary arteries (LCA, RCA) originate from the ascending aorta (Fig. 8) and supply oxygen to different regions of myocardium. The RCA supplies blood to the sinus and atrioventricular nodes, and the majority of the right atrium and ventricle. In 80% of patients, the posterior descending artery of the posterior myocardial septum is the terminal branch of the RCA ("right dominant"). The LCA, or left main artery, bifurcates to the left anterior descending (LAD) and the circumflex arteries. The LAD and important tributaries, diagonal arteries, supply blood to the anterior aspect of the ventricular septum and the majority of the left ventricle. The circumflex artery and its tributaries, obtuse marginal arteries, deliver blood to the lateral and posterior left ventricle and in the minority of patients is the dominant artery of the posterior septum ("left dominant"). Normally, little variation in coronary artery anatomy and minimal collateral circulation exists.

Pathophysiology

Atherosclerosis within the lumen of the coronary arteries is the principal etiology behind ischemic heart disease. Diabetes mellitus, hypertension, hypercholesterolemia, and smoking predispose vessel intima to injury and development of atheroma. Hemodynamically critical stenosis occurs when lumen diameter is narrowed by 50% or when 75% of total lumen surface area is obstructed. Most atheromatous lesions are located in the proximal one-third to one-half of vessel segment most commonly in the left anterior descending artery followed by the RCA, circumflex artery, left main coronary artery, and right posterior descending artery.

Myocardial oxygen demand is dependent on heart rate, myocardial contractility, and systolic myocardial wall stress. Normal oxygen extraction of myocardium is already 75% at rest; therefore, increased blood flow must occur in response to increased oxygen demand. Compensatory vasodilation allows up to five times the resting blood flow to enter the coronary circulation. However, coronary artery stenosis prevents maximum vasodilation and limits blood flow during increased demand. Anaerobic metabolism and acute ischemia at the myocyte level predominates in this situation. Substernal chest pain, angina pectoris, is the hallmark presentation in three-fourths of patients with CAD and is the manifestation of the myocardium's exquisite sensitivity to ischemia. Patients describe a "pressure" or "tightness" in the chest that is usually short in duration and often accompanied by shortness of breath, nausea, diaphoresis, and numbness or pain in left shoulder, arm, neck, or jaw. It is important to recognize that atypical and even classic anginal type pain can be caused by pulmonary processes, esophageal disorders, or pericardial disease.

Fixed atheroma is well understood as the cause of stable or exertional angina in which a typical stress induces angina that is relieved by rest and/or sublingual nitroglycerin. In contrast, unstable angina is a pattern of chest pain that becomes unpredictable, difficult to control with usual therapy, and increases in frequency, duration, and intensity. A number of etiologies have been implicated in the development of unstable angina. Progressive atherosclerosis of a fixed lesion, fissuring, ulceration, or rupture of a plaque with superimposed thrombosis, platelet aggregation, and activation or finally vasospasm superimposed on occlusive lesions set the stage for a myocardial infarction event. Thus, unstable angina is also referred to as "preinfarction angina." Variant (Prinzmetal's) angina is less well understood but is thought to be

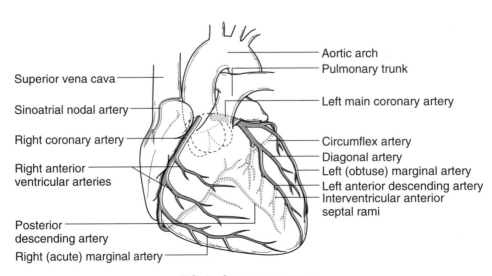

FIG. 8. Coronary anatomy.

caused by arterial spasm with or without an associated atheroma.

Acute Myocardial Infarction

Acute myocardial infarction describes myocardial necrosis secondary to ischemia. The size of infarction is dependent on the size of the coronary bed occluded, duration of occlusion, collateral supply, and metabolic demands of the myocardium at the time of infarction. Generally, two regions of infarct are described, subendocardial and transmural. The inner (subendocardial) myocardium is the most vulnerable to abnormalities of perfusion. Diffuse atherosclerosis that results in decreased oxygen delivery in the face of increased oxygen demand is the usual cause of subendocardial infarction. Conversely, transmural infarction is full thickness necrosis caused by occlusion of either a trunk or branch of a coronary artery.

Complications of Myocardial Infarction

Myocardial dysfunction can be both systolic and diastolic. Pump failure is seen when >30% of left ventricle has infarcted. In addition, because injured myocardium is less compliant, ventricular end-diastolic pressure increases. Significantly elevated left ventricular pressures may result in pulmonary edema. Similarly, elevated right ventricular pressures can result in hepatic congestion and peripheral edema. Mortality and morbidity generally parallel the extent of myocardial necrosis.

Ventricular septal rupture occurs in the setting of anterior wall or posterior septal infarction. A new onset holosystolic murmur and acute cardiogenic shock seen 3 to 5 days after infarction are common manifestations of the new VSD. Cardiac catheterization may be performed to temporarily occlude the VSD with an "umbrella"; however, the definitive treatment involves early surgical repair.

Papillary muscle rupture is a cause of early death in patients that have sustained an infarction with extensive necrosis of interventricular septum. It may occur simultaneously with a VSD and is manifested by sudden appearance of CHF and dyspnea, chest pain, and a loud apical systolic murmur secondary to mitral regurgitation. Treatment must focus on increasing forward flow by increasing myocardial contractility and decreasing systemic vascular resistance prior to urgent valve replacement.

Left ventricular rupture is the principal cause of early death in 10% of patients suffering myocardial infarction from acute occlusion of the left coronary system. It occurs 3 to 7 days postinfarction, typically in elderly females, especially those with hypertension. Severe chest pain without evidence of new infarction and cardiac tamponade demand immediate investigation. Pericardiocen-

tesis or echocardiogram will reveal tamponade but may waste precious time. Definitive treatment involves immediate surgical repair via median sternotomy.

Left ventricular aneurysms are thin outpouchings of infarcted myocardium. In contrast to ventricular rupture, it develops weeks to months after infarction and rarely ruptures. Hemodynamic insufficiency, mural thrombus, and ventricular arrhythmias secondary to reentry phenomenon are common sequelae. Surgical excision of the aneurysm is reserved for patients exhibiting thromboembolism or hemodynamic compromise.

Invasive Treatment Options for Ischemic Heart Disease

Despite the fact that patients with CAD are generally older, with comorbid medical problems, and compromised myocardial reserve, it is encouraging that these same patients will continue to see decreased symptoms and improved survival from ischemic heart disease. This is undoubtedly due to tremendous advances in medical therapy and the development of invasive therapy for CAD.

Percutaneous Transluminal Coronary Angioplasty

First performed in 1978 by Gruntzig, percutaneous transluminal coronary angioplasty (PTCA) has supplemented therapy available for CAD. A balloon tipped catheter is introduced into the coronary arterial system and placed within the atheromatous luminal stenosis using fluoroscopic guidance. Inflation of the balloon induces barotrauma that cracks and disrupts atherosclerotic plaque. Success is accomplished when the luminal diameter is >50%. Refractory or recurrent lesions may require intraluminal stenting or laser recanalization.

Coronary Artery Bypass Grafting

Coronary artery bypass grafting (CABG) dates back to 1910, when Alex Carrel performed the first experimental coronary bypass using a free carotid artery graft from the descending aorta to the LCA. The understanding of cardiopulmonary bypass detailed by Gibbon and Kirklin allowed Sabiston to perform the first clinical bypass operation in 1962 using saphenous vein from the ascending aorta to RCA. Progress was slow until Favaloro et al., in 1967, at the Cleveland Clinic published his series of patients who underwent successful aortocoronary bypass using saphenous vein.

CABG is a palliative anatomic treatment for the sequela of metabolic disease. The procedure involves bypassing beyond all significant luminal stenosis utilizing an autogenous vascular conduit from the proximal ascending aorta to distal coronary vessel. From the beginning, saphenous veins were used as the grafting conduit of choice. Since the early 1980s, however, both left and right internal mammary arteries (IMA) are being used with increasing frequency for bypass of the left and right coronary systems. Short-term patency rates approaching 90% patency in the first year are comparable between saphenous vein and IMA grafts. However, the long-term patency of the IMA graft is far superior, approaching 90% at 10 years, compared to the saphenous vein graft patency of 50% at 5 years. In select patient populations, bilateral IMA grafting has been employed with success but slightly increases the incidence of postoperative sternal infection. Currently, radial artery and gastroepiploic artery conduits are being studied, but as yet no long-term data are conclusive.

All cardiac surgical patients require intensive care unit (ICU) management for postoperative hemodynamic and respiratory monitoring. Output from mediastinal tubes and thoracostomy tubes are monitored every half hour after arrival in the ICU to evaluate for inadequate hemostasis. Atrial arrhythmias are common but can be successfully treated usually with medication alone. Clinical pathways direct standard postoperative management in an effort to facilitate transfer of stable patients out of the ICU. Unnecessary laboratory tests and radiographs are eliminated to decrease cost. Length of hospital stay after open heart surgery has been decreased, with no adverse effect on outcome.

Complications of Cardiopulmonary Bypass

The enormous advantage that cardiopulmonary bypass affords the patient undergoing cardiac surgery is only minimally tarnished by infrequent complications. A complete understanding of the pathophysiology of gastrointestinal bleeding, perforated duodenal ulcer, intestinal ischemia, pancreatitis, and acute cholecystitis following CPB is incomplete. What is clear is the occurrence of an intense inflammatory reaction stemming from a cascade of neurohumoral events in patients undergoing CPB. This in combination with the ischemia/reperfusion phenomenon has been implicated as the causes of complications after CPB. Aortic cross-clamping, especially in the presence of a calcified proximal aorta, can produce thromboembolism to the systemic vascular system. Rarely, the femoral artery is cannulated for CPB access and femoral artery rupture, pseudoaneurysm formation, and rarely, acute lower limb ischemia artery have been reported. Fortunately these complications are rare but should be remembered so immediate action is not delayed.

Several studies have compared PTCA to bypass surgery. PTCA is currently used widely for single-vessel disease and in select subgroups of patients with multives-

sel disease. Patients experience relief of angina after PTCA, cardiac and noncardiac morbidity are less than that of surgery, and an operation can be avoided, at least over the short term. However, restenosis after PTCA occurred in up to one-third of patients as quickly as 3 months post-PTCA, and more reinterventions in the form of repeat PTCA were required. A significant percentage of patients also had persistent or recurrent angina requiring antianginal medication during a 3-year follow-up period. Long-term event-free survival after PTCA appears inferior to that after surgery, particularly in the group of patients with multivessel disease. At the present time, there is agreement that bypass surgery improves short- and long-term survival in patients with left main disease, multivessel disease with involvement of the proximal LAD, or triple-vessel stenosis with or without left ventricular dysfunction. Over half of patients will experience complete relief from angina without medication after bypass and will require no further intervention. However, the perioperative morbidity and mortality are higher, and as expected the length of hospital stay is longer in surgical patients. Surgical revascularization, unfortunately, has not been shown to resolve arrhythmias that existed prior to operation.

The treatment goals of revascularization have to be individualized for each patient. The risks of procedures must be balanced against expected outcomes and future potential of reintervention. Consider that the annual risk of lethal myocardial infarctions is 11% for left main disease and 3% for each of the major coronary arteries so that the annual risk for single-vessel disease is 3%, whereas that for triple-vessel disease is 9%. Angioplasty is successful at revascularizing single vessel disease. The use of PTCA in subgroups of patients with multivessel disease but without ventricular dysfunction has been successful at reestablishing coronary circulation over the short term. Infrequently, cardiac and vascular complications occur secondary to cardiac catheterization, including, but not limited to, coronary artery dissection, thrombosis or rupture, and femoral artery pseudoaneurysm or hematoma. Angioplasty is contraindicated in the treatment of left main disease; it has limited treatment value for patients with multivessel disease involving the proximal LAD or three or more vessel disease with impaired ventricular function. Literature supports CABG as the therapy of choice in these situations because it prolongs survival. Mortality risk of patients with normal left ventricular function undergoing CABG is <2%. The complications and deaths in patients with moderate and severe ventricular dysfunction are sequentially higher. For patients with single vessel or multi-vessel disease (not involving the proximal LAD artery) and normal left ventricular function, the choice of medical therapy, angioplasty, or bypass grafting can and should be individualized.

Infective Endocarditis

Despite an increased understanding, infective endocarditis (IE) remains one of the most serious treatable infectious diseases and continues to have a significant mortality. Native valvular endocarditis usually requires preexisting valve lesions. Rheumatic disease, CHD, and mitral valve prolapse are common predisposing factors. Diabetes mellitus may increase susceptibility to IE, especially in elderly patients with underlying valvular pathology. Those who use illicit intravenous drugs are particularly prone to endocarditis of the pulmonary and tricuspid valves. The majority of these patients, interestingly, do not have underlying valve lesions. Infection of a prosthetic valve accounts for 5% to 15% of all cases.

High-velocity jetstream blood flow, particularly if through a narrow orifice, causes denuding of the endothelial surface. Upon this denuded endothelium, clumps of fibrin and platelets form the necessary prerequisite nonbacterial thrombotic endocarditis (NBTE). Any bacteremia could then infect the NBTE and result in friable vegetations. Dental procedures, lung and skin infections, gastrointestinal procedures, intravenous drug use, and infected chronic indwelling venous catheters are all common predisposing factors to bacteremia necessary to infect the NBTE. Clinical manifestations of IE range from persistent fever and malaise to septic shock and can result in hemodynamic instability from acute valvular incompetence. Septic emboli to the skin, digits, and conjunctiva as well as to end organs such as the brain, spleen, and kidney are not uncommon. The critical diagnostic finding in IE is bacteremia or fungemia, particularly if found in multiple blood samples. Indiscriminate use of intravenous antibiotics, however, may obscure this finding.

Treatment involves aggressive administration of intravenous antibiotics directed at bacteria isolated from blood cultures. In the absence of prosthetic devices, resolution is usually expected over a 6- to 10-week course of antibiotics. Hemodynamic instability from valvular incompetence should be managed aggressively with pharmacologic agents to enhance forward flow and augment myocardial contractility. Stabilizing the cardiovascular system will reduce perioperative mortality and morbidity. Absolute indications for operations include refractory heart failure related to valve dysfunction, myocardial or valvular abscess with His bundle disease or unstable prosthetic valve. Relative indications for operative therapy include multiple embolic episodes (either systemic or pulmonary), persistently positive blood cultures, or systemic fungal infection, or relapses in infection. When valves are replaced in the face of acute infection, success can be achieved but with immediate perioperative risk and an increased incidence of prosthetic valve reinfection.

Valvular Disease

Cardiac valves are endothelial-lined fibrous cusps that are interposed between the atrial and ventricular cardiac chambers (mitral and tricuspid valves) and between the ventricular cardiac chambers and aortic or pulmonary outflow tracts (aortic and pulmonary valves). Valves ensure forward flow of blood through the cardiac chambers. Principal etiologies of valvular disease are congenital heart defects and rheumatic carditis. Rheumatic disease predominantly affects the mitral valve, followed by the aortic valve, tricuspid valve, and pulmonic valve.

Mechanical prostheses such as "flap-disc" devices as well as devices made from porcine tissue or homograft are used for valve replacement. Mechanical valves can last indefinitely but have inherent properties that induce erythrocyte destruction and thrombosis, requiring prophylactic therapy for the lifetime of the graft. Bioprosthesis, although not as destructive to blood cells, frequently requires replacement as early as 7 to 10 years because of degenerative changes.

Mitral Valve Disease

Mitral valve stenosis is, in most cases, the sequelae of rheumatic carditis. Infrequently, congenital valve disease and collagen vascular disorders such as systemic lupus erythematosus and rheumatoid arthritis contribute to the pathogenesis of mitral valve obstruction. Commisures of the valve cusps fuse resulting in a fish mouth or buttonhole orifice. Reduction of valve area to 2 cm^2 requires increased left atrial pressure to maintain sufficient flow but causes virtually no clinical symptoms. A valve area of $\leq$1 cm^2 is critical stenosis. The transvalvular pressure gradient at that point can approach 20 mm Hg. Tachycardia in the presence of critical mitral valve stenosis results in congestive heart failure because decreased diastolic filling time of the left ventricle decreases cardiac output. Pulmonary venous hypertension caused by increased left atrial pressure can result in pulmonary edema and hemoptysis. Thromboembolism secondary to atrial mural thrombi can occur. A dilated left atrium of chronic mitral stenosis predisposes to electrical impulse reentry and atrial fibrillation. Osler's syndrome describes hoarseness secondary to left atrial compression of the left recurrent laryngeal nerve. Fatigue and resting dyspnea are terminal manifestations of chronic venous hypertension and cardiac insufficiency secondary to mitral stenosis. Physical examination typically reveals an opening snap with diastolic rumble. Electrocardiogram may reveal a bifid P wave or frank atrial fibrillation. Chest radiograph may demonstrate left atrial enlargement. Once symptoms have developed, the patient should be considered for either valve repair (valvulotomy) or valve replacement.

In the 1920s, digital commissurotomy and instrument performed valvulotomy were the standard surgical treatment for stenosis. The procedures were quick and simple with minimal blood loss and had excellent short-term outcome. Unfortunately, these "blind" procedures had inferior long-term results, including recurrent stenosis or regurgitation from excessive commissurotomy. Open commissurotomy became favorable in the mid-1950s because it was thought that direct visualization of the mitral valve would prevent excessive commissurotomy and thromboembolism that can occur as a result of valve manipulation. However, it was more costly, and blood loss was at times excessive. A recent trial (Reyes et al.) studied minimally invasive interventional therapy, which may provide a therapeutic alternative especially in patients with prohibitive operative risk. Long-term follow-up for this procedure has not been attained. Current data support valve replacement as the standard of care that has the best long-term results with regard to valve patency and return of cardiac function.

Mitral valve regurgitation results from dilation of the mitral ring, damage to papillary muscle, and redundant mitral valve apparatus (prolapse). In acute regurgitation, left heart failure symptoms quickly predominate. In the setting of chronic regurgitation, the left atrium through hypertrophy and increased diameter size helps maintain hemodynamic stability. Physical examination reveals a pansystolic murmur. Medical management, especially in the acute setting, is directed toward increasing myocardial contractility, increasing forward flow via peripheral vasodilation, and decreasing regurgitant flow through the cardiac chambers. Valve replacement is required when cardiovascular workload exceeds compensatory ability of the heart.

Aortic Valve Disease

Aortic stenosis occurs in ~0.9% to 2.0% of the general population. Pancarditis from rheumatic fever is responsible for the majority of cases worldwide. In the United States, calcification of a bicuspid valve outnumbers rheumatic carditis as the etiology behind aortic stenosis. In the pathogenesis of disease, thickened valve cusps progressively fuse at the commisures. Virtually all patients with rheumatic aortic valve disease have microscopic or gross involvement of the mitral valve as well. Patients with aortic stenosis secondary to childhood rheumatic carditis present in the fourth to fifth decades of life.

Nonrheumatic aortic stenosis is usually superimposed on a congenital bicuspid aortic valve. A variable progression of disease has been noted. Some patients have slow and insidious wear and tear sclerosis upon a bicuspid valve, Monckeberg's aortic sclerosis, which typically presents in the seventh decade of life. Not surprisingly, in this patient population, coexistent arteriosclerosis of coronary vessels is common. A small subgroup of patients with congenital bicuspid aortic valves exhibit rapid calcific stenosis before the age of fifteen.

Aortic stenosis causes left ventricular outflow tract obstruction. At a valve area of 1.0 cm², patients exhibit symptoms consistent with left heart failure. At 0.7 cm², critical stenosis, transvalvular pressure gradients can exceed 100 mm Hg. Left ventricular hypertrophy combined with increased left ventricular wall stress results in increased myocardial oxygen demand that can exceed oxygen delivery and result in angina regardless of the presence or absence of coronary atherosclerosis. When critical stenosis limits cerebral perfusion, syncope becomes a clinical symptom. Finally, when myocardial contractility becomes insufficient to overcome outflow tract obstruction, dilated cardiac failure develops. Congestive heart failure may be the first presentation in a child. Other manifestations of aortic stenosis include cerebral embolism and hemolytic anemia. IE can develop upon deformed valves. Sudden death due to ventricular tachyarrythmias occurs in up to 20% of patients with severe aortic stenosis.

Physical examination reveals a loud crescendo-decrescendo murmur heard over the right upper sternal border that is transmitted to the carotid areas bilaterally. Electrocardiography demonstrates a pattern of left ventricular hypertrophy. Chest radiograph is helpful only at end-stage disease when cardiomegaly and pulmonary edema may be found. Echocardiography will show the turbulent flow through the valve. Cardiac catheterization is recommended in patients with a history of angina pectoris, men older than 35 years of age, and women who are postmenopausal because of the high incidence of concomitant CAD.

The natural history of aortic stenosis is insidious with a rapid decompensation. In the adult, symptoms consistently predict mortality (Table 1). Valvotomy is reserved for pediatric patients to postpone valve replacement and potentially prevent the necessity for multiple operations. In adults, valve replacement and CABG, if appropriate, are indicated when valvular stenosis exists and symptoms are only attributable to left ventricular outflow tract obstruction. Conversely, in asymptomatic patients with valve area of ≤0.7 cm², valve replacement is mandated. Though decreased ventricular function increases perioperative risk, it does not preclude patients from operation because ventricular function may actually improve with valve replacement. For elective procedures, exhaustive efforts should be undertaken to eradicate all potential foci

TABLE 1. *Mean survival with symptoms from aortic stenosis*

	Angina	Syncope	Heart failure
Mean survival	5 years	2–3 years	12–18 months

of overt or occult infection. In particular, dentition must be cleaned and infected teeth extracted as well as skin lesions or subcutaneous abscesses resolved prior to any valve replacement. Mean 5-year survival after operation approaches 75% and is generally better if no ventricular dysfunction exists.

Aortic regurgitation results predominantly from rheumatic carditis and IE. Infrequently, ascending aortic aneurysms and connective disorders involving the aortic arch, e.g., Marfan's syndrome, can dilate the valve annulus causing aortic insufficiency (AI). Regurgitant flow from aorta to left ventricle occurs during diastole and is proportional to the size of the orifice, the pressure gradient between systemic vascular resistance and left ventricle, and the duration of diastole. In acute AI, cardiac failure develops rapidly because the left ventricle is unable to accommodate a sudden increase in end diastolic left ventricular volume. With chronic regurgitation, most patients remain compensated for long periods by left ventricular dilation and decreased systemic vascular resistance. Tachycardia develops to decrease duration of diastole. In patients with long-standing disease, physical examination detects a displaced cardiac impulse. A blowing early diastolic murmur is heard best along left sternal border. Additional aspects of physical examination of patients with AI have been described. Corrigan's pulse is a rapid distention followed by quick collapse in the carotid or radial artery during systole. Traube's sign describes "pistol shot" sounds heard over the femoral artery area. Pulsatile flow visible at the capillary level of the digits is Quincke's sign. An Austin-Flint murmur is a diastolic murmur caused by regurgitant flow on an open mitral valve leaflet.

With acute insufficiency, invasive monitoring along with pharmacological enhancement of contractility and lowering of systemic vascular resistance (SVR) facilitates forward flow blood circulation. After cardiovascular stabilization, elective aortic valve replacement can be performed. In chronic disease, valve replacement should be attempted before the left ventricle has become dysfunctional, although severely diminished contractile function (as with aortic stenosis) should not prevent valve replacement.

Tricuspid Valve Disease

As with other valvular pathologic conditions, rheumatic fever is the primary cause of tricuspid stenosis and is usually detected through evaluation of mitral or aortic valve disease. Most patients are asymptomatic; some can manifest right heart failure symptoms, including severe peripheral edema, hepatomegaly with liver dysfunction, and ascites. Surgical treatment should be performed when symptoms are present or when operative therapy for coexistent mitral or aortic valve surgery is planned. Valvuloplasty rather than valve replacement is

performed in most cases with satisfactory results. Tricuspid regurgitation, on the other hand, is almost always due to right ventricular dilation. Less commonly, tricuspid insufficiency can result from endocarditis from intravenous drug abuse or chronic indwelling central venous catheters. Most patients with tricuspid regurgitation but without pulmonary hypertension do not require surgical intervention. Fluid restriction and diuresis alleviates symptoms secondary to elevated central venous pressure. When operative management is required, valvuloplasty is usually successful. With concomitant left heart valve lesions, a complete multivalve procedure should be considered if patient clinical status is satisfactory.

Pulmonary Valve Disease

Isolated pulmonary valvular disease is exceedingly rare. Most pathological states are associated with congenital disease, i.e., TOF. Carcinoid plaques, though exceedingly rare, have a predilection for pulmonary valve leaflets. Pulmonary regurgitation is invariably a feature of chronic pulmonary hypertension and less commonly due to pulmonary artery dilation from idiopathic or collagen vascular disease, i.e., Marfan's syndrome. The Graham-Steell murmur is a decrescendo diastolic murmur heard at the third rib interspace about the left sternal border. Management of pulmonary valve disease must focus on the principal cause of the pathophysiology. In rare circumstances of intractable right heart failure secondary to isolated pulmonary stenosis or regurgitation, valve replacement should be performed.

PERICARDIUM

Parietal pericardium is a fibroserosal sac within the mediastinum that contains the heart and great vessels. The visceral pericardium envelopes the heart. Arterial supply and venous drainage come from nutrient vessels of the internal mammary vascular complex. Lymph drains to the tracheobronchial lymph node basin.

A small amount of clear pericardial fluid, plasma ultrafiltrate, bathes the heart within the pericardial sac. The accumulation of excess fluid within the pericardium defines a pericardial effusion. A vast number of causes can be classified as infectious, inflammatory, malignancy, or systemic disease. Symptoms of a pericardial effusion relate to fluid pressure on the cardiac chambers within a confined space.

Pericarditis

Pericarditis describes many inflammatory or infectious processes that can affect the pericardium and result in a pericardial effusion. Uremic "fibrinous" pericarditis is a complication of renal failure that can occur at all levels of azotemia. Purulent pericarditis, commonly from Staphylococcus or Hemophilus, can result from direct contamination or contiguous spread of a pneumonic process. Tuberculous pericarditis develops in a similar fashion. Viral pericarditis is caused predominantly by the Coxsackie A and B and Influenza A and B viruses. Neoplastic pericarditis results from infiltration of malignant cells upon the pericardium, causing an intense inflammatory reaction and exudative effusion containing malignant cells. Dressler's syndrome is pericarditis that develops usually 1 week but as long as 6 months after a myocardial infarction. Similarly, postpericardiotomy syndrome describes an inflammatory response of fever, chest pain, and friction rub without leukocytosis, wound infection, or other source of infection after undergoing cardiac surgery. Constrictive pericarditis refers to the fibrous encasement around the heart due to the secondary scar following the inflammatory reaction. Kussmaul's sign refers to the paradoxical jugular venous distention during inspiration.

What is common to all types of pericarditis is the presence of chest pain. Sometimes it is difficult to distinguish pericarditis from myocardial ischemia. Pain secondary to pericarditis, radiates to the back, is exacerbated by breathing and lying supine, and is relieved by sitting up and leaning forward. A pericardial friction rub is commonly heard on auscultation of the precordium. Fever may be present. Electrocardiography in the acute stage reveals diffuse ST segment elevation especially in the anterior leads. Echocardiography easily visualizes the pericardial effusion.

In addition to treating the principal cause of the pericarditis, drainage via either needle aspiration or pericardiotomy (pericardial "window") is performed. Indomethacin or other nonsteroidal antiinflammatory drugs usually achieve symptomatic relief in Dressler's syndrome and postpericardiotomy syndrome. A corticosteroid taper schedule can be prescribed for refractory cases. Bacterial or fungal pericarditis is treated with intravenous antibiotics. Tuberculous pericarditis is treated with antituberculosis medications. Pericardiectomy for constrictive pericarditis is usually necessary to "release" the heart and reestablish cardiovascular integrity.

Cardiac Tamponade

Symptoms present from a pericardial effusion are related to the amount of fluid and the rate at which the effusion developed. A slowly amassing collection of 1 L can be asymptomatic; however, a 100-cc collection that develops rapidly usually results in cardiovascular collapse. Cardiac tamponade describes any amount of pericardial fluid that causes cardiac insufficieny by compressing the heart. The classic findings of hypotension, jugular venous distention, and distant heart sounds, described by

Beck, are seen in their entirety in only one-third of cases. A chest radiograph demonstrates a water bottle configuration of the cardiac silhouette in large effusions. Echocardiography is fast and noninvasive, and accurately shows the effusion. Cardiovascular collapse develops because of impaired diastolic ventricular filling. Due to low pressure within the right heart system, the right atrium and ventricle are the first cardiac chambers to become compromised. Pressure equilibration occurs in eventually all cardiac chambers when the patient's hemodynamic status has become severely compromised. Pericardiocentesis should be performed only in patients in extremis by sterilely inserting a needle in the left subxiphoid area aiming for the ipsilateral shoulder. Complications of this procedure include myocardial puncture, coronary artery laceration, and pneumothorax. An emergent subxiphoid pericardial window is the definitive procedure of choice.

CARDIAC NEOPLASMS

Metastatic tumors are the most common neoplasm of the heart. The incidence of primary neoplasms of the heart is <0.5%. Most of these tumors are benign and have an excellent long-term result after treatment. Primary malignant tumors are much less frequent and have a poor prognosis after diagnosis is made. The majority of malignancies are found in adults. Echocardiography has replaced cardiac angiography as the diagnostic standard. High-resolution computed tomography scan can evaluate associated extracardiac mediastinal pathology.

Myxomas are the most common type of benign cardiac tumor in adults and occur with greatest frequency in the third to sixth decades of life. They are derived from stem cells of the subendocardium and develop as polypoid endocardial growths that project into the cardiac chamber. Although multiple tumors are possible, isolated myxomas predominate and are located in the left atrium. Malignant degeneration has been reported but is exceedingly rare. Constitutional symptoms of fever, malaise, and arthralgias are frequently present. It is thought that these symptoms are induced by an autoimmune reaction to the tumor. A left atrial tumor can exert a "ball valve" effect, which can mimic mitral stenosis. Systemic embolus occurs in up to a third of patients, primarily to the cerebrovascular system and infrequently to the peripheral arterial system or coronary arteries. The disease entity should be considered in young patients exhibiting sinus rhythm with embolic phenomenon. Likewise, when a grey gelatinous friable mass is embolectomized, it should be sent immediately to the laboratory for intraoperative tissue diagnosis. Surgical therapy is successful in the vast majority of patients if treated in a timely fashion. Because 10% of patients awaiting surgery will suffer a stroke, excision should be undertaken early. A median sternotomy is performed, and cardiopulmonary bypass is used for resection of tumor with a margin of normal endocardium.

Rhabdomyomas are the most common benign cardiac tumor in children. They are commonly associated with tuberous sclerosis that involves the central nervous system. Although the majority of rhabdomyomas eventually regress, fatal cardiac arrhythmias may intervene. Cardiac catheterization assisted–ablation of arrythmogenic foci has been performed with satisfactory results.

Sarcomas represent all malignant tumors of the heart and are extremely rare. Angiosarcomas comprise the majority of cases. Less common types include rhabdomyosarcoma, fibrosarcoma, and malignant fibrous histiocytoma. Because of the aggressive nature of the tumor, myocardial invasion leads to progressive and refractory congestive heart failure. Infrequently, a malignant pericardial effusion can result. Diagnosis is made by endovascular or open biopsy. Virtually all cases are diagnosed after distant metastasis has occurred, and no surgical therapy can be offered. Adjuvant therapy is consistently unsuccessful.

SUMMARY

It is interesting to review the rapid development of cardiac surgery. In a relatively short period of time, cardiac surgery emerged due to technological developments and advances in other medical specialties. Surgical procedures for acquired heart disease are being performed on older patients with advanced comorbid medical conditions but with better clinical results, thanks in large part to expanded understanding of cardiopulmonary bypass, myocardial protection, and intraoperative anesthesia management. Just as important is the aggressive medical management of acquired cardiac disease that has permitted patients with previously inoperable disease to undergo complex operations with improved survival. Without a doubt, cardiac catheterization and PTCA have tremendous diagnostic and therapeutic value. Neonatologists confidently stabilize the newborn with cyanotic congenital heart defects to allow complete evaluation and resuscitation before corrective or palliative surgery is performed. The future of cardiac surgery points toward increased use of advanced cardiac support for end-stage disease in preparation for cardiac transplantation and further understanding of cardiopulmonary bypass to eliminate some infrequent complications and further decrease morbidity of cardiac surgery.

STUDY QUESTIONS

1. What determines the shunt volume across an ASD, a VSD, and a PDA?
2. Trace the development of irreversible pulmonary hypertension secondary to chronic left to right shunting.
3. Describe the pathophysiology behind ischemic atherosclerotic heart disease.
4. Discuss advantages and disadvantages of the invasive treatment options for ischemic heart disease.
5. Distinguish the clinical differences between acute and chronic valvular disease. Use some examples.

SUGGESTED READING

Agathos EA, Starr A, eds. Aortic valve replacement. *Curr Probl Surg* 1993;30.

Agathos EA, Starr A, eds. Mitral valve replacement. *Curr Probl Surg* 1993;30:485–592.

Braunwald E, ed. *Heart disease.* 4th ed. Philadelphia: Saunders, 1992.

Cotran R, Kumar V, Robbins S. *Pathologic basis of disease.* 4th ed. Philadelphia: Saunders, 1989.

Kirklin J, Barrat-Boyes B, eds. *Cardiac surgery.* New York: Churchill-Livingstone, 1986.

Lytle BW, Cosgrove DM, eds. Coronary artery bypass surgery. *Curr Probl Surg* 1992;29:737–807.

Reyes VP, Rasu BS, Wynne J, Stephenson LW, et al. TUKI, 29. Percutaneous balloon valvuloplasty composed with open surgical commissurotomy for mitral stenosis. *N Eng J Med* 1994;331:961–967.

Sabiston D, Spencer F, eds. *Surgery of the chest.* 5th ed. Philadelphia: Saunders, 1990.

CHAPTER 21

Trauma Surgery

Nicholas Namias, Tammy Kopelman, and Larry C. Martin

Traumatic injury accounts for significant morbidity and mortality worldwide. Until recently, is was the leading cause of death among young adults in the United States. The financial costs of health care provided for victims of traumatic injury as well as rehabilitation for patients who have sustained permanent disability as a result of trauma are staggering. Unfortunately, individuals of all age groups, all socioeconomic classes, and all ethnic races may one day sustain devastating injury.

The "golden hour" of trauma refers to the critical time after injury during which diagnosis and treatment must be initiated to render a positive effect on patient outcome. It should be the goal of the medical student to understand the pathophysiology of various injuries. Additionally, by participating in a trauma surgery clerkship, students should learn the principles of patient evaluation and initial resuscitation during the "golden hour" of trauma. This information is useful not only for the student with aspirations for a career in surgery but for all physicians who can expect to be consulted one day to assist in the care of a trauma patient.

UNIVERSAL PRECAUTIONS

Although television and cinema have dramatized the glamour of trauma and emergency medicine, one must never forget the risks of providing health care, especially in trauma surgery. A high proportion of patients seen in emergency rooms carry hepatitis, human immunodeficiency virus (HIV), or other communicable diseases. Therefore, adherence to universal precautions is mandatory, particularly in this setting. You must maintain the protective barriers between you and the patient, e.g., eye shields, gloves, gown, mask, and handwashing after each patient contact.

PRIMARY SURVEY AND RESUSCITATION

The "ABCs"

Patient **a**irway, **b**reathing, and **c**irculation are the cornerstones of the care of the trauma patient and comprise the primary survey. If the **a**irway is not appreciated to be patent or the potential loss of airway patency is anticipated, aggressive efforts to secure the airway must be undertaken. The mouth and oropharynx must be cleared of blood, vomitus, dental prostheses, and any other foreign bodies. Patients with decreased mental status may lack the ability to maintain a patent airway. Using the chin lift or jaw thrust maneuvers may preserve airway patency until which time endotracheal intubation or cricothyroidotomy can be performed. Clinicians must recognize that if the mechanism of injury could have caused a cervical spine injury these maneuvers must be performed with in-line cervical spine traction. If an orotracheal airway is to be placed, the anterior portion of the cervical collar is removed and in-line traction delivered to avoid extending a possibly injured cervical spine. Absent spontaneous respirations necessitates assistance with **b**reathing via endotracheal intubation and mechanical ventilator. Patient survival is predicated upon adequate ventilation; without these necessities, further intervention or therapy is meaningless.

After ensuring "**a**" and "**b**," adequate **c**irculating volume must be insured. Two large-bore (18-gauge) peripheral intravenous catheters provide the best vascular access for fluid infusion in the trauma patient. Because flow resistance is directly proportional to length of the catheters and inversely proportional to the radius, fluid infusion through a long small-gauge venous catheter is inadequate for the trauma patient. Standard resuscitation fluid is crystalloid solution.

TABLE 1. *Clinical estimation of patient fluid and blood losses*

	Class I	Class II	Class III	Class IV
Blood loss (cc)	Up to 750	750–1,500	1,500–2,000	>2,000
Blood loss (% blood volume)	Up to 15%	15–30%	30–40%	>40%
Pulse rate	<100	>100	>120	>140
Blood pressure	Normal	Normal	Decreased	Decreased
Pulse pressure (mm Hg)	Normal or increased	Decreased	Decreased	Decreased
Respiratory rate (breaths/min)	14–20	20–30	30–40	>35
Urine output (cc/hr)	>30	20–30	5–15	Negligible
Mental status	Slightly anxious	Mildly anxious	Anxious and confused	Confused and lethargic
Fluid replacement requirement	Crystalloid	Crystalloid	Crystalloid and blood	Crystalloid and blood

Adapted from American College of Surgeons. *Instructor manual for advanced trauma life support.* 5th ed. Chicago: American College of Surgeons, 1993.

With few exceptions, hemodynamic instability in the trauma patient is hemorrhage until proven otherwise. Shock is succinctly defined as inadequate blood and oxygen delivery to the tissues to match the physiologic oxygen demand (Table 1). Loss of up to 15% of circulating blood volume (class I hemorrhage) is well compensated in normal individuals with no change in blood pressure and mild tachycardia. Loss of 15% to 30% of blood volume (class II hemorrhage) is reflected by oliguria (<30 cc/hr), tachypnea (respiratory rate of 20 to 30 breaths/min), tachycardia, decreased pulse pressure, and anxiety. Systolic blood pressure in class II hemorrhage, however, remains normal. Loss of >30% to 40% circulating blood volume (class III hemorrhage) is reflected by obvious clinical signs. Patients have a decrease in blood pressure and marked tachycardia. Class III hemorrhage also leads to a significant change in mental status. Blood loss of >40% of circulating volume (class IV hemorrhage) is an immediately life-threatening situation. Patients present with markedly decreased mental status, and the skin is cold and pale. Blood pressure is extremely low with obvious tachycardia. Urine output is negligible.

Fluid bolus infusion aids in determining the clinical severity of shock. For example, a prompt and lasting response to a fluid bolus suggests that the patient was hypovolemic due to hemorrhage that has since stopped. A transient response may be a sign that there is ongoing hemorrhage, and no objective response indicates severe shock most likely requiring surgical control. Blood products are usually given in class III or IV hemorrhage to combat shock, the deficit in oxygen-carrying capacity. Direct pressure on visible bleeding or simple suture of lacerations may quickly provide the necessary hemorrhage control. Recognize, however, that if indications for surgical intervention exist (as will be discussed shortly), further blood infusion should take place in the operating room rather than in the resuscitation room. Current research in the field of resuscitation includes treatment with small volumes of hypertonic saline. The consensus on the outcome of this research remains to be seen.

"D and E"

Neurologic assessment (**d**isability) and "head-to-toe" patient **e**xposure follow the ABCs. Initial neurologic assessment should document the patient's Glasgow Coma Scale (GCS), pupillary size and response, and a cursory motor and sensory examination for signs of focal neurologic injury. GCS (Table 2) serves as a standard method of evaluating mental status among the physicians and nurses, and allows for assessment of deterioration or improvement during the course of treatment. Similarly, documentation of baseline strength and sensation in all extremities is important because changes over time may indicate an underlying neurologic injury. Removal of all clothing and "log rolling" (to maintain spinal immobilization) permit vital examination of "every square inch" of the body surface. The perineum and cleft of buttock are but a few places that have hidden wounds from otherwise careful clinicians.

SECONDARY SURVEY AND DEFINITIVE TREATMENT

While maintaining vigilance over the "a,b,c's," the secondary survey and definitive therapy can proceed. As in

TABLE 2. *Glasgow Coma Scale*

Points	Eye opening	Verbal	Motor
6	—	—	Obeys commands
5	—	Oriented	Localizes pain
4	Spontaneous	Confused	Withdraws from pain
3	To command	Inappropriate	Flexor tone
2	To pain	Incomprehensible	Extensor tone
1	None	None	None

Mortality associated with Glasgow Coma Scale: 13–15, rare; 9–12, ~12%; 3–5, 60–70%.

all other specialties of medicine, patient evaluation begins with a detailed history and thorough physical examination. The subsequent diagnostic workup must be rapid, efficient, and directed to the traumatic injuries. Unnecessary tests only add expense and delay appropriate and perhaps life-saving therapy.

History

History taking is often difficult in the trauma situation. Communication with a patient in shock or with altered mental status can be difficult if not impossible and attention to the ABCs remain primary objectives ahead of patient history. When the patient's clinical status permits, a detailed history should be sought. For example, understanding the mechanism of injury is crucial in determining specific organ injury patterns (e.g., the driver of a car impacted from the left side may have left rib fractures, left pulmonary contusion, or splenic injury). Although proven to save lives, seat belts can actually be associated with specific abdominal, thoracic and spinal injuries ("seat belt injury") and deserves consideration in certain circumstances. Understanding all previous medical and surgical history is required in the acute and convalescent phases of injury. Routine medications indicate general health problems for which the patient is being treated as well as provide explanation for unexpected physiologic responses. Examples include elderly patients who routinely take beta receptor antagonists for hypertension and do not exhibit tachycardia in response to hypovolemia. History of allergies is important, as the patient is likely to receive antibiotics, pain medication and possibly intravenous contrast for radiographic studies. Previous drug use, including tobacco and alcohol, can be useful in respiratory management and prevention of withdrawal syndromes, respectively. Emergency rescue personnel are an excellent source of history and their input should be welcomed.

Physical Examination

Physical examination of the trauma patient is done rapidly and efficiently with a focus on the discovery of traumatic injuries. After the ABCs are established and stabilized, a complete secondary assessment should be performed from head to toe. The eyes are examined for size and reaction of the pupils as evidence of neurological injury. Ears are inspected with an otoscope for hemotympanum or the presence of cerebrospinal fluid leak (otorrhea), both evidence of basilar skull fracture. Facial tenderness or instability suggests facial bone fracture. With immobilization maintained, the neck is palpated for tenderness and crepitus, suggesting esophageal or airway injury and the cervical spine is palpated to elicit tenderness due to fracture. Abnormally distended external jugular veins are a sign of increased intrathoracic pressure or

central venous pressure (CVP), as in cardiac tamponade. The heart and lungs are auscultated, for evidence of intrathoracic injury which will be discussed. The abdomen is examined for contusions or seat belt marks (see above) and palpated to elicit signs of peritonitis. The pelvis is tested for stability with anterior to posterior and lateral compression forces, respectively, to seek evidence of fracture. The motor strength and sensation of extremities are evaluated. Appreciation of physical deformity indicates long bone fracture until proven otherwise. Palpable pulses are documented and unexpected asymmetry demands further study.

"TUBES AND FINGERS, A STRONG ARM, AND A LONG NEEDLE"

The old adage "A tube or finger in every body orifice" refers to the diagnostic information obtained from physical examination and therapy and effect of tubes placed in body cavities. To this day this principle still holds value. For example, nasogastric tubes are placed routinely in most victims of major trauma to evacuate the stomach and reduce the risk of aspiration. Blood in the nasogastric aspirate may indicate occult gastrointestinal injury. Deviation of the nasogastric tube in the mediastinum on chest radiograph is consistent with the presence of a mediastinal hematoma. Similarly, visualization of the nasogastric tube in the left chest on chest film is a sign of diaphragmatic rupture with herniation of abdominal viscera in the thorax. Suspected basilar skull fracture, e.g., severe midface trauma or cribiform plate fracture, may allow passage of the nasogastric tube into the cranial vault and is a contraindication to this procedure.

The urinary bladder should be catheterized in trauma patients to allow assessment of gross hematuria and monitoring of urinary output. Urinary output is the most sensitive indicator of hypovolemia and can be used to direct fluid therapy. Gross hematuria suggests kidney, ureter or bladder injury and merits further workup. Contraindication to placement of a foley catheter is evidence of urethral injury including gross blood at the urethral meatus, butterfly distribution bruising of the perineum, and "high-riding" prostate. A retrograde urethrogram is generally required to evaluate a suspected urethral injury.

A digital rectal examination should be performed on all trauma patients. Diminished or absent anal sphincter tone on digital rectal exam is a sign of spinal injury. Prostatic findings in males has already been mentioned. Pelvic examination should be performed on all women with pelvic fractures. Bony spicules palpated in the vagina alters the diagnosis to open pelvic fracture, which carries a much higher morbidity and mortality from septic complications than a simple closed pelvic fracture.

"Strong arms and long needles" makes symbolic reference to the point that certain cavities can be "tapped" for diagnostic and therapeutic reasons. The neurosurgeon can perform emergency ventriculostomy to reduce intracranial pressure in patients with signs and symptoms of life-threatening elevated intracranial pressure. Percutaneous insertion of a needle into a joint, arthrocentesis, is indicated in suspected joint capsule violation and to drain painful hemarthroses. Emergency room thoracotomy has been performed by qualified surgeons to treat life-threatening thoracic trauma.

Radiographic Studies

Radiographs taken in the resuscitation room should be limited to those that will influence the acute care of the patient. Routinely, three radiographs are obtained in blunt trauma victims: (a) lateral cervical spine radiograph, (b) a chest radiograph, and (c) pelvic radiograph. A lateral cervical spine radiograph is obtained to diagnose subluxation or fracture that requires emergent distraction and realignment. Any patient with evidence of closed head trauma, no matter how minor, should be presumed to have associated cervical spine injury until radiographic evidence proves otherwise. An anterior-posterior (AP) chest radiograph provides a wealth of information in trauma patients regarding lung injury, chest wall injury, and diaphragmatic injury. It may be required to locate a missing bullet or other projectile. Pelvic radiograph is an essential study to be obtained in the resuscitation area because clinical diagnosis of pelvic fracture is often inaccurate. Radiographs obtained in patients sustaining penetrating trauma are based upon the location of injury and the specific information obtained.

Laboratory Studies

Laboratory studies should be limited to those that will be diagnostically relevant and have clinical significance. Blood sample for type and cross-match should be obtained in patients with suspected or known hemorrhage. Selective utilization of laboratory studies such as complete blood count (CBC), arterial blood gas (ABG), prothrombin and partial thromboplastin times (PT/PTT), and serum chemistry (Na, K, Cl, CO_2, BUN, Cr, Glucose) eliminate unnecessary health care cost. Even in the care of trauma patients, cost consciousness militates against the indiscriminate ordering of laboratory studies.

SPECIFIC INJURIES

Head Injury

Head injury can be classified as closed and penetrating head trauma. The pathophysiology in penetrating or closed head injury results from swelling or bleeding. Because the skull is rigid and fixed in size, there is no compliance nor extra space to accommodate even minute

increases in brain swelling or cerebral bleeding, and as a result, intracranial pressure increases. The third cranial nerve becomes compressed as the brain herniates, explaining why a fixed and dilated pupil indicates ipsilateral brain injury. As the brain continues to swell, the intracranial pressure exceeds the cerebral perfusion pressure (mean arterial pressure minus CVP), until the metabolic demands of the brain can no longer be met by the inadequate perfusion. With persistent unrelieved intracranial hypertension, herniation of the unci (medial portions of the temporal lobes) through the opening for the brainstem in the tentorium ensues.

Specific injuries to the brain that cause increased cranial pressure include parenchymal contusions, subarachnoid hemorrhage, subdural hemorrhage, and epidural hemorrhage. During deceleration injury, such as head impact in a motor vehicle accident, even though the skull has impacted a fixed object, e.g., dashboard, the brain continues to move forward at traveling speed until it collides with the inner surface of the skull. Recoil energy then sets the brain parenchyma in reverse to impact the opposite surface of the skull. Contusions at each impact point are termed coup and contra coup injury. Methods to reduce intracranial pressure include drainage of cerebrospinal fluid via the ventriculostomy, administration of mannitol, and induction of barbiturate coma. Elevation of the head of the bed may reduce intracranial pressure, but has unpredictable effects on cerebral perfusion pressure. Hyperventilation is used only briefly in cases of impending herniation, and does not have sustained efficacy in reducing intracranial pressure.

Other injuries to the head are of significance to the trauma surgeon. Scalp lacerations can be the source of significant bleeding. An underlying skull fracture may be present as well. Closure of the laceration for hemostasis must be performed quickly prior to the patient leaving the resuscitation area. Cosmetic repair can be accomplished after life-threatening conditions have been addressed. Ocular injuries are treated by patch coverage of the eye until an ophthalmologist is available, except for chemical injuries, which are treated by continuous irrigation of the globe with large volumes of normal saline until the patient can be seen by an ophthalmologist. No attempt should be made to "neutralize" the offending agent, as this will only cause further damage from the heat given off by the exothermic reactions of neutralization. Facial fractures need early attention of a maxillofacial surgeon, for diagnosis, stabilization, and occasional release of an entrapped globe in an orbital fracture. Fractures of the posterior table of the frontal sinus are open skull fractures.

Neck

Nowhere else in the body are so many different vital structures found in such a confined space as in the neck. Respiratory, digestive, neurological, and vascular struc-

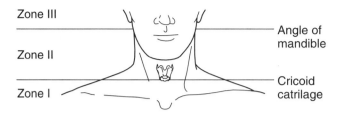

FIG. 1. *Zones of neck*

tures are all in close proximity to each other in the neck, and serious injury to any of these can be life-threatening. Trauma to the neck by either blunt or penetrating mechanisms, if accompanied by bleeding, expanding hematoma, or airway obstruction, warrants emergent neck exploration in the operating room. Otherwise, further workup by computed tomography (CT) scanning, ultrasound (US), angiography, contrast swallow, esophagoscopy, and bronchoscopy, in any combination, is utilized to evaluate neck injury, as indicated.

A penetrating neck wound is defined as violation of the platysma muscle. Penetrating neck injury is further subdivided based on location (Fig. 1). Zone I injuries are those that occur between the clavicle to the cricoid cartilage. Zone II injuries are defined as injuries between the cricoid cartilage to the angle of the mandible. Zone III injuries extend from the angle of the mandible to the base of the skull.

Previously, penetrating trauma to the neck was managed by mandatory exploration, but the high rate of negative exploration and possible morbidity from surgery placed this management protocol under heavy scrutiny. Currently, in patients sustaining penetrating trauma to Zone II but without "hard signs" (Table 3) of organ injury, mandatory versus selective exploration based upon diagnostic studies or deterioration during serial examination remains the center of controversy (Fig. 2). If selective exploration is chosen, arteriography is commonly used to evaluate the vascular system. A combination of bronchoscopy and laryngoscopy is utilized to evaluate the trachea. The esophagus remains the most dif-

TABLE 3. *"Hard signs" indicative of organ damage in penetrating neck injury*

System	Sign
Vascular—carotid artery, jugular vein	Exsanguinating hemorrhage, expanding hematoma, pulsatile hematoma
Neurologic	Brachial plexus injury, cerebrovascular accident from carotid artery injury
Esophagus	Subcutaneous emphysema, hematemesis
Airway	Subcutaneous emphysema, hemoptysis

ficult to assess, but a combination of esophagography with or without endoscopy is usually used for evaluation. Injuries in zones I and III pose a technical challenge because of bony confinements and difficult access. With an exception for obvious injuries or patients in extremis, a selective approach with arteriography, esophagography, and bronchoscopy is used to determine need for operation (Figs. 3 and 4).

Thoracic Injury

Chest injuries, whether blunt or penetrating, can involve the chest wall, the lungs and pleura, the heart and vascular structures, the esophagus, or the spine and spinal cord. Patients with penetrating chest trauma tend to have isolated chest injury, whereas blunt chest trauma patients are prone to have multiple system injuries. When faced with a patient who has suffered chest trauma, regardless of mechanism, one must give consideration first to two rapidly reversible life-threatening injuries: tension pneumothorax and pericardial tamponade. Algorithms for management of penetrating chest trauma are offered in Fig. 5.

Tension Pneumothorax

When the visceral pleura is violated (e.g., knife, bullet, fractured rib), air leaks from the lung into the pleural space. Increasing accumulation of air causes increased intrathoracic pressure, eventually resulting in mediastinal shift toward the contralateral hemithorax. Apart from the respiratory insufficiency from compressed ipsilateral lung parenchyma, hemodynamic embarrassment from extrinsic compression of the heart and vena cava results in decreased cardiac output and shock. This diagnosis must be considered in patients with diminished breath sounds ipsilateral to the side of chest trauma, distended neck veins, and hypotension. Emergent percutaneous decompression of the pleural cavity with an angiocatheter placed into the pleural cavity through the second intercostal space in the midclavicular line can be life-saving. Placement of a thoracostomy tube provides definitive therapy.

Pericardial Tamponade

The pericardium is a relatively noncompliant fibrous sac. Traumatic pericardial tamponade develops as a result of intra-pericardial bleeding and formation of a space occupying clot that impairs diastolic filling of the heart. It is usually a consequence of penetrating trauma. Rarely, blunt myocardial rupture can result in the same clinical symptoms. Elevated CVP and jugular venous distention (JVD) are initial signs of cardiac tamponade. Because the right atrium cannot fill, reduced preload decreases cardiac output. A narrowed pulse pressure and hypotension

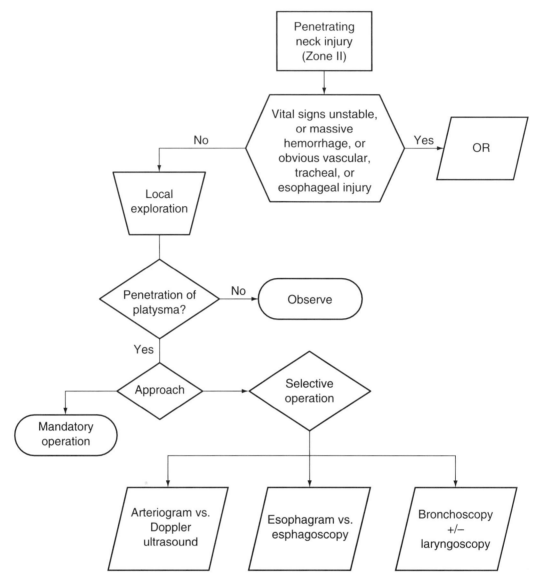

FIG. 2. Evaluating penetrating injuries to Zone II of neck

are end-stage manifestations of pericardial tamponade. Beck's triad represents the classic constellation of symptoms of pericardial tamponade: (a) distant heart sounds, (b) distended jugular veins, and (c) hypotension. An immediate subxiphoid pericardial window for decompression and evaluation of the pericardial cavity is supplanted perhaps only by emergency room thoracotomy performed by qualified personnel. Pericardiocentesis for both diagnostic and therapeutic purposes has fallen out of favor because of the significant false-positive and false-negative rate, incompleteness of therapy, and the inability to definitively treat a major cardiovascular injury. Echocardiography can demonstrate pericardial fluid with high sensitivity and specificity and can be utilized to evaluate patients sustaining precordial penetrating injury,

provided it is available and there is no evidence of hemodynamic instability.

Hemothorax

Fluid in the thorax of a trauma patient, especially those sustaining penetrating injuries, is invariably a hemothorax. Although most cases of penetrating thoracic trauma and resultant hemothoraces are self-limiting, requiring only thoracostomy tube drainage, occasionally a massive hemothorax complicates penetrating chest trauma. Massive hemothoraces are defined as immediate loss of >1,500 cc of blood upon placement of a thoracostomy tube or the persistent chest tube output of >200 cc/hr. In this situation,

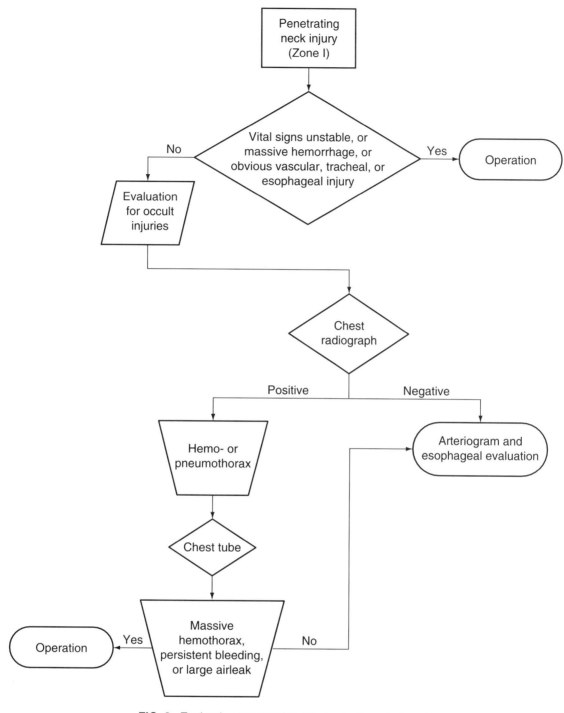

FIG. 3. Evaluating penetrating injuries to Zone I of neck

formal thoracotomy is the required treatment. Penetrating injury to the thoracic great vessels is a frequent cause of massive hemothorax, and although most patients are hemodynamically unstable and require emergent repair and revascularization, occasionally angiography is performed in stable patients to delineate the injury and direct surgical therapy.

Frequently, patients sustaining penetrating chest trauma are found by rescue personnel in extremis or without signs of life and are brought to the trauma center. Similarly, patients with penetrating chest injuries who are initially stable occasionally deteriorate rather abruptly. In these situations, emergency center thoracotomy is the patients' only chance for survival. A left anterolateral thoracotomy is performed to control bleeding or decompress a cardiac tamponade. In addition, the descending aorta is cross-clamped to increase afterload and direct blood to the brain and coronary arteries. Should the patient stabilize, formal

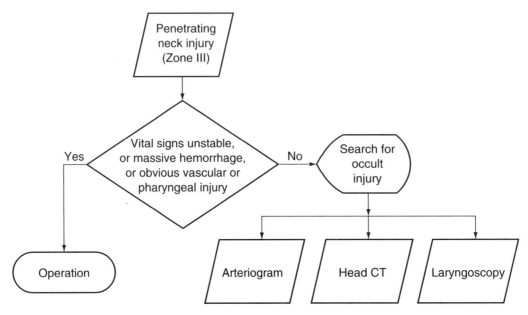

FIG. 4. Evaluating penetrating injuries to Zone III of neck

thoracotomy in the operating room is performed. The best outcomes are limited to those patients who have isolated penetrating injuries and deteriorate near or within the trauma resuscitation center.

Ruptured Thoracic Aorta

Rupture of the thoracic aorta typically occurs following high-energy blunt deceleration trauma. Ninety percent of patients who suffer this injury die in the field. Aortic disruption occurs just distal to the ligamentum arteriosum, which affixes the aorta, and results in adjacent aortic wall "blow out" during impact. Mediastinal widening, first and second rib fractures, massive hemothorax from blunt trauma, deviation of the nasogastric tube, and elevation of the left mainstem bronchus are but a few of the chest radiographic findings suggestive of ruptured thoracic aorta. Unfortunately, the chest radiograph is not specific. CT scan and transesophageal echocardiogram are noninvasive studies that document classic aortic rupture well, but angiogram remains the standard test to confirm the injury. Surgical treatment should be scheduled promptly after diagnosis is made. Missing this diagnosis is invariably fatal as the majority of patients with this injury will have a spontaneous rupture over the next few days.

Other Chest Injuries

Simple pneumothorax occurs secondary to laceration of the visceral pleura and necessitates thoracostomy tube. Frequently, a solitary finding of subcutaneous emphysema about the chest wall is secondary to an occult pneumothorax. Rib fractures are extremely common in blunt chest injury. Progressive atelectasis, hypoxemia, and possible superinfection complicating rib fractures are the result of "splinting" and suppression of cough reflex due to pain. The principles of management of rib fractures is preventing underlying pulmonary dysfunction and obliteration of pain. Elderly patients, patients with preinjury lung disease, or pain associated with multiple rib fractures require admission, pain control, and aggressive pulmonary physiotherapy. Flail chest is characterized by more than two adjoining ribs, each fractured in two places, with the patient exhibiting paradoxical chest movement on inspiration, i.e., rising on exhalation and falling on inhalation. Treatment usually involves mechanical ventilation to avoid hypoxia and hypoventilation. Radiographic evidence of a pulmonary contusion typically lags behind respiratory dysfunction and is presumed in patients with tremendous blunt injury and rib fractures. Visualization of abdominal viscera or the nasogastric tube in the thorax may indicate a diaphragmatic injury.

Esophageal injury following penetrating trauma to the chest with a trans-mediastinal trajectory must be suspected. Esophageal injury following blunt trauma is uncommon. Esophagram and esophagoscopy have a greater sensitivity combined than either test alone. Contrast-enhanced CT may also be useful. Esophageal injuries discovered within 24 hr of event are treated with repair and thoracostomy tube drainage. Those injuries discovered after this period are best treated by thoracostomy tube drainage with or without esophageal "exclusion." Inadequate drainage leading to mediastinitis is a highly lethal complication.

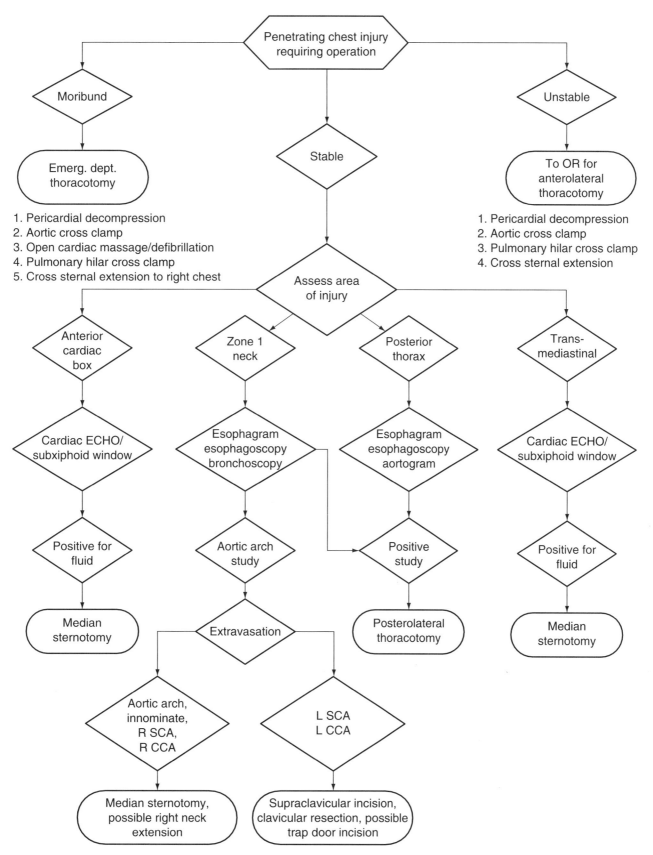

FIG. 5. Indications for operation for penetrating chest injury

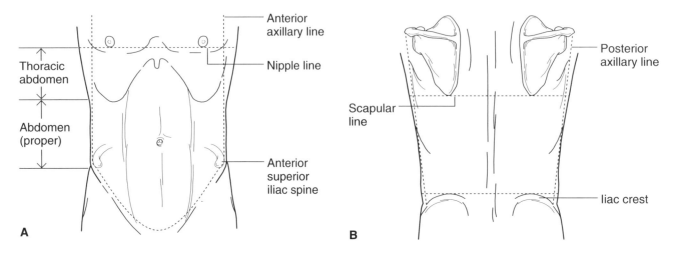

FIG. 6. *Boundaries of the abdomen, back, and flanks.*

Abdominal Trauma

Abdominal trauma is categorized as blunt or penetrating injuries. Penetrating trauma to the abdomen is subcategorized by "region"—thoracic abdomen, abdomen (proper), flank, and back (Fig. 6). The anterior boundaries of the abdomen is defined by the nipple line and inguinal ligaments anteriorly and by the scapular line and iliac crests posteriorly. The portion of abdomen shielded by ribs is considered the thoracic abdomen. Below the costal margin is regarded as the abdomen (proper). The strip of abdomen bounded by anterior and posterior axillary line is considered the flank. The back is confined by the posterior axillary lines below the tip of the scapula.

Blunt Trauma

In the blunt trauma patient without neurologic injury or altered mental status, the need for further diagnostic studies of the abdomen is dictated by clinical examination. Those with abdominal tenderness and signs of peritonitis require laparotomy for diagnosis and therapy. For those "stable" patients, however, who have equivocal signs of abdominal injury, altered sensorium or other factors which make abdominal examination unreliable, or multiple trauma for which other tests will be performed, diagnostic evaluation of the abdomen is undertaken.

Diagnostic peritoneal lavage (DPL) is a sensitive test for intraperitoneal injury from blunt trauma (Fig. 7). After placing a catheter carefully through the abdominal wall into the peritoneum, aspiration is performed to detect the presence of gross blood. A return of 5 cc of blood is considered "positive" and is an indication for laparotomy. The absence of gross blood on aspiration is followed by instillation of 1 L of crystalloid into the peritoneal cavity. An aliquot of this fluid removed by gravity drainage is sent for chemistry and cellular analysis. Standard positive criteria include 100,000 red blood cells (RBC) per mm^3 or 500 white blood cells (WBC) per mm^3, presence of bile, elevated amylase, or intestinal contents.

The only absolute contraindication to DPL is the presence of an indication for operation. There are a number of relative contraindications to the closed technique and are remembered easily as "the four **P**'s": **p**regnancy, **p**revious surgery, **p**ediatrics, and **p**elvic fracture. In pregnancy, the enlarged gravid uterus is jeopardized by blind passage of a needle. With previous abdominal surgery, adhesions may exist, affixing loops of bowel to the anterior abdominal wall that a blindly passed needle may injure. Although pediatric patients rarely require DPL for diagnosis, it is recognized that the stomach resides much lower and the urinary bladder sits higher in the abdominal cavity and is predisposed to inadvertent injury by closed DPL. Finally, pelvic fractures may have significant extraperitoneal hematomas below the anterior abdominal wall, which may be accessed during closed DPL and perhaps lead to an unnecessary laparotomy. In these situations, "open" DPL is performed through a small midline supraumbilical incision through skin. A catheter can then be placed into the peritoneal cavity under direct vision.

DPL has been proven through the years as a minimally invasive test with excellent sensitivity although with a few limitations. DPL cannot reveal contained retroperitoneal injury. Additionally, DPL tells nothing about the source of the blood. For example, hemoperitoneum may come from minor liver lacerations that have stopped bleeding and therefore positive results from DPL may lead to an "unnecessary" laparotomy. The level at which results are considered "positive" are arbitrary but chosen to ensure that injuries requiring operations are seldom

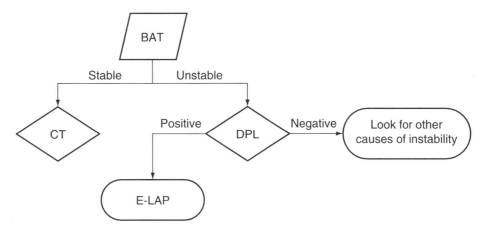

FIG. 7. Evaluating blunt abdominal trauma (BAT) using diagnostic peritoneal lavage (DPL). CT = computed tomography, E-LAP = exploratory laparotomy

missed. Occasionally, "nontherapeutic" laparotomies will be performed.

CT scan is an important study in the evaluation of abdominal trauma (Fig. 7). As a general rule, hemodynamically unstable patients with blunt abdominal trauma belong in the operating room, not in the CT scan area! Otherwise, CT is valuable in the diagnosis of pelvic injuries, injuries of abdominal solid organs, and retroperitoneal injuries. Injuries to hollow viscera of the abdomen, though, may not be accurately detected by CT.

US has been investigated recently as a diagnostic tool with high sensitivity and specificity in the evaluation of blunt abdominal trauma (Fig. 8). US reliably demonstrates free intraperitoneal fluid, which in trauma victims represents hemoperitoneum until proven otherwise. The detection of small amounts of fluid in the perihepatic, perisplenic, or pelvic regions of the body can be per-

formed in minutes in the resuscitation room. The ease and rapidity of use make it advantageous in repeat examination when necessary.

Penetrating Trauma

Patients sustaining gunshot wounds to the abdomen, with few exceptions, are taken to the operating room for emergent laparotomy after quick evaluation in the resuscitation room (Fig. 9). Occasionally, patients sustain tangential gunshot wounds without peritoneal penetration or clinical evidence of peritonitis and do not require operation. Management of stab wounds to the abdomen is based on clinical condition and DPL results. Obviously, hemodynamic instability, the presence of peritoneal signs, or evidence of evisceration are indications for immediate laparotomy, and further diagnostic tests only delay neces-

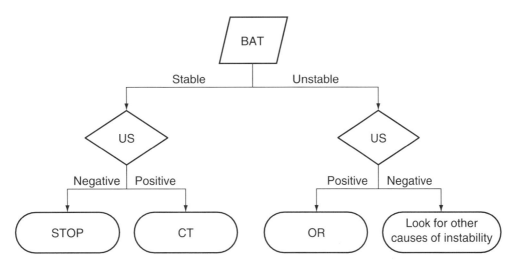

FIG. 8. Evaluating blunt abdominalusing ultrasound. BAT = blunt abdominal trauma; US = ultrasound; CT = computed tomography; OR = operating room

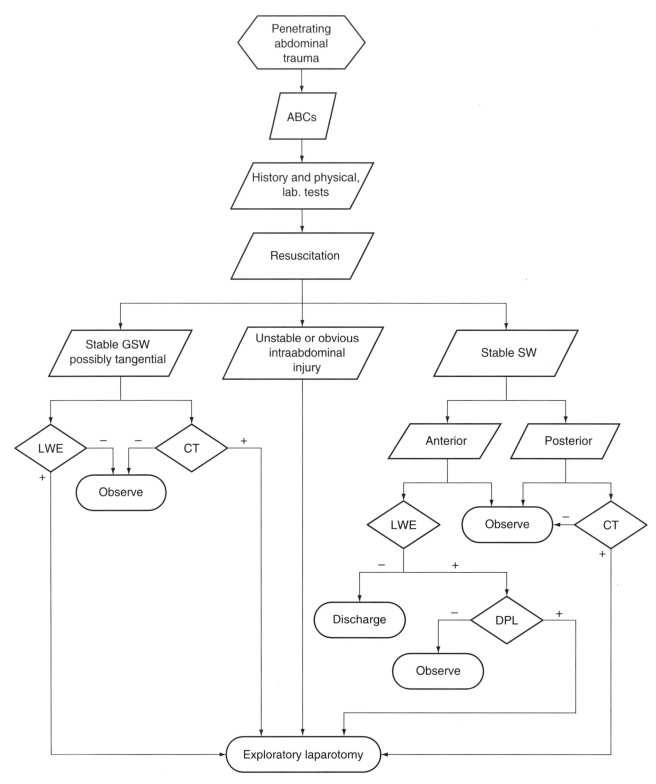

FIG. 9. Management of penetrating abdominal trauma. LWE = local wound exploraton, DPL = diagnostic peritoneal lavage, CT = computed tomography

sary surgical intervention. In stable patients with stab wounds, however, DPL has been successfully proven to determine with high sensitivity and specificity which patients had intraperitoneal injury. First, local wound exploration was performed to detect anterior fascia penetration. Patients with nonviolated anterior abdominal fascia obviously did not have intraperitoneal injury and required only closure of the wound. Violation of the anterior abdominal fascia implied peritoneal penetration and these patients underwent DPL. Performance and guidelines of DPL are as previously outlined. Because greater sensitivity is required in detecting injury from penetrating abdominal trauma, the RBC count considered positive is lower than in blunt trauma. Initial aspiration of 5 cc of gross blood is a positive result. In the absence of an initial positive aspiration, crystalloid fluid is instilled as previously described. Typically, >20,000 RBC/mm^3 or >500 WBC/mm^3 constitutes a "positive" result.

Specific Abdominal Injuries

The solid viscera include the liver, spleen, kidneys, and pancreas. The liver because of its sheer size is perhaps the most commonly injured abdominal organ following blunt trauma. US and CT scan offer excellent diagnostic capabilities with regard to liver injuries. DPL, although not diagnostic for liver injuries, is invariably "positive" with major liver injuries. Patients with evidence of hemoperitoneum and hypotension are taken emergently to the operating room for exploration and control of bleeding. Active bleeding should be controlled in a timely fashion using blunt suture technique, electrocautery, laser coagulation, or resection. Sponge packing is utilized in clinically unstable patients in whom it is not expected to control bleeding in a short period of time. Reexploration and unpacking is performed after hypothermia, coagulopathy, and hypotension have resolved. In "stable" patients, appropriate treatment is based on clinical status and radiologic classification of severity of injury. Minor parenchymal fracture noted on CT without clinical evidence of hemodynamic instability does not require exploration. Observation in a monitored setting is mandatory.

Although the spleen is a much smaller organ than the liver, it is also commonly injured in blunt abdominal trauma. The pediatric surgical literature is replete with data on successful splenic salvage following observation of patients sustaining splenic trauma. The success rate is not the same for adults. Although minor splenic injuries can be treated expectantly, most major splenic trauma is treated appropriately by splenectomy. Splenorrhaphy is appropriate in stable patients with isolated splenic injury recognizing that the priority is patient survival not splenic salvage. The relative ease of splenectomy and the minimal surgical risks far outweigh the prolonged hospital stay and probable transfusion required with expectant management of splenic trauma. Postsplenectomy patients are at increased risk for infection with encapsulated organisms, *Nisseria meningitidis, Streptococcus pneumonia,* and *Haemophilus influenza.* Antipneumococcal vaccine is given after splenectomy.

The pancreas is located in a relatively protected position in the retroperitoneum. Blunt injury to the pancreas can follow direct anterior abdominal trauma and typically occurs at the neck of the pancreas from compression over the spine and parenchymal "fracture." Penetrating injury to the pancreas is frequently associated with other intraabdominal injuries. The major concern following pancreatic trauma, whether blunt or penetrating, is extravasation of pancreatic enzymes and resultant adjacent tissue injury. If pancreatic injury is appreciated at the time of operation, peripancreatic drainage is necessary. Resection may be required. Rarely, injury to the head of the pancreas with extensive associated duodenal injury from penetrating trauma, may necessitate pancreaticoduodenectomy (Whipple procedure).

Kidney trauma involves injury to the hilar vessels, parenchyma, or urinary collecting system. Blunt parenchymal injury without evidence of urine extravasation noted on CT scan in an otherwise hemodynamically stable patient can be managed nonoperatively. Evidence of urinary extravasation or persistent bleeding from the kidney are indications for operation and repair. With an exception for uncontrollable bleeding from hilar injuries and extensive parenchymal destruction, immediate nephrectomy is rarely necessary. Kidney repair (nephrorrhaphy) can usually be performed although consideration is made to intraoperative patient status before embarking on lengthy procedures. If nephrectomy is indicated, intravenous pyelogram is obtained to document function of the contralateral kidney.

In contrast to solid visceral injuries, hollow viscera injuries invariably require operative repair. Control of peritoneal contamination and debridement of nonviable tissue are principles of surgical management.

Injuries to the stomach and small intestine are usually repaired primarily or resected with primary reanastomosis. The high volumes of gastric, biliary, and pancreatic secretions conducted by the duodenum generally necessitate extended nasogastric decompression and drainage around repair of duodenal injuries to detect unexpected postoperative leak. Extensive duodenal injury may require temporary "exclusion" along with drainage, especially if associated with pancreatic injury.

Colon injuries from low-velocity ammunition used in civilian firearms were previously managed by mandatory proximal diverting colostomy. Although there are select clinical circumstances that mandate construction of diverting colostomy, many trauma surgeons now perform primary repair or resection with primary reanastomosis without increased incidence of complications. Surgical incisions are left open following repair of colon injuries.

292 / SURGICAL SPECIALTIES

Injuries to the rectum (Fig. 10) are managed by proximal diverting colostomy, rectal disimpaction, presacral drainage, and "drugs" (antibiotics)—"the four Ds." Colostomy closure is performed after the rectal injury has healed completely.

Abdominal vascular injuries are commonly seen in penetrating trauma and infrequently in blunt trauma. Injury to retroperitoneal vasculature may result in a contained hematoma or active intraperitoneal bleeding. Portal and mesenteric vessels usually present with active intraabdominal hemorrhage. Exploration of contained hematomas is generally indicated for all cases due to trauma, the exception being pelvic hematomas from blunt trauma that are not expanding. Repair of large vessels is performed after obtaining proximal and distal vascular control. Active hemorrhage is controlled best with digital occlusion while controlling proximal and distal to the injury.

Pelvic Fracture

Pelvic fracture is a common injury associated with tremendous morbidity in blunt trauma patients. Simple pelvic fractures without evidence of active bleeding require prophylactic therapy to combat deep venous thrombosis (DVT). True "open" pelvic fractures are defined as pelvic fractures with associated violation of perineal skin or rectal/vaginal mucosa and is accompanied by mortality rates in excess of 50%. A diverting colostomy is required in open pelvic fractures to diminish bacterial contamination of fracture site. Unstable pelvic fractures include those with >4 cm pubic symphysis diastasis, vertical "shear" fracture or widening of the sacroiliac joint(s). Unstable pelvic fractures causing hemodynamic instability require immediate external fixation. Management of pelvic fractures with persistent bleeding involves stabilization, resuscitation with blood products, correction of

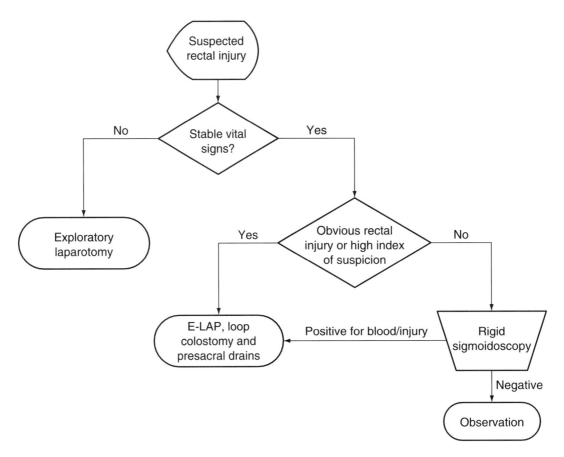

FIG. 10. Management of rectal trauma

coagulopathy, and angiography to detect arterial bleeding amenable to selective embolization. Inadvertent entry into a pelvic hematoma during operative repair of other abdominal injuries often results in uncontrollable exsanguinating hemorrhage and should be avoided.

Extremities

Soft tissue injuries require thorough irrigation and debridement (Fig. 11). Clean wounds can be repaired primarily within 6 hr of injury. Conversely, contaminated wounds are left open. If coverage of bone, tendon, and vascular structures cannot be achieved, elective reconstruction with flaps or skin flaps may be required.

Peripheral vascular injuries can be both limb- and life-threatening. Infrequently, intimal disruption can result from blunt trauma, particularly with orthopedic injuries, and must be remembered to prevent complications from limb ischemia. Gunshot wounds and stab wounds not infrequently lacerate vascular structures. In addition, gunshot wounds can result in intimal damage, contusion, and thrombosis of arteries. Hemodynami-

cally unstable patients with active bleeding from penetrating vascular injuries are taken directly to the operating room for exploration and repair. Similarly, patients with paresthesias secondary to distal extremity hypoperfusion, bruits detected by auscultation or pulsatile hematoma require prompt vascular repair. If, after debridement, arterial reapproximation cannot be performed without undue tension, an interposition graft of reversed saphenous vein or polytetrafluoroethylene (PTFE) is placed. Stable patients with "soft signs" of vascular injury, i.e., asymmetric or diminished pulse, "large" blood loss prior to arrival in emergency room, or large soft tissue hematoma, should undergo arteriography to identify and locate the injury.

Orthopedic injuries are significant for the mechanical derangement they represent, the systemic complications that ensue, and the complications that result from prolonged immobilization. Extremity deformity, particularly shortening or angulation, are signs of fracture and should be immobilized with splints until they can be reduced. Eventual function depends on anatomic reduction. Long bone fractures, particularly of the femur, can be an unrecognized source of large volume blood loss into a fascial

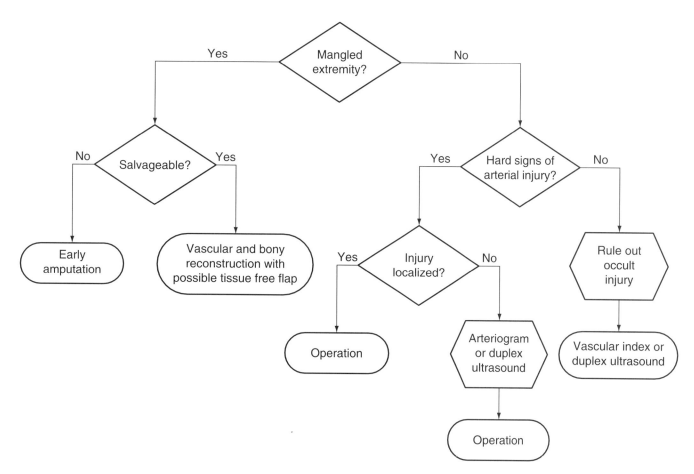

FIG. 11. Management of extremity trauma

compartment. Respiratory insufficiency following long bone fractures infrequently results from embolization of microparticles of fat (fat embolus) to the pulmonary circulation. Furthermore, prolonged immobilization from untreated fracture leads to atelectasis and predisposes patients to DVT. Early reduction and fixation, with early mobilization, are paramount in reducing the incidence of these complications.

Compartment syndrome can result from soft tissue edema and bleeding from a long bone fracture. Elevated myofascial compartment pressure impairs capillary perfusion of the nerves and muscles of the involved compartment resulting in the classic symptoms of paresthesias, pain, pallor and paralysis. A common misconception held among many clinicians is that the presence of a palpable distal pulse clinically excludes compartment syndrome. When compartment pressure exceeds systolic blood pressure (i.e., the point at which the pulse would be lost), irreversible ischemic neuropathy and myonecrosis have already occurred. Prompt fracture reduction, elevation, and icing help decrease the incidence of compartment syndrome. When the syndrome is present, fasciotomy is performed to release compartmental hypertension.

All joints are examined through active (if possible) and passive range of motion for pain and instability. Internal rotation of a lower extremity is a sign of posterior hip dislocation. Posterior knee dislocations have a high associated incidence of popliteal artery thrombosis due to intimal injury and must be remembered. Violation of the joint capsule, "open joint," is suspected with skin injury overlying a joint and, if detected, requires irrigation in the operating room and a short course of intravenous antibiotics.

SUMMARY

The approach to the trauma patient is described by the Advanced Trauma Life Support curriculum of the American College of Surgeons. Although many of the diagnostic and therapeutic interventions used to manage traumatic injury vary widely among institutions, the management issues and algorithms presented should be viewed as reasonable but not necessarily the only treatment plans. What is true, irrespective of the mechanism of traumatic injury, is the fact that clinical assessment and management must be swift and decisive to positively affect patient outcome during the "golden hour" of trauma.

STUDY QUESTIONS

1. What is the "golden hour" of trauma?
2. Describe the essentials of the initial management of a patient sustaining blunt trauma.
3. Define the specific categories of hemorrhage and the clinical manifestations of each.
4. Describe proper evaluation of a patients who has sustained a stab wound.
5. What laboratory studies and radiographic studies are absolutely necessary in the initial evaluation of a trauma patient?

SUGGESTED READING

Feliciano DV, Moore EE, Mattox KL, eds. *Trauma.* 3rd ed. Norwalk, CT: Appleton-Lange, 1996.
Shires TG, Thal ER, Jones RC, et al. Trauma. In: Schwartz SI, Shires TG, Spencer FC, eds. *Principles of surgery.* 6th ed. New York: McGraw-Hill, 1994:175–224

CHAPTER 22

Burn Surgery

Nestor de la Cruz-Munoz and C. Gillon Ward

Burn injury is considered trauma and is evaluated and treated in a similar fashion. The circumstances surrounding the burn injury can involve accident, assault, suicide, work-related incident, or abuse. The systemic response to locoregional burn injury is related to changes in cardiovascular hemodynamics, serum chemistry composition, and renal perfusion, to name a few. The long-term effects of nonfatal burn trauma are many and include permanent or temporary disability, emotional and psychological unsettling, and cosmetic disfigurement. The following is a presentation of the different classifications of burn trauma, evaluation and treatment, and some special considerations. Medical students should recognize the clinical importance of burn trauma regardless of the cause and size of injury.

Flame burns injure through different mechanisms. Direct contact obviously can cause thermal injury to skin and underlying tissue. These injury patterns are magnified with the clothing that the burn patient is wearing, which can secondarily catch fire or melt, both of which increase contact time on skin. An inhalation injury results from the inspiration of flame or smoke and generally causes upper large airway injury. It should be suspected in specific cases—e.g., flame burn in an enclosed space, carbonaceous sputum, singed facial and nasal hair, and respiratory distress without obvious thoracic trauma. One must recognize that respiratory insufficiency secondary to inhalation injury may not manifest until 18 to 36 hr after injury.

Skin contact against a hot solid object (e.g., pot, stove element) results in thermal injury. The depth of burn is proportional to duration of contact and the specific heat of the object at the time of injury. Scald burns are caused by hot liquids, including hot water, cooking oil, tar, or molten metal. The depth and severity of these types of burns are dependent on the specific boiling point of the offending agent. Tar burns usually result in deep second or third degree injury due to the high specific heat of tar.

The full extent of the injury may not be defined until 24 hrs after the burn. There is no immediacy in removing the tar as it has usually cooled by the time the patient reaches the emergency room. Although petroleum-based fluids such a gasoline or kerosene are effective in removing tar, pain and destruction to surviving tissues make these products undesirable. Commercial tar removers are used in the emergency room. Alternatively, silver sulfadiazine or neosporin ointment slowly separates tar from the wound over a 24-hr period.

Chemical burn severity is based on the type and concentration of the chemical, and the length of time that the chemical remains on the skin. There can be continued tissue damage in progress while a patient is being seen in the emergency room. Damage prevention must be accomplished by removing the patient's clothing and irrigating the affected area with a generous amount of water. Chemical neutralization may result in an exothermic reaction and worsen tissue damage. Ammonia in the form of gas or liquid deserves special consideration. If inhaled, it combines with lung water to form ammonium hydroxide. It produces a chemical burn of the airway epithelia and is often a lethal injury. Electrical burns are classified into low- and high-voltage injuries. U.S. household current is 110 V with a 60-cycle alternating current. The conduction of current through the body can produce a lethal arrhythmia. Interestingly, the burn injury from the electrical spark tends to be insignificant. Children learning to crawl occasionally chew electric cords, causing deep burns in the corners of the mouth and tongue. Major tissue destruction is usually associated with ≥500 V. There are three mechanisms to such an injury. The first is direct damage from the current, resulting in cellular coagulation. Much of the destruction is deep and away from current entrance site. One must recognize that the full extent of the injury may not manifest until 5 to 7 days postburn. Frequent early debridement is necessary. The second mechanism is from arcing of the current. The arc has a

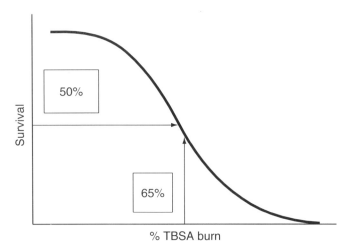

FIG. 1. LA$_{50}$ anticipated morbidity and mortality. When determining the predicted outcome of a burn, it is important to know the expected LA$_{50}$ associated with a particular injury. The chart included here applies to young adults. The curve shifts to the left at the extremes of age. As an example, a 25-year-old person with a 35% TBSA should have a 100% survival rate, provided there are no premorbid diseases. This same injury in an 80-year-old person has a mortality rate approaching 100%; the mortality rate is somewhere between these extremes for a child younger than 2 years old.

temperature of 2,500°C and causes a concentrated deep thermal injury. The third mechanism is a flame burn caused from the ignition of clothing by the arc. Electrical injuries also produce muscular injury and necrosis even though the superficial injuries do not appear substantial. The muscle damage and ensuing compartmental edema must be recognized, and escharotomy or fasciotomy may be necessary. Infrequently, electrical current causes muscle contractions that can fracture bones.

The more important factors determining morbidity and mortality are the percentage of body area burned, the age of the patient, the depth of the burns, and the presence of an inhalation injury. The total body surface area (TBSA) burned that will cause a 50% mortality of the affected patients is designated the lethal area 50% (LA$_{50}$) (Fig. 1) The LA$_{50}$ varies with patient age. The group from 3 years to 50 years tolerates burns the best, with an average LA$_{50}$ of 60% to 65% TBSA. Neonates and infants do slightly worse, with an LA$_{50}$ of 50% TBSA. LA$_{50}$ of individuals over 50 years old is ~40% TBSA; for those over 70 years old, it is as low as 25% TBSA.

EVALUATION AND TREATMENT OF THE BURN PATIENT

Patients who have sustained burn injuries are evaluated in the same manner as any other trauma patient. The primary survey and concomitant resuscitation is followed by secondary survey. Endotracheal intubation is required in patients who cannot maintain a patent airway. Suspected laryngeal edema secondary to inhalation injury mandates direct laryngoscopic evaluation of the vocal cords. If a patient is uncooperative or restless, the primary diagnosis is hypovolemic shock or hypoxia rather than pain. Two large-bore intravenous catheters are inserted, preferably through intact skin or alternatively through burned tissue if necessary. The blood pressure is evaluated and supported with a balanced salt solution.

Secondary survey begins with a complete physical examination. Particular attention is devoted to possible additional injuries. The patient may have been burned during an automobile accident, house fire with falling debris, explosion with projectiles, etc. The approximate time of the burn as well as the circumstances surrounding the burn are noted. Only after hemodynamic stability is appreciated is attention turned to the burn wound.

Special precautions are taken on behalf of the burn patient. Secondary to loss of skin barrier, core hypothermia can develop rapidly. The trauma resuscitation room are therefore warmed to assist the burn patient conserve body heat. Personnel entering the room are gowned and masked and the patient is covered with sterile drapes to reduce contamination of wounds.

Evaluating the depth and size of the burn is an important step in the assessment of the burn patient. These assessments affect many decisions in the triage and treatment of the patient. Burns are classified into degrees based upon the depth of the injury (Fig. 2). First degree burns are painful and warm, but the epidermis remains intact. This injury normally heals in <6 days. Second degree, or partial thickness, burns extend into the dermis. The epidermis usually blisters or sloughs off. This injury is further subdivided into superficial or deep second degree defined by the depth of the dermis injured. As the burn deepens, the dermal color of the wound lightens from a pink (superficial) to a white (deep) burn. Second degree burns are painful because the sensory nerve endings are injured but not destroyed and continue to send painful stimulation. Reepithelialization occurs within 2 to 3 weeks. Skin grafting can be done if the open surface area is large and subjects the patient to undue infection. Third degree, or full-thick-

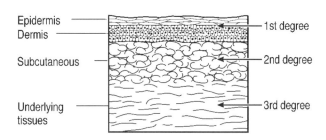

FIG. 2. Skin layers with the corresponding depth of burn.

Date of observation _____
Date of burn _____
Days post burn _____

(√) **Reason for observation**
( ) Admission
( ) Weekly check
( ) Post surgical procedure
( ) Other
(Specify _____)

Estimated % burn by area

Area	3°	Total
Head		
Neck		
Anterior trunk		
Posterior trunk		
Genitals		
Buttocks		
Upper arm		
Forearm		
Hands		
Thighs		
Legs		
Feet		
SUM		

Relative percentages of areas affected by growth (circle age used)			
Area	Age 10	Age 15	Adult
A = 1/2 head	5 1/2	4 1/2	3 1/2
B = 1/2 thigh	4 1/2	4 1/2	4 3/4
C = 1/2 leg	3	3 1/2	3 1/2

A = Autograft   H = Homograft   X = Xenograft

A

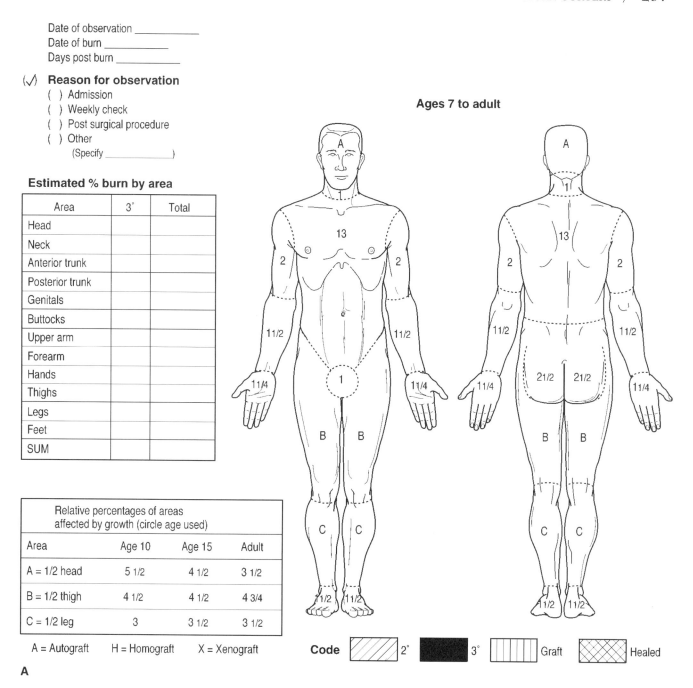

Ages 7 to adult

Code [///] 2°   [■] 3°   [|||] Graft   [XXX] Healed

FIG. 3. (A) Burn sheet for patients ages 7 to adult. This sheet can be used for calculating total body surface area of burn.

ness, burns extend through the dermis into the subcutaneous tissues. The wound may appear white. These burns are not tender because the nerve endings have been completely destroyed. Third degree burns cannot heal by secondary intention and are closed by grafting and contraction.

To estimate the size of a burn in adults, paramedics in the field and emergency room personnel use the Rule of Nines. The surface injury is estimated by assuming the head and each arm are each 9% of the TBSA; each leg and each side of the torso is 18% TBSA; and the genitalia are 1% TBSA (Fig. 3A). Estimated percent TBSA burned in children is problematic because of the proportionally large TBSA of the head (Fig. 3B). The TBSA of the head approaches normal proportions at ~9 to 10 years of age. A common injury to children is a scald burn to the head and face that can exceed 15%, often requiring admission and resuscitation.

Date of observation _____
Date of burn _____
Days post burn _____

( ) **Reason for observation**
    ( ) Admission
    ( ) Weekly check
    ( ) Post surgical procedure
  ✓ ( ) Other
        (Specify _____)

Ages Birth to 7 1/2

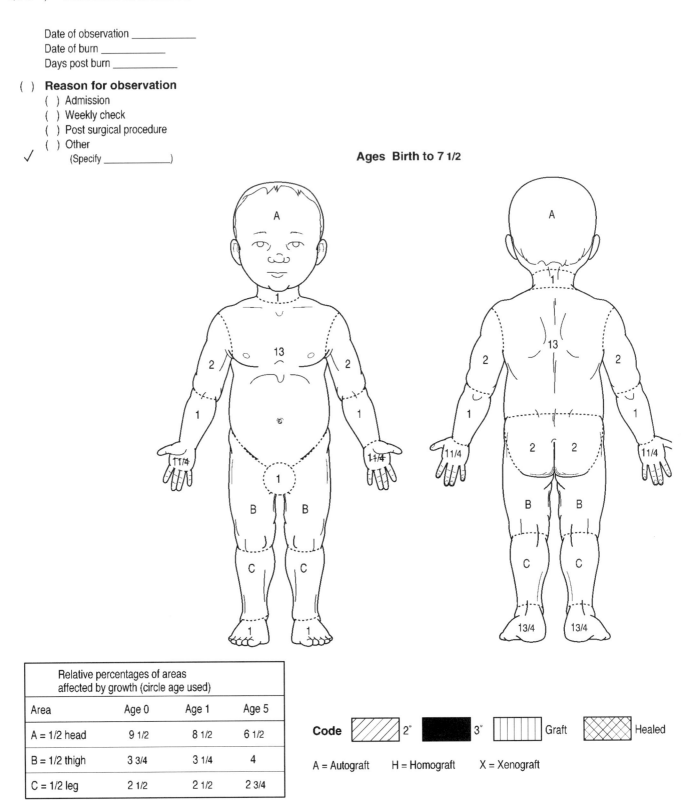

Relative percentages of areas affected by growth (circle age used)			
Area	Age 0	Age 1	Age 5
A = 1/2 head	9 1/2	8 1/2	6 1/2
B = 1/2 thigh	3 3/4	3 1/4	4
C = 1/2 leg	2 1/2	2 1/2	2 3/4

Code [2°] [3°] [Graft] [Healed]

A = Autograft   H = Homograft   X = Xenograft

B

FIG. 3. (B) Burn sheet for patients ages birth to 7.5 years.

TABLE 1. *General guidelines for patient admission for burn treatment*

10–15% total body surface area burn (TBSA)
2% TBSA, third degree burn
Suspicion of child abuse
Inability to care for wound at home
Electrical injuries
Inhalation injuries
Face, hand, feet, flexor crease involvement
History of diabetes or vascular insufficiency
Cellulitis or infected wounds
Circumferential extremity burns
Associated traumatic injuries

General guidelines for patient admission for burn treatment are listed in Table 1. While criteria for admission are individualized, admission is considered for an adult when the burn is ≥10% to 15% TBSA or if ≥2% of the TBSA is a third degree burn. An adult's second degree burn of 10% to 15% TBSA and a child's burn of 10% TBSA is not a local injury, but rather has systemic effects with fluid and electrolyte changes. Burns of >10% in children and 25% in adults are major and require intensive monitoring. Electrical injuries and the possibility of inhalation injuries receive special consideration due to the propensity to underestimate the severity of the wounds and for the patient to worsen clinically in the ensuing 24 to 48 hr. Other patients admitted to the hospital are those with burns of the hands, face, major joints, cellulitis or infection of older burns, circumferential injury, or burns associated with other traumatic injuries. The presence of co-morbid diseases such as diabetes and vascular insufficiency predisposes to poor wound healing and may require admission for meticulous wound care. The complication rate is higher than usual with these diseases.

NONWOUND ISSUES

Social issues are considered when determining need for admission. Suspected cases of child abuse require admission and evaluation by the child protection. Adult patients unable to care for the wounds at home, either due to the location of the wounds or an unsatisfactory home situation, are considered for admission.

24-HOUR FLUID RESUSCITATION: "24 HOURS AFTER TIME ZERO"

Generally, intravenous fluid resuscitation is required in adults with burns of ≥15% TBSA and in children with ≥10% TBSA burned (Fig. 4). Patients with smaller burns do not usually require intravenous rehydration. Several formulae are used to calculate the required fluids for the first 24 hr after a significant burn. The formula most commonly used is the Baxter or Parkland formula.

Fluid resuscitation encompasses a 24-hr period from the time of the burn, not from when the patient is first evaluated in the emergency room.. Cellular research by Baxter from the Parkland Memorial Hospital burn center demonstrated a systemic leak of intravascular volume into the interstitial space develops both at the site of injury and systemically. This resulted in a shift of fluid from the intravascular space to both the interstitial and intracellular space. Cardiac output is relatively low in the early postburn period despite aggressive intravenous fluid resuscitation secondary to this leak phenomenon. Sodium and water resuscitation with 4 cc of lactated Ringer's solution/kg/%TBSA burned replenishes the intravascular space. The total volume calculated is administered evenly over the first 24 hr after burn injury. There appears to be no advantage in using colloid solu-

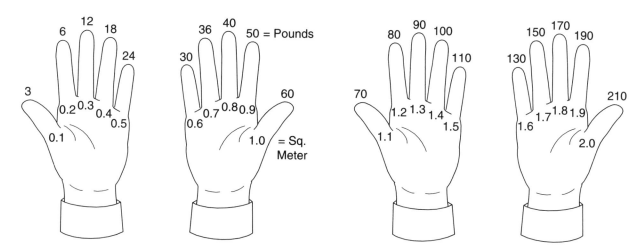

FIG. 4. The maintenance fluids for patients of different body weights are easily calculated by using an index based on surface area of burn. This is consistent with other calculations by the Burn Service because surface area of burns is a standard way of looking at patients and their trauma.

tions during the first 24 hr. It may actually increase pulmonary complications. There are other resuscitation protocols (e.g., Brooke, Moore) using different combinations of crystalloid and colloid solution, which are not discussed here.

Hypertonic solution made by adding 100 meq of sodium acetate to lactated Ringer's solution is an alternative fluid for resuscitation. It can provide the sodium required without large free water volume that accompanies high infusion rates. This is especially important in patients with large burns or circumferential wounds, in which decreased tissue edema is desired. As examples, glottic edema can compromise airway patency; similarly, peripheral edema can result in distal limb vascular insufficiency. Any required boluses for low urine output are made with standard lactated Ringer's and not with hypertonic solutions. Judicious fluid management is imperative during hypertonic resuscitation. Overresuscitation with hypertonic solution will produce hypernatremia. Hypertonic resuscitation typically produces a metabolic alkaline rebound as the acetate and lactate are metabolized to bicarbonate. The metabolic alkalosis is countered by retention of carbon dioxide.

Immediately after a large burn injury, invasive hemodynamic monitoring (e.g., central venous pressure catheters, pulmonary artery catheters) are of little value based on this increased vascular permeability and may actually induce overzealous fluid resuscitation and its complications. Except in patients with preexisting anuric or oliguric renal failure, urine output measurement via foley catheter remains the best indicator of effective fluid resuscitation. For a 150-lb adult, normal urine output is 600 to 800 cc/m² TBSA/day—i.e., ~40 to 60 cc/hr of urine (Fig. 4 depicts a method of correlating TBSA to total body weight in pounds by using digit recall). Tachycardia is common, even in the presence of satisfactory volume resuscitation because of supranormal catecholamine levels and cannot be utilized as true objective data regarding the patient's hemodynamic status. Mental status is often altered by analgesics, and is a poor subjective criterion for evaluation of peripheral perfusion. Skin turgor and capillary filing are difficult to qualitatively and quantitatively evaluate in burned skin. Changes in hematocrit occur throughout the resuscitation phase and cannot be used to quantify adequate resuscitation.

An underestimation of resuscitation requirements is common in inhalation and electrical burns because of hidden injury. A tremendous amount of fluid can be sequestered within burned pulmonary epithelia. Electrical current can have limited injury externally at the entrance site. Internally, however, entire muscle compartments can be destroyed because of the coagulation effect of electrical current. Muscle that is destroyed yields myoglobin, hemoglobin, and cellular debris that is filtered at the renal glomerulus and precipitates within the collecting tubules and can result in acute tubular necrosis. Systemic administration of sodium bicarbonate alkalinizes the urine and helps prevent precipitation of myoglobin and hemoglobin in the kidney. Diuretics are typically not needed if the resuscitation fluids are run at a rate to maintain urine output of ≥100 cc/hr to wash out myoglobin and hemoglobin from the tubules. Mannitol may be used if necessary to induce a tubular "washout"

Glucose is not necessary for adults in the first 24 hr. Early use of glucose containing solutions may induce an unwanted osmotic diuresis. Infants, on the other hand, do not have large stores of glycogen and thus serum glucose of an immature child can become dangerously low. A mixture of 5% glucose and lactated Ringer's is run in young children at a rate to produce an adequate hourly volume of urine. If glycosuria occurs, the glucose concentration is reduced to 2.5%, or 1.25% if needed. Patients may spill ketones into their urine during fluid resuscitation, but it has no apparent clinical significance.

LABORATORY STUDIES

Standard admission blood work at the time of admission includes a complete blood cell count, electrolytes, blood urea nitrogen, creatinine, and coagulation studies. An arterial blood gas and chest radiograph is performed in patients suspected of sustaining inhalation injury. A toxicology screen may document illicit drug or alcohol abuse as a contributing factor in burn injury. Withdrawal symptoms can then be anticipated and preemptively treated. Patients with major burns receive a booster of tetanus toxoid, even if they have been immunized in the past. Patients with an unclear history of immunization receive full immunization against tetanus.

WOUND CARE

A patient admitted with a large wound is covered and kept warm. Treatment begins immediately because heat and evaporative losses of water are large. Ice or iced solutions are not used. They do decrease pain and edema, but they also cause hypothermia, increase metabolic demand, and may injure marginally viable cells within the burn wound. Wounds are debrided by removing all of the loose, injured epidermis and exposing all of the burned area. An accurate TBSA burn injury can then be calculated. Wounds are covered with a topical antimicrobial and sterile dressings. The dressings are changed twice a day to prevent wound infections.

The most commonly used topical agent is silver sulfadiazine cream (Silvadene). It has intermediate wound penetration and a good antimicrobial spectrum. A common complication of silver sulfadiazine is transient leukopenia. White blood cell counts (WBC) must be followed and the cream stopped for 24 hours if the WBC falls below 2,000. Mafenide acetate (Sulfamylon) has excellent wound penetration and is used to decrease bacterial colonization of wound prior to wound excision. It should not be used on large burns because it is systemically absorbed and causes a metabolic acidosis secondary to carbonic anhydrase inhibition and is painful upon application. Dakin's solution (dilute sodium hypochlorite) is occasionally used as wet to dry dressings. It is particularly effective the day before an open wound is to receive a split-thickness skin graft. Dakin's solution is the only topical used for burn wounds known to kill the human immunodeficiency virus. This is important because burn wounds weep and shed body fluids. In small partial thickness wounds, Bacitracin ointment is often used. It is inexpensive and efficient. There are many other topicals such as silver nitrate, povidone-iodine, and Furacin, each having a specific risk-benefit profile.

Wound care is painful, and patients often require supranormal amounts of narcotic medication for pain control. A balance between the benefits of analgesia and the hazards of somnolence or respiratory depression must be maintained at all times. Medications are titrated by small incremental doses until the dressings procedure is tolerable; each day the dosing may change.

SPECIAL CONCERNS

Gastrointestinal Tract and Nutrition

Every effort is made to utilize the gastrointestinal (GI) tract before subjecting a patient to the complications associated with intravenous hyperalimentation solutions. If a patient cannot swallow, tube feeding is instituted. Due to the systemic nature of burn injury, however, intestinal ileus is common in patients sustaining TBSA burns of ≥15%. Nasogastric tube decompression and parenteral nutrition may be necessary in the interim prior to resolution of GI dysfunction.

Stress gastritis (Curling's ulcers) is common in burn patients, especially those individuals sustaining ≥15% TBSA burn. Mucosal ischemia, bile acids reflux into the stomach, and increased hydrochloric acid combined with decreased gastric mucosal cytoprotective barrier contribute to pathogenesis. Fortunately, life-threatening hemorrhage is exceedingly rare. Vitamin A is given to augment the production of mucin. Oral antacids are administered to neutralize the excess acid produced. H_2 receptor antagonists are reserved for patients with a documented history of duodenal ulcers or those patients who are refractory to gastric pH control with oral antacids. Bile acids are bound and inactivated by giving cholestyramine every 6 hr. Replenishment of intravascular volume deficits will increase splanchnic blood flow and decrease or eliminate mucosal ischemia.

TABLE 2. *Child's daily calorie requirements*

Age	Nutritional requirements
Newborn to 6 months	100 kcal/kg
6 months to 2 years	75 kcal/kg
2 years to 25 kg's	50 kcal/kg

These calculated values are doubled if the child has a

Indirect calorimetry and the Harris-Benedict formula are the most accurate methods of determining caloric needs for a burn patient. A simpler method for estimating adults requirements is by the Curreri formula:

24-hr calorie need = (25 × kg) + (45 × % burn).

The protein requirement of a patient with healing burn wounds is increased to nearly three times daily requirement. A child's daily calorie requirements can be estimated by the formulae in Table 2.

Circumferential or near circumferential injuries of the extremities require elevation and frequent neurovascular examinations. Indications of neurovascular insufficiency of the involved extremity include neurologic changes, e.g., pain, paresthesia, diminished peripheral pulses with poor capillary refill, and cyanosis. Full-thickness escharotomy should be performed to allow reperfusion of the extremity. If the circulatory compromise is not improved after the escharotomy, the muscular compartments are evaluated for fascial release (fasciotomy). Circumferential burns of the chest may restrict chest expansion and require escharotomy to improve ventilatory mechanics.

"AFTER THE 24-HOUR RESUSCITATION PERIOD"

Several events herald the emergence from the 24-hr resuscitation period. Hemoconcentration that occurred because of the systemic leak phenomenon during the first 24-hr period reverses as the vascular permeability is stabilized and systemic edema fluid slowly returns to the intravascular space. As a result, the hematocrit begins to fall from dilution but also from red cell lysis because the half-life of a red blood cell (RBC) is markedly reduced after burn injury. A diuresis phase ensues as well from increased relative intravascular volume.

Colloid can be given after the 24-hr resuscitation period with the belief that it will remain in the intravascular space. The Parkland formula loosely recommends 20% to 60% of the plasma volume as salt-poor albumin at a rate to keep a normal urine output. Other formulae suggest a combination of colloid and crystalloid solutions, all with the common goal of maintaining urine output. The increased intravascular albumin may recruit extravascular fluid into the intravascular space.

BURN SURGERY

Historically, severely burned patients underwent operative debridement after the eschar had separated from the wounds. Contemporary burn surgeons term this "late debridement." Most feel early debridement decreases the incidence of infections and sepsis by removing nonviable tissue. Studies have yet to confirm this hypothesis, but many institutions have adopted this burn wound management principle.

Tangential excision shaves injured skin until there is a viable, bleeding surface. Elements that allow secondary closure, such as hair follicles and sweat glands, are not removed. Full-thickness injuries are treated with full-thickness excisions down to the fascia. This process allows tertiary closure by autogenous skin grafting.

Heated operating rooms help the patients conserve core body temperature. Succinyl choline is *not* used for muscle paralysis, as the associated systemic hyperkalemia may cause cardiac arrhythmias. Excision of burn wounds is a procedure that entails a significant blood loss. Up to 200 cc of blood is lost per 1% TBSA burn wound excised. Multiple units of packed RBCs should be immediately available in the operating room. At each operative debridement procedure, tangential excision of >15% TBSA burn wound is not recommended.

The treatment end point for burn injury patients is wound coverage. This reduces the incidence of infection, prevents significant fluid volume shifts, and allows temperature control. If there is adequate donor site surface area, autogenous skin grafting is preferred therapy. Alternatively, homograft (cryopreserved skin) and synthetic semipermeable skin are viable options for temporary coverage. These allografts can remain viable on burn wounds for up to 1 week.

BURN SEPSIS

About half of fatalities from burn injury are secondary to overwhelming wound sepsis. The two major sources of contamination are from the patient's endogenous bacterial flora and from nosocomial organisms spread by health care personnel. Caps, masks, and gloves should be worn when wounds are undressed, and frequent hand washing cannot be overemphasized.

Prophylactic antibiotics are not used routinely except under certain circumstances (e.g., diabetic patients, immunocompromised patients, patients with an indwelling prosthesis). Antibiotics are started when there are clinical signs of a wound infection or signs of sepsis. Medications are metabolized rapidly, secreted into open wounds, and excreted at a higher rate than in a normal patient. Serum drug levels should be sampled frequently.

The majority of burn patients exhibit a low-grade fever. Clinical signs of sepsis indicating the need for

antibiotics include a progressive thrombocytopenia, glucose intolerance, disorientation, high fluid requirement to stabilize the blood pressure, paralytic ileus, and a prolonged fever. Although pulmonary and urinary tract infections are considered in the sick patient with multiple invasive lines and tubes, the burn wound is the most common source of infection. Wounds are inspected for any changes that herald a wound infection. Wound characteristics that suggest infection include conversion of deeper previously viable tissue into nonviable tissue, hemorrhagic areas, cellulitis, or early separation of the eschar. Qualitative culture swabs are sent for bacterial identification and antibiotic sensitivity. Quantitative culture biopsy is sent for a bacterial count per gram of tissue. Wounds are considered infected and not ready for grafting if the count of bacteria exceeds 10^5/g tissue. Such a bacterial count in the wound is defined as burn wound sepsis.

REHABILITATION

From the moment a burn patient is evaluated, physical and occupational therapy is started. It is important to begin as soon as possible because burn wounds tend to contract. The goal of therapy is to prevent contractures and improve function of affected joints. In the intensive care unit, where patients are mainly immobile, therapy consists of passive and active range of motion. Pressure garments, splints, and plastic face masks are used during the long rehabilitation process to decrease hypertrophic scars and joint contractures.

Patients are considered ready for discharge when their wounds are free from infection and when their open wounds do not require extensive therapy, beyond the patient's capability. If there are no support systems at home or in the community, patients may require hospitalization until all wounds are closed.

The process of therapy and scar control may take ≥2 years. As outpatients, burn patients are seen frequently to refine function and scars. Contractures are released early if there is a distortion of the anatomy. Plastic surgeons can revise the matured scars. Social workers help patients to return to society. Psychologists help patients cope with disfigurement issues.

MINOR BURNS

Patients seen in the emergency room or clinic who do not warrant admission have their wounds debrided using an intravenous narcotic for pain control. They are instructed how to clean the wound twice a day with a mild soap and water. Silvadene cream or Bacitracin ointment is used as the wound topical. Patients are instructed to recognize signs of wound infection. Range of motion exercises are taught to prevent scar contractures. A return clinic appointment is made, the timing dependent on the severity of the wounds and the need for rehabilitation therapy. Prophylactic antibiotics are not given except for special circumstances as previously mentioned.

SUMMARY

Burn injury is a systemic insult to body homeostasis that can have devastating physiologic, cosmetic, and emotional consequences. Physicians who manage burn wounds must recognize the management principles discussed here to ensure good recovery. Ideally, the end result of therapy should be the return of the patient to a functioning and fulfilling life.

STUDY QUESTIONS

1. A 73-year-old man comes into the trauma center with 97% TBSA flame burns. Most of the injury is third degree. What is your plan of treatment?
2. What kinds of burns, signs, and symptoms would make you suspicious of an inhalation injury?
3. Discuss the different topical creams and the advantages and disadvantages of each.
4. At what point should a person with circumferential burns receive escharotomy as part of treatment?
5. Compare the different resuscitation protocols.

CHAPTER 23

Surgical Critical Care

Sydney J. Vail and Joseph M. Civetta

There are three general categories of patients who can be considered for admission to the Surgical Intensive Care Unit (SICU). They are patients who require monitoring and observation, those with extensive nursing care requirements, and the truly critically ill who need constant physician care. Some patients may be admitted preoperatively for invasive hemodynamic evaluation and/or monitoring because of their significant cardiac risk factors. This evaluation permits appropriate preoperative preparation to improve cardiac, performance and to try and minimize postoperative cardiac problems including both ischemic events and low cardiac output (CO), which in turn may lead to congestive heart failure or late multiple organ dysfunction syndrome (MODS). Patient care in the SICU is a dynamic process; patients' needs are never static; neither is their care or the information that we obtained from them. Information is charted on a flow sheet, which demonstrates trends that develop during the dynamic SICU course.

DEFINITIONS AND NOMENCLATURE

Systemic inflammatory response syndrome (SIRS) is seen in association with a variety of clinical conditions. Both infectious and noninfectious disease states, including confirmed infections, pancreatitis, ischemia, multitrauma and tissue injury, hemorrhagic shock, immune-mediated organ injury, and others, can cause this clinical inflammatory process. The clinical manifestations include, but are not limited to, more than one of the following: (a) a body temperature of >38°C or <36°C, (b) a heart rate (HR) of >90 beats/min, (c) a respiratory rate of >20 breaths/min or hyperventilation with arterial carbon dioxide partial pressure ($PaCO_2$) of <32, and (d) white blood cell count (WBC) of >12,000 or <4,000 or >10% bands. Complications of SIRS are the development of shock, renal impairment, pulmonary complications, such as adult respiratory distress syndrome (ARDS), cardiac

dysfunction, and other organ system dysfunction or failure. The resulting syndrome is known as MODS; it can also result from sepsis. This syndrome is characterized by the need for supportive care to maintain homeostasis. The term "sepsis" combines SIRS with the presence of a documented infection. This is a manifestation of the patient's response to an infection. When sepsis is associated with hypotension (systolic BP of <90 or its reduction by ≥40 mm Hg from the baseline) despite adequate fluid resuscitation, along with the presence of perfusion abnormalities (i.e., lactic acidosis, oliguria, acute change in mental status), septic shock is diagnosed.

Pulmonary dysfunction can be thought of in terms of an initial lung injury, i.e., acute lung injury (ALI), which may progress to ARDS. ALI is defined by inflammation and increased capillary permeability associated with clinical, radiographic, and physiologic abnormalities that cannot be explained by, but can co-exist with, left atrial or pulmonary capillary hypertension (HTN). The recommended criteria for ALI include (a) acute onset, (b) a ratio oxygenation to arterial oxygen partial pressure/fraction of inspired oxygen (PaO_2/FIO_2) of ≤300 (independent of positive end/expiratory pressure [PEEP] used), (c) bilateral infiltrates on chest x-ray (CXR), and (d) pulmonary artery occlusion pressure (PAOP) of ≤18 mm Hg. To diagnose ARDS, add oxygenation: PaO_2/FIO_2 of ≤200 (independent of PEEP used).

BODY SYSTEMS

Pulmonary System

Patients are continuously monitored for changes in their respiratory status. Acute changes such as cardiac or respiratory arrest will require immediate ventilation, usually by endotracheal intubation. Other patients will have progression of their disease process, i.e., progressive pulmonary insufficiency due to chronic obstructive lung disease (COLD) or ARDS that will eventually require them to be intubated.

There are four basic criteria for intubation: (a) impairment of the airway, (b) inadequate airway protection, (c) inadequate pulmonary toilet, and (d) invasive forms of ventilatory support. Patients from the operating room will arrive either intubated or not depending on the operative procedure performed, anesthetic technique, and/or their level of consciousness. Patients can experience airway compromise after successful extubation. Airway edema (intrinsic), postoperative neck hematomas, subcutaneous emphysema, or other causes of extrinsic airway compromise may reduce the airway patency enough to interfere with normal oxygenation and/or ventilation.

Patients who are unable to "protect" their airway require intubation to "maintain" their airway. The patient who cannot cough adequately or has an impaired gag reflex is at risk for aspiration. Oversedation or incompletely reversed or resolved general anesthesia incurs the same risk as does an impaired mental status (new cerebral vascular accident or toxic/metabolic encephalopathy). Other causes that may require endotracheal intubation include the inability to handle pulmonary secretions (sputum). Retained secretions can be the cause of respiratory failure/arrest, collapse of previously inflated lung tissue (atelectasis), and pneumonia. Patients who demonstrate stridor, hypoxia, desaturation by pulse oximetry, hypercarbia, or obtundation require evaluation for intubation. Hypoxemia is graded as mild (PaO_2 of <80 mm Hg), moderate (PaO_2 of <60 mm Hg and SaO_2 of <90%), and severe (PaO_2 of <40 mm Hg and SaO_2 of <75%) while inspiring room air (21% O_2). Hypercarbia as a reflection of ventilatory failure is defined by a PCO_2 value of >50 mm Hg.

There are several methods to monitor patients' oxygenation and ventilation using either invasive or noninvasive modalities that include pulse oximetry, mixed venous oximetry, and arterial blood gas (ABG) analysis. Pulse oximetry is a noninvasive method of determining percent oxygen saturation of hemoglobin (Hgb) in arterial blood. This method is designated as SpO_2 to differentiate it from the saturation determined from an ABG (SaO_2). The monitoring probe can be placed on a finger, toe, ear lobe, or nasal bridge to determine oxygen saturation. Mixed venous oximetry (SvO_2), an invasive modality, can be performed through a right heart/pulmonary artery (PA) catheter continuously or intermittently depending on the equipment available. This measurement represents the flow-weighted average of the venous oxygen saturations from all perfused tissues in the body. SvO_2 is used to monitor the balance of oxygen delivery and consumption. Changes in this parameter warrant further evaluation of the four determining factors of SvO_2: (a) CO, (b) arterial oxygen saturation (SaO_2), (c) oxygen consumption (Vo_2), and (d) Hgb concentration.

The objectives of ventilatory support are to normalize alveolar ventilation (as judged by $PaCO_2$) and to achieve and maintain an adequate level of arterial oxygenation (PaO_2). These goals can be achieved in a noninvasive (nonintubated) or invasive (intubated) manner.

Noninvasive Techniques

Supplemental oxygen can be given to raise the PaO_2 and thus treat hypoxemia. However, the underlying cause of the hypoxemia must be sought and treated appropriately. Simply treating with supplemental oxygen may be masking a more severe underlying problem, i.e., alveolar hypoventilation, increased intrapulmonary shunt, and ventilation/perfusion mismatch. Acutely, oxygen therapy is aimed at increasing the SaO_2 to >90%, which corresponds to a PaO_2 of ~60 mm Hg, when the oxyhemoglobin dissociation curve is in the normal position.

Continuous positive airway pressure (CPAP) elevates airway pressure above atmospheric pressure throughout spontaneous inspiration and exhalation by using a closed system, i.e., face mask or nasal mask containing a demand valve and imposing PEEP through a valve positioned at the exhalation port. It increases lung volume and improves oxygenation by elevating functional residual volume above the closing volume, thereby preventing airway closure and alveolar collapse. This mode of support assists only spontaneous breathing; it requires an intact respiratory drive and adequate alveolar ventilation. It will improve oxygenation if hypoxemia is caused by decreased lung volume.

Bilevel positive airway pressure (BIPAP) provides inspiratory and end-expiratory lung volume augmentation without tracheal intubation. The settings of this dual-mode support are based on the degree of (a) hypoxic respiratory failure-expiratory pressure and (b) hypercapnic respiratory failure-inspiratory pressure. Like CPAP, it has a closed system containing a valve that sets two pressure levels, the expiratory positive airway pressure level, and the inspiratory positive pressure level. The unit cycles between the two modes that are adjusted (there are separate settings) to the degree of hypoxic or hypercarbic respiratory failure.

Invasive Techniques/Mechanical Ventilation

Patients who are unable to exchange O_2 and CO_2 by spontaneous ventilation require mechanical assistance. For airflow to occur, a pressure gradient must develop between the airway opening and the alveoli. In spontaneous ventilation, respiratory muscles produce a negative intrathoracic pressure. Pressure at the mouth is atmospheric, and thus a gradient for flow is generated. Mechanical ventilation produces a positive pressure gradient that enables flow to reach the alveoli. There are several modes of mechanical ventilation that will be discussed.

Intermittent mandatory ventilation (IMV) is a mode of ventilation that combines a preset number of ventilator-delivered mandatory breaths of predetermined tidal volume and patient-generated spontaneous breaths. This mode allows the patient to perform a variable amount of respiratory work depending on the set number and volume of the ventilator-generated cycles and the patient's own ability. Pressure support ventilation (PSV) augments spontaneous breaths and offsets the resistive forces imposed by the ventilator tubing and the endotracheal tube. It is designed to assist spontaneous patient breathing; therefore, an intact respiratory drive is needed. A patient without spontaneous breathing cannot be ventilated using PSV. It is used to "unload" the respiratory muscles and decrease inspiratory work of breathing. An analogy would be the use of a "spotter" during weight lifting, helping to lift extra weight that your muscles could not do alone. Spontaneous breathing maintains normal respiratory muscle function and prevents disuse atrophy. The less a patient depends on mechanical ventilatory support and sustains their intrinsic respiratory muscle strength and endurance, the sooner they can be removed from mechanical support as the initial respiratory insult that reduced compliance and increased airway resistance resolves.

With assist control ventilation (A/C), every patient breath is supported by the ventilator. The ventilator delivers a breath, either when triggered by the patient's inspiratory effort (assist) or independently, if such an effort does not occur within a preselected period (control). A disadvantage to this mode of ventilation is that the patients do essentially no work to breath; they are totally supported by the ventilator. Once patients initiate the breath (usually only 1 cm H_2O effort) and trigger the ventilator, their work is over for that cycle.

Ventilator Settings

An IMV rate is set to maintain $PaCO_2$ (35 to 45 mm Hg), usually 6 to 8 breaths/min. The rate is decreased as the patient begins to breath spontaneously.

A tidal volume of 10 to 12 ml/kg to allow adequate alveolar inflation and decrease likelihood of atelectasis. Minimal FIO_2 is given to keep PaO_2 at ≥65 mm Hg (associated with SpO_2 of 92%). PEEP is utilized to maintain positive airway pressure at end expiration to prevent distal airway collapse and used to recruit functional residual capacity (FRC), which improves ventilation to areas of low ventilation/perfusion (V/Q) ratios. Pressure support (PS) is utilized and adjusted to avoid a fatiguing respiratory "work" load (intrinsic parenchymal disease, endotracheal tube, and ventilator breathing circuit) that must be measured while adjusting PS to achieve an exhaled tidal volume of 7 to 8 ml/kg.

ABG sampling is routinely performed for patients with any acute cardiovascular or respiratory dysfunction. The

pH, PaO_2, and $PaCO_2$ are measured, and HCO_3 and SaO_2 are calculated. It is important to determine the etiology of an abnormal value and treat the patient appropriately. Adjustments of the ventilator are usually based on the ABG. As an example, low PaO_2 may be treated with increased PEEP or increased supplemental FiO_2.

Weaning From Ventilator Support

Extubation protocols determine when the patient can be safely and successfully extubated. Weaning trials need to be based on endurance criteria rather than a strength determinant at a single moment in time. Thus, gradual decrementation over time permits the patient to demonstrate the ability to assume the reloading of the respiratory muscles. Indices used in the past such as forced vital capacity (FVC) and negative inspiratory force (NIF) are not accurate predictors, for this reason. In fact, they may fail to predict those who may be extubated and prolong intubation. Also, the wide variations in criteria cited in the literature suggest that these absolute numbers do not separate patients to everyone's satisfaction. Often, in order to decrease the failure rate (increased incidence of reintubation) criteria are made more stringent (higher values for FVC and NIF), and the number of patients who could have passed by endurance criteria and have been successfully extubated would also increase; lengthening the duration of mechanical ventilation increases resource utilization, costs, and subjects patients to further risks of mechanical ventilation, including barotrauma, airway edema, and nosocomial pneumonia. In the "uncomplicated" patient, PS may be weaned by 30% changes in centimeters of water: 20 > 14 > 10 > 7 > 5, proceeding as long as tachypnea (>38) does not develop. IMV may be decreased from its initial setting (6 to 8 breaths/min) to 4 then 2 and finally 1 as the patient breathes spontaneously. The 1-IMV breath may be continued at 15 ml/kg as a sigh breath during PSV and weaning in those patients who have continued mechanical ventilation. Once patients are at "minimal settings" and the reason for intubation and mechanical ventilation has resolved, extubation is indicated. The patient is given a "trial" of CPAP and FiO_2 of 21% (room air) trial. If the patient's breathing pattern remains acceptable and rate remains ≤38, and ABG results are acceptable (e.g., pO_2 > 50 mm Hg, pCO_2 < 50 mm Hg), the patient can be extubated with a <5% incidence of reintubation.

Cardiovascular System

ICU patients are admitted with preexisting stable or unstable cardiac disease, evolving changes in their cardiac status, or expected changes secondary to their illness or operative procedure. Cardiac performance is influenced by many factors, including "preload," "contractility," and "afterload" and judged by CO, HR, stroke volume (SV), filling pressures, and systemic vascular resistance (SVR). PAOP is an estimate of left ventricular filling pressure (preload). Similarly, central venous pressure (CVP) estimates right ventricular filling pressure. Intrinsic force of myocardial contraction independent of preload and afterload describes contractility. CO and mean arterial pressure are the indices that reflect changes in inotropic activity. Afterload describes the sum of forces against which the left ventricle must act to eject blood into the aorta. It is composed of peripheral vascular (friction) resistance, arterial capacitance (stiffness), the mass of aortic column of blood, and the blood viscosity. The most commonly used measure of left ventricular afterload is the SVR.

Invasive hemodynamic monitoring at the bedside permits the acquisition of information concerning cardiorespiratory performance and the effects of therapy in critically ill patients. Arterial catheters are placed when continuous blood pressure (BP) monitoring and/or frequent arterial blood samples are needed. States in which precise and continuous BP data are necessary include acute hypertensive crisis, shock of any etiology, use of vasoactive or inotropic drugs, hypotensive anesthesia, high levels of respiratory support, and any situation in which the factors affecting cardiac function are rapidly changing. Because BP trends are as important as absolute values, direct arterial BP monitoring reminds the clinician to think about what is happening and to determine why changes are occurring.

The Swan-Ganz PA catheter is a balloon-tipped, flow-directed, multilumen instrument that is able to provide the following information: CVP, pulmonary artery systolic and diastolic pressures (PAS and PAD), mean pulmonary artery pressures (PAP), PAOP, CO, mixed venous blood gas sampling, continuous mixed venous oximetry (SvO_2), and right ventricular ejection fraction (special catheter). The indications most often used for placement of a PA catheter are listed in Table 1. The PA catheter is able to monitor the patient's present hemodynamic status and changes relative to any therapeutic intervention.

The catheter may be inserted via a central venous route, usually through the subclavian or the internal jugular veins and, with the balloon inflated, advanced until the balloon occludes a branch of the PA determined by waveform recognition (Fig. 1). It is important to follow the progress of the catheter (watching the pressure tracings during advancement and noting the distance markers on the catheter) from balloon inflation to recognition of the PAOP tracings. Catheters not in proper position can give inaccurate measurements, and those that are advanced too far can potentially rupture a branch of the PA. As the catheter traverses the right ventricle, ventricular arrhythmias can occur that are usually self-limited but should be treated if sustained. Intravenous lidocaine and a defibrillator should

TABLE 1. *Recommended indications for placement of pulmonary artery catheters*

General
  Shock unresponsive to perceived adequate fluid therapy
  Oliguria unresponsive to perceived adequate fluid therapy
  Assessment of the effect of intravascular volume on cardiac function
  Delineation of cardiovascular contribution to multiple organ system dysfunction
Surgical
  Preoperative cardiovascular assessment and perioperative management of high-risk patients undergoing extensive surgical procedures
  Intraoperative and postoperative assessment of cardiac function during cardiac or major vascular procedures
  Management of postoperative cardiovascular complications
  Assessment and management of cardiac function in patients, especially the elderly, who have suffered multisystem trauma
  Resuscitation of patients who have suffered severe burns especially if central venous pressure and urine output appear to be unsatisfactory monitoring parameters
Pulmonary
  To differentiate noncardiogenic ARDS from cardiogenic pulmonary edema
  To assess effects of high levels of ventilatory support on cardiovascular status
Cardiac
  Complicated myocardial infarction
  Unstable angina requiring intravenous nitroglycerine therapy
  Congestive heart failure unresponsive to conventional therapy, to guide preload and afterload therapy
  Pulmonary hypertension, for diagnosis and monitoring during acute drug therapy

be at the bedside of any patient having a PA catheter inserted. The first maneuver when noting sustained arrhythmias is to deflate the balloon and withdraw the catheter from the heart back into the superior vena cava (SVC). This usually corrects the problem; insertion is then reattempted. When the catheter is in the proper position (also verified by CXR) and the balloon is inflated, the PA branch is occluded, there is no forward blood flow, and the distal tip of the catheter is approximately equal to mean left atrial pressure (LAP). The correct term is "pulmonary artery occlusion pressure"—i.e., PAOP—although pulmonary capillary wedge pressure is still used, i.e., the "wedge" pressure. The balloon is deflated; a PA tracing reappears, and the balloon is reinflated slowly until the PAOP tracing reappears. With the balloon inflated, the catheter tip is in effect one end of a continuous valveless column of blood ending in the left atrium; in the absence of flow, there is no pressure gradient; thus, the PAOP approximates LAP. In the absence of mitral valve disease or premature valve closure, the LAP reflects the left ventricular end-diastolic pressure (LVEDP). LVEDP will

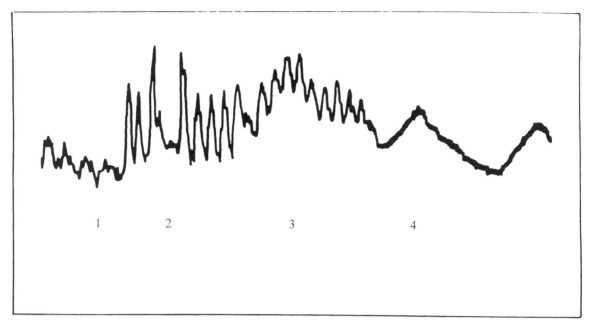

FIG. 1. A recording of a pulmonary artery catheter passed from the right atrium to the PAO position. Note the RA pressure tracing *(1)* is followed by RV pressures *(2)*, pulmonary artery pressures *(3)*, and finally, PAO "wedge" pressures with ventilator induced pressure variation *(4)*.

reflect left ventricular end-diastolic volume (LVEDV), although the exact relationship depends upon left ventricular compliance. The LVEDV reflects the end-diastolic stretch of the ventricular wall muscle fibers, which represents the true preload. Thus, changes in PAOP are frequently used as the estimate of changes in left ventricular preload. CO is determined using the thermodilution technique. When CO and HR are known, the SV can be calculated, recalling the equations: CO/HR = SV.

Interventions

The primary determinants of SV are preload, afterload, and contractility. Hemodynamic intervention begins with attempts to increase SV by increasing preload with intravascular volume if PAOP is low. Fluid is administered rapidly while changes in PAOP and CO/SV are monitored. If tissue perfusion remains inadequate after optimizing preload, SV augmentation may be accomplished by increasing myocardial contractility with inotropic drugs or decreasing afterload with vasodilators or both. Once it has been determined that the hypotension is not due to inadequate intravascular volume (low PAOP or preload) or decreased afterload, which may be treated by increasing SVR, an inotropic agent is started. The goal of inotropic therapy is to increase CO and SV. This, in turn, increases BP, which reflects the ejection of the SV into the vascular area, to provide adequate coronary and end-organ perfusion.

Adrenergic agonists stimulate the heart through their β_1 effects and act on the peripheral arterial vasculature through both α_1 and β_2 receptors. Epinephrine has dose-dependent effects on the heart and peripheral vasculature. At lower doses (0.04 to 0.1 μg/kg · min), the β effects predominate, including increased HR, CO, and SV, and decreased SVR. With higher doses, SVR increases due to α effects plus increased venous return. Myocardial oxygen consumption is also increased, and myocardial ischemia may result if the increase in consumption is greater than the increased supply produced by the higher CO and perfusion pressure. Continuous ST-segment monitoring of myocardial ischemia is absolutely necessary with the use of epinephrine. Adverse cardiac events, such as myocardial infarction, congestive heart failure, or arrhythmia, are associated with epinephrine-related myocardial ischemia. Norepinephrine has potent β_1 effects and increases myocardial inotropy; its α effects lead to vasoconstriction, which reduces renal and mesenteric perfusion while increasing LV afterload. BP increases, but CO may decrease due to increased afterload. This agent also increases myocardial oxygen consumption and can aggravate myocardial ischemia. Isoproterenol has potent β effects and no effect on α receptors. Peripheral vasodilatation occurs with β_2 stimulation, and increases in HR, contractility, and CO occur with β_1 stimulation. This drug does not increase coronary perfusion pressure and causes an increase or persistence in anaerobic myocardial metabolism and ventricular irritability. Dopamine is titrated to the desired hemodynamic response. At low doses (1 to 4 μg/kg/min) dopaminergic (DA-1) receptors are stimulated to increase renal blood flow. There is also stimulation of mesenteric, cerebral, and coronary DA-1 receptors causing vasodilatation. DA-2 receptor stimulation inhibits norepinephrine release, thereby causing vasodilatation. Doses of 5 to 10 µg/kg/min have β_1 effects that result in increasing CO, SV, and BP, whereas doses of >10 µg/kg/min have α_1 effects, and increase SVR and cardiac filling pressures. Dobutamine, a synthetic catecholamine, has mostly β_1 adrenergic effects, and minimal vasoconstrictive and chronotropic effects.

The beneficial effect of vasodilators is produced by their ability to reduce LV work that is mediated by reducing SVR (afterload) or increasing venous capacitance. With reduction of afterload, myocardial tension and time of contraction are both reduced: each is associated with myocardial oxygen consumption. Nitroglycerine is used to reduce preload and LAP, and increase coronary flow. Nitroprusside affects both preload and afterload by its arterial and venous dilatation. Adequate intravascular volume must be maintained and BP carefully titrated to avoid hypotension and decreasing myocardial oxygen delivery.

Cardiac Arrhythmias

Cardiac arrhythmias are categorized by point of origin (e.g., supraventricular or ventricular) and rate (e.g., bradycardia or tachycardia).

Supraventricular Arrhythmias

Sinus rates of >100 beats/min are defined as sinus tachycardia and can be due to fever, pain, hypoxia, hypovolemia, anemia, anxiety, medication, and shock. Treatment is aimed at the underlying cause. Sinus rates of <60 beats/min are termed "sinus bradycardia" and can be due to drugs, increased intracranial pressure, hypothyroidism, carotid sinus massage, and sinus node dysfunction. Treatment is indicated if the patient is symptomatic due to hypoperfusion or reduced CO. Atropine is the initial drug of choice, given intravenously (0.5 to 1 mg) in the acute setting. Isoproterenol can be used as a continuous infusion, beginning with 1 µg/min and titrated to effect. If drug therapy fails to treat the bradycardia, an external pacemaker or transvenous pacing catheter may be used. Premature atrial contractions (PACs) are characterized by premature abnormal P waves, usually followed by a normal QRS complex (AV nodal conduction can be variable). Premature junctional contractions (PJCs) initiate a premature normal QRS complex without a preceding P wave. Atrial flutter is characterized by an atrial rate of 250 to 350/min and either 2:1, 3:1, or 4:1 AV conduction. A "saw tooth" pattern of P waves is typically seen on rhythm strip or electrocardiogram (inferior leads most pronounced). Performing carotid massage usually slows AV conduction enough to reveal flutter waves. If the patient is hemodynamically unstable, synchronized cardioversion is indicated. Rapid ventricular responses can be treated with digitalis, calcium channel blockers, and type Ia antiarrhythmic agents (Quinidine, Procainamide, Disopyramide). Atrial fibrillation is characterized by complete loss of organized atrial activity with a ventricular response rate of between 100 and 200 beats/min, usually. Hemodynamically unstable patients should have synchronized cardioversion performed, starting at 50 joules. Digitalis and esmolol are given to control the ventricular response by slowing conduction through the AV node.

Ventricular Arrhythmias

Premature ventricular contractions (PVCs) originate below the level of the AV node, are characterized by an early wide complex not preceded by a P wave, and are followed by a compensatory pause. Frequent (>6 to 8/min), multifocal, or multiple couplets or triplets require intervention, such as intravenous lidocaine or procainamide. Ventricular tachycardia (VT) is diagnosed when more than three consecutive PVCs at a rate of >100 beats/min is seen. This dysrhythmia requires rapid recognition and treatment due to the possibility of deterioration to ventricular fibrillation (VF). Ventricular flutter is a rapid form of VT (>200 beats/min) that can deteriorate to VF if not treated, whereas VF is chaotic ventricular activity. Please refer to the ACLS protocols by the American Heart Association for treatment algorithms.

Hypertensive Emergencies

Severe HTN is defined as a diastolic pressure of >120 mm Hg. This level of HTN is associated with end-organ injury, including the central nervous system (encephalopathy or intracranial hemorrhage), renal insufficiency, and heart failure or myocardial ischemia. Continuous arterial pressure monitoring is a necessity to allow titration of therapy. The goal of treatment is to reduce mean arterial pressure [MAP = DBP + 1/3 (SBP - DBP); DBP = diastolic pressure; SBP = systolic BP] to 120 mm Hg over 1 to 2 hr or reduction in MAP by 20%. Sodium nitroprusside, at an initial rate of 0.5 to 1.0 µg/kg/min and titrated to desired BP, is a first-line agent. It is a direct vasodilator, with an immediate onset of action and a short duration of action.

Shock

Shock is defined as "an acute clinical syndrome initiated by hypoperfusion, resulting in severe dysfunction of organs vital to survival." This definition (of 1992) is not that different from one described in 1872 by Samuel D. Gross. He refers to shock as a "rude unhinging of the machinery of life." The clinical presentation of shock varies because each organ system is affected differently, depending on the severity of the perfusion defect, the underlying cause, and prior organ dysfunction. Shock is classified as hypovolemic, cardiogenic, and mixed.

Hypovolemic shock can result from hemorrhagic—e.g., gastrointestinal (GI) bleeding, trauma, internal bleeding—and nonhemorrhagic causes—e.g., diarrhea and vomiting, renal losses, diabetes insipidus, burns, pancreatitis, and peritonitis). Cardiogenic shock is commonly the result of myocardial infarction, cardiomyopathy, valvular disease/dysfunction, cardiac trauma, massive pulmonary embolus, and cardiac arrhythmia. Mixed shock can occur with sepsis, toxic shock, trauma without hypovolemia, neurogenic shock, and anaphylactic shock.

The vital organs most often affected by shock are the brain, heart, and kidneys. The brain is able to autoregulate its perfusion until the MAP is <60 to 70 mm Hg. The most common clinical manifestation to decreased cerebral perfusion is a change in mental status. Cardiac dysfunction that is due to shock can perpetuate further shock and lead to worse cardiac dysfunction (tachycardia, rhythm changes, congestive failure). Oliguria due to a decrease in glomerular filtration rate (GFR) during shock is a common renal manifestation. A metabolic acidosis (lactic acidosis) and arterial hypotension are two systemic manifestations of shock. Lactic acidosis is due to tissue hypoxia and anaerobic metabolism, often complicated by inadequate hepatic function to metabolize the increased lactate. Management includes primary resuscitation (airway, breathing, circulation), repletion of intravascular volume, increasing tissue perfusion to limit cellular hypoxia, and defining the etiology and providing specific therapy.

Renal System

The kidneys function to excrete metabolic wastes and regulate water, electrolyte, and acid/base balances. They are involved in BP regulation through the renin-angiotensin system, red blood cell production with secretion of erythropoietin, and calcium homeostasis through production of the active form of vitamin D.

Acute renal failure (ARF) occurs as an abrupt decline in renal function (decreased GFR) to cause retention of nitrogenous waste. This definition does not reflect the amount of urine produced. ARF can be manifest as oliguric (<400 ml/day) or nonoliguric (>400 ml/day) renal failure. Causes of renal failure are classified as prerenal, renal, or postrenal. All three present as increases in BUN and Cr (azotemia), in either the oliguric or nonoliguric forms. Prerenal azotemia is caused by decreased renal perfusion that is typically associated with an absolute decrease in intravascular volume or decreased CO. Renal azotemia is caused by glomerular disease, interstitial nephritis, renovascular disease, and acute tubular necrosis (ATN) in the general population. In the ICU, multiple specific and interrelated factors are more common

including sepsis, nephrotoxic agents (especially aminoglycosides and amphotericin), intravenous contrast media, shock/hypovolemia, immunosuppressive agents, and the hepatorenal syndrome. Postrenal azotemia is usually due to obstruction to urine flow after the level of the renal collecting system.

A relatively specific test to determine prerenal ARF is to calculate the fractional excretion of sodium (FE_{Na}), the fraction of filtered sodium that is ultimately excreted by the nephron.

$$FE_{Na}\% = (Urine_{Na} \times Plasma_{Cr}/Plasma_{Na} \times Urine_{Cr}) \times 100,$$

where Na is sodium and Cr is creatinine. A value of <1% is consistent with prerenal causes and >1% consistent with renal causes of ARF. Clinical examination and other available information (CVP, PAOP, CO) can usually rule out prerenal etiologies, a Foley catheter rules out lower tract obstruction (if urine is obtained), and a renal ultrasound can rule out a hydronephrosis (upper tract obstruction) as the cause of ARF.

The major determinants of outcome from ARF are the precipitating events and preexisting disease. Probably the most important treatment for patients with ARF, however, is stimulating urine output if they are oliguric. Repleting intravascular volume, monitoring of PAOP, reversal of hypotension and hypoxemia, use of diuretics, and renal-stimulating doses of dopamine are all therapeutic options available to treat oliguric ARF. Compared with patients with oliguric ARF, patients with nonoliguric ARF have less hemodialysis (HD) use and improved survival. The mortality rate from ARF is ~50%; in nonoliguric patients, it is ~25%, but in oliguric ARF, the mortality rate rises to ~70%. During ARF, complications from drug, fluid, and nutrition therapy are common; early recognition with proper management can avoid major complications. HD is often necessary when the patient has hypervolemia, significant metabolic acidosis, uremic symptoms, hyperkalemia, or other metabolic derangements. Dialysis can be performed intermittently with the potential complication of hemodynamic instability. Continuous methods of dialysis and ultrafiltration offer gradual removal of fluids and solutes and provide continuous blood purification and greater hemodynamic stability.

Alimentary Tract

Following general anesthesia and/or abdominal surgical procedures, normal GI peristalsis is interrupted via direct GI tract trauma or increased splanchnic nerve sympathetic discharge. Typically, small bowel organized peristalsis returns first (12 to 24 hr), gastric peristalsis second (24 to 48 hr), and colonic peristalsis last (~48 to 72 hr). This process may fail because of adynamic ileus, gastric dilatation, intolerance of normal GI secretions or enteral feeds, and abdominal distention. GI distention causes patient discomfort and forces the diaphragm cephalad to decrease intrathoracic lung volumes that can impair normal ventilation.

Salivary, gastric, biliary, pancreatic, and intestinal secretions account for ~8 to 10 L/day of fluid. GI tract dysfunction can lead to losses of fluid and electrolytes: obstruction with vomiting leads to dehyration with a hypochloremic and hypokalemic metabolic alkalosis; diarrhea leads to progressive hypovolemia and a metabolic acidosis. Therapy is aimed at restoration of fluid and electrolyte balances and treating the underlying pathology.

The stomach becomes the reservoir for upper tract secretions. Placement of a nasogastric tube relieves gastric distention, obtains accurate gastric output assessment, and allows monitoring of the character of the effluent (bilious, bloody, feculent). If enough volume is evacuated by suction, a hypochloremic metabolic alkalosis can develop. Causes for a prolonged ileus in the ICU patient include narcotic analgesics, electrolyte imbalances, intraabdominal inflammation, sepsis, MODS, and shock states.

Clinical examination/assessment of the abdomen is often difficult because patients have impaired mental status (sedation, analgesics, primary or secondary disease processes) or recent abdominal surgery with perioperative pain. When infection is suspected, an intraabdominal source should be considered after abdominal surgery when the patient's status deteriorates and other more obvious sources (wound infection, pneumonia, urinary tract infection (UTI), device-related bloodstream [catheter or line] infection) have been ruled out. Metabolic and electrolyte imbalances, mechanical ventilation, malnutrition, and shock associated with hypoperfusion are associated with complications such as mesenteric ischemia, pancreatitis, bowel obstruction, acute cholecystitis (calculous or acalculous), and hollow viscus perforation. All cause signs and symptoms of an acute abdomen; prompt diagnosis and treatment are essential to reduce morbidity and mortality. Therefore, these conditions must be suspected in order to be detected in a timely fashion.

GI tract bleeding in the critically ill must be diagnosed, managed, and resuscitated quickly and simultaneously. Approximately 70% of all GI bleeding stops spontaneously, with an associated 8% to 10% mortality. Management is directed first at prevention, then at treatment of the consequences of GI blood loss. In the critically ill, endoscopic evident gastritis or ulceration has been documented in 75% to 100% of patients, although clinically evident bleeding occurs in only ~20%. Hematemesis, bloody nasogastric aspirate, melena, and hematochezia all indicate GI bleeding. Indications of major blood loss include resting tachycardia, orthostasis, acidosis, azotemia (without previous renal disease), transfusion requirement beyond expected operative losses, hematochezia from an upper GI source, failure to clear bright red blood during gastric lavage, and continued bleeding or rebleeding during endoscopy.

Patients at greatest risk are those with burns, sepsis, major trauma, and MOSD/MOSF. Prophylactic therapy significantly reduces the risk of acute upper GI bleeding. Available agents include antacids, H_2 blockers, and cytoprotective agents (sucralfate). Neutralization of or prevention of acid secretion has been associated with increased incidence of nosocomial pneumonia, especially in long-term ventilated patients; therefore, cytoprotective agents are preferred. Prompt, adequate, and complete resuscitation may be the most important preventative maneuver as "stress gastritis" appears to be the result of mucosal ischemia. Empiric therapy for treatment of upper GI bleeding is aimed at raising gastric pH or inducing vasoconstriction of bleeding vessels with somatostatin or vasopressin. Definitive therapy is directed at the point of bleeding: endoscopy to perform sclerosis or cautery, angiography for identification of bleeding vessel with embolization or directed vasoconstrictive agent infusion, or surgery to remove the bleeding source and prevent acid secretion.

Surgical Nutrition

Nutritional support requires a set plan initiated on admission to the SICU. Each patient is assessed for their risk of developing, or degree of preexisting, malnutrition (inadequate nutrient intake for ~7 days or weight loss of ≥10% of preillness body weight). Preexisting diseases resulting in a reduced caloric intake and chronic malnutrition are common, especially in patients with bowel obstruction, pancreatitis, cancer cachexia, chronic illness, chronic pain, and perioperative nothing-by-mouth (NPO) status. Increased metabolic demands, i.e., sepsis, burns, multiple trauma, and multiple operative procedures, place the patient at risk for acute malnutrition.

Patient's history, examination, and laboratory tests make up the nutritional assessment that determines present status and requirements. Obvious muscle wasting, reduced serum albumin (half-life of 21 days), prealbumin (half-life of 2 days), and transferrin (half-life of 8 days) are all indicators of acute or chronic malnutrition. An estimate of daily caloric needs is 20 to 30 kcal/kg/day of nonprotein calories, with protein requirements of 1.5 to 2.5 g/kg/day, depending on the level of individual stress.

Nutrition is delivered by two routes: enteral and parenteral. The enteral route is preferred as it is physiologic, maintaining normal anatomy, as well as neural, endocrine, immune, and humoral states in terms of gut interactions. The parenteral route is utilized when enteral nutrition is not practical or possible secondary to the lack of GI integrity or compromised function. Enteral nutrition is administered orally if possible to patients with low risk of aspiration and intact cough and gag reflexes. Other patients will require placement of a feeding tube by either an invasive or noninvasive technique. Techniques include bedside nasogastric/nasoenteric (duodenal or preferably jejunal), fluoroscopic nasogastric/nasoenteric, percutaneous fluoroscopic tubes (PFG/PFJ), percutaneous endoscopic tubes (PEG/PEJ), and surgical gastrostomy or jejunostomy.

The rate of administration, more than the osmolarity or type of feeding, influences how the patient will tolerate enteral nutrition, the major side effect being diarrhea and/or malabsorption. Elemental diets are utilized in the patient who has minor or moderately depressed gut absorptive function; these diets contain amino acids or short-chain peptides instead of intact proteins, oligosaccharides or monosaccharides as a source of carbohydrates, and long- or medium-chain triglycerides for fat content. Polymeric diets are used in the patient with an intact absorptive capacity; they are composed of whole proteins, oils, and corn syrup to provide the protein, fat, and carbohydrate calories.

Most current methods of nutritional management often fail to provide a fuel source for the intestinal mucosa, especially when using total parenteral nutrition (TPN). It is known that the GI tract plays a significant role in modulation of the metabolic, humoral, and immune responses of the body during stress and critical illness. Glutamine is the primary energy source for the small intestinal epithelium. Glutamine is the most abundant amino acid in the body, but levels rapidly decrease with illness and stress. Patients with sepsis have impaired metabolism of glutamine that may affect breakdown of the gut mucosal barrier and lead to translocation of bacteria. Therefore, the diet must be supplemented with enteral glutamine (enteral feeding reduces septic morbidity rates when compared to parenteral nutrition).

TPN is delivered through a central venous access catheter and is given when the GI tract cannot be used for nutritional support. The cost of TPN is considerably more than enteral feeding and has significant complications associated with its use. Complications include technical (catheter failure), infection (potentially leading to catheter-related sepsis), metabolic (glucose, fluid, electrolyte, and acid/base imbalances), and nutritional (deficiency or excess of macronutrients, minerals, vitamins, and trace elements). Its efficiency, though now considered less than enteral feedings, is unquestioned; it offers nutrition to the patient who otherwise could not be given nutritional support. All types of nutritional support need to be modified when the patient has hepatic, renal, pancreatic, respiratory, short bowel syndrome, or other functional/structural problems. The nutritional support staff should be consulted, and vigilance must be maintained to avoid complications in both the enterally and parenterally fed patient.

Infectious Disease/Fever

Fever is a disorder of normal thermoregulation that is controlled in the anterior hypothalamus. The most important role for fever in the critically ill patient is to provide an early warning sign for infection or inflammation. The most accurate location for taking a temperature and following a temperature trend is a core location (via a sensor on the distal end of a PA catheter) followed by an esophageal or bladder temperature probe. Rectal temperature recording is a better noninvasive mode than an oral or axillary method.

When a patient develops a temperature of >2° above the highest temperature in the preceding 24 hr, a fever workup is initiated. The first step of the workup is a careful review of the history, including recent procedures and operations along with a detailed and directed physical examination. A directed approach most likely will lead the examiner to the etiology of the fever; the "shotgun" approach of ordering multiple laboratory and radiographic studies does *not* take the place of a carefully performed assessment of the patient. Although it may ultimately determine the infectious source, it is inefficient, wasteful, time-consuming, and thus counterproductive in this cost-sensitive era. "Panculturing" a patient is popular jargon but poor practice.

Patients in the unit have many potential sources of fever: prolonged intubation that can cause colonization with pathogenic bacteria leading to tracheobronchitis or predisposing the patient to pneumonia; nasogastric or nasoenteric tubes that induce sinusitis by causing swelling of the ostia; indwelling urinary catheters that can predispose to UTIs or pyelonephritis; invasive arterial or venous catheters associated with entrance site infections/cellulitis or catheter-related sepsis (bacteremia with the same organism cultured from the catheter); surgical incisions or other operative sites that can become infected; and use of broad-spectrum antibiotics that allow the patient to become superinfected by fungi because of the suppression of bacterial growth, just to name a few of the nosocomial (hospital-acquired) infections that lead to increased length of stay, utilization of resources, and increased morbidity and mortality rates. Ventilator-associated pneumonia has the highest mortality rate of the nosocomial infections.

Early fever (<48 hr) in the postoperative patient is most likely from atelectasis following a general anesthesia and reduced FRC. Rapid resolution of the fever is usually seen after improving pulmonary toilet (increasing FRC with coughing, deep breathing, and use of an incentive spirometer to open collapsed distal airways). Other than a directed physical examination, no further workup is usually necessary for early postoperative fevers.

Late fevers (48 hr) require a more organized and detailed investigation to determine the etiology. Wound infections are diagnosed if there are erythema, tenderness, edema, and drainage noted in the operative site. Crepitance around a surgical site could be a sign of necrotizing fasciitis or *Clostridium* infection that represents a surgical emergency requiring immediate debridement. Pyuria noted in the foley drainage system should raise suspicion for a UTI. Purulent sputum, infiltrates on CXR, leukocytosis, and a predominant bacteria species by gram stain from tracheobronchial secretions support the diagnosis of pneumonia.

Transcutaneous vascular catheters that have inflammatory changes at the skin entry site are likely to become infected. If a transcutaneous vascular access catheter is suspected as the source of fever, it can be exchanged over a guidewire for a new one and the intracutaneous segment (not the catheter tip) sent for quantitative culture (Civetta, JM). This segment is the part of the catheter that traverses the skin and subcutaneous tissues to enter the vascular system. If this segment culture reveals >15 colony-forming units, it is considered positive for infection, the replaced line is removed, and a new site is used for central access. Today, we utilize "protected" catheters (antibiotic/antibacterial impregnated catheters) that reduce the incidence of catheter-related infections. The risk of infection for arterial catheters is related to the site of insertion. The axillary site has greater potential for infection than the femoral, which has a higher rate of infection than the radial artery.

When treating suspected infections, the antibiotics used should be chosen to treat the suspected organism(s) involved. Ideally, the empiric antibiotics (chosen before the culture results are known) will be effective against the subsequently identified organisms. The likelihood can be increased by collecting and calculating susceptibility of all organisms cultured within the specific ICU. Prolonged therapy with broad-spectrum antibiotics increase the risk for superinfection, especially with fungi; the most limited but efficacious antibiotic should be used, and prophylactic antifungal therapy should be started empirically whenever broad-spectrum antibiotics are used. Widespread and sometimes indiscriminate use of antibiotics can lead to the development of resistant organisms that are resistant to all antibiotics. This problem is of increasing importance: vancomycin-resistant enterococcus and multiple drug-resistant *Pseudomonas aeruginosa* have been identified in many hospitals in the last few years.

We utilize antibiotics in three general ways: (a) prophylactic (<48 hr) to prevent bacterial invasion, (b) empiric (<96 hr) when infection is obvious or highly suspected but organism(s) are not yet identified, and (c) therapeutic (>7 days) when treating a known organism/disease process. Antibiotic therapy should be considered a dynamic process, with continued review of laboratory information and assessment of the patient's response, which may dictate changes in therapy. Transmission of infectious agents or materials from patients to health care workers (and back to other patients) has prompted the use of Universal Precautions. Protective eyewear/face shields, masks, gloves, impervious gowns, surgical caps, needle safety devices, etc., reduce exposure to infectious agents. The cornerstone of preventing patient-to-patient transmission of organisms is handwashing, before and after patient contact.

SUMMARY

The three major objectives of monitoring critically ill patients are (a) to assure that the patient remains stable, (b) to provide an early warning system for untoward events, and (c) to evaluate the efficiency and efficacy of interventions performed. The experience in the SICU is an opportunity to treat the most critically ill patients—a challenge at the least and an accomplishment in the end.

Not all patients will recover. If the time arrives that we realize that cure is no longer possible, we do not give up in despair. Rather, we change our goal to a new and equally vital one: caring for the patient and family. Our time should be spent in communication, explanation, and clarification rather than ordering new drugs, tests, or procedures. Effective clinical decision-making still depends primarily on the processor: a knowledgeable and caring physician. When life cannot be prolonged with value for the patient, our role changes to foster the patient's dignity at the time of death. If we do not recognize when death is inevitable, continued efforts prolong the patient's dying—an unworthy and intrusive process. Rather, we should withdraw care, and respect the patient's autonomy and wishes, whether expressed in an advanced directive or through a proxy or family member. Understanding when further care and treatment are futile and serve no obvious purpose other than to interfere with the process of dying is of paramount importance in the care of the critically ill.

STUDY QUESTIONS

1. List the four determining factors of Sv_{02}.
2. Following a successful CPAP trial and extubation, the patient incurs a ____% risk of reintubation.
3. List at least seven of the indications for placement of a PA catheter.
4. The primary determinants of SV are HR, blood viscosity (Hct), and contractility. True or false?
5. The most important treatment for patients with oliguric ARF is (choose one): (a) increasing CO; (b) increasing overall volume status; (c) stimulating urine output; (d) initiating early HD; (e) renal transplant.

SUGGESTED READING

Bernard GR, Artigas A, Brigham KL, et al. Report of the American-European Consensus Conference on Acute Respiratory Distress Syndrome: definitions, mechanisms, relevant outcomes, and clinical trial coordination. *J Crit Care* 1994;9:72.

Civetta JM, Taylor RW, Kirby RR, eds. *Critical care.* 3rd ed. Philadelphia: Lippincott-Raven, 1997.

Members of the Amercan College of Chest Physicians/Society of Critical Care Medicine Consensus Conference Committee. Definitions for sepsis and organ failure and guidelines for the use of innovative therapies in sepsis. *Crit Care Med* 1992;20:864.

Simeone FA. Shock, trauma and the surgeon. *Ann Surg* 1963;158:759.

CHAPTER 24

Pediatric Surgery

Marc Davison, Claudio Oiticica, and Donald M. Buckner

When William Ladd created a separate surgical service at the Boston Children's Hospital in the 1930s, it was the first surgery service dedicated specifically to surgical disease of childhood in this country. It was felt by some, however, that pediatric surgery should not be a subspecialty as there were already too many subspecialties in surgery. The expanded knowledge regarding congenital and acquired childhood diseases as well as the tremendous clinical advances in prenatal care, neonatal intensive care, and well baby care have increased survival of critically ill pediatric patients, some of whom may not have survived in the previous era. Accordingly, pediatric surgery has kept pace with the rapid developments in pediatric clinical management and has indeed proved itself worthy of designation as a surgical subspecialty. In 1975, an examination for the Certificate of Special Competence in Pediatric Surgery was the first of its kind given.

There is an old adage in pediatrics: A premature infant is not a small newborn, a newborn is not a small infant, an infant is not a small child, and a child is not a small adult. Aside from the obvious anatomic differences as to size, the physiologic and embryological differences can be daunting. This chapter attempts to give but a taste of some of the differences. If medical students glean from this chapter a reasonable understanding and a healthy respect of pediatric surgical disease, they and their future patients will be well served.

COMMON PEDIATRIC SURGICAL DISEASES

Appendicitis

Appendicitis occurs in all ages but is the most common cause of an acute surgical abdomen between the ages of 5 and 35. Statistically, the incidence of disease prior to puberty is equal between males and females. Around puberty, the male to female ratio regarding disease inci-

dence is 2:1; however, after the age of 25, the incidence of disease between males and females normalizes again. Obstruction of the appendiceal lumen is the fundamental mechanism behind the pathogenesis of acute appendicitis. Lymphoid hyperplasia and fecalith are the most common etiologies in the pediatric age group. Parasites infrequently cause appendicitis in Third World countries.

With regard to the topic of appendicitis, a few concerns with respect to pediatric patients must be considered. Although patient history and physical examination are all that is required in evaluation of patients with presumed acute appendicitis, often a clinical diagnosis is not as straightforward as many clinicians would wish because of several factors. First, the inability to obtain adequate history from either the patient or parents frequently presents a formidable challenge to both pediatricians and pediatric surgeons with regard to diagnostic accuracy. Second, the lack of a well-developed omentum, especially in young children, can allow free perforation and dissemination of appendiceal contents within the peritoneal cavity. This progression of events occurs much faster than in adults, and upon examination of the abdomen, atypical findings may sway clinical assessment away from the diagnosis of appendicitis. Third, the differential diagnosis of abdominal pain in children includes, but is not limited to, gastroenteritis, mesenteric adenitis, pneumonia, and pancreatitis, all of which are diseases managed with nonoperative measures. Finally, abdominal pain in children many times is a nonspecific associated finding with other illnesses, which can further confuse clinical judgment.

Despite the many variations in clinical presentation, the presence of classic signs and symptoms as well as progression of disease is common, fortunately. Pain begins as periumbilical discomfort, which, over time, shifts to the right lower abdominal quadrant at McBurney's point (Fig. 1). Voluntary guarding and rebound tenderness are typically localized to the right lower quad-

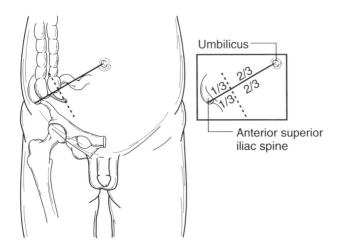

FIG. 1. Relation of appendix to abdominal wall.

rant. Generalized peritonitis characterized by a diffusely tender, perhaps rigid abdomen associated with a leukocytosis of >20,000 cells/mm³ blood and fever suggests that perforation of the appendix has occurred.

If patient examination and history are equivocal, abdominal flat plate and upright radiograph may indicate a right lower quadrant pathologic process in development (e.g., right lower quadrant ileus, fecalith). Abdominal sonogram may aid in diagnosis by demonstrating a distended noncompressible appendix. A contained fluid collection in the right lower abdominal quadrant in the face of a patient history typical for appendicitis suggests the presence of a periappendiceal abscess.

Once the diagnosis is established, appendectomy is performed expediently after administering adequate intravenous fluid resuscitation and intravenous antibiotics through a muscle-sparing incision about McBurney's point. The exception to this dictum is the presence of a periappendiceal abscess. These patients typically have no evidence of systemic sepsis and have a well-defined right lower quadrant mass that is nontender on physical examination despite a clinical history consistent with recent appendiceal inflammation. Acute appendicitis complicated by periappendiceal abscess is treated by percutaneous drainage followed by interval appendectomy, usually 6 to 12 weeks after the initial event. Broad-spectrum antibiotics are administered to combat bacteremia during manipulation of the infected periappendiceal fluid collection. Antibiotic therapy is then tailored to specific bacteria cultured from abscess cavity once these results are known.

Phimosis, Paraphimosis, and Circumcision

The glans penis and foreskin (prepuce) develop during the third month of pregnancy, and by the fifth month

of gestation, fusion between the epithelium of the glans and foreskin has occurred. Separation of the glans and foreskin begins shortly after birth, although only a small minority of infants have retractable foreskin at birth. The foreskin of one-fourth of uncircumcised male infants becomes retractable at 6 months of age usually because of routine gentle retraction and cleansing of the preputial space. These continued efforts will allow the foreskin to be freely retractable in 90% of males by age 4. Forceful retraction should not be performed as it is painful and unnecessary.

In 1870, 5% of American males were circumcised. Advocated as a cure for many illnesses, 25% of males were circumcised by 1900. During World War II, tropical diseases of the foreskin in American servicemen promoted the trend toward routine circumcision, and by 1960, 95% of males were circumcised at birth. Thereafter, routine circumcision was questioned, and in 1971, the Committee on the Fetus and Newborn of the American Academy of Pediatrics proclaimed that "there is no valid medical indication for routine circumcision in the neonatal period." Although circumcision is the most common surgical procedure performed in children today, the current rate of routine circumcision has fallen to 605 to 70% of American male infants. The annual cost of routine circumcision approaches $50 million per year.

Circumcision is defined as surgical excision of the foreskin to the level of the coronal sulcus. Indications for circumcision are many and include those listed in Table 1. Phimosis is defined as a stenosis of the preputial ring such that the foreskin cannot be fully retracted. Paraphimosis is a partially stenotic preputial ring that is retracted and incarcerates the glans penis at the level of the coronal sulcus. The ensuing edema of the prepuce can result in a tourniquet effect and subsequent ischemia of the glans penis. Acute incarceration from a paraphimosis constitutes a surgical emergency requiring release of the preputial ring and perhaps a circumcision. Inflammation and infection of the glans (balanitis) and prepuce (posthitis) from colonized smegma that collects within the preputial space are indications for circumcision. Religious reasons for circumcision remain as an indication for circumcision.

In infants, special clamps (e.g., Gomco, Mogen clamp) are applied for excision of foreskin. In older children and adults, resection and freehand sleeve suturing technique is performed. Complications are rare but include bleeding, infection, and retained foreskin.

TABLE 1. *Indications for circumcision*

Phimosis
Paraphimosis
Balanitis
Religion

Inguinal Hernia and Hydrocele

Between the seventh and eighth months of gestation, testes descend into the scrotum associated with a diverticulum of peritoneum, the processus vaginalis (Fig. 2). Normally, that portion of the processus immediately surrounding the testis becomes the tunica vaginalis, while the remainder of the processus becomes obliterated. If the latter segment remains patent, a communication exists between scrotum and peritoneum. A hernia is simply a patent processus vaginalis through which bowel or other intraabdominal contents protrude. One that contains peritoneal fluid alone defines a communicating hydrocele.

The incidence of inguinal hernia in infants and children is estimated between 10 and 20 per 1,000 live births. Males outnumber females by a 4:1 ratio. The vast majority of inguinal hernias in infants and children are the indirect type because of a persistent processus vaginalis. A large majority of hernias are diagnosed on the right side, 10% are found bilateral, and 35% are isolated to the left groin. The higher incidence of right-sided hernias is probably related to the later descent of the right testis and delayed closure of the processus vaginalis. Direct and femoral hernias are exceedingly rare as these are considered acquired rather than congenital hernias. There is a sixfold increase in incidence of indirect hernias in premature infants.

Typically, a visible bulge in the infant's groin during periods of increased intraabdominal pressure is noted while bathing or changing the diaper. Frequently, similar maneuvers to induce valsalva (e.g., crying) are required to visualize the hernia on clinical examination. The differential diagnosis for inguinal masses includes hydrocele, retractile testis, undescended testis, varicocele, or testicular tumor. With exception for a hydrocele, palpation generally distinguishes these other entities. Hydroceles typically illuminate within the scrotum, but often cannot be distinguished from hernia contents as even bowel in a neonate will transilluminate. If a hernia is irreducible, it is said to be incarcerated. Commonly associated symptoms include localized pain, emotional irritability, nausea and vomiting. Unreleased incarceration may compromise blood supply to the contents of the hernia sac leading to ischemia and eventually necrosis (strangulation).

Hydroceles are observed for a minimum of 18 months. Enlarging or symptomatic hydroceles are electively repaired by proximal ligation of the patent processus vaginalis. Noncommunicating hydroceles are usually self-limiting. In contrast, hernias that spontaneously reduce should be repaired shortly after diagnosis to prevent potential complications. Inguinal hernias are approached through a small groin incision and repaired by high ligation of the processus vaginalis. Unlike in adults, no formal reinforcement of the inguinal floor is required.

Incarcerated hernias require prompt evaluation. Reduction is attempted with mild sedation and the infant in the Trendelenburg position. If successful, the patients are admitted and semi-elective repair can be performed. Reduction of ischemic or necrotic bowel is exceedingly rare but nonetheless possible so serial abdominal examinations should be performed, preferably by the same clinician, to monitor the development of peritonitis. This interval period also allows for intravenous rehydration and lessening of tissue edema that may compromise operative results. Unfortunately, attempts at reduction are occasionally unsuccessful and emergent surgical reduction and repair is required. When strangulation of hernia contents is apparent immediate surgery is warranted.

Even in the absence of a visible contralateral hernia most pediatric surgeons routinely explore the opposite side due to the high incidence of bilateral inguinal hernias. Indications for selective contralateral groin exploration include males younger than 2 years of age, all female patients, all patients with associated disorders, and all patients with clinical evidence of contralateral hernias. Recurrence, although rare, occurs most often in premature infants, those with connective tissue disorders, and those patients whose hernias were initially incarcerated.

Pyloric Stenosis

Pyloric stenosis is a very common acquired disorder of infancy that affects 0.3% of babies born in the United States. Caucasians, especially those from northern Europe, are particularly prone to disease. Males outnumber females by a 4:1 ratio. For reasons unclear, first-born children are more likely to be affected.

Pyloric stenosis develops from progressive hypertrophy of the pyloric muscle. Gastric outlet obstruction manifests as projectile nonbilious vomiting typically between 3 and 6 weeks of age. Symptoms becomes progressively more severe and, if untreated, results in dehydration and electrolyte imbalances (e.g., hypochloremia, hypokalemia, metabolic alkalosis).

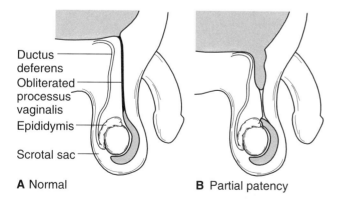

Ductus deferens

Obliterated processus vaginalis

Epididymis

Scrotal sac

A Normal   **B** Partial patency

FIG. 2. Processus vaginalis.

Classic findings during examination reveals a palpable, mobile mass in the epigastric area the size of an "olive," which represents the hypertrophied pylorus musculature (Fig. 3). Gastric distention prevents easy palpation of a distinct mass so a thin silastic nasogastric tube should be passed safely to decompress the stomach prior to examination. When pyloric stenosis is suspected and a mass is not palpable, ultrasound or upper gastrointestinal series with contrast may demonstrate pyloric channel narrowing.

Treatment begins with preoperative rehydration and correction of electrolyte imbalances. The infant is given nothing by mouth and usually preoperative nasogastric decompression is not necessary. A Fredet-Ramstedt pyloromyotomy cracks the pyloric muscle, sparing the mucosa. Postoperative feeding is begun the morning after surgery, consisting of small diluted feedings, and gradually the volume frequency and concentration are increased.

Cryptorchidism (Undescended Testis)

The testes form from the medial portion of the urogenital ridge. Under hormonal influence and the gubernaculum, the male gonads descend through the internal inguinal ring, through the inguinal canal, and finally into the scrotum (Fig. 4). Failure of descent, cryptorchidism, is thought to be due to inadequate hormone levels or the failure of the end organ to respond to adequate hormone levels. In infants born at term, the incidence is rare, but in premature infants, the occurrence approaches 5%. Fifty percent occur on the right, 25% on the left, and 25% occur bilateral. The differential diagnosis of an empty hemiscrotum includes atrophy, agenesis, ectopic, retractile, and undescended testes. Undescended testes must be differentiated from an retractile testis, which can be pulled into a scrotal position and does not require surgery. Bilateral

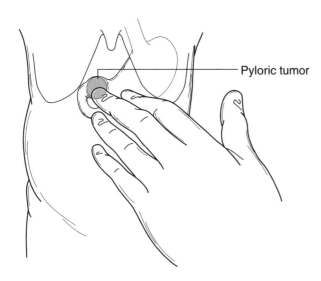

FIG. 3. Palpation for hypertrophied pylorus.

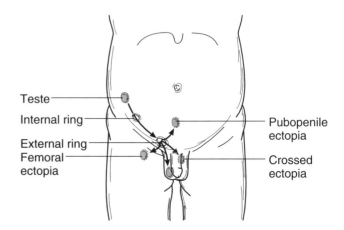

FIG. 4. Developmental migration of testicle with possible sites of ectopic location.

undescended testis should lead the physician to do a workup for urinary tract anomalies. Undescended testes are invariably associated with ipsilateral inguinal hernias.

An undescended testis left untreated is associated with decreased fertility and increased incidence of testicular malignancy (up to 40 times greater risk). Interestingly, the descended contralateral testis is at increased risk for malignancy as well. Although the risk of malignancy is unchanged with surgery, examination for testicular masses is possible with the testis in the scrotum. The most common type of malignancy is a seminoma and usually occurs after age 20. An additional problem associated with undescended testis is increased risk of trauma (due to testicle located at the pubic tubercle).

Once diagnosis is made, the optimal time for surgical repair is between 1 and 2 years of age. Lengthening of the spermatic cord and fixation of the testis within the scrotum, orchiopexy, is attempted in one procedure. At our institution, we utilize the Dartos pouch technique. Occasionally, staged procedures are required to achieve this result. A high retroperitoneal or intraabdominal testis may require transposition of the internal ring to obtain adequate length of the spermatic cord structures. Alternatively, the spermatic cord vasculature may be divided, and collateral blood supply from the inferior epigastric vessels can suffice in supplying blood and nutrients to the testis. Orchiectomy may be indicated if the testis does not reach the scrotum after all attempts have failed provided a second testis is present.

Testicular Torsion

Testicular torsion refers to rotation of the testis with torsion of the spermatic cord within the scrotum. It occurs most commonly between late childhood and early adolescence but may occur at any age of life. Inadequate fixation of the testis within the scrotum is the accepted etiology. Patients present with acute onset testicular or scrotal pain that radiates to the groin and is sometimes associated with nausea, vomiting, and lower abdominal pain. The affected testis is elevated in the hemiscrotum and exquisitely tender. Associated scrotal erythema and edema is typical. Antecedent history of similar episodes of lesser intensity with spontaneous resolution may be indicative of prior torsion-detorsion episodes. Prehn's sign describes exacerbation of pain with elevation of the testis and is very suggestive of testicular torsion.

The acute scrotum can be caused by trauma, torsion of appendicular structures, or epididymitis. The exclusion of testicular torsion, which requires surgical therapy, is a principal concern in these patients. If patient history and physical examination convincingly suggests testicular torsion or diagnostic studies are consistent with clinical suspicion, emergent scrotal exploration is clearly indicated and should be undertaken. However, in patients in whom clinical presentation suggests pathology other than torsion, additional testing may be sought. Doppler ultrasound studies and nuclear scintigraphy of the testis may demonstrate adequate testicular blood flow or epididymitis, respectively. In these specific cases, surgery would be appropriately avoided. When equivocal results are obtained from these or other studies, observation is not considered appropriate management especially in the presence of persistent scrotal pain. Early operative intervention in the setting of clinical uncertainty is supported by the fact that testicular salvage rates and fertility are inversely proportional to the duration of torsion.

Surgical detorsion and orchiopexy is the standard of care. Additionally, because of the high incidence of bilateral anatomic predisposition to torsion contralateral orchiopexy is commonly performed. Orchiectomy is reserved for clinically nonviable testes.

Gastroesophageal Reflux

Normally, the lower esophageal sphincter is a physiologic valve and acts as a barrier to the reflux of gastric contents into the esophagus. The three components that contribute to the physiologic valve at the lower esophageal sphincter are the esophageal hiatus, the angle of His, and the high-pressure distal esophagus. Asymptomatic small-quantity reflux is considered common. However, symptomatic reflux is pathologic and can result in respiratory dysfunction, poor nutritional status, and esophageal inflammatory signs. In the neurologically impaired pediatric patient, delayed gastric emptying may be the cause of reflux. Reflux is also seen in a majority of patients who have undergone repair of congenital diaphragmatic hernia and in a small minority of patients who have been treated for pyloric stenosis, esophageal atresia (EA), tracheoesophageal fistula (TEF), and intestinal malrotation.

Complications of symptomatic reflux include the following: Repeated micro- or macroaspiration can lead to coughing, choking, reactive airway disease, aspiration pneumonia, and bronchopulmonary dysplasia. Sudden cases of apnea have been explained by occult gastroesophageal reflux (GER). Given the propensity to poor caloric intake, severe malnutrition does not allow satisfactory growth and development and is typical of chronic disease. Esophagitis from chronic reflux can be associated with anemia. In long-standing untreated cases, stricture, esophageal shortening and Barrett's esophagus can develop. Satcliff-Sandifer syndrome describes iron-deficiency anemia and voluntary contortions of head, neck, and trunk in an attempt to improve distal esophageal peristalsis in the presence of GER.

The presence of symptoms or the suspicion of reflux warrant diagnostic studies. Barium esophagram is highly sensitive to detect an incompetent lower esophageal sphincter. If the results of this study are equivocal, but the patient history is suggestive of disease, 24-hr esophageal pH monitoring or manometry studies can be performed. Endoscopy with biopsy is utilized in cases of advanced GER to evaluate integrity of esophageal mucosa.

After the diagnosis is confirmed, nonoperative therapy is instituted. Assuming a more upright position during feedings, and reducing the volume and increasing the viscosity of oral intake are regarded as positional therapy. Antacids (e.g., cimetidine, ranitidine) and prokinetics (e.g., bethanechol, metoclopramide) constitute medical therapy. Failure to resolve symptomatic episodes of reflux or poor nutrition and unsatisfactory advances in growth development are some indications for surgery (Table 2). Figure 5 relates currently accepted protocols regarding antireflux surgery correlated with clinical disease. GER associated with large hiatal hernias often do not resolve with nonoperative therapy. The Nissen fundoplication is a 360-degree esophageal wrap and is considered the standard against which all other procedures are compared. Thal fundoplication is an anterior 270-degree wrap (Fig. 6). Both procedures reestablish the angle of His and reconstructs an intraabdominal lower esophageal sphincter. A gastrostomy tube

TABLE 2. *Indications for surgery in gastroesophageal reflux*

Absolute
  Apneic episodes
  Recurrent/persistent pneumonitis
  Esophagitis
  Failure of medical therapy
Relative
  Atypical asthma
  Croup
  Paroxysmal night coughing
  Choking episodes
  Chronic vomiting

SELECTION OF ANTIREFLUX OPERATION

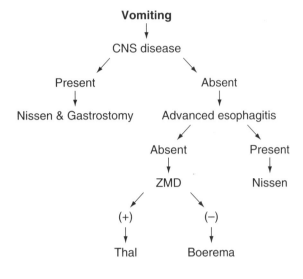

Vomiting

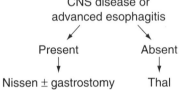

**Reflux-induced
Respiratory Symptoms/Disease**

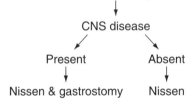

**Advanced Esophagitis/Peptic
Stricture/Barrett's Epithelium**

FIG. 5. A general algorithm for the selection of antireflux operation in infants and children based on the complication of gastroesophageal reflux disease, associated central nervous system (CNS) disease, and the prolonged (+) or normal (−) value for the mean duration of acid reflux episodes during sleep (ZMD) derived from extended esophageal pH monitoring. (From Filston H, ed. Pediatric surgery. *Surg Clin North Am* 1992;72:1381.)

is placed to act as a postoperative vent for the stomach. When the patient's gastric emptying is clinically normal, small gastrostomy tube feedings are started and slowly advanced. At seven days, a barium swallow is performed to ascertain the functional status of the fundoplication procedure. If there is no indication of swallowing difficulty or impedance to flow through the lower esophageal sphincter, oral feedings are begun.

Intussusception

Intussusception is a common cause of intestinal obstruction in the pediatric age group and is due to a portion of proximal bowel invaginating into distal bowel (Fig. 7). It is most often observed between 5 and 10 months of age and is slightly more common in males. Typically, a lead point initiates the intussusception. In younger children, the lead point, although infrequently identified, is often attributed to lymphoid hyperplasia of the Peyer's patches in the terminal ileum from an antecedent viral infection. In older children, the lead point is commonly a Meckel's diverticulum. Other causes include polyps, intestinal duplication, lymphomas, submucosal hemorrhage, lymphosarcomas, and inspissated feces. The most common segment of bowel to intussuscept is the ileocolic region. Ileoileal and colocolonic segments have also been observed.

Clinically, children exhibit a sudden onset of crying and irritability followed by vomiting and currant jelly stools. Usually there are multiple attacks, but, fortunately, between episodes, the child appears well. Subsequently, however, after repeated attacks, the child may become somnolent and lethargic. On examination, a sausage-shaped abdominal mass may be palpated in right upper quadrant and an absence of bowel is appreciated in the right lower quadrant (Dance's sign). If not corrected, the intussuscepted segment of bowel may become incarcerated and eventually ischemic from vascular insufficiency.

Barium enema is utilized to detect and often treat intussusception. An abrupt cut off in barium contrast at the leading edge of the intussusception is diagnostic. Hydrostatic reduction is attempted with a 1-m high column of barium. Reduction is complete when barium flows freely into the proximal bowel. If reduction is incomplete, the procedure can be repeated perhaps two to three times. Success rates range from 40% to 80% in reported studies. Recurrence after successful reduction is unusual but not rare, so children are frequently admitted for 24-hr observation.

Failure to reduce the intussusception or the presence of peritonitis mandates surgery. Exploration is carried out through a right lower quadrant muscle-splitting incision and reduction is attempted in a retrograde fashion and if reduction is successful, appendectomy is performed. If unsuccessful, resection with primary anastomosis and appendectomy are performed.

COMMON CONGENITAL ANOMALIES REQUIRING SURGERY

Congenital Diaphragmatic Hernia

The diaphragm begins to form at 3 weeks of gestation and is derived from four embryological precursors: the

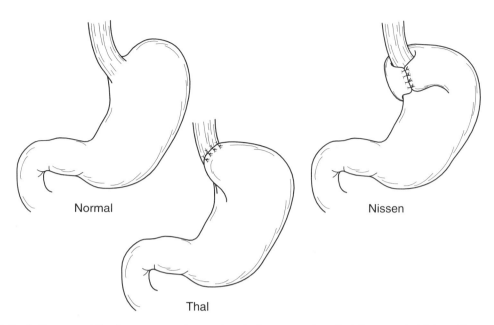

FIG. 6. A diagram of the two commonly used antireflux operations in infants and children. The normal stomach also is depicted for comparison.

septum transversum, dorsal mesentery of the esophagus, paired pleuroperitoneal membranes, and muscle of the lateral and dorsal body walls (Fig. 8). These structures unite and coalesce over a period of weeks and become the immature diaphragm. Closure of the pleuroperitoneal canal occurs as the final step in development. Failure of closure results in diaphragmatic hernia, also known as the hernia of Bochdalek.

At 10 to 12 weeks of gestation, the midgut returns to the abdominal cavity. In neonates with congenital diaphragmatic hernia, the defect is located in the left posterolateral diaphragm in 90% of cases. Thus, a segment of intestines and perhaps solid organs will herniate into the chest if a defect is present. The resulting mass effect of the bowel in the ipsilateral as well as contralateral hemithorax results in pulmonary hypoplasia and pulmonary hypertension. The extent to which the lungs mature correlates directly with predictable survival.

This congenital defect is infrequent and occurs approximately once in 2,500 live births. Thirty percent to 50% of such newborns are stillborn, and of those who are alive at birth, there is an overall predicted mortality of 50%. Females outnumber males by a 2:1 ratio. Associated anomalies are common and include major central nervous system, cardiac, and chromosomal abnormalities.

Prenatal diagnosis is often established with ultrasound. In the newborn, diagnosis must be considered in a cyanotic neonate with respiratory insufficiency, a scaphoid abdomen and decreased breath sounds auscultated in the affected hemithorax. Diagnosis is confirmed with chest radiograph, which demonstrates bowel in the chest and mediastinal shift toward the contralateral thorax.

Until recently, the diagnosis of a congenital diaphragmatic hernia was indication for emergent surgery. With tremendous progress in neonatal intensive care as well as the utilization of advanced ventilatory support, neonatologists concentrate more on respiratory stabilization, intravascular rehydration, and nasogastric decompression prior to operative therapy. When the newborn is clinically stable, the surgical procedure is approached through the abdomen. Surgical repair of the hernia is performed after replacement of the intestines and organs to within the abdominal cavity.

The excessive morbidity from pulmonary hypoplasia has opened a new frontier of research, open fetal surgery. Although purely experimental, the reduction of the congenital diaphragmatic hernia and repair of the diaphragm was successfully performed in the majority albeit small number of patients. However, the incidence of intraoperative fetal demise as well as associated premature fetal delivery with poor outcome have tainted the relative successes of this investigation. This new development in pediatric surgery is still in its fundamental

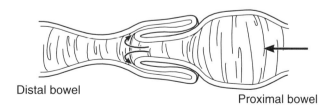

Distal bowel

Proximal bowel

FIG. 7. Intussusception of the bowel.

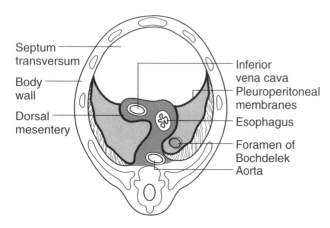

Septum transversum

Body wall

Dorsal mesentery

Inferior vena cava

Pleuroperitoneal membranes

Esophagus

Foramen of Bochdelek

Aorta

FIG. 8. Coronal view of embryological development of the upper portion of the diaphragm. Left foramen of Bockdalek shown in color.

stages and further research combined with careful patient selection and advances in technology are requisite to achieving positive results.

Congenital Intestinal Atresia

Congenital intestinal obstruction is infrequent and occurs in approximately one in 2,700 live births. Males and females appear to be equally affected. Failure of canalization of the intestinal lumen, intestinal atresia, is the most common cause of neonatal obstruction and must be considered in newborns with persistent bilious vomiting.

Duodenal atresia is categorized by location either proximal or distal to the Ampulla of Vater and are distinguished by examining the gastric contents for the presence of bile. Morphological subtypes include mucosal diaphragm, solid fibrous cord, or segmental agenesis (Fig. 9). At the third week of gestation, when the biliary and pancreatic ducts are forming, the duodenum is a solid core of epithelium. Over the next 3 to 4 weeks, the duo-

denum undergoes vacuolization and recanalization with reconstitution of the lumen. Failure of recanalization results in obstruction often associated with developmental malformation of the pancreas and terminal part of the biliary tree. Segments of small bowel atresia can occur from the ligament of Treitz to the ileocecal junction. Colonic atresia is rare and accounts for <5% of all cases of intestinal atresia. The morphologic subtypes of atresia in the small bowel and colon are similar to those described for duodenal atresia. Jejunoileal and colonic atresias, in contrast, are thought to result from ischemic injury to the bowel after the midgut has returned to the colonic cavity.

Small bowel obstruction in utero manifests as polyhydramnios and is characteristic of duodenal and proximal jejunal atresia. Distal ileal or colonic obstruction, generally, does not result in clinically evident polyhydramnios. Persistent vomiting in an infant after birth and nasogastric aspirate that reveals >25 cc of bilious gastric contents is very suggestive of intestinal atresia. Absence of gas and intestinal contents distal to the obstructed segment results in a scaphoid abdomen. Abdominal radiographs may indicate the site of obstruction in patients with presumed intestinal atresia. For example, the presence of gastric air accompanied only by duodenal air, the so-called "double bubble," is the sina qua non of duodenal atresia. Similarly, abdominal films of babies with proximal jejunal atresia show only a few air-fluid levels and no gas in the lower part of the abdomen. Barium enema differentiates intestinal obstruction from Hirschsprung'sdisease, meconium plug syndrome, or meconium ileus. Contrast material by mouth is avoided if possible.

Surgical intestinal reconstruction is mandatory. Duodenoduodenostomy is performed for duodenal atresia unless a wide gap exists between the two ends of the duodenum, in which case duodenojejunostomy is performed. For jejunoileal atresias, the dilated tip of the proximal bowel resected as is the tip of the distal segment, and an end-oblique anastomosis is performed. Patients with colon

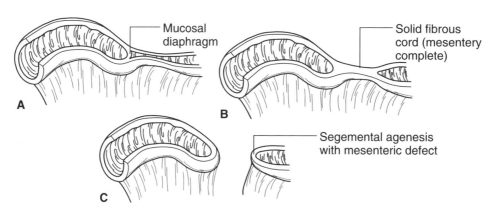

Mucosal diaphragm

Solid fibrous cord (mesentery complete)

A

B

Segemental agenesis with mesenteric defect

C

FIG. 9. Different types of morphological subtypes of intestinal atresia.

atresia should always have a temporary end colostomy with resection of the dilated proximal segment. Gastric decompression may be accomplished by the insertion of a gastrostomy tube.

Biliary Atresia

Neonatal jaundice is caused by a number of clinical entities, including immature hepatic function, sepsis, metabolic errors, and hemolysis. Jaundice is the typical presentation of biliary atresia also, and although babies are well otherwise, jaundice persists and worsens. In these cases, neonatologists and pediatricians generally pursue a number of diagnostic tests to exclude or confirm those diseases mentioned. Ultrasound is important to visualize the presence or absence of intrahepatic and extrahepatic bile ducts and a gallbladder. Hepatic scintigraphy, hepatobiliary scan for PIPIDA, distinguishes hepatocellular disease (no hepatic uptake) from biliary atresia (normal hepatic uptake without excretion into bile ducts and intestines).

Diagnosis mandates operative biliary reconstruction. Unfortunately, it is difficult to impossible to find discrete bile ducts to which biliary enteric anastomosis can be created. In 1968, Kasai reported a series of patients with biliary atresia in whom biliary reconstruction was performed. Dissection of the hilum of the liver was performed until biliary leak from small biliary radicles was created. A defunctionalized limb of jejunum was opened longitudinally and fashioned to Glisson's capsule to allow bile to drain into intestines (Fig. 10).

Although the Kasai procedure is considered one of the greatest advances in pediatric surgery, it does not cure disease. Despite living to adulthood, the majority of patients still have persistent jaundice requiring periodic intervention and a small minority progress to biliary cirrhosis and portal hypertension. Transplantation, with decreased perioperative mortality and improved long-term graft survival, is the treatment for end-stage biliary atresia. Preemptive liver transplantation in infancy has been proposed as preventive medicine; however, it is not widely accepted because of the inherent long-term morbidity of immunosuppression and because of the limited donor supply. Currently, biliary-enteric reconstruction provides favorable palliation of disease, and although multiple biliary interventions are sometimes required, these are generally well tolerated. The prohibitive morbidity of immunosuppression as a consequence of liver transplantation is avoidable.

Esophageal Atresia and Tracheoesophageal Fistula

At 3 weeks of gestation, a respiratory diverticulum forms at the ventral aspect of the pharyngeal foregut (Fig. 11). The diverticulum elongates and gives rise to the trachea and lung buds. The ventral trachea and dorsal esophagus are separated by a septum formed by the fusion of the lateral walls of the common tracheoesophageal channel. Failure of complete formation of this septum results in a TEF. The etiology of EA is less clear.

The following symptoms and signs should alert the physician to the possible diagnosis of EA and TEF. Polyhydramnios appreciated antepartum in combination with postpartum drooling, coughing, choking, regurgitation of saliva or food, and aspiration are all consistent with proximal EA. Cyanosis with eating and progressive respiratory distress is very suggestive of a proximal TEF, which permits the passage of liquid into the trachea. In either case, respiratory distress, atelectasis, and pneumonia often result. Additional associated pathology include esophageal dysmotility secondary to Auerbach's plexus deficiency and tracheomalacia from compression by a thickened esophageal upper pouch during development.

The different types of EA and associated TEF are depicted in Fig. 12. Gentle placement of a thin silastic feeding tube into the proximal esophagus helps categorize the anomaly. Care is taken not to persist in the presence of resistance. A chest radiograph will demonstrate the feeding tube in the hypopharynx area in patients with proximal EA. Absence of gas in the abdomen represents type A EA. Gas in the stomach but not in small bowel

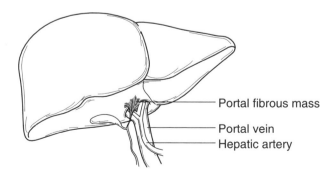

FIG. 10. The portal fibrous mass characteristic of biliary atresia.

Portal fibrous mass
Portal vein
Hepatic artery

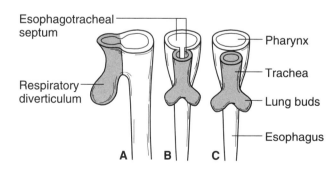

Esophagotracheal septum
Respiratory diverticulum
Pharynx
Trachea
Lung buds
Esophagus
A   B   C

FIG. 11. Embryological development of the respiratory diverticulum and the esophagus. (Adapted from Sadler F, ed. *Langman's medical embryology.* 5th ed. Baltimore: Williams and Wilkins, 1985.)

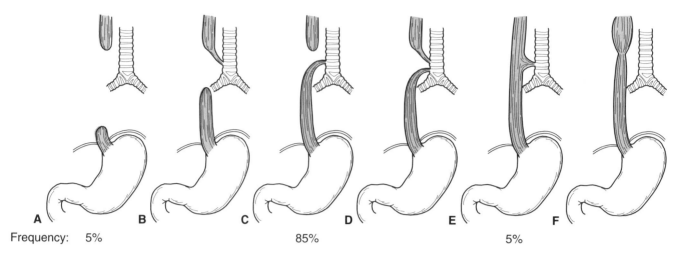

Frequency: 5%   85%   5%

FIG. 12. Different types of esophageal atresia with tracheoesophageal fistula.

may represent a distal fistula with associated duodenal atresia. Bronchoscopy can be used to clarify anatomy.

Associated anomalies occur in half of affected patients. The majority of congenital defects affect the cardiac system. Other anomalies include but are not limited to vertebral, anal, renal, radial, and limb deformities. It is understandable that these infants with associated anomalies have a higher mortality rate.

In healthy babies with classic type C EA/TEF, early attempt at primary repair and closure of the fistula is advocated. Cases complicated by pneumonia or significant atelectasis may require proximal pouch decompression, intravenous antibiotics and gastrostomy tube placement for enteral feedings. Primary repair is delayed until life-threatening problems have resolved. In babies with associated anomalies that are life threatening or with persistent pneumonia and sepsis, or in neonates who are small for gestational age, division of the TEF and placement of gastrostomy tube is performed urgently to allow clinical resolution. After stabilization, primary repair can be attempted. In patients with a long gap between the esophageal ends (type A), the proximal pouch may be stretched with a dilator, as may the distal pouch via gastrostomy for a period of 6 weeks prior to surgery. At surgery, circumferential esophagomyotomy of the proximal pouch may increase esophageal length to provide for a tension-free anastomosis. Alternatively, an esophageal tongue flap may be created for extra length.

Long-term prognosis and survivability are excellent. In the care of a skilled surgical team and intensive postoperative nursing care, nearly 100% of all healthy babies as well as preterm babies afflicted with TEF survive. In ill babies, the long-term survival is still good, with an overall mortality of <7%. Complications include anastomotic leak, recurrent fistula, reflux, and tracheal compression (via the aorta or innominate artery).

Imperforate Anus

The anorectum develops during the fourth week to sixth month of fetal life. The urorectal septum divides the primitive distal urinary system from the hindgut portion destined to become the anorectal region (Fig. 13). An

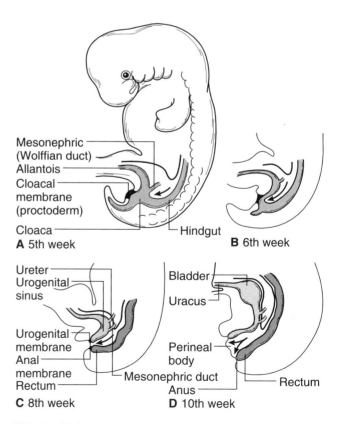

FIG. 13. Embryologic development of the rectum and anus.

ectodermal depression overlying the anorectal canal, proctodeum, eventually regresses yielding the anal canal opening. The margin of anal pit (ectoderm) and hindgut (endoderm) becomes the dentate line of the anorectal canal. When the anal membrane fails to open, simple imperforate anus develops. Complex cases involve maldevelopment of the urorectal septum resulting in abnormal communication between urogenital tract and hindgut (Fig. 14).

The incidence of imperforate anus and other anorectal anomalies is approximately one in 4,000 live births. Males predominate slightly over females and there is a high incidence of associated anomalies. This disease has been classified by Pena according to sex and distance from anal pit. In the male, rectourethral fistula represents the most frequent defect in which a fistula opens into the bulbar prostatic part of urethra. Just above the fistula the rectum and urethra share a common wall. Lower urethra fistulas are associated with good quality pelvic muscles, a well-developed sacrum, and a prominent anal dimple. The reverse is true for higher fistulas. In females, a vestibular fistula is the most common defect in which the bowel opens immediately behind the hymen in vestibule of female genitalia. Muscles, nerves, and sacrum are usually normal and prognosis is good after reconstruction.

Surgical reconstruction is required for all variations in anorectal anomalies. For low lesions, creation of a neoanus and minimal posterior mobilization to reconstruct the fistula within the limits of the external sphincter may be all that is required. For high malformations, complex reconstruction, including creation of neourethra, neovagina, or neoanorectum, is required and is accompanied by a higher early and late complication rate. Postoperative complications include diarrhea, constipation, anal incontinence, anorectal strictures, and recurrent fistula.

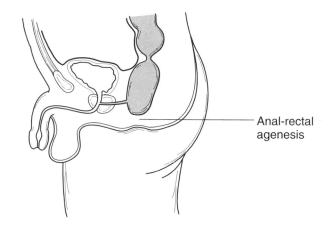

FIG. 14. Anorectal agenesis with rectourethral fistula.

Anal-rectal agenesis

Hirschprung's Disease

Hirschprung'sdisease is the result of absence of ganglion cells in the myenteric plexus of the intestine. In the vast majority of cases this disease is limited to the rectosigmoid region although any portion of the colon and other intestinal segments may be involved. Due to aganglionosis, normal peristalsis does not occur and a functional bowel obstruction supervenes. Although the exact mechanism is not clear, proposed explanations of the absence of ganglion cells include failure of migration of enteric neuroblasts, failure of differentiation of precursor cells (neutral crest cells) into neuroblasts, and destruction of neuroblasts after migration.

Clinical presentation in newborns with Hirschsprung's disease varies. Classically, failure to pass meconium in the first 18 hr of life in a full-term neonate born at term increases suspicion for disease. Abdominal distension and vomiting develops thereafter. Other newborns may exhibit signs and symptoms of necrotizing enterocolitis (fever, leukocytosis, abdominal tenderness). Other diagnoses that should be considered include intestinal atresia, functional constipation, and idiopathic intestinal dysmotility syndromes.

In patients that fail to pass meconium shortly after birth, simple perianal examination must be performed to exclude imperforate anus. Abdominal radiograph is utilized to exclude intestinal atresia. If no contraindications exist in these patients with suspected Hirschsprung's disease, a barium enema is performed that will demonstrate a "cone-shaped" transition zone between proximal dilated and distal nondilated bowel. Rectal biopsy is the gold standard diagnostic test and demonstrates neural hypertrophy and absence of ganglion cells. Rectal manometry may be a helpful supplementary diagnostic tool should other tests prove equivocal or be unavailable.

Surgical treatment is required in all cases. The overwhelming majority of patients are newborns at diagnosis and, with exception for selected cases, a staged procedure is undertaken. A proximal end ostomy is constructed to permit bowel decompression and allow hypertrophied proximal bowel to normalize prior to definitive reconstruction. Furthermore, nutrition can be maximized and emergence of enterocolitis of Hirschprung's can be eliminated. Definitive surgical procedures are performed between 6 months and 1 year of age. Swenson reported a series of patients in whom he performed resection of the aganglionic colon and reconnected normal colon to the anus in pull-through fashion. A similar procedure called the Soave-Boley procedure involves complete excision of the mucosa and submucosa of the distal aganglionic colon and anastomosis of ganglionic colon at the anus pulled through the rectal muscular sleeve. These procedures and others not mentioned have been extensively studied and shown to have similar results. In recent years, primary pull-through operations without prior ostomy have been advocated by some pediatric surgeons in selected cases. Postoperative complications are infrequent and include anastomotic leak, stenosis, and enterocolitis.

Omphalocele and Gastroschisis

The abdominal wall is formed from embryologic folds: cephalic, caudal, right lateral, and left lateral. These structures unite surrounding the umbilical arteries, vein and yolk sac. Failure of closure of the anterior abdominal wall at the umbilicus results in anatomical defects (Fig. 15).

Omphalocele is defined as a protruding mass of bowel in the central abdomen covered by a membrane. The size of the abdominal wall defect varies. Malrotation of bowel is frequently associated with moderate to large size defects. Patient with an omphalocele often have associated chromosomal anomalies, including trisomy 13, 18, or 21. Other anomalies include prune belly syndrome and Beckwith-Wiedemann syndrome.

Gastroschisis describes a similar protrusion of intestines through a small abdominal wall defect in the right periumbilical region. Unlike omphalocele, however, the bowels lack a covering and are exposed. Malrotation of the bowel is invariably present and often associated with intestinal atresia. Preterm diagnosis is established by elevated alpha-feto protein and by ultrasound. Vaginal delivery is tolerated well in full-term newborns with either gastroschisis or omphalocele. Upon delivering, the exposed abdominal organs are protected with wet saline gauze and either saran wrap or plastic bag.

Patients with gastroschisis require preoperative nasogastric tube decompression prior to emergent surgical intervention to reperitonealize the bowel. Primary closure can be effected in ~50% of patients. For patients in whom this cannot be accomplished due to disparity between abdominal cavity and the viscera, a silastic covering is constructed. In these cases, sequential procedures to reduce the abdominal viscera to containment within the peritoneal cavity are done at the bedside with definitive closure of abdominal wall performed in the operating room usually within 7 to 10 days. The survival rate of patients with gastroschisis in whom appropriate treatment is rendered exceeds 90%.

Patients with omphalocele do not require emergent surgery. However, a preoperative evaluation for the above-mentioned anomalies should be performed. Patients with small defects are brought to the operating room for elective primary closure. For large defects, mercurochrome is applied to the sac and primary delayed closure is performed. Surprisingly, a higher mortality rate approaching 30% is associated with omphalocele presumably a reflection of the severity of associated congenital anomalies.

Other Intestinal Anomalies

Meckel's Diverticulum

Meckel's diverticulum represents the most common congenital anomaly of the intestine and is found in **2%** of the general population, within **2** ft of the ileocecal valve on the antimesenteric border, and usually no more than **2** in. in length ("rule of 2's"). Although Meckel's diverticula can produce obstruction or perforate, hemorrhage is the most important presentation.

These lesions are caused by incomplete obliteration of the embryologic vitelline duct (Fig. 16). Males are affected more than females. Patency to the skin results in an enterocutaneous fistula while a fibrous band may result in intestinal volvulus. Ectopic gastric mucosa is commonly found in the diverticulum and often results in peptic ulcers of adjacent mucosa. These ulcers can be complicated by massive gastrointestinal hemorrhage

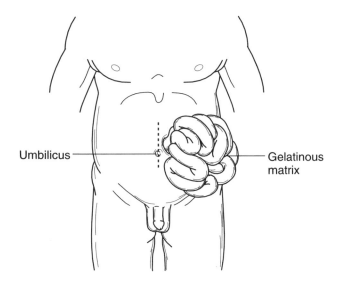

FIG. 15. Gastroschisis that occurs lateral to the umbilicus.

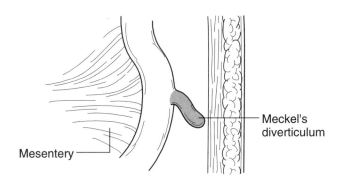

FIG. 16. Meckel's diverticulum, which usually appears ~2 ft from ileocecal valve on the antimesenteric border.

although children rarely are evaluated at the time that active bleeding is occurring. Bleeding is typically severe in children younger than 2 years of age.

Diagnostic studies (e.g., upper gastrointestinal barium series, endoscopy, barium enema, and proctoscopy) are invariably negative. In 1970, Jewett reported the sodium pertechnate radionuclide localization of Meckel's diverticulum. Lesions associated with bleeding are widely resected, usually including the ulcer located in adjacent mucosa. Resection of asymptomatic Meckel's diverticula can be performed but is controversial. Postoperative recovery is invariably excellent.

Intestinal Malrotation

In the fourth week of embryonic life, the midgut herniates into the umbilical cord and elongates. During this period, an initial 90-degree counterclockwise rotation occurs during elongation. At ~10 to 11 weeks, the intestines return to the abdominal cavity, undergoing 180 degrees of further counterclockwise rotation (Fig. 17).

Incomplete intestinal rotation usually presents clinically in the neonatal period as intestinal obstruction. Early in the course of disease, bilious vomiting occurs a short period after consuming oral feeding. Thereafter with worsening symptoms, intolerance to oral feeding and intractable bilious vomiting predominates. Upper gastrointestinal series with dilute barium contrast demonstrates the intestinal anomaly. Surgical exploration should be undertaken after adequate intravascular resuscitation has been administered and electrolyte abnormalities corrected. Operative dissection and replacement of bowel into appropriate anatomic lie is not always as easy as anticipated. Long-term functional recovery is seen in the majority of patients. Postoperative adhesive small bowel obstruction is infrequent but not rare.

COMMON PEDIATRIC NEOPLASMS REQUIRING SURGERY

Wilms' Tumor (Nephroblastoma)

Nephroblastoma, or Wilms' tumor, is the most common renal malignancy and the second most common abdominal tumor in children. Peak incidence is between 2 and 4 years of age with an annual incidence of eight per 100,000 children younger than 15 years of age. There is a slight female preponderance of disease. This tumor is often associated with various congenital anomalies, including aniridia, cryptorchidism, hypospadias, hemihypertrophy, Drash's syndrome, and Beckwith-Wiedemann syndrome. The tumor occurs in both kidneys in only 5% of patients. The female preponderance is increased in those with bilateral tumors.

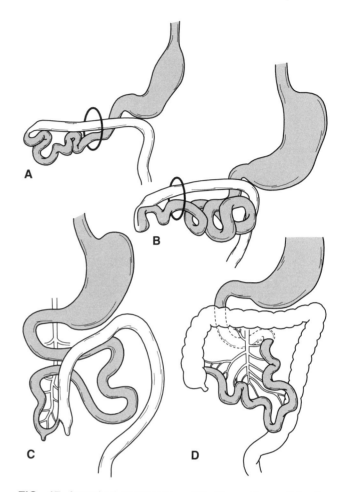

FIG. 17. Intestinal malrotation. (A) Elongation within the umbilical cord. (B) Intestines begin to rotate as they return into the abdominal cavity. (C) Counterclockwise rotation of the intestines. (D) Final resting place of the cecum in the right lower quadrant.

An asymptomatic abdominal mass is the typical clinical presentation of nephroblastomas. Examination of the abdomen occasionally reveals a large, palpable subcostal mass. Hematuria and hypertension may be associated renal symptoms. Symptoms of pain, fever, and anemia may represent tumor necrosis and bleeding. Extension of the tumor into the renal vein and inferior vena cava can result in hepatosplenomegaly, ascites, cardiac murmur, varicocele, or gonadal metastases.

The differential diagnosis in this clinical setting is extensive and includes hydronephrosis, multicystic kidney disease, kidney duplication, neuroblastoma, teratoma, and rhabdomyosarcoma. Although many diagnostic studies can be utilized to evaluate asymptomatic abdominal masses, computed tomography (CT) scan of the abdomen and pelvis yields the most information. Clinical staging can be obtained which guides therapy (Table 3). Tissue biopsy is not indicated because surgical extirpation of the tumor is required.

TABLE 3. *Staging of Wilms' tumor*

Stage	Description
I	Unilateral disease, limited to kidney
II	Disease extends beyond kidney but is excisable
III	Locoregional spread of disease, e.g., local invasion, lymphadenopathy
IV	Distant metastasis
V	Bilateral kidney involvement

In patients with unilateral disease, a radical nephrectomy is performed, and surgical staging information is obtained. In patients with bilateral disease (stage V) or excessively large tumors appreciated by CT scan, neoadjuvant chemotherapy is offered. If bilateral disease is noted at laparotomy, surgical excision is avoided but tissue biopsy of the lesion is obtained and regional lymph nodes are sampled for grading and staging of the tumor. A second-look laparotomy is performed 6 weeks to 6 months after chemotherapy to attempt curative resection of the remaining tumor. Studies support the use of adjuvant chemotherapy (dactinomycin, vincristin, doxorubicin) in stage III and IV disease.

Histopathology (Table 4) is the most important prognostic indicator. Other negative prognostic indicators are listed in Table 5. Overall, 3-year survival after diagnosis in tumors with favorable histology is 93%. In comparison, 3-year survival rates in patients with poorly differentiated tumors is 62%.

Neuroblastoma

Neuroblastoma is the fourth most common malignancy and the most common solid abdominal tumor in children younger than 1 year of age. The tumor is encountered once in 14,000 live births. Pathogenesis of neuroblastoma begins with dysplastic changes of the neuroblast cell. Neuroblast cells, derived from neural crest cells, migrate to the sympathetic chain and adrenal gland and mature into ganglion cells. Dysplastic change of neuroblast cells into a ganglion neuroblastoma or ganglioneuroma may occur spontaneously.

Although the varying clinical presentation is dictated by the location of the tumor and not its metabolic activity, neuroblastomas develop only in sympathetic nervous tissue. The adrenal gland is the most common site of dis-

TABLE 4. *Grading of Wilms' tumors*

Grade	Description
1	Well-differentiated glomerular/tubular tissue
2	<50% tumor well-differentiated
3	Anaplastic/sarcomatous tissue
4	Atypical: leiomyomatous, myxomatous, hemangiomatous lesions

TABLE 5. *Poor prognostic indicators in Wilms' tumor*

Undifferentiated tumors
Age of >2 years
Size of >375 g
Tumor extension beyond renal capsule
Locoregional and distant metastasis

ease. Tumors in neck and abdomen often present as a palpable mass whereas thoracic lesions present commonly with neurologic deficits. Those in the paracaval and paraaortic area are irregular and infiltrating. The most common presentation is that of a large abdominal mass. Fifty percent of patients have metastases at the time of diagnosis. Associated symptoms include myoclonus, opsoclonus and secretion of vasoactive intestinal polypeptide. The majority of neuroblastomas are biochemically active, most secreting catecholamine metabolites, some secreting acetylcholine. These clinical manifestations represent a more malignant course.

Should patient history and physical examination suggest the presence of a neuroblastoma, laboratory studies, including complete blood cell count, serum liver transaminases, blood urea nitrogen, serum creatinine, and urinary catecholamine excretion, are helpful screening tests. Diagnostic imaging includes abdominal radiograph, skeletal radiograph with orbital views, bone scan, and CT scan. Bone marrow aspirate is essential to document widespread disseminated disease.

The major staging systems (Tables 6 and 7) in use include those of Evans, Pediatric Oncology Group, and International Neuroblastoma Staging System (INSS). The Evans system uses tumor extending across the midline as a poor prognostic indicator, whereas the Pediatric Oncology Group system uses involvement of regional lymph nodes and age. The INSS is an attempt at a comprehensive staging system.

Surgical resection is clearly indicated for localized disease. For locoregionally advanced disease, however, therapy has evolved from review of past clinical experience.

TABLE 6. *Evans classification of neuroblastoma*

Stage	Description
I	Tumor confined to organ of origin (completely excised)
II	Tumor extends beyond organ of origin but not beyond midline; regional lymph nodes may be involved
III	Tumor extends beyond midline to encroach on tissues on opposite side (exclude overhanging tumor)
IV	Distant metastases (skeletal, other organs, soft tissues, distant lymph nodes)
IV-S	Localized primary tumor not crossing midline with remote disease confined to liver, subcutaneous tissues and bone marrow, but without evidence of bone cortex involvement

TABLE 7. *International neuroblastoma staging system (INSS)*

Stage	Description
1	Localized tumor confined to organ of origin; complete excision possible microscopic residual disease, ipsilateral and contralateral lymph nodes without malignant involvement
2A	Unilateral disease with residual macroscopic disease after excision, ipsilateral and contralateral lymph nodes without malignant involvement
2B	Unilateral tumor with residual macroscopic disease after excision, ipsilateral lymph nodes with evidence of malignant involvement; contralateral lymph nodes remain free of disease
3	Tumor infiltrating across midline or contralateral lymph nodes with evidence of malignant involvement or midline tumor with bilateral lymph node malignant involvement
4	Dissemination of tumor to distant lymph nodes, bone, bone marrow, liver, and/or other organs
4S	Localized primary tumor as defined for Stage 1 or Stage 2A but with dissemination limited to liver, skin, or bone marrow

Critical scrutiny of previous experience which suggested that complete excision of tumor was necessary for curative intent revealed this information to be misleading. Indeed, radical resection can be performed in the majority of cases but occasionally with substantial morbidity or even mortality. Reevaluation of these data hinted that residual disease was present postprocedure and that patient survival did not correlate with complete resection. Recent literature supplemented by the excellent response of these lesions to established chemotherapy protocols does not support radical resection as primary therapy and many contemporary pediatric surgeons sacrifice residual disease for decreased morbidity.

Inspecting these tumors after surgical resection, reveals large, lobular, and purplish red tissue. Upon palpation, these lesions blanch with a halo of surrounding erythema which is thought to be related to release of acetylcholine. As mentioned, current therapy has evolved and is dictated by the clinical stage of disease. Surgical extirpation with adjuvant chemotherapy and radiation therapy is indicated in a majority of patients. Five-year survival is excellent for stage I disease and approaches 100%. In comparison, 5-year survival is <15% for stage IV disease.

SUMMARY

Advances in pediatric medicine have paralleled and complemented the progress in pediatric surgery. Clinical success ranges widely from treatment of common inguinal hernias to multiple complex congenital anomalies. Certainly, both have contributed to the increased survival and well-being of today's newborn. Apart from these advances, though, is the recognition of pediatrics as a unique field. It is well recognized that the devastating diseases of childhood and infancy can have equally catastrophic emotional and psychological disturbances for both patient and parents. Fortunately, it is the compassion and caring qualities exemplified by many of these clinicians that can effectively treat disease while calming fears and apprehension. Pediatric surgery working with pediatric medicine is more than saving a young life: it is about saving a whole lifetime.

STUDY QUESTIONS

1. Describe the pathogenesis of congenital inguinal hernias. Differentiate between an inguinal hernia and a hydrocele.
2. Describe the typical clinical history of infants with pyloric stenosis and the appropriate clinical management for this disease.
3. What is a hernia of Bochdalek and how does it develop?
4. Outline the pathogenesis of TEF. What are the different types of TEF, and which is the most common?
5. Characterize the pathology behind Hirschprung's disease and appropriate clinical management.

SUGGESTED READING

Filston H, ed. Pediatric surgery. *Surg Clin North Am* 1992;72:1105–1123.
Markley M, Oiticica C, Buckner D, et al. *The University of Miami manual of pediatric surgery.* Miami: University of Miami, 1995.
Raffensperger J, ed. *Swenson's pediatric surgery.* 5th ed. Norwalk, CT: Appleton and Lange
Skinner M, Grosfeld J. Inguinal and umbilical hernia repair in infants and children. *Surg Clin North Am* 1993;73:439–450.
Smith EI, Haase GM, Seege RC, et al. Surgical perspective on the current staging in neuroblastoma: the International Neuroblastoma Staging System proposal. *J Pediatr Surg* 1989;24:386.

CHAPTER 25

Neurosurgery

Brian Wieder and Barth A. Green

Patients with neurosurgical disease often present formidable clinical challenges. Although the complexities and vagaries of the central nervous system (CNS) are not completely understood, the exact location of pathology is frequently determined from simple patient history and physical examination. With a basic understanding of neuroanatomy, the first challenge is lesion localization, "anatomic diagnosis." The second challenge, "etiologic diagnosis," is surmounted, recalling neuropathology common to the various functional areas. Differential diagnosis is streamlined by applying known epidemiological and presenting patterns for various CNS diseases. Finally, the nervous system has a extremely limited capacity for regeneration, and therefore, proactive, rather than reactive, management is imperative in neurosurgical patients. Recognizing signs and symptoms of imminent catastrophe after diagnosing neurosurgical disease can prevent irreversible neurologic damage and promote successful patient outcomes.

ANATOMY AND ETIOLOGY OF NEUROSURGICAL DISEASE

Anatomy

After a detailed patient history is obtained, a thorough physical examination is performed, with particular attention to the nervous system. Exhaustive discussion regarding a detailed neurologic examination is covered in many excellent texts and will not be repeated here. The fundamental segments of the neurologic examination include mental status, cranial nerves, motor, sensory, reflexes, coordination, and ophthalmoscopy.

Neurological findings invariably localize the pathologic lesion(s). Deficits of a single functional area are most likely caused by a single lesion. Deficits of several functional areas are caused either by multiple lesions or a large lesion affecting adjacent areas. A lesion may also cause local deficits and vascular compression, causing distant effects in the territory of the vessel. Diffuse deficits are usually caused by a systemic disease process rather than a focal lesion.

Etiology

Patient demographics, onset characteristics, precipitating events, duration, and progression of symptoms have diagnostic implications. They help characterize the disease process as vascular, infectious, neoplastic, degenerative, congenital, traumatic, hormonal, or metabolic. For example, acute onset implies a vascular or traumatic etiology. In contradistinction, symptoms of long duration and slow progression imply a more benign process, while the reverse is true of malignant processes. Symptom onset following illness implies infectious or paraneoplastic disorders.

DIAGNOSTIC STUDIES

Without a doubt, advances in imaging technology have greatly improved diagnostic precision in the field of neurosurgery. Although considered archaic by many contemporary neurosurgeons, plain skull radiography provides a quick and cost-effective means of diagnosis. Shift of the pineal gland ≥3 mm, skull fracture, vascular marking, and calcification all have localizing value when better diagnostic technology is not available. Computed tomography (CT) scan is the best imaging modality of bony lesions, intracranial calcification and acute bleeding and is usually quicker, less expensive, and more readily accessible than other technologies. Magnetic resonance imaging (MRI) technology is rapidly advancing and has overtaken CT scan as the primary diagnostic modality for neurosurgical disease. Single photon emission CT (SPECT) is another imaging technique that is gaining favor among neurosurgeons. Positron emission tomography (PET) is limited by its cost and need for an on-site cyclotron, but yields important information concerning function, blood flow, protein synthesis, and receptor binding. Neurosonology has several applications, including noninvasive assessment of blood flow and anatomy data of the extracranial arteries. More recently, transcranial ultrasound has been applied in the assessment of intracranial blood flow velocity and in early detection of vasospasm in patients with subarachnoid hemorrhage (SAH). Angiography remains the gold standard in diagnosis of neurovascular disease. It elucidates vascular anatomy and offers access for endovascular treatment.

Lumbar puncture is indicated for diagnosis of SAH, meningeal processes, and drainage of cerebrospinal fluid (CSF). It is contraindicated to perform lumbar puncture in any patient with possible intracranial hypertension secondary to a CNS mass lesion. Immediate herniation and death might ensue. CT scan must be obtained prior to lumbar puncture to rule out this possibility.

RECOGNITION AND INITIAL MANAGEMENT OF NEUROSURGICAL EMERGENCIES

The initial physician to asses the patient regardless of specialization must be facile in neurologic evaluation. Recognition of imminent neurologic disaster mandates emergent treatment that can prevent irreversible neurologic demise. Appreciation of such situations, however, is often clouded by intoxication, illicit substance use, prescribed pharmacological agents, and baseline neurologic dysfunction. Therefore, it is imperative to maintain a high clinical index of suspicion.

Endotracheal intubation is indicated in patients that are unable to protect their airway and in those with inadequate ventilation. Indeed, the performance of diagnostic procedures in uncooperative patients may be facilitated by intubation and short-term paralysis with sedation. Additionally, hyperventilation decreases intracranial pressure (ICP) by causing vasoconstriction of intracranial blood vessels. Excessive hyperventilation, however, can lead to cerebral ischemia and should be avoided. Intubation in neurosurgical patients is performed using pharmacological aids that avoid unnecessary ICP elevations associated with valsalva, hypercapnia, or noxious stimulation.

In patients with an obvious neurological deficit, performance of a quick but thorough neurological examination is critical particularly prior to the administration of nervous system altering agents. This combined with a precise history will determine the most probable location and etiology of disease. Accurate interpretation of vital signs in neurosurgical patients is also important. As will be explained later, bradycardia may herald the onset of cerebral herniation. Alternatively, bradycardia is not always reflective of impending herniation. It may reflect

loss of cardiac adrenergic input secondary to disruption of sympathetic pathways as in those with spinal cord injuries above T_5. However, such patients are usually hypotensive. Hypotension with relative bradycardia implies spinal cord injury rather than hypovolemia. Neurogenic shock demonstrates increased cardiac output and is easily distinguished from low cardiac output states seen with cardiogenic and hypovolemic shock. Neurogenic shock may mimic early septic shock, but other data usually readily distinguish each entity.

SPECIAL CONCERNS IN NEUROSURGICAL PATIENT MANAGEMENT

Elevated Intracranial Pressure

At equilibrium, intracranial contents occupy a fixed volume (V) within the cranial vault equal to the sum of

$$V_{br} + V_{blood} + V_{fl} + V_{csf},$$

where br is brain, fl is interstitial fluid, and csf is CSF. The brain assumes 70% of intracranial volume while blood, cerebral spinal fluid, and interstitial fluid share the remaining 30% in relatively equal proportions. According to the Monro-Kellie doctrine, volume increases in one component of the cranial vault necessitates a compensatory volume decrease in the other components of the cranial vault, an increase in the ICP or both. Despite limited compliance of intracranial structures, these subtle changes maintain ICP in the adult between 5 and 10 mm Hg. As these homeostasis mechanisms fail, however, ICP rises. Increased ICP reflects mass such as tumor or hematoma, cerebral edema, intracranial arterial or venous hypertension, or hydrocephalus. Persistently elevated ICP, particularly when refractory to maximum treatment protocols, carries a poor prognosis.

Symptoms of intracranial hypertension may be subtle. The earliest sign is usually headache. However, in patients with depressed mental status, irritability, restlessness, and combativeness may be the only clues. Other manifestations include abducens nerve palsy or diplopia, vomiting without nausea, and, in later stages, stupor, apnea, and abnormalities in vital signs. Some symptoms are related to brain shift and herniation more than elevated pressures. Papilledema implies pressure elevation for >24 to 48 hr.

ICP monitoring is indicated in patients with Glasgow coma score (GCS) of <8 with evidence of intracranial pathology. Such degrees of unresponsiveness prevents early recognition of subtle deterioration suggestive of worsening pathology. Furthermore, a monitor may be inserted in those who historically or radiographically demonstrate a high probability of developing intracranial hypertension, e.g., hydrocephalus. Finally, transient ICP fluctuations occur without evidence of neurological deterioration. However brief, elevated ICP should be promptly relieved to prevent untoward neurologic sequelae.

Noninvasive monitors extrapolate ICP from measurements of the anterior fontanel and are used in neonates. Invasive direct or indirect systems obtain ICP measurement from intraventricular, intraparenchymal or extraaxial locations to monitor these changes. Intraventricular systems also enable withdrawal of CSF as a method of "venting" pressure. Coagulopathy can be corrected and should not preclude monitor placement if necessary. In situations of imminent herniation, this may not be possible and a subarachnoid monitor may be a viable option.

The pathophysiology related to increased ICP is complex. Primarily, cerebral blood flow and cerebral perfusion pressure (CPP = mean arterial pressure − ICP) decreases because of the compressive forces on the intracranial vasculature. As CPP falls to <40 mm Hg (normal, >50 mm Hg), cerebral oxygen delivery is compromised. The resultant ischemia and edema exacerbates the already increased ICP.

As eluded to previously, the continuous monitoring of vital signs is imperative. Harvey Cushing recognized that hypertension with bradycardia and bradypnea (Cushing's response) correlates to impending cerebral herniation. Brain herniation is a catastrophic result of increased ICP. It is defined by the protrusion of brain matter beyond the normal confines of its containment. Imaging studies or other diagnostic tests are not indicated because these only delay appropriate therapy. Immediate surgical decompression (craniotomy) or CSF evacuation (venticulostomy) may be life saving in otherwise unsalvageable patients.

Treatment of Elevated ICP

Initial intracranial hypertension management includes avoidance of unnecessary stimulation during intubation, coughing, pain, and suctioning. Head elevation has not conclusively been shown to be beneficial, but its use is widespread. Similarly, fluid restriction is a traditional part of ICP control, but supportive data is lacking. Hypotension, hypovolemia, and hypoosmolality should be avoided. Over hydration promotes cerebral edema and also should be avoided. Volume deficits may be corrected with glucose-free normal saline or blood products. Hyperglycemia aggravates intracranial hypertension as excess glucose leaks across faulty blood-brain barriers to act as an extravascular osmole.

Hyperventilation

Recent studies show that hyperventilation may be best suited for acute ICP reduction in transient elevations. Maintenance of P_aCO_2 at 30 mm Hg ± 2 and adequate oxygenation (P_aO_2 >80 mm Hg) prevents pH-mediated cerebral vasodilatation and promotes respiratory alkalosis–induced vasoconstriction, which decreases ICP. The complication of prolonged hyperventilation is cerebral ischemia secondary to blood flow reduction. Positive end-expiratory pressure improves oxygenation and, despite elevations in central venous pressure, generally does not cause significant ICP elevations. Ventilator changes are done gradually as rebound ICP increases occur with abrupt cessation of hyperventilation. Carbon dioxide associated vasomotor reactivity may be disrupted in patients sustaining closed head trauma who tend to exhibit tachyphylaxis to hyperventilation therapy.

Osmotic Diuretics

Sucrose, albumin, urea, and mannitol are all used in treatment of intracranial hypertension. Mannitol is the most effective at recruiting fluid across a "leaky" blood-brain barrier to within the vascular space, thereby decreasing ICP. Mannitol, however, also has a limited effective period because of the inherent mannitol leak across the blood-brain barrier and induction of fluid shift that counteracts mannitol's effect. This can lead to a rebound phenomenon when mannitol is not discontinued gradually.

Within 15 minutes after intravenous administration of a standard mannitol dose (0.25 to 1.0 g/kg of body weight), ICP reduction should be appreciated. Normal serum osmolality of 290 to 300 mOsm can be safely elevated to 310 to 315 mOsm, above which renal failure and decreases cerebral blood flow secondary to high blood viscosity predominates. Loop diuretics have a synergistic effect with mannitol.

Corticosteroids

Although the mechanism of action and the most effective dose is not known, dexamethasone has been shown to decrease vasogenic edema from cerebral tumors. As yet, it has not been shown to be effective in trauma or infarction. Hyperglycemic ketoacidosis, aseptic necrosis of the hip, immunocompromised status, and other factors complicate its use. Intravenous administration of 10-mg loading dose followed by 4 to 6 mg every 6 hr is a typical dosing schedule.

Cerebrospinal Fluid Removal

CSF removal from a ventriculostomy, "venting," or other drainage system is the fastest means of relieving increased ICP. Naturally, though, it has the most transient effect and repetitive venting is often necessary. Sterile technique is essential.

Barbiturates

In patients with elevated ICP refractory to standard management protocols, barbiturates are used. Judicious administration results in decreased cerebral metabolic and oxygen demand, free radical elimination, decrease cerebral blood flow through vasoconstriction and prevention of cerebral edema. Typical pentobarbital doses are in the range of 3 to 10 mg/kg loading dose, with a 0.5 to 3.0 mg/kg hourly intravenous maintenance. Cerebral perfusion pressure, however, can fall precipitously as cardiac contractility and mean arterial pressure decrease. Invasive intravascular monitoring is usually required for continuous monitoring. Although its use in patients with closed head trauma is common, the efficacy of barbiturate therapy remains controversial.

Temperature Control

Hypothermia is currently a topic of aggressive scientific investigation. Core body temperatures of <30°C decrease ICP, cerebral metabolic demand and blood flow and has been advocated as the technique providing the best neuroprotection. It is not without complications, the most significant including cardiac arrhythmia and coagulopathy. Its use, therefore, has been discontinued until studies utilizing moderate hypothermia (33°C to 34°C) demonstrate neuroprotection without accompanying morbidity. In contradistinction, hyperthermia by as little as 1°C influences outcome adversely and must be avoided. Cooling measures (e.g., hypothermia blanket, iced saline gastric lavage/enema, etc.) should be utilized if needed.

Fluid and Electrolyte Concerns

Judicious fluid management is mandatory in neurosurgical patients. Cerebral edema is worsened by hypervolemia, hypoosmolality, and fluids containing glucose. Respiratory alkalosis created by hyperventilation decreases ionized calcium levels predisposing to cardiac arrhythmias. Furthermore, alkalosis results in hypokalemia by both intracellular potassium shift and potassium ion loss for hydrogen ions conservation to correct respiratory alkalosis. Pharmacologic agents used in managing neurosurgical patients, including loop diuretics, osmolar agents, and steroids, can induce hyperglycemia and hyperosmolar diuresis, nonketotic coma, and hypokalemia. Hyponatremia is often seen in neurosurgical patients due to increased serum levels of antidiuretic hormone and atrial-natriuretic factor. Sodium repletion with hypertonic saline is appropriate. Fluid restriction may induce hypovolemia and vasospasm. Diabetes insipidus is a frequent complication of closed head trauma and requires prompt treatment with replacement of lost free water. Desmopressin or pitressin (synthetic antidiuretic hormone) may be required.

Respiratory System Concerns

Pulmonary function deserves special consideration in neurosurgical patients. Consideration of particular neurologic deficits helps establish individualized proactive respiratory management plans. Depressed mental status and cranial nerve injury inhibits airway patency. Spinal cord injury may reduce ventilatory capacity. Neurogenic pulmonary edema resulting from excess sympathetic tone or loss of parasympathetic tone may require supportive ventilation, osmotic diuresis, ICP control, or sympatholytic agents. Not surprisingly, patients with CNS injury are 10 times more likely to develop a fatal pulmonary embolism than the general surgical population. Deep venous thrombosis prophylaxis is initiated as soon as possible. Often extensive nervous system injury may preclude anticoagulation. Such cases may require inferior vena caval filter. Diagnostic prowess and compulsive general care are the tools of prevention of pulmonary complications.

Seizures

Posttraumatic seizures are common in the early postinjury period. Immediate control prevents hypoxia or ICP elevations. Prophylactic antiseizure therapy is considered standarad, although long-term therapy is not indicated unless cortical damage has occurred. Such seizures are rarely epileptogenic.

Other Concerns

Nutritional supplementation in neurosurgical patients is beyond the scope of this chapter. As with other disease processes, early alimentation, especially via the enteral route improves outcome. Avoidance of hyperglycemia, however, is essential. Bowel and bladder regimens, decubitus prevention, and prevention of nosocomial infections in comatose, paralyzed, and otherwise debilitated and immunocompromised patients require a considerable amount of time in neurosurgical units.

HEAD INJURY

Head injured patients often present with concomitant intoxication, illicit substance use, or multisystem trauma. Prior to the administration of sedative agents, rapid initial assessment of the time course, mechanism of injury, and neurologic condition are essential. A tailored examination even in unresponsive patients yields valuable information.

Specific attention is focused on identifying signs of herniation, including pupil dilation or Cushing's response,

TABLE 1. *Glasgow coma scale*

Points	Eye opening	Verbal	Motor
6	—	—	Obeys commands
5	—	Oriented	Localizes pain
4	Spontaneous	Confused	Withdraws from pain
3	To command	Inappropriate	Flexor tone
2	To pain	Incomprehensive	Extensor tone
1	None	None	None

Mortality rate associated with Glasgow coma scale: 13–15, rare; 9–12, ~12%; 3–5, 60–70%.

and "localizing signs" such as gaze preference, anisocoria, cranial nerve palsies, paralysis, unilateral reflex abnormalities, or sensory levels. A dilated pupil implies ipsilateral mass lesion with uncal compression of the ipsilateral oculomotor nerve with 85% sensitivity. Clinical signs of herniation indicate a neurologic emergency, and, provided patient airway, breathing, and circulation are established, nothing should delay emergent neurosurgical intervention.

If no evidence of impending herniation is appreciated then complete assessment begins. A thorough cranial nerve examination should be performed, especially in unresponsive patients. The optic and oculomotor nerves are assessed by examining pupil size and response to light. Oculocephalic or oculocaloric response assesses oculomotor, trochlear and abducens nerve function, together with vestibular nerve and brain stem integrity. Oculocephalic testing is contraindicated until cervical injury is excluded. Corneal response requires an intact afferent limb (trigeminal nerve) and efferent limb (facial nerve). The "gag" response indicates intact glossopharyngeal (afferent limb), and vagal nerve (efferent limb) function, which implies an intact brain stem. Motor, sensory, and reflex examinations document the best response and symmetry. Bilateral deficits imply spinal cord injury. Unilateral deficits imply brain or peripheral nerve injury. A significant number of exceptions to these trends occur.

Finally, serial examinations of pertinent systems are essential as changes in neurologic status demands reassessment of treatment plans. The GCS does not replace the neurologic examination but objectively measures neurologic integrity and documents progress or regress of clinical condition (Table 1).

Scalp Injury

Clinicians should not underestimate scalp injuries. Patients have exsanguinated from untreated scalp lacerations. Digital inspection of the underlying bone and galea is mandatory. Simple scalp lacerations without fracture or violation of the galea are closed quickly to eliminate the uncertainty of hemostasis prior to proceeding to diagnostic testing. After shaving and thorough irrigation, foreign debris and devitalized tissue are removed, and reapproximation of skin is performed using continuous nonabsorbable monofilament suture. If the galea has been violated, reapproximation of the galea with absorbable suture is performed prior to skin closure. A large moist gauze dressing and sterile compressive head wrap is placed over scalp avulsions until debridement in the operating room can be performed. Microvascular reanastomosis of preserved skin avulsions may be attempted if the clinical status of the patient permits.

Skull Fracture

Skull fractures are either open (skin and galea violated) or closed (skin or galea intact), simple or comminuted, and nondisplaced or depressed. Additionally, they may disrupt major vascular channels such as the middle meningeal artery or dural sinuses. Nondisplaced closed fractures in neurologically normal patients require no specific treatment other than neurologic observation for 24 hr. Open, but nondisplaced fractures, are irrigated, debrided, and closed urgently with appropriate antibiotics administered. Depressed or contaminated fractures are elevated and debrided in the operating room and closed after inspection of the dura. If the dura has been violated, it too must be debrided and closed. Emergent intervention in contaminated fractures is considered standard of care.

Basilar skull fractures may cause periorbital ecchymosis (raccoon's eyes), postauricular ecchymosis (Battle's sign) rhinorrhea, otorrhea, hemotympanum, or bleeding from the external auditory canal. If the temporal bone is involved then hearing deficits and facial weakness may ensue as a result of injury to cranial nerves VIII and VII, respectively. Lower cranial nerve deficits imply occipital bone fractures. Profuse auricular bleeding indicates internal carotid artery or sigmoid sinus disruption. In such cases, the ear is packed with gauze, and emergent diagnostic cerebral angiography is performed. Rhinorrhea and otorrhea are treated with head elevation. Lumbar CSF drainage is performed for persistent leaks. Although controversial, prophylactic antibiotics against gram-positive organisms can be administered.

Epidural Hematoma

Typically, epidural hematomas are the result of skull fractures and bony laceration of the middle meningeal artery. Arterial hemorrhage into the extradural space leads to rapid hemispheric compression and mass shift (Fig. 1). Ipsilateral pupillary dilation and contralateral hemiparesis are due to uncal herniation. Coma and death quickly ensue if the hematoma remains untreated.

Brief loss of consciousness, followed by a variable lucid interval and then a rapid neurological demise is the classic presentation of an epidural hematoma. Neurologic

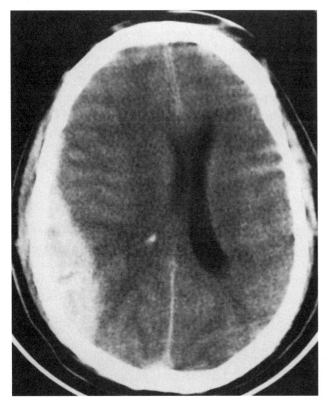

FIG. 1. Classic convex-shaped acute epidural hematoma. Note the midline shift and effacement of lateral ventricle.

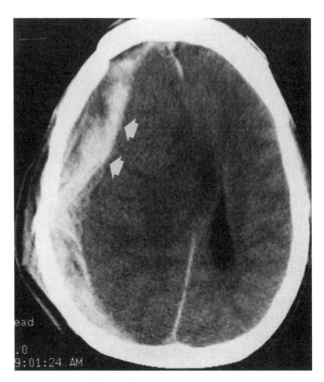

FIG. 2. Subdural hematoma.

decompensation obligates emergent decompression. Diagnostic testing only delays life-saving intervention. Fortunately, this injury is readily curable if recognized and treated expeditiously. Immediate intubation, hyperventilation, administration of mannitol, exploratory burr holes ipsilateral to the dilated pupil and skull fracture, and contralateral to hemiparesis should be performed. Clinical examination incorrectly localizes the hematoma in 10 to 15% of cases secondary to Kernohan's notch phenomenon. The herniating uncus, in this case, pushes the brain stem, contralateral cerebral peduncle, and contralateral third cranial nerve against the contralateral edge of the tentorial incisura rather than directly compressing the ipsilateral structures resulting in ipsilateral hemiparesis and a dilated pupil contralateral to the hematoma. Thus, if no hematoma is encountered initially the procedure is repeated on the contralateral side. Once the hematoma is identified, formal craniotomy and evacuation of hematoma is performed. Successful recovery is seen in the majority of patients where treatment is expeditious.

Subdural Hematoma

When bridging veins between the cortex and dura tear, a subdural hematoma develops (Fig. 2). In the elderly and alcoholics, who typically have some degree of brain atrophy, these bridging veins are under tension and can be avulsed with minimal trauma. Closed head trauma, however, with cortical laceration or rupture of intracerebral hematoma and bleeding into the subdural space remains the most common pathogenesis of subdural hematomas.

Differentiation of fluid densities by CT scan determines the age of subdural blood. Hypodense fluid collections imply chronic or subacute hematoma with less viscosity. Subdural hematomas can grow over several weeks secondary inward osmotic draw of fluid and recurrent small hemorrhage accumulation. These patients present with progressive headaches, irritability, confusion, and lethargy. In contrast, hyperdense fluid collections, especially in the face of recent trauma, are acute hematomas until proven otherwise.

In contrast to epidural hematomas, subdural hematomas occasionally can be observed if no absolute indication for evacuation exists. Acute subdural hematomas causing altered mental status or neurological deficits are evacuated via craniotomy. The postoperative prognosis, however, is not as favorable as epidural hematomas because of the commonly associated cortical insult. Subacute hematomas are easily evacuated and clinical improvement is expected after evacuation. Chronic subdural hematomas are usually >3 weeks old, and burr hole drainage of the low-viscosity "crank case oil" appearing collection is usually curative. Redrainage and rarely craniotomy may be necessary for difficult cases.

Intracerebral Hematoma

Intracerebral hematomas result from shearing or contusive injury to intracerebral vessels. Contusions underlie an area of blunt trauma (coup) or lie opposite the area of trauma (counter-coup). Frequently, intracerebral hematomas can rupture into the subdural space causing subdural hematomas. Symptomatic mass effect necessitates surgical evacuation.

Penetrating Brain Injury

Penetrating injuries require immediate craniotomy for debridement of devitalized tissues and evacuation of hematoma. All foreign bodies and bony fragments are removed if easily accessible. In general, the higher the projectile velocity the greater the parenchymal damage. Anticonvulsant prophylaxis and proper antibiotic coverage is provided.

Depressed Mental Status in the Presence of a Normal CT Scan

Surprisingly, a large number of patients following closed head trauma exhibit depressed mental status without evidence of injury on CT scan. Common explanations in these situations include intoxication; other substance influence, postictal, or postconcussive states. Fortunately, such patients rapidly improve within very short periods of time or with substance reversal. If improvement does not occur, diffuse axonal shearing injury, anoxic brain injury, or fat emboli syndrome may be the source of neurologic deficit. These processes all carry a much poorer prognosis for recovery.

SPINAL CORD INJURY

Spinal cord injury is the fourth leading cause of traumatic death in the United States. Motor vehicle accidents cause ~40% of these injuries resulting from penetration, concussion, vertebral fracture, or dislocation. Spinal cord injury without radiologic abnormality can result from cervical hyperextension of a stenotic vertebral canal. Early diagnosis, reduction of misalignment, function preservation, decompression, stabilization, and prevention of complications are standard management principles.

Bony deformity, spinal tenderness, bilateral sensory or motor deficits, and hypotension with bradycardia is indicative of, but not always present in, spinal trauma. Examination of extremity motor strength and tone, voluntary and resting rectal tone, all aspects of sensation, deep tendon, and pathologic reflexes, and inspection with palpation of the spine is requisite. Often, examination is made difficult by concurrent extremity fractures, hemo-

dynamic instability, altered mental status, or other more immediately life-threatening injures. In situations where thorough examination is not possible, spinal cord injury is presumed until proven otherwise.

Complete transection of the spinal cord causes immediate spinal shock, a loss of all motor and sensory function, areflexia, and flaccidity below the injury. Edema or hematoma ascending above C_4 or direct cord insult at this level affects respiratory capability. Injury above the T_5 level diminishes sympathetic tone resulting in bradycardia or hypotension. In the absence of hypovolemia or hemorrhagic shock, treatment with vasopressor and chronotropic agents is appropriate. Over the next 4 to 6 weeks, spinal shock resolves, giving way to classic upper motor neuron spacticity and hyperreflexia. Such injuries carry a poor prognosis for functional recovery.

Hemi-cord injury results in ipsilateral hemiparalysis, loss of light touch, and proprioceptive sensation below the lesion and contralateral loss of pain and temperature sensation beginning several levels below the level of the lesion, termed "Brown-Sequard syndrome." Partial deficits, rather than the classic constellation of neurologic findings, are more common.

Central cord syndrome—i.e., compression of the cervical spinal cord with hyperextension of a stenotic or spondylotic cervical canal—is quite common. Motor and sensory deficits in the distal upper extremities, more than the lower extremities, often with dysesthetic pain, is the classic pattern. Patients often improve with medical treatment (corticosteroids), but occasionally cervical spinal decompression is required for patients with refractory symptoms.

Anterior cord syndrome describes anterior spinal cord injury affecting anterior horn cells and spinothalamic tracts, while dorsal column function, e.g., touch, vibration, and proprioception, remains intact. Hyperflexion or axial compression with direct cord trauma or disruption of the anterior spinal artery blood flow is the predominant mechanism and functional prognosis is poor.

Conus syndrome can involve both the cord (conus medullaris) and its exiting nerve roots (cauda equina). Bowel and bladder dysfunction and sacral anesthesia are heralding symptoms. Motor dysfunction soon follows and may either be upper or lower motor neuron in nature, owing to both spinal cord tract and anterior horn compression. Cauda equina syndrome manifests predominantly as lower motor neuron findings. Bowel and bladder symptoms occur later than in conus syndrome. Motor dysfunction occurs early and is lower motor neuron in nature.

Diagnosis

Plain spine radiography is the imaging gold standard for traumatic spine injury. Radiographic evaluation of all spinal segments must include antero-posterior and lateral views. For cervical spine evaluation, oblique and odontoid views are usually required for visualization of C_1 to T_1 vertebra. Incomplete visualization is unacceptable. Flexion and extension views are obtained only if neck pain and neurologic deficit are absent. Although cervical CT scan is being used more frequently in the assessment of acute spine trauma, it is probably better used in complementary evaluation of fractures identified by plain radiography. MRI has replaced myelography in assessing cord compression. It offers the benefit of direct cord visualization, but is time consuming and cumbersome in acutely injured, intubated, or uncooperative patients.

Clinical Management

Patients with suspected spinal cord injuries are immobilized until injury is excluded. Padded backboards prevent interim decubitus formation. Intravenous corticosteroids (methylpredisolone) are administered if <8 hr have elapsed since injury. Contraindications to corticosteroid use include injuries >8 hr old, penetration of viscous organs, and contaminated wounds. Cervical misalignment is immediately reduced with skull tong traction under radiographic confirmation. Muscle relaxants or operative reduction may be necessary. Indications for emergent surgery include inability to reduce fractures, neurologic deterioration, and worsening compression from a herniated disc, hematoma, or bone. Acute decompression of neurologically stable patients is controversial. Penetrating injuries are debrided and closed. Supportive care, e.g., nutritional, intravascular volume resuscitation, and ventilatory support, is provided as needed. Psychologists, and physical, occupational, and respiratory therapists complete the multidisciplinary approach to patients with spinal cord injuries.

PERIPHERAL NERVE INJURIES

Peripheral nerve injuries fall into three categories. Temporary functional loss (i.e., "leg falls asleep") represents functional deficit without axonal disruption or neuropraxia. Axonotomesis describes axonal degeneration with preservation of the myelin axonal sheath as a result of persistent nerve compression. Neurotomesis describes traumatic disruption of axons, myelin and supportive tissue. Neurologic deficit(s) indicate the anatomic location of the injury. Acutely, electromyography is often normal and not indicated. However, several weeks after injury if neurologic deficit persists, it is abnormal and quantitates the degree of denervation.

Only patients with neurotomesis require emergent surgery but only after management of all other potentially life- or limb-threatening injuries. Primary reanastomosis is possible in patients with sharp nerve transections and clean wounds. In contaminated wounds or in extremities with tremendous blunt injury, nerve ends are identified and fixed to fascial layers to preserve length. Once the wound is infection-free, bluntly damaged nerve ends are debrided and reanastomosed. Nerve grafting is performed if primary reanastomosis is not possible.

During the recovery period, physical therapy is crucial to maintain range of motion, flexibility, and strength. Extended distance between injury and effector muscle predicts poor long-term functional prognosis.

NEUROLOGIC CHILD ABUSE SYNDROMES

Multiple injuries separated by time and space and unusual injuries for age are common "clues" to occult child abuse. Suspicious lesions include stellate, bilateral or multiple skull fractures, subdural hematomas, cranial soft tissue trauma, and spinal cord injury in the absence of an obvious explanation (i.e., motor vehicle accident). Highly suspicious lesions include interhemispheric subdural hematomas, chronic extraaxial collections, leukomalacia, skull fractures of various ages, and subarachnoid or retinal hemorrhage. The battered child syndrome describes multiple systemic and blunt head injuries occurring over time. Often, behavioral clues support clinical suspicions. Shaken baby syndrome describes a single episode of violent shaking, resulting in acute subdural, SAH, or retinal hemorrhages. Battered child syndrome may accompany this. All physicians should maintain a high index of suspicion with regard to suspected child abuse.

NEOPLASTIC DISEASE OF THE CENTRAL NERVOUS SYSTEM

Primary or metastatic tumors can involve the brain, spinal cord, peripheral nerves or their coverings. About 17,500 new CNS neoplasms are diagnosed annually in the United states. Epidemiological factors and presenting patterns facilitate differential diagnosis. Biological behavior is of great importance with regard to the rate of symptom onset, resectability, response to adjuvant therapy, and long-term prognosis. Classifications and grading systems objectively characterize biologic behavior. The list of tumor types is extensive, and only select pertinent topics are included here.

Central Nervous System Neoplasms

Epidemiology and Etiology

In children and young adolescants, nervous system tumors are second only to leukemia in cancer frequency. Up to three-fourths of childhood CNS tumors are infratentorial, whereas the reverse is true in adults. In general, childhood tumors carry a much better long-term prognosis than adults. In adults (15 to 54 years), CNS tumors account for the third and fourth highest cancer-related death rates among men and women, respectively. However, meningiomas and schwannomas show female predominance. The incidence of metastatic tumors increases with increasing age, but the likelihood that a primary tumor is benign also increases. Although therapeutic advances have improved survival rates, the incidence of nevous system neoplastic disease continues to rise.

To date, CNS tumorogenesis correlates solely with environmental factors, including radiation, environmental toxins, and viral inoculation. With rare exceptions, genetic associations have not been identified. As well, links to tobacco use and alcohol consumption have not been found. The increased incidence of meningioma with previous head trauma is disputable.

Clinical Presentation

The focal mass effect from CNS tumors shifts the brain to regions of lower pressure; thus, tumor growth rate and location determine clinical presentation. During the inital course of disease, patients classically complain of headaches, and visual blurring, diplopia, vomiting, irritability, and photophobia secondary to intracranial hypertension. A depressed level of consciousness is a late clinical sign. As brain parenchyma is forced out of its normal anatomic confines, herniation or obstructive hydrocephalus ensues.

In the evaluation of patients with suspected intracranial masses, ophthalmoscopy is essential. Papilledema or loss of retinal venous pulsations implies intracranial hypertension. Optic pallor implies optic nerve compression, and optic discitis implies lymphoma. Tumors can be irritating leading to positive symptoms (i.e., seizures) or destructive resulting in negative symptoms (i.e., functional loss). Focality of these clinical symptoms can help localize the tumor. Stigmata of endocrinopathy may be present with pituitary tumors or with tumors secreting adrenocorticotropic hormone or antidiuretic hormone.

Diagnosis

Contrast-enhanced and nonenhanced CT scan of the brain is widely chosen as the initial study of choice. MRI, however, is rapidly surpassing CT scan as the diagnositic gold standard in the evaluation of intracranial masses. Both studies provide anatomic information useful for planning surgical approach and evaluating treatment progress. In difficult cases, nuclear imaging studies help differentiate among infection, tumor, or postradiation injury. In instances with vascular involvement or high tumor vascularity, angiography may be indicated.

Management

Diagnosis of CNS tumors obligates the appropriate use of medical, surgical, chemotherapeutic, or radiation therapy modalities. Medical management can reduce vasogenic edema by administration of corticosteroids and reduce ICP via hyperventilation protocols as previously discussed. Judicious fluid management and control of steroid- or stress-induced hyperglycemia are primary concerns. Surgical management may include ventriculostomy for ICP monitoring and relief of hydrocephalus, biopsy, debulking, or gross total removal. Steriotactic gamma knife radiosurgery is a new adjuvant or, in some instances, primary therapeutic modality that concentrates radiotherapy on tumor tissue minimizing normal brain exposure. Its benefit is limited with large or multifocal lesions and proper indications are still being defined.

Spinal Tumors

Spinal tumors represent 15% to 20% of CNS tumors. They are either intramedullary (in the cord), intradural extramedullary (outside the cord but within the dural sac), or extradural. Intramedullary tumors are rarely metastatic. They are generally benign and cause compression rather than invasion of the spinal cord. A total of 33% of adult spinal tumors are intradural. Greater than 80% of these are primary glial tumors. Virtually all extradural tumors are either schwannomas, neurofibromas, meningiomas, or filum ependymomas.

Nerve root tumors present with progressive radiculopathy. Cervical region tumors present with predominantly upper extremity symptoms, neck pain or suboccipital pain. Night pain upon recumbancy that improves during the day is suggestive of tumor. Thoracic tumors present with spastic myelopathy and numbness of the lower extremities. They produce pain mimicking cardiac disease or refer pain to the viscous organs. Right T7 level tumors may refer pain to the gallbladder, and right T11-12 level tumors have led to unnecessary appendectomies. Tumors of the conus and cauda equina present with conus or cauda equina syndromes.

Intramedullary tumors classically present with nonradicular, nonradiating segmentally localized pain. Often a suspended dissociated sensory level or central cord syndrome is found on examination. Bowel and bladder dysfunction occur earlier than with extramedullary tumors. Extramedullary tumors are predominantly slow-growing eccentric tumors, with asymmetric upper motor neuron presentations. Bowel and bladder symptoms occur relatively late. Other spinal cord dysfunction may arise depending on tumor location within the canal. Malignant or metastatic tumors demonstrate a more rapid course.

Childhood

Childhood spinal cord tumors account for only 4% to 10% of CNS tumors. However, intramedullary tumors are somewhat more probable than in adults. Intradural low-grade astrocytomas, ependymomas, and dermoids/epidermoids prevail, while neuroblastomas sarcomas and primitive neuroectodermal tumors are the characteristic extradural neoplasms. Local pain, torticollis, loss of milestones, gait changes, and change in handedness are often the earliest clues.

Management

Plain radiographs demonstrating vertebral body erosion, enlarged neuroforamina, loss of normal curvature, or eroded pedicles imply tumor. Plain and contrast MRI is the imaging modality of choice for suspected spinal tumors. Myelography or CT myelography are useful alternatives; however, they do not image cord parenchyma. In cases where vertebral angulation or severe bony compression is evident, the spine is considered unstable and is immobilized. Corticosteroids are indicated for acute loss of function. Bowel and bladder care, decubitus precautions, pulmonary toilet, and preservation of function are paramount. Biopsy or tumor removal is undertaken with microdissection under magnification. Meningiomas and shwannomas can be resected for cure. Malignant or metastatic tumors presenting with acute symptom onset are decompressed emergently if postoperative prognosis indicates acceptable quality of life. Other tumors, although benign, are difficult to resect completely, and adjuvant therapy may be recommended. Instability is managed with internal fixation and fusion or external bracing.

Peripheral Nerve Tumors

Peripheral nerve tumors include neoplasms derived from the neural crest, including dorsal roots, cranial nerves, and autonomic nerves. Neurofibromas, schwannomas, traumatic neuromas, and malignant peripheral nerve sheath tumors predominate. Classically, patients present with an initially painless mass that gradually enlarges causing local or radiating pain with deficits in the nerve distribution. Spinal root tumors present with radicular symptoms. Lower motor neuron deficits are found. Tapping over a soft tissue mass may lead to radiating disesthesia (Tinnel's sign). Cutaneous stigmata of neurofibromatosis (café au lait spots) may exist.

Cranial nerve tumors present with cranial nerve dysfunction. A common example is the acoustic schwannoma, which commonly involves the eighth cranial nerve in the cerebello-pontine angle. It presents with poor speech discrimination and high-frequency hearing loss. A typical history includes turning the television progressively louder or switching telephone use from one ear to the other as the deficit worsens.

Surgical excision of schwannomas is curative. However, accessibility and relationships to important neural or vascular elements may preclude total excision. Leaving remaining tumor is often preferable to functional sacrifice, as malignant degeneration is rare and slow growth is the rule. Neurofibromas can not be resected without sac-

rifice of the parent nerve. Malignant degeneration does occur; thus, incompletely resected lesions are followed closely. Malignant nerve sheath tumors are treated with wide resection, occasionally necessitating amputation of involved limbs. Radiation is usually of minimal value.

NEUROVASCULAR DISEASE

Cerebrovascular disease is the third leading cause of death and morbidity in the United States. Vascular disease of the nervous system is categorized as atherosclerotic, inflammatory, malformative, degenerative, traumatic, or acquired. Classically, vascular disease presents with acute onset of symptoms, reflecting ischemia, thromboembolic phenomenon, or hemorrhage.

Atherosclerotic Disease

The systemic pathologic process of atherosclerosis commonly affects the arteries of the extracranial and intracavernous distribution. Larger intracranial arteries are affected at bifurcations, while smaller intraparenchymal arteries are rarely involved, except in hypertensive, diabetic, or hypercholesterolemic patients. Symptoms result from embolism, vessel rupture, or stenosis. Emboli commonly originate from ulcerated carotid bifurcation plaques or cardiac mural thrombi. Hemorrhagic infarction or hemorrhagic transformation of ischemic infarction can occur. Ischemia usually results from stenosis and can be displayed as a spectrum of clinical symptoms. Transient ischemic attacks (TIA) are symptoms that resolve within 24 hr, whereas reversible ischemic neurological deficits (RIND) resolve between 24 hr and 3 weeks. Cerebral infarction represents irreversible neurologic damage. Uncontrolled reperfusion of an ischemic infarct infrequently undergoes hemorrhagic conversion.

Patients with hypertension, cardiac arrhythmias or murmurs, carotid bruits, previous strokes, or peripheral are individuals at high risk for cerebrovascular disease. Fortunately, TIA or RIND and not stroke are the typical clinical presentation of vascular disease. Carotid disease commonly presents with transient sensory deficits, although hemiparesis or aphasia can occur. Amaurosis fugax, fleeting monocular blindness described by patients as a "sheet being drawn over one eye," is another classic example of reversible neurologic symptoms from carotid disease due to microemboli shed into the optic artery. Transient diplopia, vertigo, circumoral numbness, dysarthria, dysphagia, and blindness are suggestive of vertebrobasilar artery disease.

It is clear that patients with ischemic symptoms should undergo evaluation for carotid disease. Recent literature now suggests that all asymptomatic high-risk patients should undergo screening for carotid disease as well since carotid endarterectomy in asymptomatic patients with >60% stenosis has been shown to decrease stroke risk. The screening procedure of choice is carotid duplex ultrasound. Carotid angiography is confirmatory. Magnetic resonance arteriography (MRA) is improving and provides a diagnostic alternative in patients unable to undergo conventional angiography.

Appropriate therapy for carotid artery disease is currently evolving. Carotid endarterectomy is indicated in symptomatic patients with >70% stenosis or asymptomatic patients with >60% stenosis. Indications in patients with lesser stenosis but with ulcerative plaques are still not clear. The best management of vertebrobasilar stenosis, either medical or surgical, has not been well studied. Treatment plans and surgical approach must be individualized considering premorbid clinical status and comorbid medical disease.

With regard to the treatment of acute stroke, a multidisciplinary approach, termed at some institutions "brain attack," is being instituted at major stroke centers. In this approach, a team of neurologists, neurosurgeons, and interventional neuroradiologists attempt to minimize infarct volume and preserve functional tissue with aggressive acute resuscitation, controlled reperfusion of ischemic brain, limitation of cerebral metabolic demands, and antagonism of irreversible cell dysfunction. Thrombolytic therapy, hypervolemic hemodilution, anticoagulation, hypothermia, barbiturates, calcium antagonists, amino acid antagonists, and free radical scavengers are all being used. It has become evident that education of emergency medical personnel in early recognition of stroke may allow preemptive initiation of the "brain attack" system so that time is not wasted. Program organizers have coined the adage, "Time is brain."

Prevention of cerebral ischemia has been a topic of great debate. Control of risk factors, including hypertension, tobacco use, diabetes, hypercholesterolemia, and cardiac disease, are established primary stroke prevention measures. Antiplatelet aggregating agents such as aspirin and, to a greater extent, Ticlopidine decrease stroke risk by as much as 50% and constitute secondary stroke prevention.

Vascular Malformations

Four types of vascular malformations exist, arteriovenous malformations (AVM), venous angiomas, capillary telangectasias, and cavernous malformations. Capillary telangectasias and venous angiomas are common but rarely clinically relevant. AVM, in contrast, represent direct artery-to-vein shunts without intervening capillaries and have a high risk of rupture because of high flow and thin endothelium. Incidence of rupture is ~4% per year. Spontaneous hemorrhage is the most common presentation, although seizures, hydrocephalus, or other deficits may manifest. Surgical extirpation with brain preservation is the treatment objective. Utilizing steriotactic gamma knife radiosurgery for small AVM in surgically dangerous areas is being performed. Endovascular

embolization can make surgery safer, but its use as a primary treatment modality has not been promising due to vessel recanalization. Occasionally, operative risk of AVM excision significantly outweighs lifetime risk of rupture and surgery is not offered.

Cavernous malformations (angiomas) are tufts of sinusoidal channels with no intervening brain. Small localized hemorrhage presents as seizure or focal neurologic deficit, but since rebleed rates are low, diagnosis is not an absolute indication for surgery. Resection is considered for accessible lesions, causing intractable seizures or recurrent hemorrhage. Gamma knife radiation has been shown to successfully treat these lesions in the majority of cases.

Intracranial Aneurysms

SAH from aneurysm rupture is second in frequency only to traumatic SAH (Fig. 3). Intracranial aneurysms are classified as berry, mycotic, or fusiform. Berry aneurysms are acquired and occur predominantly at bifurcating arterial branches within the circle of Willis. More than 90% involve the anterior circulation. A small minority of berry aneurysms are multiple, with female predominance. Mycotic aneurysms are usually bacterial and rarely fungal in etiology. They typically occur on distal arterial branches, especially of the middle cerebral

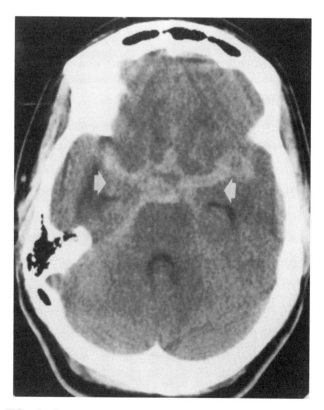

FIG. 3. Acute subarachnoid hemorrhage from ruptured intracerebral artery aneurysm.

artery. Fusiform aneurysms are likely atherosclerotic and commonly occur at the vertebro-basilar junction.

Mass effect or embolic phenomenon can be the initial presenting symptoms of intracranial aneurysms, especially in giant (>2.5cm) aneurysms, but SAH predominates in the vast majority of cases. The "worst headache ever," possibly with loss of consciousness or depressed mental status, is classic patient history. Examination may reveal meningismus or focal neurologic deficits. Posterior communicating arteries commonly cause ipsilateral oculomotor nerve compression with palsy or pupil dilation. Intracavernous aneurysms cause cranial nerve III, IV, and VI palsy. Basilar apex aneurysms may compress the brain stem. Supracavernous carotid aneurysms may compress the optic nerve. The Hunt and Hess scale clinically grades the severity of neurological damage in SAH (Table 2).

CT scan demonstrates SAH that has occurred within 24 hr with 90% sensitivity. Rupture site can often be predicted by SAH location. Middle cerebral aneurysms are more likely to cause subdural or intraparenchymal bleeding, while intraventricular hemorrhage is usually caused by communicating artery aneurysm rupture. If the result of CT scan is negative or inconclusive but patient history overwhelmingly suggests SAH, then lumbar puncture is performed. Confirmatory diagnosis relies upon the presence of hemoglobin breakdown products producing a pinkish or yellow CSF. The first and last collection tubes are sent for both cell count and characterization of the supernatant to exclude false-positive results from traumatic lumbar puncture. A lab time delay allows hemoglobin breakdown of red blood cells from traumatic puncture and also gives false-positive results. If SAH still cannot be excluded after lumbar puncture, urgent four-vessel cerebral angiography is indicated. Three-fourths of patients with nontraumatic SAH demonstrate one or more aneurysms angiographically. Vasospasm, thrombosed aneurysm, or inadequate study are infrequent causes of false-negative results.

The preferred treatment for angiographically confirmed aneurysms is surgical ligation. Patients with grade I or II symptoms undergo elective surgery at the earliest convenient time. Surgical timing is less clear in patients with grade III or IV symptoms; however, experience suggests earlier surgical intervention provides for better patient outcome. The best treatment for patients in deep coma with decerebrate posturing (grade V), is controversial. What is clear, though, is that successful management is predicated upon exclusion of the aneurysm from parent artery circulation prior to rerupture or vasospasm. Rerupture rates of 4.1% in the first 24 hr, 19% by 2 weeks, and 30% by the end of the first month with a 50% to 70% mortality are representative, and indication for urgent surgical intervention appears clear. However, critical vasospasm, which typically occurs 7 to 10 days after the index hemorrhage but can be present either clinically or radiographically from 4 days to several months following rupture, makes surgical intervention treacherous. The "window of opportunity," during which time operative morbidity is lowest and expected patient outcome is best, coincides with the period of greatest clinical stability and the period of minimum rerupture and vasospasm generally accepted to be <4 days after the index hemorrhage. Angiography may be delayed until which time clinical vasospasm has resolved.

Pre- and Postoperative Management

Preoperative control of blood pressure, correction of coagulopathy, and pain relief provided in a quiet, relaxing environment are mandatory. Stool softeners prevent strain and nimodipine modulates vasospasm risk. Any unnecessary disturbance, including phlebotomy, catheter insertion, or rectal medications, can precede rerupture, with a mortality rate of >50%. Clinical vasospasm is treated aggressively with hypervolemic hemodilution and artificial hypertension in an attempt to increase cerebral blood flow. Such treatment carries high risk in patients with unsecured aneurysms, but lack of treatment carries a similarly poor prognosis. Endovascular aneurysmal occlusion may be indicated in such cases. Failure of medical management is an indication for emergent cerebral angioplasty.

Primary Intracerebral Hemorrhage

Hypertensive hemorrhages are the most common cause of spontaneous intracerebral hemorrhage. The prevailing locations in decreasing order of frequency are the putamen, cortex, head of the caudate, thalamus, and pons. Clinical presentation mimics patients with SAH: acute headache and severe neurologic deficits or altered mental status. A history of uncontrolled hypertension with severe hypertension on admission are distinctive clinical symptoms. CT scan is invariably diagnostic, demonstrating high-density contrast intraparenchymal hemorrhage. Surgical evacuation in all cases has not shown benefit over

TABLE 2. *Hunt and Hess grade for subarachnoid hemorrhage*

Grade	Symptoms
I	Asymptomatic, or minimal headache and/or slight nucal rigidity
II	Moderate to sever headache, nucal rigidity, no neurological deficit other than isolated cranial nerve palsy
III	Drowsiness, confusion, mild focal deficit
IV	Stupor, moderate to severe hemiparesis, possible early decerebrate tone, and vegetative disturbances
V	Deep coma, decerebrate posturing, moribund appearance

medical therapy. Exceptions include lobar or cerebellar vermian hemorrhages with severe mass effect, acute hydrocephalus, or brain stem compression. In such cases, emergent ventriculostomy or surgical evacuation prevents death. Amyloid angiopathy is a vascular disorder of the elderly that results in lobar hemorrhages. When mass effect is severe, surgical evacuation is performed.

DEVELOPMENTAL ANOMALIES OF THE CENTRAL NERVOUS SYSTEM

Hydrocephalus

The choroid plexus located in the lateral, third, and fourth ventricles produces the majority of CSF at a rate of 0.33 cc/min CSF circulates through the ventricles, sub-arachnoid space, and the spinal canal prior to reabsorption at the arachnoid granulations along dural sinuses. Hydrocephalus is defined as abnormal accumulation of CSF in the ventricular system (Fig. 4) and occurs in approximately three per 1,000 live births. The hydrodynamic dysfunction which leads to hydrocephalus can be caused by obstruction of ventricular circulation, failure of absorption, or rarely from over secretion.

Congenital hydrocephalus can be diagnosed in utero by prenatal ultrasound. Common etiologies include hind brain malformations such as Dandy Walker and

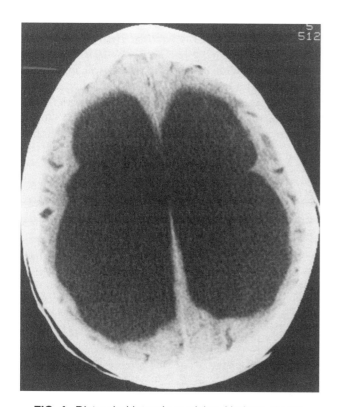

FIG. 4. Distended lateral ventricles. Hydrocephalus.

Chiari malformation, infections such as toxoplasma or cytomegalovirus, and cerebral aqueductal stenosis. Postnatal hydrocephalus is more common than the congenital variant and is usually caused by tumor, hemorrhage, or meningitis.

Patterns of presentation depend on age of onset. Before age 2, rapid exponential head growth or size greater than the 98th percentile is usual. Cranial sutures splay to compensate for the increased intracranial volume and a bulging anterior fontanel typically accompanies the enlarged head. Bradycardia, apnea, or downward ocular deviation imply brain stem compression and imminent herniation. After the age of 2, headache, vomiting, and depressed mental status are the initial symptoms, as suture fusion by this age prevents cranial expansion.

CT scan or, preferably, MRI confirms the diagnosis and may provide etiologic clues. In brain stem compression, however, emergent ventricular drainage based on clinical suspicion is life saving. Bypassing the hindrance to flow, either with shunt systems (e.g., ventriculoperitoneal shunt) or rerouting CSF through new surgically created channels, is the preferred treatment.

Myelomeningocele

Myelomeningocele, is the most common of the midline fusion abnormalities, and results from failure of closure of the embryologic neural tube. Consequently, ectoderm-derived bone, muscle, ligament, and skin that ordinarily cover the spinal cord posteriorly remain in a lateral position, giving a bifid bony appearance—thus, the name spina bifida. The unfused neural plate is exposed in the midline of the back. Varying degrees of neurologic dysfunction occur below the level of the lesion. There is a strong association with other congenital anomalies, including Chiari malformation, hydrocephalus, scoliosis, and club foot deformity. Urgent surgical closure prevents meningitis and protects remaining neural function. Broad-spectrum antibiotic coverage is administered, and a moist dressing is placed until surgical closure can be performed.

DISEASES OF THE SPINAL CORD

The spinal cord extends form the medulla to the conus medullaris, which lies at the L_1-L_2 disc space. Nerve roots continue as the cauda equina until they leave the vertebral canal. There are 31 pairs of spinal nerves: eight cervical, 12 thoracic, five lumbar, five sacral, and one coccygeal. Each spinal nerve exits the vertebral canal through neural foramen. In the cervical region, the nerve root exits the canal through the neural foramen above the vertebral body of the same level. In the thoracic, lumbar, sacral, and coccygeal levels, the root exits below the same numbered vertebral body.

Symptoms result from either disease of the spinal cord (myelopathic), the roots (radiculopathic), or both. Myelopathy describes pathology of the spinal tracts, and upper motor neuron findings, including hyperreflexia and spasticity, are typical. Radiculopathy implies deficit or pain in a nerve root distribution and are lower motor neuron disorders demonstrated by atrophy and hyporeflexia. The most common pathologies of myelopathy or radiculopathy that require surgery include herniated cervical or lumbar disc disease, spinal canal stenosis, degenerative changes, spinal cord cysts and tumors, and nerve root tumors. Annual financial expense accrued in disability and legal costs approaches $50 billion.

Herniated Vertebral Disc

By far the most common cause of either myelopathy or radiculopathy is herniated disc disease. Peak incidence of herniated disc disease occurs between 30 and 40 years of age. Men are more commonly affected than women. Associated risk factors include smoking, pregnancy, obesity, and repetitive heavy lifting and twisting. Intervertebral levels L_5-S_1 and L_4-L_5 are under the greatest load and are the most mobile and thus are most predisposed to disc herniation. Because of the relatively strong central portion of the posterior longitudinal ligament, lumbar disc herniations commonly project lateral. Cervical levels are the second most common area of disc herniation. Central cervical disc herniations are more common than in the lumbar region. The thoracic region is a rare site for disc herniations. Central disc herniations produce myelopathy in the cervical region and cauda equina syndromes in the lumbar region. In general, lateral disc herniation compresses nerve roots one level below; i.e., an L_5-S_1 disc herniation causes S_1 root compression. Acute, intermittent, or progressive radiating pain, reflex abnormalities, and sensorimotor deficits reflect the exact level of the compression (Table 3). Radiography confirms the anatomic diagnosis.

Although diverse and controversial treatment modalities exist, it is generally accepted that surgery is required for intractable radicular pain, failure of nonoperative management, or recurrent incapacitating episodes affecting quality of life. Furthermore, cauda equina syndrome, presence of foot drop or severe quadriceps weakness, or bowel and bladder dysfunction represent neurosurgical emergencies. Discectomy, using either minimally invasive technology or traditional open methods, are equally successful. Probability of functional recovery is inversely proportional to duration of symptoms.

Other Common Etiologies of Spinal Disease

Degenerative spinal changes can lead to articular slip (spondylolisthesis) or degenerative stenosis (spondylosis). Localized arthritic pain, radicular pain due to bony compression of nerve roots, or myelopathy can develop. Management strategies of these aging processes are both complex and a source of much debate.

Nerve roots are affected by the same tumors as the peripheral nervous system, namely schwannomas, neurofibromas, and malignant peripheral nerve sheath tumors. They are also affected by tumors of adjacent tissues, including bony tumors, metastases, lipomas, ependymomas, and other tumors. Tumor removal is the goal when feasible.

INFECTIONS OF THE CENTRAL NERVOUS SYSTEM

Bacterial Infection of the Central Nervous System

Bacterial infection of the CNS occurs when a breach in anatomic and immunologic host immune defenses occurs. Skin, bone, meninges, and the blood-brain barrier constitute the anatomic barrier. Bacteria can spread to the CNS by destroying anatomic barriers, foreign body penetration,

TABLE 3. *Segmental innervation testing*

First degree level	Assisting levels	Reflex	Muscle	Action tested
C2,3,4	—	—	Diaphragm	Diaphragm elevation
C5	C6	Biceps	Deltoid	Abduct arm of >90°
C6	C5, C7	Brachioradialis	Biceps, extensor carpi radialis	Elbow flexion, wrist extension
C7	C8	Triceps	Wrist flexors, finger extensors	Wrist flexion, finger extension
C8	T1	—	Finger flexors	Finger flexion
T1	C8	—	Interossei	Finger abduction
L1	L2,3	—	Iliopsoas	Hip flexion with knee flexed
L2	L3,4	—	Quadriceps, adductors	Knee extension
L3	L2,L3	—	Quadriceps, adductors	Knee extension
L4	L5	Patellar	Tibialis anterior	Dorsiflexion
L5	L4	—	Extensor digitorum longus	Toe extension
S1	L5, S2	Ankle jerk	Gastrocnemius	Plantar flexion
S2,3,4	—	Anal wink, bulbocavernosus	Anal sphincter	Voluntary rectal tone

TABLE 4. *Antibiotics with blood-brain barrier penetration*

Good penetration
  Sulfa drugs
  Metronidazole
  Rifampin
  Pyrazinamide
  Isoniazid
  Chloramphenicol
Fair penetration
  Penicillins
  Third generation cephalosporins
  Vancomycin
Poor penetration
  Aminoglycosides
  Tetracycline
  Clindamycin
  First generation cephalosporins

TABLE 5. *Predominant bacterial meningitis organisms*

Age group	Organisms
Neonatal	*Group B streptococcus, Escherichia coli, Listeria*
Young children	*Group B streptococcus, Escherichia coli, Listeria, Hemophilus influenzae, Pneumococcus*
Adolescents	*Neisseria meningitidis, Hemophilus influenzae*
Adults	*Neisseria meningitidis, Pneumococcus*
Elderly	*Pneumococcus*

or, less commonly, hematogenous dissemination. Normal anatomic barriers also exclude antibiotics from CNS entry. Therefore successful antimicrobial therapy mandated development of antibiotics that penetrate anatomic defenses (Table 4). Immunologic components represent the second tier of host defense. Immune defense failure permits progression of infection.

Primary Invasion

Osteomyelitis, usually resulting from trauma or surgery, can spread into the CNS if underlying dural violation exists and cause epidural or cerebral abscess formation. Spinal cord compression from an abscess is a surgical emergency. *Staphylococcus aureus* (43%) and *Staphylococcus epidermidis* (20%) are the usual pathogens. Treatment includes decompression, debridement, and prolonged antibiotics. Initially, vancomycin for gram-positive coverage and agents effective against gram-negative organisms is recommended until gram stain or culture results permit focused antimicrobial therapy.

Mechanical Penetration

Traumatic or iatrogenic penetration of the anatomic barrier during lumbar puncture, ventriculostomy, or surgery can introduce skin or respiratory flora into the CNS. Meningitis, ventriculitis, or abscess can result. The primary management is prevention. Meticulous wound debridement and closure, and sterile technique during procedures are paramount.

Streptococcus pneumoniae, Hemophilus, *Neisseria meningitidis,* and *Staphylococcus aureus* are common pathogens of posttraumatic meningitis. Klebsiella, *Staphylococcus epidermidis,* enterobacter, and pseudomonas are common postoperative microbes causing CNS infection. Vancomycin and ceftazidime are recommended in both situations.

Gram-positive cocci (*Staphylococcus epidermis, Staphylococcus aureus, Streptococcus viridans,* Enterococci) most frequently infect prosthetic shunts and indwelling ventriculostomy catheters. In most cases, antibiotics and removal of the infected catheter is curative. Temporary catheters may be required for hydrocephalus management or administration of intrathecal antibiotics. Vancomycin is the appropriate therapy in most cases.

Cerebritis or abscesses are frequently "sterile" by in vitro analysis; however, when an organism is isolated, Staphylococcus, Streptococcus, and coliform organisms dominate. Biopsy is recommended before antibiotics are administered. Broad-spectrum antibiotics are administered until culture results permit focused treatment. Patients with large abscesses may require surgical drainage, excision, and supportive care.

Hematogenous Spread

Meningitis commonly results from blood-borne colonization of the CNS. Typical clinical symptoms include headache, vomiting, stiff neck, fever, lethargy, and confusion. Findings can be subtle in neonates and the elderly; therefore, a high index of suspicion is required to make the diagnosis. Certain findings imply a specific organism. The presence of splinter hemorrhages about the skin, for instance, implies *Neisseria meningitidis,* whereas previous respiratory infection implies *Hemophilus influenzae.* Different organisms predominate in different age groups (Table 5). Empiric antibiotic therapy is initiated immediately after emergent lumbar puncture.

Other CNS Infections

Virus can enter the CNS by any of the mentioned routes as well as by following nerve roots, penetration through the cribiform plate, or other, not fully understood routes. In general, treatment is nonoperative, although the neurosurgeon may be called upon for diagnostic biopsy or management of intracranial hypertension. Fungal infections usually spread to the CNS by direct erosion through the sinuses or by hematogenous spread. Hemorrhage and destruction require debridement to optimize medical therapy. Neurocysticercosis and human immunodeficiency virus (HIV) deserve special consideration.

Neurocysticercosis

The most common parasitic disease is cysticercosis and can affect those who eat any fecally contaminated food. The ova of the adult pork tapeworm, taenia solium, is occasionally ingested by humans. These ova then penetrate the intestinal wall, enter the blood stream, and come to rest in the hosts muscle, brain, and eyes. Early in their life cycle, they may not produce symptoms except if mass effect causes ventricular CSF outflow obstruction or compresses eloquent structures. When they die, however, an intense immune reaction produces seizures, chemical meningitis, and focal deficits. CT scan is the best diagnostic test. Eosinophilia and positive complement fixation tests show low sensitivity and specificity. Treatment with praziquantel kills the organism but can exacerbate symptoms as the dying parasite causes further inflammation. Surgical removal is indicated for intractable seizures or obstructive hydrocephalus.

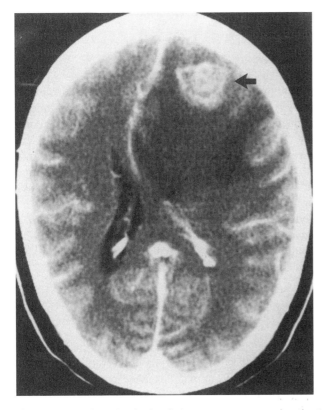

FIG. 5. Ring-enhancing lesion in immunosuppressed patient consistent with toxoplasmosis.

Human Immunodefficiency Virus

More than 50% of HIV-infected patients will eventually develop CNS-related disease. Familiarity with presentation patterns and advanced imaging have improved noninvasive diagnostic abilities. Most disease processes are managed with radiation or chemotherapy. The most common mass lesions in patients with AIDS are lymphomas and toxoplasmosis. Occasionally, craniotomy is required to confirm diagnosis or debulk mass effect. *Toxoplasma gondii* is the most common HIV-related CNS infection and occurs in up to one-fourth of patients (Fig. 5). The currently recommended treatment is Sulfadiazine combined with pyrimethamine.

SUMMARY

Physical examination of the nervous system is an integral part of the routine physical examination. There are few organ systems in the body that give such accurate clues as to the exact anatomic location and etiologic diagnosis. Physicians with a basic understanding of neuroanatomy and the neurologic examination can rapidly decipher the nature, severity, and urgency of the pathologic process. The early recognition of neurologic emergencies and proactive management will be life saving.

STUDY QUESTIONS

1. Describe the modalities for treating increased ICP and the appropriate indications for each.
2. Describe the propper evaluation and management of a patient with suspected cervical spine injury.
3. True or false?: Scalp lacerations in the absence of any other injury are not life-threatening injuries and can be closed after adequate irrigation and debridement as soon as time permits.
4. Following a high-speed motor vehicle accident, a patient with multisystem trauma and significant blood loss presents after pharmocolgic sedation for intubation in the field. His sedation precludes complete examination. His blood pressure is 90/50, with a pulse of 60; his hematocrit is 27%. He has no internal injuries but multiple extremity fracures. The bleeding from the left lower extremity is contolled. What other injuries are implied by the information that you have here?

SUGGESTED READING

Greenberg MS, ed. *Handbook of neurosurgery.* New York: Greenberg Graphics Publishing, 1990.

Lindsay K, Bone I, Callander R. *Neurology and neurosurgery illustrated.* 2nd ed. New York: Churchill and Livingstone, 1991.

Youmans J, ed. *Neurological surgery. Vols. I–V.* 4th ed. Philadelphia: Saunders, 1996.

CHAPTER 26

Orthopedic Surgery

L. Stacy Mitchell, Mark Brown, and Gregory A. Zych

BASIC SCIENCES

Bone

Bone is made up of organic and inorganic substances. The organic component accounts for ~40% of the dry weight of bone, and the remaining 60% is made up of inorganic (mineral) substrates. Collagen, which gives bone its tensile strength, is composed primarily of type 1 collagen and makes up 90% of the matrix. The structure of collagen consists of a porous triple helix of tropocollagen that allows mineralization and eventual calcification. Proteoglycans, which are partially responsible for the compressive strength of bone, are made up of a hyaluronic acid core protein bound to disaccharide polymers (glycosaminoglycans). The remainder of the organic component of bone consists of glycoproteins (i.e., osteonectin and fibronectin), phospholipids, and phosphoproteins, which aid in bone formation and promotion of increased bone density. The inorganic composition of bone is largely due to the presence of various salts that are responsible for the mineralization of the matrix. Calcium hydroxyapatite is the predominant inorganic constituent that gives bone its compressive strength.

Bone formation occurs by two different methods. The first, enchondral ossification, is heralded by the creation of bone from a previously laid down cartilage model. This event is brought on by the invasion of vascular channels into the cartilage anlage, where osteoprogenitor cells differentiate into osteoblasts to form bone. The cartilage model grows through appositional (width) and interstitial (length) growth. The second type of bone formation is called "intramembranous ossification." Bone formation of this type occurs without a preexisting cartilage model. Although not entirely understood, this method of bone formation is thought to occur by the aggregation of mesenchymal cells into condensed layers or membranes. Mesenchymal cells that are adjacent to blood vessels differentiate into osteoblasts and create centers of ossification for the eventual formation of bone.

Bone repair is the process by which an injured bone heals after a fracture. Hematopoietic cells that are found in the fracture hematoma are capable of secreting growth and chemotactic factors that will promote a subsequent inflammatory response. Cells, such as osteoblasts and fibroblasts, will become present at the bone ends to begin the next phase of bone repair, primary callus formation. This phase begins usually within the first 2 weeks, and the eventual amount of callus formation at the fracture site is indirectly proportional to the degree of immobilization. Remodeling, which begins during the second half of the repair stage, takes place based on numerous factors (i.e., fracture size/site, bone quality, and mechanical stress) and can last up to 7 years after clinical healing has occurred.

Musculoskeletal Structure

Cartilage is found in various places in the body and performs numerous functions. For the purpose of this chapter, cartilage will be considered in its relationship to bones and joint function. Articular cartilage is composed of ~65% water, 15% to 20% collagen (mainly type 2), 10% to 15% proteoglycan, and 5% chondrocytes. Articular cartilage decreases friction, distributes load evenly, and provides various metabolic functions. Injuries to articular cartilage from trauma, infection, and aging can lead to inflammation of the joint (arthritis).

Ligaments are structures that link one bone to another, providing joint stability. These tissues are mainly composed of type 1 collagen. Injuries to ligaments may destabilize a joint secondary to compromise of joint strength or damage to nerve tracts (mechanoreceptor) found within ligaments.

Tendons are composed primarily of type 1 collagen and function to attach muscle to bone. Insertion into bone

347

exists by way of terminal calcified structures known as "Sharpey's fibers." Tendon injuries are usually a result of trauma but can also be associated with, if not attributed to, increasing age. Although the exact etiology and mechanism is poorly understood, an age-related paucity of neighboring blood vessels has been noted in cadaveric specimens. Tendon repair is noted to be weakest at 7 to 10 days, regains most of the premorbid strength at 4 weeks, and achieves maximal strength between 6 and 12 months. Early, protected range of motion during this period is thought to decrease potential unwanted scarring and increase tendon strength at the level of Sharpey's fibers.

Muscle is composed of functional units of contraction known as "sarcomeres." A stimulating action potential causes thick (myosin) filaments to slide against the thin (actin) filaments within the sarcomere and provide the kinetic basis for muscle contraction. This action potential takes place secondary to a release of calcium that is stored in the sarcoplasmic reticulum. Muscle contraction occurs from insertion toward origin. Isometric contraction occurs when tension is generated, but the overall muscle does not shorten. In isokinetic contractions, maximal tension is generated in a muscle at a constant speed over the full range of motion. "Isotonic contraction" refers to the existence of constant tension throughout the entire range of motion. A muscle contraction in which the muscle shortens is known as a "concentric contraction." In an eccentric contraction, the muscle actually lengthens as the muscle fibers contract. Slow twitch fibers have increased mitochondria, enzymes, and triglycerides but low concentrations of glycogen and ATPase. Energy production and utilization is predominantly oxidative in nature. These slow fibers are incapable of generating quick bursts of strength contractions but are slow to fail in repetitive contractions. In contrast, fast twitch fibers are larger and stronger than slow twitch fibers. Contractions are quicker, and there is a higher ATPase concentration within fast twitch fibers compared to slow twitch fibers. Energy production and consumption occurs in predominantly an anaerobic fashion.

Intervertebral discs within the spine provide shock absorption and stability during motion. They consist of a central gel-filled structure called the "nucleus pulposus," surrounded by the annulus fibrosis. Intervertebral discs are composed of 85% water, proteoglycan, and collagen (types 1 and 2). A herniated disc, which often occurs at the L4-L5 disc space, can cause compression to spinal nerves, roots, or the cord. Radicular pain and parathesias are felt in the buttocks and lower extremities. Most herniations occur in the posterolateral space, where the posterior longitudinal ligament is the weakest. Central prolapse usually results in back pain only and could precipitate a potential loss of bowel and bladder function (cauda equina syndrome). This occurrence is considered a surgical emergency and is discussed later.

Oncology

Orthopedic oncology includes both benign and malignant lesions of the musculoskeletal system and the surrounding neurovascular structures. The most common benign tumor in children and adults is a lipoma. Most malignant lesions of the musculoskeletal system are the result of metastasis. Multiple myeloma is the most common primary bone malignancy in adults. Sarcomas are defined as malignant neoplasms of mesenchymal-derived tissue and are the least common of all malignant lesions. Sarcomas may be fatty, fibrous, muscular, nervous, or synovial, or of vascular origin. Rhabdomyosarcoma, a malignant tumor of striated muscle, is the most common sarcoma of soft tissue origin. In the pediatric population, leukemia is the most common malignancy, seen with metastasis to bone accounting for the largest cause of musculoskeletal tumors. Although considered rare, osteosarcoma is the most common primary bone malignancy of children. Ewing's sarcoma, a tumor of round cell origin, is the second most common bone malignancy in children. Treatment of neoplastic lesions of the musculoskeletal system may involve surgical fixation and/or adjuvant radiation therapy.

PEDIATRIC ORTHOPEDICS

Embryological development of the musculoskeletal system begins between 4 and 6 weeks of gestation. During this time, limb buds derived from mesenchymal tissue (mesoderm) form the upper extremities and lower extremities. Bony elements of the skeletal axis and extremities are formed primarily from enchondral ossification. Some bones develop via intramembranous ossification.

Birth trauma has decreased over the past few decades due to improved obstetrical management. However, injuries to the musculoskeletal and nervous systems still occur during delivery. There is an increased risk of injuries of the brachial plexus with breech births, forceps deliveries, prolonged labor, and shoulder dystocias. Treatment of brachial plexus palsies is centered around passive range of motion exercises by the therapist. Most brachial plexus palsies resolve without surgical intervention.

Pediatric Orthopedic Conditions

Torticollis is a congenital deformity of the head and neck resulting from contractures of the sternocleidomastoid muscle. The exact etiology of this disorder is unknown. It may be associated with various cervical spine abnormalities. This condition will usually resolve with gentle passive stretching. Surgery is usually reserved for cases that persist beyond 1 year despite aggressive neck-stretching exercises.

Metabolic bone diseases are a heterogeneous group of disorders that are primarily caused by a deficiency of a substrate, product, or metabolite that is required to produce normal bone. In rickets, called "osteomalacia" in adults, problems arising from the lack of vitamin D, its expression, or its absorption lead to imbalances in calcium and phosphorus metabolism. Classically, this disorder is characterized by brittle bones, bowing of long bones, transverse radiolucent bone lines on x-ray (Looser's lines), dorsal kyphosis ("cat back"), enlargement of costal cartilages (rachitic rosary), and cupping/widening of the physis. Osteogenesis imperfecta, caused by a defect in collagen formation, is highlighted by brittle bones, ligamentous laxity, tooth defects, and short stature. Pathologic fractures are very common. Most fractures are managed with nonoperative intervention. The presence of blue sclera is a feature of this condition but is only found in 20% to 30% of these patients. Osteopetrosis is a disorder caused by osteoclastic dysfunction. Dense bones ("marble bone disease"), a rugger jersey spine, and an Erlenmeyer flask–shaped distal femur are demonstrated on radiography. Treatment of osteopetrosis may include bone marrow transplantation.

Hematopoietic disorders often lead to abnormalities in the musculoskeletal system. Sickle-cell anemia is particularly, although not solely, prevalent in the African-American population, affecting ~1% of individuals. A sickle-cell crisis caused by dehydration can lead to bone ischemia and infarction. Growth disturbances, dactylitis (hand and foot swelling), osteonecrosis of the femoral and humeral heads are common features of this disease. Osteomyelitis, as well as septic arthritis, are also frequent findings in sickle-cell anemia. Salmonella species are often cultured from aspirates of bone and joint infections and are as prevalent as Staphylococcus (generally considered the primary infectious agent in patients without sickle-cell disease). Hemophilia, a sex-linked recessive disorder, is caused by decreased serum levels of either factor VIII or IX. Recurrent hemarthroses, intramuscular hematomas, formation of blood cysts, and squaring of the patellas are classic orthopedic manifestations of this disease. Leukemia, the most common malignancy of childhood, is associated with bone demineralization, lytic lesions, and joint sepsis.

Cerebral palsy is a nonprogressive neuromuscular disorder of unknown etiology. This condition is thought to occur in the perinatal period resulting from injury to the immature brain. Proposed etiologies include perinatal infections (e.g., TORCH—i.e., toxoplasmosis, rubella, cytomegalovirus, and herpes simplex), prematurity (most common), anoxia, and head trauma. The classification of cerebral palsy can be done on the basis of topography or physiology. Using the topographical method of classification, involvement of upper and lower extremities on the ipsilateral side of the body is known as "hemiplegia." "Diplegia" refers to functionally more paraplegia of the lower extremities than the upper extremities. In quadriplegia, there is equal involvement of all four limbs. The prognosis for ambulation is best in patients with hemiplegia. Using the physiologic method of classification, patterns of movement are described as spastic, athetoid, ataxic, rigid, or a combination. In the spastic patient, hypertonicity and hyperreflexia are noted to exist with restricted movements. Athetoid patients are seen to have a frequent dance-like succession of involuntary motions. Patients with the ataxic form of cerebral palsy demonstrate a wide-based gait, dysmetria, dysarthria, and dysdiadocalkinesis. In the rigid type, the patient exhibits a waxy, cogwheel pattern of movement. The patient's extremity appears to be fixed in position during an examination. Surgery is reserved for patients who are >3 years of age, possess good intelligence, have voluntary motor control, or have the spastic form of cerebral palsy.

"Myelodysplasia" refers to disorders of the spinal cord that are present at birth. The etiology is unknown. A primary defect in development or hydrocephalus may be responsible. In spina bifida occulta, a defect occurs in the vertebral arch. The cord and meninges are confined to the spinal column without protrusion through the defect. A meningocele describes herniation of meninges (sac) through the vertebral arch defect without protrusion of neural elements. In myelomeningocele, spina bifida exists with protrusion of both meninges and neural elements. "Rachischisis" refers to the presence of neural elements through the bony defect without its protective meningeal covering. Classification of this disorder is based on the lowest neurological level of motor function. Many abnormalities of the lower extremities are associated with myelodysplasias. Hip dislocations are most common with L3-L4 level disease. Ambulation requires at least an L4 functional level. Changes in neurologic function can be associated with hydrocephalus (most common), tethered cord, and hydromyelia. About 70% of myelodysplastic patients have hydrocephalus demonstrated by CT scan.

Pediatric scoliosis is defined as rotation and lateral deviation of the spine. Most cases are idiopathic and will be the focus of this discussion. The spine of a patient with scoliosis clinically and radiographically appears to take an S-shaped configuration. The curve description is based upon the location of the curve's apex. The most common type of curve seen is a right thoracic curve. The next most common type of curve is a right thoracic and left lumbar curve ("double major"). The left lumbar curve or right lumbar curve patterns are infrequently seen. In adolescent patients, left thoracic curves are rare and should be evaluated with an MRI scan to rule out cord abnormalities. Increased curve progression is seen with skeletal immaturity, larger curves, and younger age. Treatment is based on the degree of curve, skeletal maturity, and curve progression. Serial observation is the mainstay of treatment for scoliotic curves of <25 degrees.

Bracing of the trunk is most often used for curves between 25 and 40 degrees in the immature patient. The use of truncal bracing has been found to be most effective when the orthosis is worn 23 hr/day. Curves of >40 degrees are typically treated with operative intervention.

Disorders of the cervical spine in children can occur independently but are often found in association with other congenital abnormalities. Klippel-Feil syndrome is a failure of normal segmentation of cervical somites. The radiographic studies in these patients reveal multiple fused cervical segments. Clinically, patients with this disorder often demonstrate the classic triad of a low posterior hairline, decreased range of neck motion, and a short webbed neck. Congenital scoliosis, renal aplasia, Sprengel's deformity, heart defects, and brain stem abnormalities are often associated with this disorder. Treatment is usually limited to physical therapy with surgical intervention reserved for chronic pain or myelopathy due to cervical instability. Scheuermann's disease is defined as increased thoracic kyphosis (>45 degrees), with ≥5 degrees wedging at three sequential vertebrae. This condition is often found in association with various other spinal abnormalities. Complaints of occasional back pain in an adolescent male with poor posture is the typical patient presentation. The patient is unable to correct his hyperkyphosis with hyperextension of the trunk. The mainstay of treatment is physical therapy and bracing. Surgery is usually reserved for skeletally mature symptomatic patients with kyphotic deformity of >65 degrees.

Sprengel's deformity is a congenital undescended scapula that is often seen with hypoplasia, internal rotation, omovertebral connections, and winging. This condition is associated with scoliosis, renal disease, and Klippel-Feil syndrome. Patients with this condition often show a decreased range of shoulder motion. Surgery may sometimes be needed for cosmesis and severe limitations of motion.

Developmental dysplasia of the hip (DDH) describes abnormal development or hip instability secondary to capsular laxity and mechanical factors. Often considered to result from intrauterine position, the exact etiology of this condition is unknown. This disorder is usually seen in first-born children, females, breech births, and children with a family history for hip dysplasia. This condition affects primarily the left hip but is often found bilaterally. DDH may be seen in association with other musculoskeletal abnormalities such as torticollis and metatarsus adductus. Diagnosis of DDH can be made clinically by a trained examiner or with the use of radiographs or ultrasound. Treatment is based upon the ability to achieve or maintain a stable hip reduction. Most patients with DDH respond well to reduction in a specialized (Pavlik) harness. While in this harness, the hips are flexed at ~100 degrees and with mild abduction. The use of the harness is usually limited to patients less than 6 months old, reducible hips, patients with capsular/ligamentous integrity, and patients with an intact L-5 neurological level. Patients with irreducible hip dysplasia or those who fail to maintain concentric hip reductions following harness treatment require surgical intervention.

"Legg-Calvé-Perthe's disease" refers to osteonecrosis of the proximal femoral epiphysis. This condition is considered to be an aseptic, self-limiting disease of unknown etiology. This disorder is usually seen between 4 and 8 years of age and is more prevalent in males. Clinically, patients may present with a limp and complain of hip or knee pain. This condition often mimics septic arthritis and therefore an infectious process must be excluded. Children younger than 8 years of age have a better prognosis for reduced morbidity of the hip joint. Treatment may range from bed rest and traction to the use of abduction braces, or even surgery. Concentric containment of the femoral head inside the acetabulum with maintenance of hip motion is the goal in all of these treatment modalities.

Slipped capital femoral epiphysis (SCFE) is a disorder of the hip usually seen in adolescent males. SCFE is more common seen in African-American obese males with a family history of SCFE. Approximately 20% to 30% of these cases are bilateral. The exact etiology is unknown. In this disorder, the proximal femoral epiphysis (head) is noted to remain in the acetabulum, while the femoral neck is displaced laterally and anteriorly. These patients clinically present with a limp and complains of hip or knee pain. The location of pain varies usually with the duration of symptoms. An acute slip (<3 weeks) is usually treated with closed reduction and percutaneous pinning. Chronic slips (>3 weeks) may respond to closed reduction or simply pinning in situ. Various surgical procedures can be performed based on the degree and chronicity of displacement. Forced reduction before pinning must never be performed. Osteonecrosis, chondrolysis, and degenerative arthritis of the hip may occur secondary to the disorder itself or its treatment.

Clubfoot deformity is a common childhood foot disorder. In this deformity, the hindfoot is noted to be in varus (forefoot in adduction) and the hindfoot held in a plantar flexed (equinus) position. The entire hindfoot is rotated medially around the talus, which remains in place. Clubfoot deformities are seen more commonly in males and half are bilateral. Initial treatment of this disorder consists of closed manipulation and serial casting. Approximately up to 85% of clubfoot deformities respond to conservative treatment. Surgical intervention may be needed for failure of conservative measures or in refractory cases.

Muscular dystrophy is an inherited condition of early childhood that is characterized by progressive motor weakness. Several varieties of this disease exist. Duchenne's muscular dystrophy is the most common form. It is considered a sex-linked recessive abnormality that affects predominantly young patients. Clinically, these patients are noted to ambulate with a clumsy gait and possess impaired motor skills. Pseudohypertrophy of the calves and lumbar lordosis are also common findings. Patients with muscular dystrophy are often seen using their hands to walk up their legs in order to obtain an upright position (Gower's sign). Laboratory studies reveal elevated levels of creatine phosphokinase (CPK). Muscle biopsy demonstrates areas of frank necrosis, scarring, and connective tissue infiltration. Historically, most patients with Duchenne's muscular dystrophy died before reaching their late teens from associated cardiac and pulmonary complications. Treatment of this condition centers around keeping the patients ambulating with therapy, bracing, and surgical release of contractions.

Osteomyelitis and septic arthritis in children requires an early diagnosis and prompt treatment to decrease the potential risk of musculoskeletal deterioration. Pathogenesis of osteomyelitis in children is thought to occur due to a rich metaphyseal blood supply and a thickened periosteum. Septic arthritis is largely due to the presence of transphyseal vessels and intracapsular containment of the metaphysis (i.e., hips and shoulders) seen in children younger than 3 years of age. The most common route of infection in osteomyelitis is through hematogenous spread. Osteomyelitis can also result from direct inoculum (trauma) or direct local extension. Septic arthritis often develops from a neighboring osteomyelitis. The most common organism isolated in osteomyelitis for all ages is the Staphylococcus species. Group B Streptococcus and *Escherichia coli* are highly prevalent in osteomyelitis found in neonates and may exceed Staphylococcus. *Hemophilus influenzae* is also quite common from ages 3 months to 4 years. *Neisseria gonorrhea* is more prevalent in the adolescent population. In septic arthritis, Staphylococcus is the most common organism present. From ages 6 months to 6 years, *H. influenzae* is the second most prevalent organism. *N. gonorrhea* is found second to *Staphylococcus aureus* in the teenage population. Patients with osteomyelitis and septic arthritis usually present with complaints of warmth, pain, and increased tenderness over the involved area. The child may limp or refuse to ambulate secondary to pain. In septic arthritis, the child will usually demonstrate a decreased range of motion with extreme pain being elicited by passive extremity manipulation by the examiner. Laboratory analysis, such as a white blood cell count and erythrocyte sedimentation rate (ESR), may be helpful in making the diagnosis. Radiographs and bone scans may be useful in localizing areas of suspicion in a young or uncooperative patient. Aspiration of a suspected joint must be performed before any administration of empiric antibiotic therapy is instituted. Osteomyelitis may be treated with antibiotics unless a collection of pus exists or radiographic changes are seen. Under these circumstances, surgical intervention for drainage and debridement must be performed. Treatment of septic arthritis, except for the hip joint, can either be managed with ser-

ial aspirations/irrigation or with surgical drainage. Surgical intervention is required for septic arthritis of the hip joint and for other joints that fail to respond to serial aspirations/irrigation.

Transient synovitis is the most common cause of hip pain in children. This condition may be associated with allergic reactions, viral illness, or trauma. The exact etiology of this condition is unknown. This occurrence is self-limiting and can be managed with activity restriction and nonsteroidal antiinflammatory drugs (NSAIDs). This clinical entity is a diagnosis of exclusion and can only be made after all other infectious or rheumatological processes have been excluded.

Juvenile rheumatoid arthritis (JRA) is characterized as a persistent arthritis lasting >6 weeks to 3 months after all other possible etiologies have been excluded. The diagnosis is confirmed by one of the following conditions: presence of the rheumatoid factor, intermittent fever, rash, pericarditis, iridocyclitis, tenosynovitis, cervical spine involvement, or morning stiffness. Iridocyclitis, which is most commonly seen in the pauciarticular form of this disease (30%), must be screened for with frequent slit-lamp ophthalmic examinations to prevent blindness. JRA is more common in females and is often seen in various syndromes with visceral involvement. Chronic joint synovitis in this disorder leads to destruction of the articular cartilage. Treatment of this disorder includes splinting, salicylates, and, occasionally, joint synovectomy procedures.

Rheumatic fever is a disease of the immune system that may represent an autoimmune process. This disorder is seen in children from 4 to 16 years following a Streptococcal infection. The hallmark of this condition is migratory arthritis, carditis, fever, subcutaneous nodules, and a pink rash seen on the trunk and extremities (erythema marginatum). Treatment includes salicylates and antibiotics.

Pediatric Fractures

Fractures in children are distinctly different than fractures in adults (Fig. 1). The periosteum in children is thicker than that found in the adult. Because of this phenomenon, incomplete ("greenstick") and torus ("buckle") fractures in children are more likely to occur. Greenstick fractures result from the propagation of the offending

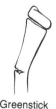

Greenstick

FIG. 1. Greenstick fracture. (From Harwood-Nuss AL, Linden CH, Luten RC, Shepherd SM, Wolfson AB. *Clinical practice of emergency medicine.* 2nd ed. Philadelphia: Lippincott–Raven, 1996:1212.)

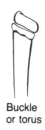

FIG. 2. Buckle or torus fracture. (From Harwood-Nuss AL, Linden CH, Luten RC, Shepherd SM, Wolfson AB. *Clinical practice of emergency medicine.* 2nd ed. Philadelphia: Lippincott–Raven, 1996:1212.)

force through the periosteum and cortex on one side(tension side) while leaving the opposite periosteum and cortex (compression side) intact. A torus fracture (Fig. 2) is the result of an impaction injury to a bone and primarily affect the metaphyseal region of the bone. Because of the various responses of the metaphyseal bone to compressive stress, the bone buckles instead of creating a complete fracture. Bones in the skeletally mature patients are more rigid than the skeletally immature patient and are more apt to demonstrate complete fractures. Pediatric fractures heal quicker and require less immobilization than their counterparts. Fractures that occur around the physis (growth plate) can cause several problems including growth arrest, bony deformities, and limb- length discrepancies. The importance of fractures involving the physis can not be over emphasized. The nomenclature

most often used for physeal injuries is based on the Salter-Harris classification system. Although modifications have been made by various authors, the focus of this discussion will be on types I through IV (Fig. 3). In a type I injury, a transverse fracture through the physis occurs. A type II injury is defined as a fracture that goes through the physis but also has a metaphyseal fragment. In a type III injury, there is a fracture through the physis and epiphysis. The type IV features a fracture that involves the physis, epiphysis, and the metaphysis. Type I and II fractures, when treated with the appropriate anesthesia, are most often managed by closed reduction and casting. Salter-Harris type III and IV injuries both have an intraarticular component and therefore will usually require surgical correction.

Child Abuse

Child abuse should be suspected in young patients (usually younger than 3 years old) with unexplainable fractures and bruises. Fractures resulting from child abuse usually occur in the long bones of the upper and lower extremities. A skeletal survey may be needed to assess the pediatric patient for old, previously untreated, or additional fractures. In the United States, mortality approaches 10% because of unrecognized repeated child abuse. All suspected cases of child abuse must be reported by the physician or hospital to the local child protection agency.

ADULT ORTHOPEDICS

The scope of adult orthopedics encompasses various conditions and numerous disease entities. This section is limited to those disorders that are most commonly encountered by the general orthopedist.

Joint Disease

Osteoarthritis, also termed "degenerative joint disease," is the most common form of noninflammatory arthritis. The exact etiology of osteoarthritis is unknown. Predisposing factors may include past trauma, previous joint sepsis, congenital disorders, and older age. Clinically, patients with osteoarthritis demonstrate a painful range of motion, swelling, and crepitus over the affected joint(s). Microscopically, articular cartilage destruction is noted with decrease in the number of chondrocytes. Radiographic examination may reveal joint space narrowing, subchondral cyst formation, and the presence of juxtaarticular osteophytes. Conservative management of osteoarthritis includes weight loss, exercise, activity modification, ambulatory aids, and NSAIDs. Surgical intervention, including joint replacement, debridement,

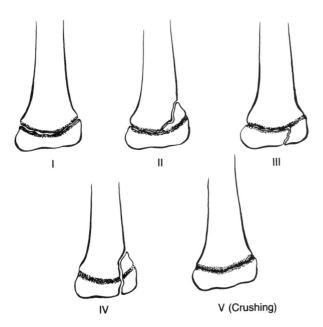

FIG. 3. Salter-Harris classification. Nomenclature of representative fractures involving the growth plate in children. (From Harwood-Nuss AL, Linden CH, Luten RC, Shepherd SM, Wolfson AB. *Clinical practice of emergency medicine.* 2nd ed. Philadelphia: Lippincott–Raven, 1996:1213.)

and even arthrodesis (fusion), may be used in the management of osteoarthritis.

Rheumatoid arthritis is the most common form of inflammatory arthritis. Females are more often affected than males with this disease. The etiology of this disorder is unknown but may represent an autoimmune process. The hallmark of this disorder is the destruction of cartilage and bone, with the involvement of the surrounding soft tissues. Patients with rheumatoid arthritis routinely complain of aching and stiffness in the morning involving the shoulder and pelvis. Physical examination is often unremarkable, and laboratory tests are usually not helpful in the diagnosis of this disease. Treatment of rheumatoid arthritis is largely symptomatic. A multidisciplinary approach including drugs, ambulatory aids, activity modification, physical therapy, bracing, and sometimes surgery may be needed to minimize pain while maximizing joint function.

Ankylosing spondylitis is an inflammatory arthritic condition that occurs at the insertion sites of ligaments into bones. Ankylosing spondylitis typically affects the sacroiliac joints more than any other joints. Uveitis may also be present. Males with the HLA-B27 immunohistologic marker comprise the majority of patients. This condition is associated with numerous spinal abnormalities, pulmonary fibrosis, and hip deformities. Treatment of this disorder is with NSAIDs, physical therapy, and, in some cases, surgery.

Reiter's syndrome is an inflammatory condition that affects young males. The classic triad of nongonococcal urethritis, conjunctivitis, and oligoarthritis is often seen in this disorder. Ulcers on the penis, mouth, and extremities are frequently seen on physical examination. The treatment of the arthritic component in this syndrome includes NSAIDs and physical therapy.

Gout is an inflammatory disorder of uric acid metabolism. The hallmark of this condition is the deposition of urate crystals (tophi) into joints that is believed to trigger a deleterious immune response. Gout is usually seen in males between the ages of 40 and 60 years. The classic area of involvement is the great toe, but gout can affect any joint. Radiographically, periarticular erosions with sclerotic borders are seen. The urate crystals demonstrate a thin, tapered, strongly negative birefringent appearance to polarized light. The mainstay of treatment is the use of indocin, allopurinol, colchicine, and dietary modification.

Calcium pyrophosphate deposition disease (CPPD) is an inflammatory disorder of pyrophosphate metabolism. This disease is also known as "pseudogout" because it is seen in older patients and often mimics gout-like attacks. Radiographs reveal linear calcifications in the hyaline cartilage and the menisci in knees. The crystals in CPPD demonstrate blunt, rhomboid-shaped rods that are weakly positive birefringent. The mainstay of treatment consists of the use of NSAIDs and physical therapy. Refractory cases may necessitate the need for joint debridement.

Surgical Treatment of Joint Disease

Joint replacement surgery, arthroplasty, is used to treat various forms of arthritis that produce incapacitating pain. The arthritis may have resulted from a rheumatological condition, trauma, congenital deformity, tumor, osteonecrosis, or a previous joint infection. In the United States, most joint replacement surgery is performed on the hips and knees but only after conservative treatment has failed. Nonoperative therapy for arthritis includes weight loss, use of ambulatory aids (i.e., walker or cane), activity modification, physical therapy, NSAIDs, and, occasionally, joint injections with steroids. The entire joint may be replaced (i.e., femoral head and acetabulum) and is termed "total joint arthroplasty." Less frequently, only a part of a joint (i.e., femoral head) is replaced, and this is referred to as a "hemi-arthroplasty." Joint arthroplasty may be performed with or without the use of bone cement based on the patient's age, associated medical conditions, or the surgeon's preference. Other procedures such as joint resection, arthrodesis (fusion), or osteotomies may be considered in these patients. The average time from the index procedure to the first revision arthroplasty is often between 7 and 10 years. The longest period of relief following arthroplasty is usually experienced after the initial procedure. Less favorable results are seen after each subsequent revision. Due to the aforementioned findings, joint replacement surgery is usually advocated for patients >65 years of age. Perioperative complications involving joint replacement surgery include deep venous thrombosis (most common), joint sepsis, pulmonary embolism, nerve injury, large blood loss, and intraoperative hypotension when inserting cement. Long-term complications include component loosening, implant failure, dislocations, late infections, and local heterotopic ossification. The latter problem may be treated prophylactically with perioperative indomethacin or postoperative radiation therapy.

Compressive Neuropathies

Compressive neuropathies are a heterogeneous group of conditions that stem from nerve ischemia. The precipitating factor leading to this ischemic phenomenon is mechanical entrapment of a nerve due to various anatomical, developmental, or metabolic abnormalities. Other factors such as compartment syndromes, tumor or bony spur formation, infections, and iatrogenic causes can also be associated with compressive neuropathies. Although many nerve entrapment syndromes have been described, this section focuses on those seen with compression of the median and ulnar nerves. Carpal tunnel syndrome is the most common type of compressive neuropathy. In this condition, the median nerve becomes compressed within the carpal tunnel which is formed by the carpal canal and the overlying transverse carpal ligament. The median nerve travels in the carpal tunnel with the long flexor tendons that are approaching their insertion sites on the thumb and the remaining digits. Carpal tunnel syndrome is thought to occur from the swelling of these tendons (flexor tenosynovitis) within the confined carpal tunnel. This occurrence is often associated with repetitive function occupations (i.e., typists and jack hammer operators), pregnancy, diabetes, thyroid disease, amyloidosis, and alcohol abuse. Diagnosis is confirmed by a classic history (pain, paresthesia, and motor weakness in the area of the hand supplied by the median nerve), atrophy and weakness of the thenar (thumb) eminence, Tinel's and/or Phalen's sign, or an electromyogram/nerve conduction velocity (EMG/NCV) test. The ulnar nerve most often becomes entrapped at either the elbow (cubital tunnel) or the wrist (ulnar tunnel). Compression at these two sites often results from repetitive trauma, previous fractures, vascular abnormalities, or neighboring growths. Lipomas (fat) and ganglion cysts are more likely associated with ulnar tunnel syndrome from compression of the ulnar nerve while in Guyon's canal. The symptoms resulting from entrapment of the ulnar nerve at either site include pain and parathesias at the compression site or in the area of the hand represented by the nerve's sensory distribution. Wasting of muscle and motor weakness in the hypothenar group may also be noted. Diagnosis for ulnar nerve compression is once again by history, physical examination, and possibly with the aid of an EMG/NCV test. Treatment options for these entrapment neuropathies include splinting, activity modification, and surgical release or transposition of the nerve.

Polymyositis

Polymyositis is an inflammatory condition of muscles resulting in tenderness and induration. This condition is usually seen in adult females who complain of muscle aches without any history of recent trauma or febrile illness. Patients with polymyositis can develop photosensitivity. Laboratory results demonstrate elevated levels of C-reactive protein, ESR, and CPK. Tissue biopsy reveals a predominance of inflammatory cells that is pathognomonic for polymyositis. Treatment of this condition may require systemic corticosteroids.

Dupuytren's Disease

Dupuytren's contracture of the hand is a locally aggressive proliferative dysplasia of connective tissue in the palm of the hand. It is similar to the plantar fibromatosis found in the foot known as "Ledderhosen's disease." The exact etiology for either entity is unknown. Dupuytren's contractures in association with seizure disorders, diabetes, smoking, alcohol use, and a genetic predisposition have been described. The clinical picture of both Dupuytren's and Ledderhosen's disease features progressive

areas of focal nodularity with cords of thickened tissue and contractures. Dupuytren's contractures may occur as a separate disorder or in tandem with fibromatosis of the feet or the penis (Peyronie's disease). Treatment options include stretching, physical therapy, or a subtotal surgical resection of the involved tissue. Neurovascular compromise may occur with operative intervention. Recurrence in this condition is not uncommon after surgical resection.

Special Situations

Hand Infections

S. aureus is the usual infectious agent in hand infections. Some infections, do however, consist of anaerobic or polymicrobial organisms. Infections around the nail bed (i.e., paronychia/eponychia) are the most common types of hand infections. Deep space infections typically occur in the immunocompromised (i.e., AIDS, diabetes) patients. "Infectious flexor tenosynovitis" refers to the presence of suppurative fluid in the flexor tendon sheath. Patients with this condition present with the affected digit held in a flexed position and complain of severe pain from passive extension by the examiner. Surgical irrigation and debridement with intravenous antibiotics is the mainstay of treatment. Human bites most often reveal S. aureus as the offending organism, but potential Eikenella corrodens infection should be treated empirically with penicillin or amoxicillin. Pasteurella multocida must also be considered in hand infections from cat and dog bites. Pasteurella is also sensitive to ampicillin or amoxicillin.

Reimplantation Surgery

Reimplantation surgery for traumatic amputations can only be undertaken if the severed extremity has not been mangled or severely crushed. Other factors such as patient age, body part severed, overall patient condition, ischemic-time duration, and mechanism of injury must be carefully considered before reimplantation begins. Certain areas of the hand and specific injury types respond poorly to reattachment attempts and are routinely found to be unsalvageable. An example is severe ring avulsion injuries occurring between the metacarpal necks and the base of the middle phalanges in digits 2 through 5. The amputated segment and the residual limb must first undergo debridement followed by reassessment for replantation potential. Once reimplantation is chosen, realignment and stabilization of the bone followed by the repair of extensor and flexor tendons are performed. After completion of the bone and tendon procedures, sequential repair of the artery, nerve, and vein are then performed. The best results of success following replantation surgery are generally seen in children.

Compartment syndrome

A compartment syndrome is defined as an elevated pressure within a confined soft tissue space that can compromise neurovascular integrity of structures and muscles in that space. Compartment syndrome may be a complication of burns, fractures, arterial injuries, blunt or penetrating trauma, and intravenous fluid extravasation. Physical examination reveals a swollen extremity. Paresthesias, pain, and paresis are early signs of decreased circulatory perfusion of an extremity. A common misconception among clinicians is the notion that presence of a palpable pulse excludes compartment syndrome. On the contrary, the presence of a palpable pulse signifies only that the compartment pressure has not risen above systolic blood pressure but is high enough to obliterate capillary blood flow and cause cellular ischemia at the muscular and neuronal level. Compartment pressures can be measured using various methods and normally do not exceed 30 to 40 mm Hg or come within 20 to 30 mm Hg of the patient's diastolic blood pressure. The treatment of choice for a compartment syndrome is an emergent fasciotomy. When performed within 4 to 6 hr from the onset of symptoms, reperfusion of the limb and favorable results are expected. Clinical diagnosis should not await the presence of symptoms, and efforts should always focus on early surgical intervention.

Adult Fractures

The treatment of fractures in skeletally mature patients (adult) differs from that in the skeletally immature (pediatric) patients because the growth plates are closed. Detailed information regarding the mechanism of injury can often determine the type of fracture sustained (i.e., open versus closed) as well as the energy intensity absorbed during the injury. Fracture management is dictated by the mechanism of injury as well as location and severity of the fracture. Other important factors include any preexisting medical condition and associated injuries incurred by the patient.

Management Principles

The hallmark of initial orthopedic intervention after assessment includes fracture reduction, immobilization, and elevation (at or slightly above heart level). In addition, early intermittent icing is recommended to prevent excessive swelling. Finally, the neurovascular integrity of the distal extremity must be assessed frequently after the reduction and immobilization have been performed.

The decision to utilize intramedullary nailing, internal fixation, external fixation, percutaneous pinning, or casting depends on multiple factors. Specifically, the management of orthopedic injuries in trauma patients must follow the strict rules set forth in the ATLS guidelines. A patent airway, reestablishment or maintenance of pulmonary function, and provision of hemodynamic stability must all be achieved before orthopedic intervention is initiated. Open fractures, spinal cord injuries, joint dislocations, traumatic amputations, impending or established compartment syndromes, and unstable pelvic fractures are orthopedic emergencies and should be treated accordingly.

Closed fractures are treated by urgent closed reduction or open reduction and internal fixation (ORIF). In certain situations, prolonged traction may be indicated, e.g., multiple trauma patient who is clinically unstable. Open fractures are defined as fractures that occur with a concomitant communication between the fracture site and the outside environment. Open fractures must undergo irrigation and debridement (ideally within 4 to 8 hr), reduction, and stabilization. Postoperative wound management is of critical importance. Generally, 48 to 72 hr of broad spectrum intravenous antibiotics are administered. An additional 48 to 72 hr of intravenous antibiotics is needed following each subsequent irrigation and debridement procedure. Intraoperative cultures may be obtained after the completion of the irrigation and debridement process, but their usefulness in fracture and wound management has been disputed.

Upper Extremity Fractures

Fractures that occur at the distal diaphyseal-metaphyseal junction of the radius with dorsal angulation of the distal segment is known as a "Colles fracture" (Fig. 4). Typical presentation is a swollen, painful wrist that has developed from a fall onto an extended upper extremity. This fracture can often be treated by cast or brace management if reduction can be adequately maintained with these devices. Colles fractures that are highly comminuted, unstable, or have a significant intraarticular component are best treated with ORIF, with or without external fixation. Isolated ulnar and humeral shaft fractures are usually managed with a fracture brace. Fractures affecting both the radial and the ulnar shafts of the same extrem-

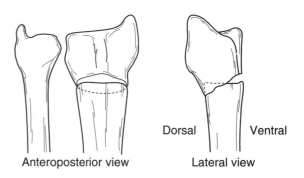

Anteroposterior view Dorsal | Ventral Lateral view

FIG. 4. Colles fracture.

ity are historically unstable and are usually treated with ORIF. Most clavicle, scapula and proximal humerus fractures can be managed with immobilization and careful, periodic observation alone. Clavicle and scapula fractures in trauma patients imply a significant energy absorbed by the body. Associated thoracic and abdominal injuries may be present. A sling may be worn briefly by patients with these injuries. A warning should be given to these patients regarding progressive shoulder stiffness with prolonged sling use.

Lower Extremity Fractures and Pelvic Fractures

Fractures of the femoral head or neck that occur in patients under the age of ~55 years are considered surgical emergencies. These injuries are best treated within 4 to 6 hr to avoid avascular necrosis of the femoral head secondary to compromise of its blood supply. Fractures of long bones, particularly the shaft of the femur predispose these patients to a myriad of complications including deep venous thrombosis and fat embolization. The hallmark of fat embolization is hypoxemia without evidence of pulmonary or chest injury and petechiae about the conjunctiva, axilla, and chest wall. Supportive care is usually sufficient treatment for fat embolization. Most contemporary orthopedic surgeons favor early intramedullary nailing of femoral and high-energy tibial shaft fractures to permit early ambulation and remove the imposed risks that predispose to pulmonary complications. Fibular shaft fractures, when occurring as an isolated injury, require no internal or external fixation. Fractures that occur in or around joints such as the ankle and knee typically require some form of ORIF.

Pelvic fractures are a tremendous cause of patient morbidity and mortality in the trauma patient. Open pelvic fractures imply associated break in the skin or epithelium about the pelvis, e.g., perineum and vagina. General orthopedic management principles are combined with a diverting colostomy to prevent continuous soilage of the fracture wound. Unstable pelvic fractures are those that exhibit at least two fractures of the pelvic ring. An open book is an example of an unstable fracture. Up to 4 L of blood can be contained within the pelvis in the presence of pubic symphyseal diastasis of >4.0 cm. The management of acute, unstable pelvic fractures may require the emergent application of an external pelvic fixator to prevent exsanguination into the pelvis. Infrequently, patients with persistent hemodynamic instability with evidence of active bleeding but minimal pubic diastasis may benefit from angiographic diagnosis of pelvic arterial bleeding and undergo selective embolization for control of hemorrhage. Elective ORIF of pelvic and acetabular fractures is often performed for various fracture patterns and joint incongruencies.

Spinal Cord Injuries

Injuries of the spinal cord in the adult age group typically occur as a result of blunt trauma. As a general rule, fractures of the spinal column rarely involve just a single vertebral segment. Radiographs of the entire spine are usually obtained once a fracture or dislocation has been detected at any spinal column level.

Cervical spine fractures are the most frequently missed injuries in the mentally impaired or uncooperative patient. The altered mentation of these patients may be due to head or body trauma, alcohol intoxication, substance abuse, or psychogenic shock. The immediate placement of cervical collar and patient immobilization on backboards by the rescue personnel have helped to diminish the unfortunate sequela of unrecognized spinal cord injuries. A thorough history must be obtained from all trauma patients, rescuers, and eye witnesses at the scene of the injury. Once the patient has been delivered to the trauma center, a careful inspection of the face, thorax, and abdomen must be undertaken to assess the probability of a concomitant spinal injury. A physical examination of trauma patients is considered incomplete without determining the neurological status of the patient. Severe facial trauma should alert the examiner as to the high probability of cervical spine involvement. Seatbelt marks found on restrained backseat passengers should raise suspicion of lower thoracic or upper lumbar spinal column (distraction) injuries. Burn marks seen on patients caused by the use of shoulder belts implies underlying rib, spleen, and thoracic spine injuries. Patients who sustain calcaneal fractures after falling or jumping from great heights have associated compression fractures of the lumbar spine in ~10% of cases.

Traumatic spine injuries may lead to spinal shock, which usually resolves spontaneously in 72 hr. More severe spine injuries may result in complete or incomplete loss of spinal cord function at or below the level of the injury. Several forms of incomplete spinal cord syndromes have been described. Central cord syndrome, the most common type of all incomplete cord injuries, represents an insult to the central cord gray matter. Patients with this syndrome have more motor and sensory loss in their upper extremities as compared to their lower extremities. The prognosis for recovery in these patients is considered fair. Anterior cord syndrome, the second most common type of incomplete injury, results from compromise of the anterior two-thirds of the cord with sparing of the dorsal columns-medical lemniscus tract. These patients demonstrate a greater loss of lower than upper extremity function. The prognosis for recovery with this syndrome is poor. The last type of incomplete cord injury in this discussion will be the Brown-Sequard hemisection syndrome. As the name implies, 50% of the cord is involved, resulting in loss of ipsilateral proprioception, motor, and two-point touch while causing a contralateral loss of pain, temperature, and crude touch. The prognosis for this injury is the best of all incomplete cord lesions. Treatment of spinal column and cord injuries includes the use of cervical collars, halo vests, skeletal traction, and surgery where indicated.

SUMMARY

Evaluation of patients with orthopedic disease requires careful investigation into associated medical disorders and previous orthopedic conditions. Age can be helpful in arriving at a diagnosis. Regarding traumatic musculoskeletal injuries, the mechanism of injury is an essential detail that must be obtained as part of the initial assessment. Management of orthopedic injuries involves reduction, immobilization, and elevation. Clinicians must evaluate for frequently associated injuries that may take precedence over orthopedic injuries. Nevertheless, the complications of untreated orthopedic injuries such as deep venous thrombosis, fat emboli, and compartment syndrome must be prevented by prioritizing all traumatic injuries and treating in a timely and efficient manner.

STUDY QUESTIONS

1. What is the pathophysiology behind compartment syndrome?
2. What is the first symptom of impending compartment syndrome?
3. What are the principles of managing orthopedic injuries?
4. Describe fat emboli syndrome.
5. What is the pathogenesis of carpal tunnel syndrome?

SUGGESTED READING

Miller MD, ed. *Review of orthopaedics.* 1st ed. Philadelphia: Saunders, 1992.

Morrissy RT, ed. *Lovell and Winter's pediatric orthopaedics.* 3rd ed. Philadelphia: Lippincott, 1990.

Rockwood CA Jr, Green DP, eds. *Fractures in adults.* 3rd ed. Philadelphia: Lippincott, 1991.

Rockwood CA Jr, Wilkins KE, King RE, eds. *Fractures in children.* 3rd ed. Philadelphia: Lippincott, 1991.

CHAPTER 27

Organ Transplantation

Willem Van der Werf and Joshua Miller

The techniques for vascular anastomosis developed by Alexis Carrel in 1903 made solid organ transplantation possible. The first kidney transplant was performed in Boston in 1954 by Joseph Murray at the Brigham Hospital between identical twin brothers. This was the beginning of the evolution of transplantation. Today, >10,000 kidney and 1,000 liver transplants are performed each year in the United States. Clearly, however, the demand for organ transplantation far exceeds the donor organ supply. Advancements in immunosuppression marked by the use of steroids and azathioprine (Imuran) in the 1960s and 1970s, cyclosporin in the 1980s, and many new drugs in the 1990s, including FK506 (Prograf) and RS 61443 (Cellcept), have allowed better organ survival while decreasing the side effects of immunosuppression, such as infection and the degenerative effects of high-dose steroids.

IMMUNOLOGY OF TRANSPLANTATION

The immunologic response following organ transplantation is based on the genetic relationship between the donor and the recipient. Transplants are classified by this genetic relationship and the location in the body into which the organ is transplanted. An orthotopic transplant is placed into the normal anatomic position such as in a heart transplant and in most liver transplants. A heterotopic transplant is placed into a different anatomic position such as in kidney transplants that are anastomosed to the iliac vessels in the pelvis. An autograft is tissue transferred from the normal location to a heterotopic location in the same patient, such as a parathyroid gland transplanted to the sternomastoid muscle or a skin graft from a normal donor site. An isograft or syngeneic graft is transplanted between identical twins or between highly inbred (genetically identical) rodents. An allograft is transplanted between individuals of the same species who are not genetically identical. A xenograft is transplanted between individuals of different species such as a baboon liver transplanted to a human recipient. In addition, xenografts can be further classified depending on the presence of preformed natural antibodies. A discordant xenograft, such as a pig to human liver transplant, is usually rejected within several hours, primarily mediated by preformed or natural antibodies. Concordant xenografts are phylogenetically closer, such as baboon to human, and preformed antibodies do not exist, resulting in prolonged graft survival.

The rejection response begins when the recipient is exposed to the foreign antigens of the transplanted tissue. It is considered biologically inevitable in the absence of modulating therapy or immunologic interventions. The antigens involved are called "histocompatibility antigens" and determine the pace of the rejection. Alloantigens in humans are proteins that are coded by genes located on several chromosomes. A group of histocompatibility antigens that are most important in transplantation are the expression of a single chromosomal region called the "major histocompatibility complex" (MHC) located on chromosome 6. In humans, the MHC products are called "human leukocyte antigens" (HLA), because they were first studied on leukocytes. The HLA antigens in humans are further classified into class I and class II antigens. In general, class II antigens can trigger a strong allogeneic lymphocyte response involving proliferating T helper cells, whereas class I antigens are the targets of T cytotoxic cell functions. The class I antigens are coded by those regions of the MHC called "HLA-A," "HLA-B," and "HLA-C." These antigens are, in general, expressed on all nucleated cells. The class II antigens are expressions of the MHC genes located in the HLA-D (HLA-DR, HLA-DP, and HLA-DQ) region of the MHC. They are expressed on B lymphocytes, activated T-cells, certain endothelial cells, dendritic cells, and monocytes (macrophages). The expression of class I and II MHC antigens can be upregulated by a variety of pathophysiologic conditions involving cytokines (including graft rejection) such that they can be detected on virtually all types of cells. The MHC genes and their proteins are linked to many diseases involving the immune system. There are many more histocompatibility antigens that have not been clearly identified in the human, including even histocompatibility antigens associated with a gene on the Y chromosome, which for now are called "minor histocompatibility antigens." The identification of the HLA antigens by seroloical and newer DNA technology has allowed the matching of donor and recipient. A perfect match occurs when all detectable HLA antigens are identical between donor and recipient, a rare event. Obviously, only identical twins would be truly a perfect match for all of the human histocompatibility antigens.

Upon recognition of the alloantigen, the recipient will mount an immunologic response. The alloantigen is first processed by a type of macrophage, the antigen-presenting cell (APC), which presents the antigen on its surface in association with self class II antigens that are important for T-cell recognition (indirect method of recognition). A unique feature of alloimmunity is that T-cells of the recipient can recognize antigen in association with donor class II antigen on the donor APC (direct method of recognition). The binding between the T-cell and the APC leads to activation and release of interleukin-1 (IL-1) by the APC and interleukin-2 (IL-2) by the T-cell.

Release of these cytokines causes amplification of the immune response by activating and recruiting other T-cells, as well as B-cells. The type of T-cell involved in recognition of the alloantigen is the CD^{4+} helper T-cell. By releasing the powerful cytokine, IL-2, the CD^{4+} helper T-cell is able to activate CD^{8+} cytotoxic T-cells, which recognize class I antigens on the donor endothelial cells and cause cell destruction and rejection. Cyclosporine is one immunosuppressive agent that prevents activation of the CD^{4+} helper T-cell and thus prevents production of IL-2.

CLINICAL IMMUNOSUPPRESSION

As mentioned, the first kidney transplant was performed between identical twins in 1954 by Joseph Murray at the Peter Brent Brigham hospital in Boston. In 1962, Murray and Hume performed the first kidney transplant from a cadaver donor using Imuran and corticosteroids for immunosuppression. The success of cadaver and living related transplants has required strategies to prevent the immune system from rejecting the transplanted organs while still maintaining the ability to fight off infections. Common infections related to immunosuppression are considered opportunistic and include cytomegalovirus,

TABLE 1. *Immunosuppressive techniques*

	Mechanism	Major side effects	When used	Miscellaneous
Steroids	Lympholytic and inhibits interleukin-1 release from macrophages	Gastritis, bone symptoms, cataracts, acne, Cushing's syndrome, diabetes	Baseline immuno-suppression and rejection	—
Azathioprine (Imuran)	An antimetabolite that inhibits nucleic acid synthesis and thus nonspecifically affects all dividing cells	Bone marrow depression (decreased white cell, red cell, and platelet count)	Baseline immuno-suppression	Check white blood celll count
Cyclosporine (Sandimmune or neoral)	Blocks secretion of interleukin-2 by T-helper (CD4+) cells	Nephrotoxicity, hypertension, hyperkalemia, hirsutism, hepatotoxicity, diabetes	Baseline immuno-suppression	Check levels frequently
FK-506 (Tacrolimus or Prograf)	Similar to cyclosporine but at least 10-fold more potent	Nephrotoxicity, hypertension, diabetes, allopecia, GI symptoms	Baseline immuno-suppression	—
RS 61443 (Mycophenolate mofetyl or Cellcept)	An antimetabolite more specific than Imuran effecting the de novo pathway of purine nucleic acid synthesis	Bone marrow depression, GI symptoms	Baseline immuno-suppression	—
ALG or ATG	Polyclonal antilymphocyte or antithymocyte immunoglobulins prepared by immunizing an animal against human lymphocytes or thmocytes	—	Induction immediately after transplantation or rejection	—
OKT3	A monoclonal antibody directed against the CD3+ receptor on T-cells	—	Induction or rejection	—

herpes viruses, candida, Pneumocystis carinii and a variety of other fungi, and parasitic and bacterial organisms not normally considered pathogens. In addition, immunosuppression is associated with an increased incidence of certain malignancies, such as lymphomas and skin cancers. There are a variety of protocols for immunosuppression. The mechanisms of action and side effects of these agents should be clear (Table 1). Since all the immunosuppressive agents have side effects, they are used in combinations in an attempt to reduce the dose of each so as to minimize respective specific toxicities. Antilymphocyte globulin (ALG) and OKT3 are commonly used for induction immediately after transplantation in a self-limited therapeutic course as well as in similar interval courses to treat rejection episodes. A combination of methylprednisolone, azathioprine (Imuran), cyclosporin A (Neoral), and FK-506 (Prograf) are commonly used for maintenance therapy. Intravenous or high-dose oral steroids are also frequently effective in treating rejection episodes.

ORGAN DONATION AND PRESERVATION

Transplanted organs come from either cadaver donors or living related donors. Living related donations are possible for kidney, bone marrow, segmental pancreas, segmental liver, and even single lung transplants. A suitable cadaver donor must be pronounced brain dead prior to retrieval of the organs. Donors have usually sustained irreversible brain injury from trauma, brain tumors, anoxic injury, or cerebrovascular accidents. Contraindications to donation include preexisting localized conditions effecting the function of the organ, such as cirrhosis, pulmonary disease, or long-standing diabetes, and systemic conditions such as malignancy other than primary brain tumors, prolonged warm ischemia from cardiac arrest or hypotensive episodes, presence of antibodies against human immunodeficiency virus (HIV), viral hepatitis, or other ongoing systemic infection. The criteria for brain death are listed in Table 2. Once the criteria for brain

TABLE 2. *Criteria for brain death*

Prerequisite
  All appropriate diagnostic and therapeutic procedures have been performed, and the patient's condition is irreversible.
Criteria (to be present for 30 min at least 6 hr after the onset of coma and apnea)
  Coma
  Apnea (no spontaneous respirations)
  Absent cephalic reflexes (pupillary, corneal, oculoauditory, oculovestibular, oculocephalic, cough, pharyngeal, and swallowing)
  No electrical activity on electroencephalogram
Confirmatory test
  Absence of cerebral blood flow by radionuclide brain scan

TABLE 3. *Useful preservation durations*

Organ	Limits of preservation time
Kidney	72 hr
Liver	24 hr
Pancreas	24 hr
Heart	6 hr
Heart-lung	6 hr
Lung	6 hr
Eyes (cornea)	Several months
Skin	Indefinite
Bone	Indefinite

death are established, consent for organ donation is obtained through a previously signed donor card, drivers license, or a will, accompanied by permission from the family or legal guardian.

The solid organs commonly retrieved from the cadaver for transplantation include the heart, lungs, kidneys, liver, and pancreas. Intestinal transplants are now also occasionally being performed for a variety of conditions on very sick patients in conjunction with liver transplantation. Once these organs are removed, they are preserved to allow time for tissue typing and cross-matching (frequently performed before organ retrieval), selection and preparation of the recipient, and transport of the organ to the recipient. Hypothermia, which slows metabolic activity and decreases oxygen demand, can be achieved by perfusing the organ with a cold hyperosmotic hyperkalemic preservation solution, the UW solution developed at the University of Wisconsin, or Collins solution. The organs are either packed on ice or connected to a pulsatile perfusion machine (kidney only). The useful preservation times are listed in Table 3.

KIDNEY TRANSPLANTATION

Most patients with end-stage renal disease have had a period of dialysis prior to renal transplantation, but more transplants are being performed preemptively before dialysis is instituted. There are two methods of dialysis: hemodialysis and peritoneal dialysis. In hemodialysis, blood passes through semipermeable tubes, removing the toxic substances and restoring electrolyte, fluid, and acid-base balance. Hemodialysis requires vascular access that will deliver large amounts of blood to the dialysis machine. In the acute situation, a double lumen dialysis catheter (Udall) is inserted into the central venous system via the internal jugular or subclavian vein. For chronic dialysis, a subcutaneous arteriovenous (Brescia-Cimino) fistula, usually between the radial artery and the cephalic vein at the wrist, is preferred, but polytetraflouroethylene (PTFE) arteriovenous grafts (Gortex or Impra) in the upper or even the lower extremity can be used to establish

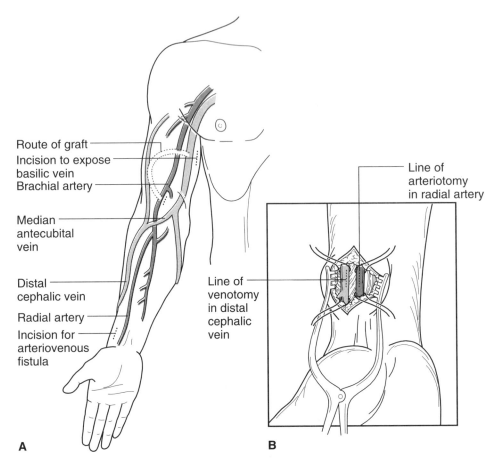

FIG. 1. AV fistula and graft. **(A)** Arteriovenous graft construction using artificial conduit. **(B)** Exposure of radial aspect of forearm for construction of Brescia-Cimino arteriovenous fistula between the radial artery and cephalic vein.

Labels in figure: Route of graft; Incision to expose basilic vein; Brachial artery; Median antecubital vein; Distal cephalic vein; Radial artery; Incision for arteriovenous fistula; Line of venotomy in distal cephalic vein; Line of arteriotomy in radial artery; A; B

high blood flow (Fig. 1). Peritoneal dialysis uses the peritoneum as the filtering membrane and involves placement of a CAPD (continuous ambulatory peritoneal dialysis) catheter transabdominally. Large amounts of dialysate are infused, allowed to equilibrate, and then drained. Complications of access grafts or peritoneal catheters include infection or thrombosis of grafts and catheters and graft aneurysms.

Although dialysis provides life-sustaining treatment, the need to go to the dialysis center two to three times per week for 3 to 5 hr prevents the patient from leading a normal life. Kidney transplantation offers the patient with end-stage renal disease the best chance for optimal medical, psychological, social, and vocational rehabilitation, and in the patient younger than 45 years is associated with a greater life expectancy than chronic dialysis. Most patients believe the freedom from dialysis is worth the risk of major surgery and lifelong immunosuppression.

The technique of living related donor nephrectomy involves a flank incision and retroperitoneal approach. The peritoneum is retracted, a long segment of ureter is

dissected down from the kidney with its blood supply intact and transected. The renal vein is isolated, which on the left involves ligating the lumbar, ovarian or testicular, and adrenal venous branches. The renal artery is isolated and then the artery and vein are transected close to the vena cava and aorta. Major complications are rare and life expectancy of the living related donor is not altered. The cadaver donor nephrectomy is usually done in conjunction with the retrieval of the liver, pancreas, and heart.

Nephrectomy of the recipient's diseased native kidneys may be indicated to control hypertension, prevent proteinuria in the nephrotic syndrome, and to eliminate a source of infection, hemorrhage, or even malignancy. Nephrectomy is usually performed at least several weeks prior to the transplant, but in children can be frequently done simultaneously with the transplant.

The recipient operation begins with dissection of the iliac vessels via a retroperitoneal approach through a lower quadrant oblique incision. The renal vein of the renal transplant is anastomosed end to side to the iliac

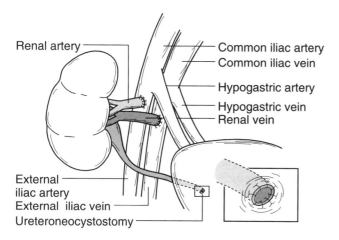

FIG. 2. Kidney transplant.

TABLE 4. *Complications of renal transplants*

Early
  Hemorrhage
  Lymphocele
  Acute rejection
  Thrombosis
  Ureter anastomotic leak
  Infection
  Acid pepcid disease
  Impaired wound healing
Late
  Chronic rejection
  Infection
    Bacterial
    Fungal
    Viral
  Ureteral obstruction
  Anastomotic stenosis
  Diabetes
  Avascular necrosis of the long bones
  Cushing's syndrome
  Cataracts
  Pancreatitis
  Cancer

vein, and the renal artery is anastomosed end to side to the external or common iliac artery or occasionally end to end to the internal iliac artery (Fig. 2). In small children, the aorta and vena cava are used in the anastomosis. The ureter is connected to the bladder by either an extravesical Liche ureterovesicostomy, in which the connection is made from the outside of the bladder, or the intravesical Leadbetter-Politano ureterovesicostomy.

The early postoperative management of the renal transplant patient involves optimizing renal perfusion, correcting electrolyte abnormalities, and immunosuppression. Urine output is measured hourly and can be replaced with one-half normal saline with 5% dextrose, and the patient frequently requires potassium and calcium replacement. Diabetic patients are maintained on glucose and insulin drips to control their blood sugar. Although there is much variation in management, most transplant centers use cyclosporine, azathioprine (Imuran), and methylprednisolone for immunosuppression. Additional immunosuppressive agents routinely used at some centers and becoming more popular include FK506 (Prograf) and RS 61443 (Cellcept). ALG and OKT3 usage is more variable.

A number of possible complications may occur in the renal transplant patient. Kidney loss may be the result of ischemia, acute or chronic rejection, technical malfunction, or recurrent renal disease. Frequent measurements of blood urea nitrogen and creatinine, sonograms, nuclear renal scans, and renal biopsy help differentiate the etiologies of graft failure. Table 4 lists several of the complications.

Although renal transplants are associated with many possible complications, the rate of permanent disabilities is low and the 1-year graft survival ranges from 75% to 85% for cadaveric grafts and 85% to 95% for living related grafts. With improved immunosuppressive agents, these results should improve in the future.

PANCREAS TRANSPLANTATION

In 1966 Kelly and Lillehei performed the first whole pancreas transplant, bringing the possibility of glucose homeostasis to all type I diabetics with the hope of preventing the secondary effects of diabetes such as blindness, renal disease, peripheral vascular disease, and coronary artery disease. Most pancreas transplants are performed in conjunction with a renal transplant; however, isolated pancreas transplants are done at a number of transplant centers and are becoming more common as the results improve. The donor pancreas is retrieved with its blood supply from the splenic and superior mesenteric arteries, and its venous drainage via the portal vein. Anastomosis is to the iliac vessels in the recipient. The pancreatic duct drains either enterically via a segment of donor duodenum that is left intact and connected to a Roux-en-Y limb of recipient jejunum or anastomosed to the bladder via a duodeno-cystostomy. The latter is more commonly performed (Fig. 3) because the urine amylase can be measured and a decrease is considered an early indicator of rejection. Pancreas transplants allow the diabetic patient to live without insulin injections and free from diet restrictions. Currently, the grafts have an ~70% to 80% 1-year survival. Rejection, arterial thrombosis, infection, and autolysis by pancreatic enzymes still prevent the widespread application of pancreas transplants to the early diabetics. A different approach is to transplant only the insulin-producing cells, islet cell transplantation. The islet cells are isolated from the exocrine portion of the pancreas and injected into the portal vein to be lodged within the liver. There have been isolated reports of success.

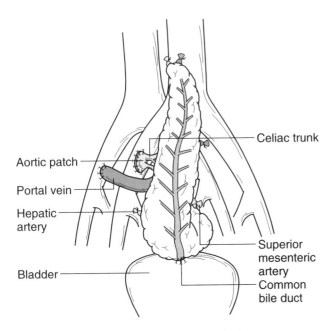

FIG. 3. Pancreas transplant.

TABLE 5. *Indications for liver transplant*

Adult
  Chronic active hepatitis
  Acute hepatitis B
  Biliary cirrhosis
  Laënnec's cirrhosis
  Sclerosing cholangitis
  α_1-antitrypsin deficiency
  Hemachromatosis
  Budd-Chiari syndrome
  Acute yellow atrophy
  Hepatocellular carcinoma
Children
  Biliary atresia
  Biliary cirrhosis
  Chronic active hepatitis
  Neonatal hepatitis
  Congenital metabolic disorders

LIVER TRANSPLANTATION

Human liver transplantation has been virtually made a therapeutic reality through the tireless innovative work of Thomas Starzl starting in 1968. However, the cyclosporine era in the early 1980s made the procedure a practice that could be applied in many transplant centers. Liver transplants involve using a whole liver from a cadaver or segmental liver from a living related or cadaver donor. The graft is usually placed in the normal anatomic (orthotopic) position, although the liver transplant can also be placed in a heterotopic position as an auxiliary transplant. In general, patients are candidates for liver transplantation if they have end-stage liver failure, as defined by a life expectancy of <1 year. There are a number of diseases that cause liver failure for which transplant is performed (Table 5). The most common causes are chronic active viral hepatitis progressing to cirrhosis, biliary cirrhosis, and sclerosing cholangitis in adults and biliary atresia in children.

Starting with the recipient hepatectomy, there are technically challenging aspects to the liver transplant since extensive blood loss may be encountered because of venous collaterals from the patient's portal hypertension and scars from previous operations. Via a bilateral subcostal incision, the liver is mobilized, and the suprahepatic and infrahepatic vena cava, the portal vein, hepatic artery, and bile duct are temporarily occluded. The liver is removed. Many surgeons utilize temporary shunts during the anhepatic phase from the portal vein and inferior vena cava to the superior vena cava in order to prevent splanchnic or renal congestion. The liver graft is then anastomosed to the vena cava, the portal vein, the hepatic artery, and common bile duct or Roux-en-Y jejunal limb (Fig. 4). In children, the bile ducts are frequently too small to be directly connected to the recipient ducts and are thus drained into the jejunum via a Roux-en-Y choledochojejunostomy. In small children, reduced liver grafts are used when the size discrepancy is too large. Liver segments can be removed with the vascular and biliary supply intact from either a cadaver or living related donor and transplanted in a similar fashion.

Complications involve hemorrhage, vascular thrombosis, rejection, biliary leaks or strictures, coagulopathy, infection, and failure of the renal, respiratory, and cardiovascular systems. Immunosuppressive drug therapy is similar to that for renal transplants. The liver appears to be better tolerated than the kidneys from an immunologic viewpoint. The overall 1-year graft and patient survival are 75% to 85%, depending on patient selection.

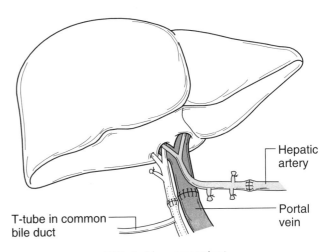

FIG. 4. Liver transplant.

CARDIAC AND PULMONARY TRANSPLANTATION

The first human heart transplant was performed by Christiaan Barnard in 1967 in South Africa but was popularized by Shumway and colleagues at Stanford University. The acceptance of cyclosporine in 1982 led to improved success and rapid growth of cardiac transplantation. The most common indications for heart transplantation are ischemic, viral, alcoholic, and postpartum cardiomyopathies. Patients are selected if they are predicted to survive <1 year and there is no alternative therapy. The donor operation is performed in conjunction with the liver and kidney teams, while a second team is preparing the recipient for transplant. The heart is removed by dividing the superior and inferior vena cava, the pulmonary veins, and proximal aorta. The recipient cardiectomy is performed in a similar fashion leaving posterior portions of both atria intact, which are then sutured to the donor left and right atrium followed by the aortic and pulmonary artery anastomosis. Immunosuppression is similar to renal and liver transplants with protocols varying at each transplant center. Rejection is monitored by routinely performing weekly endomyocardial biopsies in the first month, then periodic biopsies thereafter. Rejection episodes are treated with pulsed steroids or OKT3 for rejection resistant to steroids. The 1-year survival is ~80%.

Heart-lung, single lung, or double lung transplants have been performed successfully in patients with end-stage pulmonary failure since the 1970s. A variety of techniques have been developed over the years to prevent the breakdown of the poorly perfused bronchial anastomosis. Immunosuppression is similar except that steroids are reduced to help the bronchial anastomosis heal. Results have improved over the past 10 years to the point of routine clinical acceptance.

SMALL BOWEL TRANSPLANTATION

Intestinal transplants have been developmental in life-saving therapy for shortgut syndromes and have now approached clinical usage in a few major transplant centers. The procedure was initially developed by Toto and Tzakis at the University of Pittsburgh in the late 1980s and is utilized ~50% of the time with a concurrent liver transplant because of coexisting liver failure due to long-term intravenous hyperalimentation therapy. Immunosuppressive methods involve newer and more potent combination of agents, including Prograf, Cellcept, and even bone marrow infusion from the cadaver organ donor.

SUMMARY

The field of organ transplantation has had a remarkable impact on patient care as we acquire the ability to replace destroyed or nonfunctional organs. The integration of laboratory and clinical research has advanced the understanding of immunology, autoimmunity diseases, human tissue typing, and antibiotic therapy against opportunistic infections. The future of transplantation will involve improved techniques in allotransplantation as well as the exploration of possibilities of xenotransplantation.

STUDY QUESTIONS

1. Define the following terms: orthotopic transplant, heterotopic transplant, autograft, isograft, allograft, discordant xenograft, and concordant xenograft. Give examples for each term.
2. How does the MHC play an important role in transplantation?
3. What is the mechanism of action for each of the following immunosuppressive agents: steroids, azathioprine (Imuran), cylosporin, FK-506 (Prograf), RS 61443 (Cellcept), ALG, and OKT3?
4. Briefly describe the recipient operation for renal, pancreas, and liver transplant.
5. Name at least five diseases for which liver transplantation is often performed.

SUGGESTED READING

Black PM. Brain death. *N Engl J Med* 1978;299:393–412.

Murray JE. Human organ transplantation: background and consequences. *Science* 1992;256:1411–1416.

Starzl TE, Miller C, Broznick B, Makowka L. An improved technique for multiple organ harvesting. *Surg Gynecol Obstet* 1987;165:343–348.

CHAPTER 28

Urology

Henri T. Pham and Mark S. Soloway

The specialty of urology was recognized by Hippocrates, who stated, in the oath for physicians, "I will not cut, even for the stone, but leave such procedures to the practitioners of the craft." Since the time of Hippocrates, the field of urology has expanded tremendously, encompassing such subspecialties as urologic oncology, endourology, male infertility, impotence, neurourology, pediatric urology, female urology, and reconstructive urology. It is not uncommon for a contemporary urologist to be overwhelmed by the diversity of current urologic practice and to seek the assistance of subspecialists. Rather than superficially cover every aspect of urology, this text presents the anatomy, physiology, and pathophysiology pertinent to common urologic disorders.

BASIC ANATOMY AND PHYSIOLOGY

Kidneys

By the 36th week of gestation, the glomeruli are fully developed and the kidneys have ascended to the level of 12th thoracic vertebral body. In adults, the kidney is a retroperitoneal organ weighing ~130 to 150 g. The right kidney is positioned posterior to the liver, the ascending colon, the hepatic flexure of the colon, and the second portion of the duodenum. The left kidney is posterior to the spleen, stomach, distal pancreas, jejunum, splenic flexure of the colon, and the descending colon. The blood supply of the kidneys arises from a single renal artery originating directly from each side of the aorta in 75% of individuals. In the remaining 25%, the arterial blood supply may be from an additional one to three accessory renal arteries. The venous return of the right kidney is to a solitary renal vein leading directly to the inferior vena cava. A solitary left renal vein also serves as a terminus for the venous return of the left adrenal (adrenal vein), the left testis (gonadal vein), and a lumbar vein. Because the left renal vein is directly below the superior mesenteric artery, extrinsic compression of the left renal vein increases the venous pressures of the left gonadal vein. Thus, clinically evident varicoceles (dilated scrotal testicular veins) occur more commonly on the left side. The intrarenal anatomy can be divided into the renal cortex, the renal medulla, and the extraparenchymal collecting system.

The kidneys' main function is excretion of urine. Urine formation can be divided into three distinct processes: filtration, concentration, and secretion. Filtration is the first step in urinary excretion occurring in the renal cortex via the glomeruli. Filtration is affected by renal blood flow, filtration coefficient, and the efferent arteriolar pressure. Urinary concentration occurs in the collecting tubules through water reabsorption down its gradient regulated by antidiuretic hormone. The gradient for passive water reabsorption is established by the loop of Henle countercurrent exchange mechanism. Finally, any metabolites that are not filtered are actively secreted throughout the tubules. In addition to urine production, the kidneys maintain homeostasis of body fluids, electrolytes, and acid-base levels as well as vitamin D metabolism, and renin and erythropoietin secretion. Nearly one-fifth of the total cardiac output is delivered to the kidney to support renal metabolic function.

RENAL PELVIS AND URETER

The renal calyces, pelvis, and the ureter (Fig. 1) function as a conduit for urine to travel from the kidney to the bladder. Urine from the collecting tubules drain into the minor calyces (calyces 8 to 12), which join to form the major calyces. Three major calyces unite at the level of the renal pelvis where the ureter originates. The renal pelvis may be positioned within the renal parenchyma or outside the substance of the kidney, thereby giving it a dilated appearance. In normal kidneys, the cross-section diameter of the renal pelvis is approximately two to four

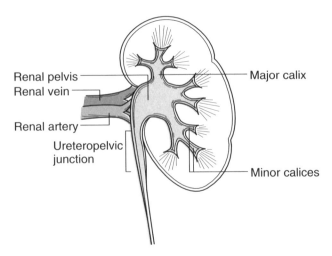

FIG. 1. Renal calices, pelvis, and ureter (posterior view).

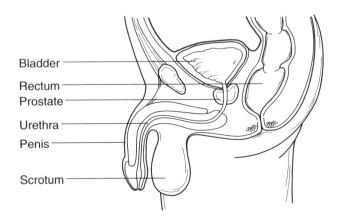

FIG. 2. Relationship of the bladder, prostate, seminal vesicles, penis, urethra, and scrotal contents.

times that of the ureter. The ureter begins at the level of the distal renal pelvis. This junction is a common site of congenital ureteral obstruction and also a frequent site where a urinary calculus may lodge. The proximal and mid ureter courses over the psoas muscle until it enters the true pelvis where it crosses over the common iliac vessels. Beyond the level of the common iliac vessels, the ureter deviates medially until it inserts into the bladder. In the female pelvis, the ureter runs posterior to the uterine artery ("water under the bridge").

Histologically, the ureters and the renal pelvis are very similar, with circular smooth muscle walls lined by transitional epithelium. The arterial blood supply of the renal pelvis and the proximal ureter is derived from the renal artery. The mid ureter is supplied by small vessels directly from the aorta, whereas the distal ureter receives blood from branches of the iliac arteries. Urinary drainage from the kidneys is facilitated by the rhythmic peristalsis of the ureters. The driving force for the sequential contractions arises from the pacemaker cells within the proximal collecting system. Electrical activities from the pacemaker cells are transmitted to the ureteral smooth muscle cells via cell to cell conduction channels (nexuses).

BLADDER

The bladder (Figs. 2 and 3) serves as a low pressure reservoir for urine and has a normal capacity of ~400 cc. The shape of the distended urinary bladder is nearly spherical which aids in low pressure storage of urine. The bladder is the most anterior organ in the pelvis, just adjacent to the symphysis pubis. In males, it is attached to the prostate inferiorly and lies anterior to the rectum. In females, the bladder is anterior to the proximal vagina and uterus. The arterial blood supply of the bladder is from the branches of the hypogastric arteries: the superior, middle, and inferior vesical arteries. Bladder

innervation is from the second, third, and fourth sacral nerve roots. The synergistic activity of the bladder detrussor muscles and the external urinary sphincter is coordinated by the pontine mesencephalic reticular formation. Suprasacral spinal cord injury, which disrupts this communication between the bladder and the sphincter, results in inefficient, high-pressure voiding, which may compromise long-term renal function.

The ureters insert at the distal posterior lateral aspect of the bladder in an area called the trigone. Upon insertion at the bladder, the ureters travel within a submucosal tunnel for a distance of 1 to 2 cm prior to opening into the bladder. This effectively forms a physiologic flap valve mechanism which prevents the reflux of urine from the bladder to the kidney. Children with congenital anomalies affecting this tunnel (shortening) are predisposed to recurrent urinary tract infections (UTIs) and renal deterioration from chronic vesicoureteral reflux.

Histological examination of the urinary bladder wall reveals that it is composed of smooth muscle layers with myofibril fascicles spaced in varying distances, depend-

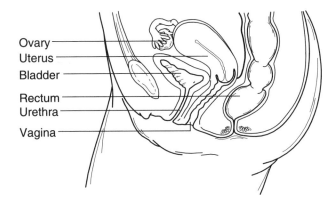

FIG. 3. Relationship of the bladder, urethra, uterus and ovary, vagina, and rectum.

ing on the level of distention. Transitional epithelium lines the bladder lumen. At the area of the trigone and the bladder outlet (bladder neck), striated muscle layers are found and are thought to facilitate urinary continence.

PROSTATE

The prostate (Fig. 2) is an accessory male sex organ with the primary function of enhancing fertility. In the normal young male, the prostate is ~20 g, with the external appearance described as that of a horse chestnut. The prostate surrounds the proximal aspect of the urethra and is contiguous with the bladder (bladder neck). It lies posterior to the symphysis pubis and is anterior to the rectum. The vas deferens enter the prostate at its base at the ampullae of the vas where they are also joined by the seminal vesicles. The ampulla of the vas continue within the substance of the prostate as the ejaculatory ducts where they open into the lumen of the prostatic urethra at the utricle. The intraprostatic anatomy can be divided into four distinct zones as described by McNeal (Fig. 4). The zones of clinical importance are the transition zone and the peripheral zone. Benign prostatic hyperplasia (BPH) is found in the former and cancer is primarily found in the latter. The prostate derives its main blood supply from a branch of the hypogastric artery, the inferior vesical artery. The lymphatic drainage is primarily to the obturator and external iliac chain of lymph nodes. Histologically, the prostatic stroma consists of connective and elastic tissues and smooth muscle fibers in which epithelial glands are embedded. This stroma is covered by a thin fibrous capsule. The secretion of the epithelial glands is via the excretory ducts which open into the ventral prostatic urethra.

Prostatic secretions make up ~30% of the ejaculate volume. Some of the prostatic secretory products include zinc, citrate, spermine, cholesterol/lipids, plasminogen activator, and seminin. These substances assist in sperm protection and transport, and semen liquefaction, all necessary for insemination.

TESTIS AND EPIDIDYMIS

The testis and epididymis (Fig. 5) are closely associated organs responsible for the production and maturation of sperm. The testicle originates as an intraabdominal organ at the fifth week of gestation. Shortly after the fifth week of gestation, the testicles merge with mesonephric tubules that are in close proximity to form the epididymis. By the 32nd week of gestation, the testicles have completed their descent and are intrascrotal organs.

The post pubertal testis measures ~4 × 3 × 2.5 cm. Under its capsule called the tunica albuginea, the testis is a conglomerate of many convoluted seminiferous tubules. The seminiferous tubules consist primarily of Sertoli (supporting) cells and spermatogenic cells. The stroma that surrounds the tubules contains Leydig cells which produce testosterone. The epididymis is composed of very convoluted tubules and is attached to the posterior superior aspect of the testis. The superior aspect of the epididymis (globus major) receives efferent tubules from the testis and the inferior aspect (globus minor) is contiguous with the vas deferens.

Figure 6 depicts the blood supply of the testis, which comes from the testicular (gonadal) artery that arises directly from the aorta bilaterally just inferiorly to the renal artery. The arterial supply of the epididymis is the artery of the vas deferens, which originates from the hypogastric artery. At the level of the internal ring of the inguinal canal, the spermatic artery and the artery of the vas deferens converge. The venous return is via the Pampiniform plexus of

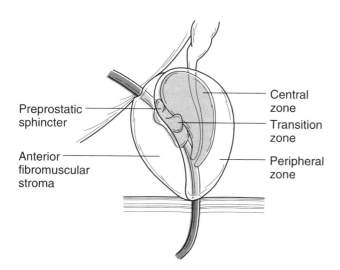

FIG. 4. Anatomy of prostate gland.

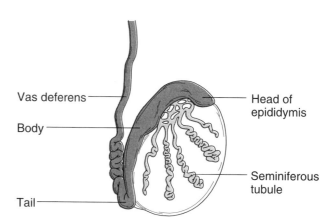

FIG. 5. Anatomic relationship of the testis, epididymis, and vas deferens.

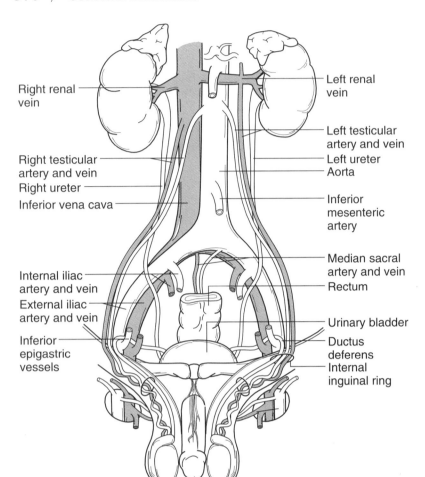

Right renal vein

Left renal vein

Right testicular artery and vein

Left testicular artery and vein

Right ureter

Left ureter

Inferior vena cava

Aorta

Inferior mesenteric artery

Internal iliac artery and vein

Median sacral artery and vein

External iliac artery and vein

Rectum

Inferior epigastric vessels

Urinary bladder

Ductus deferens

Internal inguinal ring

FIG. 6. Overview of the genitourinary anatomy. (Adapted from Gray JW, Skandalakis JE. *Atlas of surgical anatomy for general surgeons.* Baltimore: Williams and Wilkins, 1985.)

the spermatic cord. At the level of the internal ring, the pampiniform plexus forms the gonadal vein. The left gonadal vein drains into the left renal vein while the right gonadal vein empties directly into the vena cava just inferior to the right renal vein.

At puberty, the surge of follicle stimulating hormone (FSH) and testosterone stimulates spermatogenesis to occur in the seminiferous tubule epithelium in the testis. Although sperm is fully matured after a period of 64 days in the testis, they are not functional until they have migrated through the epididymis. Thus, epididymal maturation is an important phase of spermatogenesis and male fertility.

SPERMATIC CORD

The spermatic cord contains the vas deferens, the artery of the vas deferens, the spermatic artery, the pampiniform plexus of veins, lymphatic vessels from the testis, nerve branches from the genitofemoral nerve as well as from the sympathetic hypogastric plexus and the remnant of the processus vaginalis. The spermatic cord forms as the testis makes its descent into the scrotum

from the abdominal cavity. It begins at the level of the internal ring and ends distally where it meets the testis. Occasionally, the processus vaginalis does not close after the descent of the testis. Depending on the extent of closure, this may give rise to either a communicating hydrocele (partially closed) or indirect inguinal hernias (completely open). The spermatic cord is invested within layers of the external spermatic fascia, cremasteric fascia, and internal spermatic fascia.

VAS DEFERENS

The vas deferens serves as a conduit for the transport of sperm. It is a very thick and muscular tubular structure of ~3 mm in diameter lined by columnar epithelium. The vas deferens originates at the distal end of the epididymis and then travels proximally within the spermatic cord. As with the spermatic cord, it enters the inguinal canal via the external ring. As the spermatic cord enters the abdomen at the internal ring, the vas deferens deviates medially and caudally, looping over the origin of the inferior epigastric artery. It travels under the bladder until it opens into the base of the prostate at the ampullae of the vas. At the ampulla, the vas deferens becomes the ejaculatory duct where it converges with the duct of the seminal vesicle and travels within the substance of the prostate until it opens into the prostatic urethra at the utricle.

PENIS

The penis serves as support for the male urethra and is the male copulatory organ. It is made of three main structures: two dorsally located corpora cavernosa and a ventrally positioned corpus spongiosum. The corpora cavernosa consists of highly vascular spongy erectile tissue covered by a double layer of thick fascia known as "Buck's fascia." The two corpora cavernosa deviate laterally at their proximal ends where they are attached to the inferior pubic rami. The corpus spongiosum begins as the glans penis and travels ventrally under the groove created by the paired corpora cavernosa. Proximally, the corpus spongiosum expands and is attached to the fascia of the urogenital diaphragm, the perineal membrane. The urethra travels within the substance of the corpus spongiosum. The arterial supply to the penis is from the paired internal pudendal artery, which is a branch of the hypogastric artery. The venous return is via the superficial and deep dorsal vein of the penis.

Penile tumescence (erection) is dependent upon parasympathetic innervation originating from the pelvic plexus (sacral nerves 2 to 4) traveling via the cavernous nerves dorsolateral to the prostate to reach the penile hilum. With stimulation, the parasympathetic discharge causes relaxation of the smooth musculature of the arterioles of the penis, thereby augmenting blood flow and causing engorgement. At the same time, the small emissary veins of the corpora cavernosa are easily collapsed with early tumescence creating further rigidity. Sympathetic discharge at orgasm restores tone to the arterioles, thereby establishing detumescence. Deep pelvic surgeries such as radical prostatectomy may disturb this delicate innervation leading to impotence.

URETHRA

The male urethra can be divided into four regions: the prostatic, membranous, bulbous, and pendulous or penile urethra. The prostatic urethra begins at the level of the bladder neck and travels within the substance of the prostate and ends at the level of the urogenital diaphragm. The membranous urethra, as its name implies, travels within the confines of the perineal membrane, where the external urinary sphincter is located. The prostatic urethra and the membranous urethra are referred to as the posterior urethra. The anterior urethra travels within the substance of the corpus spongiosum. The bulbous urethra runs in the portion of the spongiosum that is dilated, the bulb. The remaining urethra distal to the bulb that travels under the groove of the corpora cavernosa is the penile urethra. The male urethra is covered by pseudostratified columnar epithelium except at the level of the prostatic urethra where it is lined by transitional epithelium similar to that of the bladder. The blood supply to the male urethra is from branches of the internal pudendal arteries.

The female urethra is typically ~4 cm in length and 8 mm in diameter. It courses adjacent and anterior to the distal one-half of the vagina and opens at the level of the vaginal introitus. The distal aspect of the female urethra is covered with squamous epithelium, whereas the proximal end is covered with transitional and pseudostratified epithelium.

EVALUATION OF COMMON UROLOGIC SYMPTOMS

Hematuria

Hematuria is a frequent urologic symptom with many etiologies. It has been classically taught that the timing of hematuria can localize the source. Hematuria at the beginning of voiding suggests an anterior urethral etiology, whereas terminal hematuria is due to prostate or bladder neck etiology. Total hematuria is from the level of the bladder or above. The presence or absence of pain accompanying hematuria narrows the differential diagnosis further. Painless hematuria should be considered cancer of the urinary tract until proven otherwise; although BPH, glomerulonephritis, papillary necrosis, renal arterial-venous malformation, infection, and nonobstructing stones can present with similar symptoms. Acute onset of flank or lower quadrant abdominal pain with microscopic hematuria is usually due to an obstructing renal or ureteral stone.

The evaluation of a patient with hematuria begins with the urinalysis. The extent of the hematuria and the presence of white blood cells, bacteria, and casts are all important information. An intravenous urogram (IVU), previously known as an "intravenous pyelogram" (IVP), should be performed provided that the patient does not have iodine allergy or renal insufficiency. The IVU assesses renal excretion, obstruction, and the presence of filling defects which may be due to tumor or radiolucent stones. Renal ultrasonography or radionuclide renal scan does not substitute for the IVU. Should the patient be allergic to iodine, a retrograde urogram should be performed by a urologist in the operating room. Because the IVU does not reliably detect bladder lesions, a cystourethroscopy should be performed on all patients evaluated for hematuria.

Flank Pain/Abdominal Pain

Flank pain and abdominal pain may be caused by musculoskeletal or gastrointestinal pathology. However, the sudden onset of flank pain or abdominal pain associated with hematuria is nearly always due to an obstructing ureteral or renal calculus. The excruciating pain associated with renal colic is due to acute distention of the renal capsule or the ureter. The rapid expansion of the renal capsule can trigger the sensation of nausea and cause vomiting. Classically, renal colic does not cause involuntary guarding or rebound tenderness (peritoneal signs). Occasionally, however, the pain is so severe that a complete abdominal examination may not be possible and renal colic may mimic an acute abdomen. Slower onset of flank pain associated with hematuria, pyuria, and dull costovertebral angle tenderness suggests pyelonephritis. Men with suprapubic pain and inability to void may have urinary retention from prostatic hypertrophy or acute prostatitis. Suprapubic pain associated with urinary frequency and dysuria typically is due to UTI with cystitis.

Beyond the patient history and physical examination, the most important laboratory test is the urinalysis. The presence of red blood cells in the urine dictates the need for an IVU to exclude urolithiasis. A normal ultrasound of the kidney does not rule out obstruction, because an acute blockage may not produce visible dilatation of the upper urinary tract. A negative plain radiograph of the abdomen does not exclude the presence of radiolucent stones. Suprapubic pain with a distended bladder should be treated with foley catheter decompression and an evaluation of the prostate should be initiated.

Testicular Pain/Mass

A painless and firm mass in the testis is cancer until proven otherwise. Testicular mass associated with pain is much more difficult to evaluate. A large and acutely tender testis in a young male (<30 years) should alert the physician to the diagnosis of torsion of the spermatic cord when trauma is excluded. In an elderly man with a slow onset of testicular pain, epididymo-orchitis is nearly always the etiology. More uncommon etiologies of a painful testis include tumor, hydrocele, varicocele, mumps orchitis, and nonbacterial orchitis (orchalgia).

The evaluation of an acutely painful testis in a young male should include either a testicular nuclear scan or Doppler ultrasonography to evaluate intratesticular blood flow. Painless testicular masses are evaluated with gray-scale scrotal ultrasonography to look for solid tumors of the testis. Urinalysis and urine culture are important in guiding appropriate antimicrobial therapy when the diagnosis of epididymo-orchitis is entertained.

Voiding Symptoms

Nocturia is excessive urination at night. This is a typical symptom of a patient with BPH and is due to incomplete bladder emptying. Congestive heart failure as well

as diabetes may also cause this condition. Occasionally, no pathology may be found responsible for nocturia and this symptom may simply be a manifestation of the aging bladder.

Decrease force of stream or urination may be due to anatomic obstruction, physiologic obstruction from a lack of coordination of urinary sphincter and bladder (dyssynergia) from spinal cord lesion or from neurologic conditions affecting the detrussor muscle of the bladder decreasing its contractility.

Urgency is the sudden desire to void. This may be due to bladder irritability from infection, chronic bladder outlet obstruction (prostate), or neurologic disease causing a decrease in upper motor neuron inhibition (hyperreflexia) such as a stroke or an upper spinal cord injury.

Terminal dribbling is the inability to completely stop urinary flow at the end of micturition. This is usually due to incomplete bladder emptying usually associated with prostatic hyperplasia.

Dysuria is a burning sensation associated with voiding. Common etiologies are UTI, sexually transmitted diseases (STD), and, less commonly, carcinoma in situ (CIS) of the urinary bladder.

The complete evaluation of voiding symptoms requires a detailed history as well as a complete examination with emphasis on neurological function. In the male patients, a prostate examination is mandatory to evaluate for cancer, BPH, and prostatitis. In female patients, a complete pelvic examination is needed to exclude vaginitis, urethral diverticulum, and cystocele (prolapse of the bladder), which can interfere with voiding. Laboratory workup for all patients includes urinalysis to evaluate for infection and basic serum chemistry to rule out renal insufficiency and diabetes.

Urethral Discharge

Urethral discharge associated with dysuria is usually due to urethritis from STD. Gonococcal as well as Chlamydial cultures should be performed and the patient should be treated empirically before culture results are known. Sexual contacts should be informed.

COMMON UROLOGIC EMERGENCIES

Acute Scrotum

The common etiologies of the painful scrotum include epididymitis, orchitis, torsion of the appendix testis, blunt or penetrating trauma, testicular tumor, and torsion of the spermatic cord. Of all of the causes of the acute scrotum mentioned above, torsion of the spermatic cord is the only true surgical emergency. Thus, the initial workup of patients with acute scrotal pain is aimed at excluding torsion of the spermatic cord. The age of the patient and the history of the present illness is extremely important in determining the etiology. In young men (<30 years) with a sudden onset of pain after strenuous exercise or pain during sleep that wakes him up, the diagnosis of torsion should immediately be pursued by Doppler ultrasound, radionuclide testicular scan, or surgical exploration (when noninvasive tests are not available) to evaluate intratesticular blood flow. In older men (>50 years) with a slow, insidious onset of pain with associated dysuria, epididymitis is almost certain. Trauma can be easily elicited from the history. Testicular tumors is as common in older men as it is in the younger population, and a physical examination revealing an irregular, firm mass that may or may not be tender requires surgical exploration. Torsion of the appendages of the testis mimics torsion of the spermatic cord and requires the same evaluation.

The treatment of acute torsion of the spermatic cord is an emergent surgical exploration and detorsion of the spermatic cord with bilateral fixation of the testicles. A nonviable testis found during exploration requires orchiectomy. Penetrating trauma to the testis requires exploration and blunt trauma to the testis may or may not require exploration depending on the integrity of the testis. A testicular mass requires exploration through an inguinal approach with orchiectomy if the mass appears neoplastic intraoperatively. Torsion of the appendix testis is a self-limiting process and requires only reassurance. In the elderly population (>50 years), epididymitis is treated empirically with antibiotics that cover gram-negative organisms and modified according to urine cultures. In the younger age group, sexually transmitted organisms should be suspected and antibiotic coverage should include gonococcus and chlamydia.

Fournier's Gangrene

Fournier's gangrene, also known as "necrotizing fasciitis of the genitalia," is a fulminating gangrenous disease of the male genitalia. Patients typically present with erythema and edema of the genitalia with or without crepitus. What appears to be pitting edema and generalized edema with minimal tenderness can rapidly progress to gangrene that may spread quickly along the fascial plane. Within a short period of time, this process may extend up to the axillae or down to the perineum. Predisposing factors are concurrent infection, diabetes or other systemic disease, genitourinary tract disease, and trauma.

Treatment of Fournier's gangrene involves prompt surgical debridement and broad-spectrum antibiotics active against gram-positive, gram-negative, and anaerobic organisms. Early recognition by the referring physician and immediate surgical intervention by the operative team is crucial as mortality rates have been reported to be as high as 45%.

Acute Urinary Retention

Acute urinary retention is a very distressing problem that primarily affects men. Common etiologies are BPH and urethral stricture disease. Occasionally, urinary retention is due to bladder dysfunction from diabetic cystopathy or neurologic disorder (such as multiple sclerosis or spinal cord injury).

The initial treatment for this condition is the placement of a urethral catheter. In older men with BPH, the use of a Coude catheter (urethral catheter with a curved tip) facilitates placement as the angle of the prostatic urethra is accentuated by BPH. In young men or in older men in whom the Coude catheter fails to enter the bladder, urethral stricture disease should be suspected and a history of previous gonococcal urethritis is often present. The diagnosis of urethral stricture is made by either endoscopy (urethroscopy) or retrograde urethrogram. The treatment for BPH is discussed elsewhere in this chapter. The treatment for urethral stricture is dilatation or endoscopic incision under direct vision for short lesions. Long strictures require open surgical repair. In patients with diabetes or neurologic disorders, a full physiologic evaluation of the bladder (urodynamic study) should be obtained.

Priapism

Priapism is the persistence of an erection in the absence of sexual stimulation. The most common etiologies for priapism are sickle cell disease and idiopathic. Less commonly, priapism may be due to leukemia, solid tumor infiltration with thrombosis, and medication (e.g., trazodone). Prolonged erection causes ischemia and fibrosis of the spongy erectile tissue with eventual loss of sexual potency.

Because of the risk of impotence due to prolonged priapism, treatment should be initiated as soon as possible. For patients with sickle cell disease, initial treatment consists of hydration, systemic alkalinization, analgesia, and transfusion to increase hemoglobin to >10 mg/dl. All other etiologies should be treated initially with an α-adrenergic agonist injected directly into the corpora cavernosa of the penis. Aspiration of the corpora cavernosa and irrigation should be performed if injection of an α-adrenergic agent fails. Surgical shunting procedure is indicated when conservative treatments fail.

NEPHROLITHIASIS

Renal stones have afflicted humans for >7,000 years. Despite the knowledge that we have acquired about the pathogenesis of renal stones over the years, nephrolithiasis remains a common disease throughout the world. The peak age incidence of renal calculi is between the third and fifth decade, with a male to female ratio of 3:1. Blacks have a low incidence of renal stones. Climatic and seasonal factors are also important with the highest occurrence documented in the "stone belt states" (southern and southeastern states of the United States) during the summer months.

Etiology

Many theories exist to explain the formation of renal calculi. The widely accepted modern theory can be summarized in two steps: crystallization and crystal aggregation. For crystallization to occur, there must a state of supersaturation that is determined by either excess excretion of solute or inadequate excretion of water. Because there are known organic inhibitors of crystallization, there must be a relative decrease in the concentration of these inhibitors. For aggregation of crystals to occur there must be relative stasis which is affected by anatomy as well as rate of urine formation.

Composition

Most of the renal stones are made of calcium compounds and are therefore radiopaque. In decreasing order of occurrence, renal stones are composed of the following: mixed calcium oxalate and phosphate (34%), pure calcium oxalate (33%), magnesium ammonium phosphate (15%), uric acid (8%), pure calcium phosphate (6%), and cystine (3%).

Clinical Presentation

The majority of patients with symptomatic renal stones present with acute onset of flank pain due to obstruction and pressure on the renal capsule. As the stone travels down the ureter, pain may localize or may radiate to the ipsilateral inguinal region or testis. Stones impacted in the intravesical portion of the ureter frequently give rise to urinary frequency and urgency as well as vague suprapubic pain. Frequently, renal colic is accompanied by nausea and vomiting. Renal or ureteral colic is differentiated from peritonitis when a patient moves around despite excruciating pain, unable to find a comfortable position.

The physical examination of the patient with acute renal colic often reveals flank or costovertebral angle tenderness. A mid or distal ureteral stone usually causes mild ipsilateral lower quadrant tenderness. There is never involuntary guarding, rebound tenderness, or rigidity of the abdomen.

Evaluation

Initial laboratory evaluation should include a urinalysis (UA), complete blood count (CBC), and a basic serum chemistry. Microscopic hematuria occurs in ~90% of the time in patients with renal colic. Urinary pH can be indicative of the type of stone (e.g., pH of <5.5 decreases solubility of uric acid). A mild leukocytosis is often present and, in the absence of fever, does not indicate infection. The serum electrolyte panel detects abnormalities seen with severe dehydration from vomiting and lack of oral intake.

Flank pain associated with hematuria suggests a renal stone and an IVU is indicated, provided that the patient is not in renal failure or has an iodine allergy. The IVU provides critical information regarding the location and size of the stone and the extent of obstruction (complete versus partial). This information is essential in making decisions regarding treatment. Renal ultrasound as well as radionuclide scan provide very limited information and should not be the first line diagnostic study when there are no contraindication to the IVU.

Treatment

It is well documented that ~80% of patients who have passed stones or had stones removed will reform stones within a 10-year period if the primary metabolic cause is not treated. A total of 95% of renal stone patients have an identifiable physiochemical abnormality that predisposes them to recurrent calculus formation. The medical treatment of stone disease can have significant side effects, and therefore a shotgun approach is not recommended. Furthermore, empiric treatment can potentially have greater side effects and may not be effective.

Selective medical therapy refers to the treatment of the specific metabolic abnormality. Metabolic aberrations seen include hypercalcuria, primary hyperparathyroidism, hyperoxaluria, hypocitraturia, hyperuricosuria, and cystinuria. This requires a detailed metabolic workup. A simplified initial laboratory evaluation includes serum for basic chemistry, calcium and uric acid level, urine culture, and 24-hr urine collection for calcium, oxalate, uric acid, sodium, phosphorus, citrate, creatinine, pH, cystine, and total volume. With the improvement in specimen preservation, this full metabolic evaluation can be easily completed on an outpatient basis.

Treatment of nephrolithiasis from metabolic disorders obviously depends upon the precise etiology. Hypercalcuria can be secondary to over absorption or due to renal leak of calcium. Absorptive hypercalcuria is treated with either dietary modification or calcium binding resin, depending on the severity of the defect. Renal leak hypercalcuria is best treated with hydrochlorothiazide, which decreases the excretion of calcium. Primary hyperparathyroidism (resorptive hypercalcuria) is managed by surgical removal of the parathyroid adenoma.

Similarly, hyperoxaluria has different etiologies. Enteric hyperoxaluria is due to inflammatory bowel disease, short bowel syndrome, or intestinal bypass surgery. Malabsorption leaves a large amount of unabsorbed fatty acid that binds with intraluminal calcium. As a result, intraluminal oxalate that normally binds with calcium and is excreted in the stool is absorbed systemically. When it is excreted in the renal system it binds to calcium and precipitates in the renal tubules. Treatment of this condition includes a low-fat diet supplemented with medium-chain triglycerides and a diet low in oxalate. Primary hyperoxaluria is an autosomal recessive disorder manifested as a deficiency of a liver enzyme causing an accumulation of oxalate. This condition leads to nephrocalcinosis and eventual renal failure. The use of inhibitors of stone formation such as magnesium and phosphate have been of some benefit. Dietary hyperoxaluria is managed by dietary abstinence of foods high in oxalic acid (e.g., citrus fruits, cranberries, tea, cocoa, almonds, cashews, carbonated beverages, green leafy vegetables).

Hypocitraturia is a relative deficiency in urinary citrate, an endogenous inhibitor of stone formation. The etiology of this condition is metabolic acidosis due to varying reasons. The treatment for this condition is systemic alkalinization with sodium bicarbonate, sodium citrate, or potassium citrate.

Hyperuricosuria leads to uric acid stone formation and can be treated with allopurinol, a xanthine oxidase inhibitor. Hyperuricosuria with uric acid formation can also be treated with urinary alkalinization regimen similar to that for hypocitraturia as uric acid stones are more soluble at pH above 6.5.

Cystinuria is an autosomal recessive inborn error in metabolism causing impaired reabsorption of cystine, ornithine, lysine, and arginine (i.e., COLA). Of the four amino acids not reabsorbed, only cystine has a low solubility leading to crystallization and stone formation. Treatment is aimed at increasing solubility by alkalinization and preventing supersaturation by increasing hydration. Cystine can also be bound to substances such as D-penicillamine or mercaptopropionylglycine to enhance its solubility.

In the presence of infection and obstruction due to the calculus, the goal of treatment is to minimize stone manipulation and to bypass the obstruction. This can be easily achieved with the cystoscopic placement of an indwelling ureteral stent. If the cystoscopic stent placement is unsuccessful or if the patient is septic, a percutaneous nephrostomy tube placement is warranted. In the absence of infection, renal or proximal ureteral stones of <2 cm can be treated noninvasively with extracorporeal shock wave lithotripsy. Renal stones of >2 cm are preferably treated with percutaneous nephrolithotripsy. Mid to distal ureteral stones can be retrieved with a ureteroscopic stone basket or shattered by ureteroscopic lithotripsy (laser or electrohydraulic). In the absence of high-grade obstruction, immediate surgical intervention is not necessary. Stones of <4 to 6 mm causing partial or

no obstruction may be allowed to pass spontaneously. In 1996, there are very few indications for the open surgical removal of renal or ureteral stones.

BENIGN PROSTATIC HYPERPLASIA

BPH is the most common disorder seen by urologists. Until the recent expansion in medical treatment modalities for BPH, transurethral resection of the prostate (TURP) was the most common operative procedure performed in a hospital. Most men above the age of 50 have some form of BPH, and histological evidence of BPH begins as early as the third decade of life. Autopsy series have shown that, by the age of 90, 90% of men have histologic evidence of BPH. Thus far, only two factors have been shown to cause progression of BPH: the testis and aging.

Histopathology

BPH occurs only in the transition zone of the prostate, the region that is immediately adjacent to the lumen of the prostatic urethra. Therefore, the digital rectal examination (DRE) of the prostate, which only palpates the peripheral zone of the prostate, does not accurately predict prostate size or correlate with the patient's urinary symptoms. According to McNeal, the formation of BPH involves two distinct steps: the formation of the nodules and the enlargement of the nodules. Histologic examination of a typical BPH nodule reveals a fibromyoadenomatous pattern of hyperplasia.

Symptoms

Prostatic enlargement does not produce any symptoms until there is obstruction of urinary outflow. Patients with BPH exhibit subjective symptoms which are categorized as either obstructive or irritative. Obstructive voiding symptoms include a decrease in force and caliber of the urinary stream, hesitancy in initiating flow, post void dribbling, sensation of incomplete bladder emptying, and urinary retention. Irritative symptoms such as frequency, urgency, and nocturia are primarily due to a loss of bladder compliance due to long standing obstruction. When patients are objectively evaluated with pressure flow studies, the only symptoms that consistently predict obstruction are hesitancy and decrease in force and caliber of urinary stream. Patients with neurologic abnormalities such as spinal cord compression or multiple sclerosis can have complaints that mimic BPH and a thorough history exploring previous neurologic illness or injury is crucial. Furthermore, patients with right-sided heart failure typically have nocturia and patient with uncontrolled diabetes mellitus often have bladder dysfunction and polyuria that may present as urinary frequency similar to BPH. Finally, patients with a history of STD-related urethritis or urethral trauma may have urethral stricture disease, which presents identically to BPH.

Physical Examination

Most patients with BPH do not exhibit any striking physical abnormality, unless there is profound obstruction causing renal insufficiency. A thorough physical examination should include a detailed neurologic examination and a DRE of the prostate. Increase in the deep tendon reflexes or lower extremities weakness should be carefully investigated. The DRE should document the size of the prostate, presence of prostatic nodules or rectal mucosal lesions, and the anal sphincter tone.

Treatment

A patient with mild to moderate symptoms without any of the above findings can be treated with expectant therapy, medical treatment, or surgery. Expectant treatment alone has a 30% chance of improvement. The selection of the treatment type must be based on the patient's health status, degree of symptomatology, age, and disabilities. To quantify the extent of the patient's symptoms, the American Urologic Association created a scoring system to objectify urinary symptoms as much as possible. The scoring system allows for quick assessment of the patient's current symptoms as well as the degree of progression. For a patient with mild symptoms, watchful waiting and reassurance is reasonable. The patient with moderate symptoms should be counseled on the side effects and morbidities of medical versus surgical treatment. The final decision is based on the patient's preference. For the patient with uremia, urinary retention or severe symptoms unresponsive to medical therapy, surgery is indicated.

Medical therapy consists of the α-receptor antagonists (prazosin, terazosin, dozasosin) or the 5-α reductase inhibitor (finasteride). α blockade decreases the tone of the prostatic capsule and the bladder neck. Side effects of α-receptor antagonists are orthostatic hypotension and generalized fatigue. Finasteride exert its action by blocking the conversion of testosterone to its active form, 5-dihydrotestosterone. A reduction in the active form of testosterone decreases prostatic size with minimal side effects. A review of numerous phase III trials reveals that α-receptor antagonists are slightly more effective in relieving symptoms and improving urinary flow rate.

TURP for BPH is the gold standard of therapy, against which all other treatment modalities are compared. For prostates of >100 g, open surgical enucleation is the preferred procedure due to the high risk of

bleeding and free water absorption of the endoscopic procedure when confronted with such a large gland. Newer forms of surgical treatment have evolved to eliminate the morbidity associated with the TURP and include the various LASER ablation procedures, high-frequency thermal ablation, and electrocautery vaporization. These new procedures decrease operative blood loss and length of hospital stay significantly but have less efficacy in relieving symptoms and improving urine flow rate when compared to TURP. Results of phase III trials of these newer surgical modalities are not yet available for analysis.

COMMON UROLOGIC MALIGNANCIES

Prostate Cancer

Prostate cancer is the most common cancer in men and is the second most common cause of cancer-related mortality in male patients. Prostate cancer is the only cancer in which there is a tremendous dichotomy between histologic cancer and clinically evident cancer. When the prostate is examined at autopsy, 40% of men in their seventies and 67% in their 80s have histologic evidence of cancer. In contrast, clinically evident prostate cancer results from only 3% of histologic cancer. Similar to the dichotomy between histologic and clinical cancers is the disparity in the progression rate seen in prostate cancer. To decide which patients will progress and therefore require treatment is precisely the dilemma that a urologist faces everyday when he evaluates prostate cancer patients.

Pathology

Over 95% of prostate cancer is adenocarcinoma arising from the prostatic glandular epithelium. Based on the zonal anatomy of McNeal, 75% of prostate cancers arise from the peripheral zone and the remaining 25% from the transition zone. The peripheral zone is the region that is palpated during a DRE of the prostate. Histologic grading of prostate cancer correlates closely with clinical progression and is based on the system of Gleason. The Gleason grading system ranges from 1 to 5 and is based on glandular architecture, with 5 being most anaplastic. A biopsy specimen is usually given two separate grades, due to the heterogeneity of the cancer, and a score is given. The highest score is 10, with the worst prognosis, and the lowest is 2. There are many staging systems for prostate cancer, with the primary tumor/regional nodes/metastasis (TNM) classification being the most commonly used (Table 1). Both the stage and the grade of the tumor are important prognostic indicators.

TABLE 1. *Abbreviated TNM staging system for prostate cancer*

Stage	Description
T_{1a}	<5% of TURP specimen with well-differentiated tumor
T_{1b}	>5% of TURP specimen or any extent of poorly differentiated tumor
T_{2a}	Tumors occupying 1 lobe and <1.5 cm in size
T_{2b}	Tumors occupying 1 lobe but >1.5 cm in size
T_{2c}	Tumors involving both lobes of any size
T_3	Tumors with extracapsular extension
T_4	Tumors invading adjacent structures
N+	Tumor present in regional lymph nodes
M+	Distant metastasis

T, tumor stage; N, lymph node; M, distant metastasis.

Diagnosis

Prostate cancer is asymptomatic until it invades the bladder or becomes metastatic to the bones. Rarely does prostate cancer cause hematuria or obstruction when it is organ confined. Thus, early detection of prostate cancer is dependent upon the physician. Early detection of prostate cancer consists of DRE of the prostate in conjunction with the measurement of serum prostatic specific antigen (PSA) level. The PSA or DRE alone is insufficient screening, and a substantial number of cancers will be undetected when evaluated in this manner. The American Cancer Society recommends that all men above the age of 50 with at least 10 years of life expectancy undergo yearly evaluation, which includes both a DRE and serum PSA. Men with a family history of prostate cancer or African-Americans, who have a threefold higher incidence of prostate cancer, should begin this process at the age of 40. Patients with multiple medical problems, which significantly reduce their life expectancy, are not candidates for early detection.

The final diagnosis of prostate cancer relies on the pathological diagnosis made by a transrectal ultrasound guided biopsy of the prostate. The indications for a biopsy of the prostate are a PSA level above 4 ng/ml or an abnormal examination of the prostate. Signs of prostate cancer from the DRE include asymmetry, firm nodules, and diffuse induration. A patient with an enlarged but smooth prostate does not need further workup unless the PSA level is abnormal.

Treatment

Organ-Confined Disease

Once the diagnosis of prostate cancer is made, the treatment decisions are based on the clinical stage of the cancer. Patients with an initial serum PSA of >10 ng/ml should undergo a radionuclide bone scan to rule out osseous metastasis. A serum PSA level of <10 indicates a low probability of bony metastasis. A CT scan of the abdomen and pelvis is not reliable in detecting nodal metastasis from prostate cancer and is therefore not routinely performed.

Organ-confined disease is defined as a patient with a negative bone scan and a DRE of the prostate not suggestive of extracapsular extension. Only patients with organ-confined disease are candidates for local therapy with curative intent. Currently, the proven treatments for organ-confined disease are radical prostatectomy and external beam radiation therapy. Comparison based on historical, nonrandomized series have shown nearly equal actuarial survival and disease specific survival. Side effects of surgery are sexual impotence and urinary incontinence. Morbidities of external beam radiation therapy are sexual impotence, radiation cystitis, proctitis, and urethral stricture.

Advanced and Metastatic Disease

Nearly 50% of patients have advanced prostate cancer at the time of diagnosis. Despite such a large percentage, treatment for this subgroup remains, as it has been for the past 40 years, palliative. Standard treatment for advanced or metastatic prostate cancer is androgen ablation. This can be in the form of surgical castration or a medical alteration in the hypothalamic-pituitary-gonadal axis via a monthly depot injection of luteinizing hormone releasing hormone (e.g., leuprolide, goserelin). The end result of either form of therapy is a temporary arrest in cancer growth which improves progression free survival without a significant impact on overall survival. Because the adrenal produces a small amount of androgen, nonsteroidal antiandrogens have also been used in conjunction with castration to improve progression free survival even further. Bone pains from metastatic deposits, when unresponsive to hormonal ablation, are treated with palliative localized radiation therapy and analgesics.

Bladder Cancer

Bladder cancer is the fourth most common cancer in men and the eighth most common cancer in women. Bladder cancer is also the fourth leading cause of cancer-related mortality in men. Men are three times more likely to be diagnosed with bladder cancer than women. The median age of diagnosis is between 67 and 70 years old.

Current literature suggests that bladder cancers are induced by chemical carcinogens. Malignant transformation in the transitional epithelial cells is induced by an alteration in its genome by carcinogens. Common chemicals implicated as carcinogens are aniline dyes, cigarette smoke, phenacetin (an analgesic), saccharin, and the chemotherapy agent cyclophosphamide. It is known that cigarette smokers have a fourfold higher incidence of bladder cancer as compared with nonsmokers. Other factors that predispose individuals to bladder cancers are pelvic irradiation and chronic cystitis, especially when associated with Schistosoma haematobium infection.

Pathology

Most bladder cancers are transitional cell carcinoma (TCC), which account for 90% to 95% of all bladder cancers. TCC may be papillary, sessile, or flat by gross or endoscopic examination. TCC is graded by the degree of anaplasia (grade 1 to 3), with 1 being well differentiated and 3 being poorly differentiated. The accurate grading of TCC is of great importance as the rate of progression to invasive and metastatic disease is directly correlated to its grade. For example, grade 1 TCCs have <5% chance of progression, whereas grade 3 TCCs have 45% to 50% chance of progression to metastatic disease.

Primary adenocarcinoma and squamous cell carcinoma (SCC) of the bladder are responsible for <7% of bladder cancers in the developed countries. In Egypt, where schistosomiasis is endemic, SCC is the primary pathology in >75% of bladder cancer cases. Both adenocarcinoma and SCC of the bladder are generally highly aggressive.

The current widely used staging system for bladder cancer is the TNM classification (Table 2). Both the grade and the stage of bladder cancers are directly correlated with prognosis.

Diagnosis

The most common initial presentation of bladder cancer is painless hematuria. Less frequently, bladder cancer patients may also present with dysuria, urinary frequency, suprapubic pain, or hydronephrosis. Currently, the most sensitive method for bladder cancer detection is cystourethroscopy, which can be performed in the office setting. Because the source of hematuria may arise from anywhere between the kidney and the urethral meatus, a

complete hematuria workup must include an IVU. Urinary cytology, obtained either as voided specimen or by bladder irrigation with saline, is highly sensitive in detecting CIS of the urothelium (a subclass of grade 3 TCC) and should be routinely sent, because CIS is frequently not visualized well by endoscopy or IVU.

Once the office endoscopy is suggestive of a bladder tumor, the pathological diagnosis is obtained by an outpatient operative procedure known as the "transurethral resection of bladder tumor" (TURBT). For superficial cancer of the bladder, the TURBT is both diagnostic and therapeutic. If the bladder tumor appears to invade the bladder wall, the biopsy should include the muscle of the bladder wall for staging purposes. Invasion into the bladder wall musculature indicates high-stage disease requiring aggressive therapy.

Treatment

The treatment of TCC of the bladder is highly dependent upon the grade and stage of the tumor. For grade 1 tumors limited to the mucosa, the TURBT alone is sufficient. If repeated recurrences are problematic for the patient, intravesical chemotherapy (thiotepa or mitomycin), which is well tolerated, may be offered. For grade 2 to 3 superficial tumors (stage Ta or CIS), a course of intravesical chemotherapy (mitomycin) or immunotherapy with Bacillus Calmette-Guerin is highly recommended. Close surveillance with endoscopy and urinary cytology is critical for superficial bladder cancer of any grade as recurrences are common.

Invasive TCC denotes cancer that has invaded the lamina propria (stage T1), into the bladder wall smooth musculature (stage T2-T3a), or beyond the bladder (stage T3b-T4). Many treatment options are available for this subgroup of bladder cancer patients and can be categorized as bladder-sparing or bladder replacement. Bladder-sparing approach is ideally suited for elderly, poor risk patients, or patients with minimally invasive and small solitary cancers with no associated hydronephrosis. Common bladder-sparing treatments include TURBT alone, partial cystectomy, radiation therapy, and combined radiation and chemotherapy. Approximately 50% of patients treated with bladder preservation regimens ultimately require salvage radical cystectomy. In well-selected patients, the bladder-sparing approaches may offer nearly equal survival rates while enhancing the quality of life when compared to radical surgery. Bladder replacement therapy candidates are patients with bulky, deeply invasive tumors, especially when associated with diffuse CIS or invasion of the prostatic urethra. Bladder replacement therapy consists of a radical cystectomy and a lower urinary reconstruction that may be in the form of an ileal conduit, continent intestinal pouch, or an intestinal neobladder. In men, radical cystectomy involves removal of

TABLE 2. *Abbreviated TNM classification for bladder cancer*

T$_{is}$	Flat, nonpapillary, anaplastic tumor limited to mucosa
T$_a$	Tumor limited to mucosa
T$_1$	Tumor invades lamina propia
T$_2$	Tumor invades superficial muscle
T$_{3a}$	Tumor invades deep muscle
T$_{3b}$	Tumor invades perivesical fat
T$_4$	Tumor invades adjacent organs
N	Regional lymph node(s) involved
M	Distant metastasis

T, tumor stage; N, lymph node; M, distant metastasis.

the bladder and the prostate and in women it involves the removal of the bladder, uterus, ovaries, urethra, and the anterior one-third of the vaginal wall. Despite radical surgery, 50% of patients with invasive bladder cancer progress to metastatic disease within 2 years of diagnosis.

Bladder cancer metastasizes to regional lymph nodes and distant organs. The combination chemotherapy regimen consisting of methotrexate, vinblastine, adriamycin, and cisplatin (i.e., MAC) is currently most effective against metastatic TCC. Objective complete response ranges between 15% and 50% of cases. Unfortunately, the durable response rates have been limited, and <10% of patients treated for metastatic TCC with M-VAC are alive at 5 years of follow-up.

Renal Cell Carcinoma

Renal cell carcinoma (RCC) accounts for 85% to 90% of all malignant tumors of the kidney and ~3% of all adult malignancies, excluding skin cancer. Although generally considered to be a cancer of the elderly population with the mean peak incidence in the sixth decade, RCC can be found in young adults and even in children as young as 6 months of age. RCC often occurs sporadically but can also occur in hereditary form. Von Hippel-Lindau (VHL) disease and hereditary nonpapillary RCC are both inherited in an autosomal dominant fashion. These familial syndromes present frequently with bilateral and multifocal RCC in patients who are generally younger. Other disorders associated with higher incidence of RCC include tuberous sclerosis, autosomal dominant polycystic kidney disease, and acquired renal cystic disease. Although no clear factors have been implicated in carcinogenesis of RCC, molecular geneticists have discovered that a deletion or rearrangement of the short arm of chromosome 3 is found in the majority of patients with these tumors. This region of the chromosome 3 contains the VHL gene, a new tumor suppressor gene.

Pathology

The majority of RCCs arise from the epithelial cells of the proximal tubules with a smaller number originating in the distal tubules or collecting ducts. Histologically, most RCC are of the clear cell type due to a cytoplasm rich in lipids and glycogen which are removed in the process of fixation, thereby giving this appearance of lucency. Granular cells are less common and are due to abundance of mitochondria. In RCC, tumor grade is generally not useful as prognostic indicator. Tumor stage is the only factor that determines treatment and prognosis. Many staging systems have been devised but the currently widely accepted system is the TNM classification (Table 3).

TABLE 3. *Abbreviated TNM classification for renal cell carcinoma*

T_1	Tumor of ≤2.5 cm limited to the kidney
T_2	Tumor of >2.5 cm limited to the kidney
T_3	Tumor extends into major veins or invades adrenal gland or perinephric tissues but not beyond Gerota's fascia
T_4	Tumor invades beyond Gerota's fascia
N	Regional nodal metastasis
M	Distant organ metastasis

T, tumor stage; N, lymph node; M, distant metastasis.

Diagnosis

RCC may present in many different ways and has been referred to as the great mimic. Historically, the classic triad of flank pain, flank/abdominal mass, and hematuria is suggestive of RCC. Today, with the frequent use of CT scan and ultrasound, many renal masses are discovered incidentally. However, when RCC presents clinically, hematuria is the most common complaint, followed by elevation in erythrocyte sedimentation rate, abdominal mass, anemia, flank pain, hypertension, and weight loss (Table 4).

Patients who present with hematuria should be evaluated as described previously, which includes an IVU. When the suspicion of RCC is entertained, a CT scan of the abdomen without and with intravenous contrast is indicated. The CT of the abdomen not only visualizes renal masses but also provides staging information that is pertinent in therapeutic decision making. An enhancing, exophytic parenchymal mass is suggestive of RCC. Other findings that should be looked for in the CT scan are renal vein/vena cava involvement, hilar adenopathy, and liver metastasis. Once a renal mass has been identified on the CT scan, a metastatic workup should be performed, including a plain chest radiograph and serum alkaline phosphatase and calcium levels. An elevated serum alkaline phosphatase may be indicative of bony metastasis and requires confirmation with a radionuclide bone scan.

Treatment

Radical nephrectomy remains the only effective treatment for localized RCC, involving the en-bloc removal of

TABLE 4. *Common clinical presentation of renal cell carcinoma*

Hematuria
Elevation in erythrocyte sedimentation rate
Abdominal mass
Anemia
Flank pain
Hypertension
Weight loss

the kidney with the perinephric fat, including Gerota's fascia. Occasionally, tumor thrombus may extend into the renal vein or the vena cava, or as high cephalad as the right atrium. Tumor thrombus involving the renal vein or vena cava requires vena cava exploration and removal of the tumor thrombus. When the thrombus extends into the heart, vena cava exploration and intracardiac exploration must be performed under total circulatory arrest with systemic hypothermia. The prognosis of localized RCC is very good. When RCC invades adjacent organs such as the colon, pancreas, spleen, or liver, surgical excision is rarely curative.

RCC is not responsive to chemotherapeutic agents. Immunotherapy remains the only form of treatment for metastatic RCC. Interleukin-2 is the only FDA-approved drug that yields only a 15% complete response rate with variable duration of remission from 7 to 76 months.

COMMON PEDIATRIC UROLOGIC DISORDERS

Undescended Testis

By the 32nd week of gestation, the testicles have completed their descent into the scrotum. Testicles that are not intrascrotal at birth are considered undescended. The overall incidence of undescended testicles is 3.4% to 5.8% in term boys and 9.2% to 30.0% in premature boys. The position of the undescended gonad may be intraabdominal, canalicular (inguinal), or ectopic. Retractile testicles are not truly undescended and can usually be manipulated down into the bottom of the scrotum on physical examination. The etiology of undescended testicles is not fully understood but animal models have suggested a decreased in intratesticular or serum testosterone level is causative.

The rationale for early treatment of undescended testicles are based on the following factors: improving fertility, decreasing malignant potential, decreasing the risk of torsion, and psychological. Treatment may be either medical or surgical. The only medical therapy involves the administration of parenteral human chorionic gonadotropin (hCG). hCG is thought to stimulate Leydig cells, thereby increasing serum testosterone which in turn promotes testicular descent. Success rates for this treatment range from 14% to 50%. Retractile testicles have a near 100% descent rate and hCG stimulation has been suggested as a mean of differentiating retractile testis from undescended ones, thereby avoiding unnecessary surgery.

Surgery for the undescended testicle (orchidopexy) is performed when there is no response to hormonal stimulation or when the possible side effects of hormonal stimulation (e.g., change in bone age and enlargement of the penis) are unacceptable. Orchidopexy for canalicular testis is a simple procedure with a high success rate. For the abdominal testis, laparoscopy is initially performed to confirm the existence of the gonad. Once visualized, the abdominal testis may require multiple operations for scrotal placement.

Vesicoureteral Reflux

Primary vesicoureteral reflux (VUR) occurs as a result of a lack of adequate length of the ureter within the bladder wall, resulting in a weakened physiologic flap valve mechanism. The consequence of this is retrograde movement of urine from the bladder up into the ureter and kidney with voiding. VUR predisposes children to recurrent pyelonephritis which eventually leads to renal scarring and dysfunction. Primary VUR is a congenital condition with an overall incidence of 0.4% of the normal population. The peak age of presentation is between the age of 3 to 6 years with 85% being females. Patients with VUR universally present with febrile UTI, which leads to a diagnostic evaluation revealing reflux. Thus, all children with febrile UTI documented by a positive urine culture obtained from a suprapubic tap or a catheterized specimen should be evaluated with a renal ultrasound and a contrast voiding cystourethrogram. A urine culture obtained by placing a bag over the perineum is suboptimal and misleading.

The treatment of VUR can be either medical or surgical, and the selection of which mode of therapy is often influenced by the grade of reflux. VUR is graded from 1 to 5, with grade 5 having severe hydroureteronephrosis and ureteral tortuosity. Medical treatment for VUR consists of daily low dose of antibiotics (ampicillin or Bactrim) until the reflux has resolved by radiographic studies. Surgical treatment involves ureteral reimplantation, which effectively creates a longer submucosal tunnel for the affected ureter, thereby strengthening the flap valve mechanism.

All children diagnosed with VUR should be placed on immediate antibiotic prophylaxis, regardless of when surgery will be performed. Based on the International Reflux Study for Children, there was no statistically significant difference between the randomized medical and surgical arms when the extent of renal scarring was compared. The surgical group, however, had a much lower rate of febrile pyelonephritis. Thus, an indication for surgery is breakthrough infection despite antimicrobial prophylaxis. Relative indications or ureteral reimplantation are lack of compliance with prophylaxis or follow-up and the lack of resolution of reflux with prolonged follow-up.

Hypospadias

Hypospadias is a congenital anomaly associated with a deficiency of the distal ventral urethra resulting in an abnormally proximal urethral opening. The malpositioned urethral meatus can be anywhere from the glans penis to the perineum. Distal hypospadias, with the opening typically at the level of the coronal sulcus, is the most common form and is seen in ~65% of the cases. Besides the proximally positioned meatus, the hypospadiac penis typically has a ventral curvature (chordee) and a hooded prepuce due to a lack of ventral fusion of the foreskin. The incidence of hypospadias is reported to be ~1 in 300 male children. Hypospadias is commonly associated with undescended testis and inguinal hernia (9.3%). In the severe forms of hypospadias with ambiguous genitalia, a karyotype analysis should be performed to evaluate true genotypic sex of the child. Female pseudo hermaphrodites, a genotypic female with ambiguous genitalia and associated hypospadias, should be screened for congenital adrenal hyperplasia as it is a life threatening condition in neonatal life.

Corrective surgery for hypospadias is aimed at improving body image and restoring fertility potential. The ideal time for hypospadias surgery is between 8 months and 1 year of age. Distal hypospadias surgery typically involves reconstruction of the glans penis to accommodate the neomeatus at the new tip. More proximal hypospadias requires reconstruction of the ventral urethra using a skin flap from the prepuce. Thus, newborn circumcision should not be performed in a male infant with hypospadias.

Ureteropelvic Junction Obstruction

Ureteropelvic junction (UPJ) obstruction is a common congenital anomaly affecting the junction where the proximal ureter inserts into the renal pelvis. It is the most common cause of neonatal hydronephrosis and a palpable abdominal mass. Historically, only 25% of children with this condition were recognized before the age of 1 year. Today, with the advent of prenatal ultrasonography, most of the cases are recognized in utero.

UPJ obstruction may be due to a functional obstruction or an anatomic one. Functional obstruction is due to an increase in collagen deposit adjacent to the smooth muscle bundles in the ureter. The increase in collagen deposit interferes with normal ureteral peristalsis, creating an adynamic segment. Thus, there is functional obstruction despite a patent lumen. Anatomic obstruction is frequently due to an aberrant lower pole renal vessel crossing the region of the UPJ causing extrinsic pressure on the lumen.

Once hydronephrosis is recognized by renal ultrasound and vesicoureteral reflux has been ruled out, the study of choice for the evaluation and confirmation of a UPJ obstruction is the diuretic radionuclide renal scan. The renal scan allows for accurate quantification of obstruction as well as the split renal function which ultimately will determine the need for surgical intervention.

Whatever the etiology of UPJ obstruction may be, the end result is a restriction to urinary outflow from the kidney, which may lead to renal parenchymal loss and a decrease in renal function. The goal of surgery is to restore urinary flow and to preserve renal function. The standard procedure for congenital UPJ obstruction is a dismembered pyeloplasty, which involves the excision of the obstructed ureteral segment, the excision of the redundant and dilated renal pelvis, and the reanastamosis of the proximal ureter to the reshaped renal pelvis. Success rate of surgery is >95%, with minimal morbidity.

SUMMARY

Advances in surgical techniques, pharmacology, diagnostic modalities, and pharmacology have tremendously changed the field of urology in the past decade. In the years to come, urology will continue to evolve in an attempt to improve the quality of life of patients with urologic diseases. Some of the treatment modalities presented in this text will soon be obsolete. However, the basic concept of managing urologic diseases will not change, and it is hoped that the information presented here will be of value.

STUDY QUESTIONS

1. Describe the anatomic relationship of the kidneys to the surrounding intraabdominal organs.
2. Describe the diagnostic evaluation for patients with hematuria.
3. Who are candidates for early detection of prostate cancer, and what does early detection for prostate cancer include?
4. What are signs of BPH?
5. What is invasive bladder cancer, and what are the treatment options?

SUGGESTED READING

Gillenwater JY, Grayhack JT, Howards SS, Duckett JW, eds. *Adult and pediatric urology.* St. Louis: Mosby–Year Book, 1996.
Glenn JF, ed. *Urologic surgery.* Philadelphia: Lippincott, 1991.
Tanagho EA, McAninch JW, eds. *Smith's general urology.* Norwalk, CT: Appleton and Lange, 1992.
Walsh PC, Retik AB, Stamey TA, Vaughan ED, eds. *Campbell's urology.* Philadelphia: Saunders, 1992.

CHAPTER 29

Otolaryngology

Shishir Sheth and Francisco J. Civantos

In 1924, otolaryngology, more commonly known as "ear, nose, and throat surgery," became the second organized U.S. surgical specialty. Otolaryngologists treat a wide variety of conditions involving the head, neck, and upper aerodigestive tract. Otolaryngology-related complaints are the cause for >60% of patient visits to primary care physicians. The great breadth of the specialty, however, has promoted subspecialization. A clear understanding of the anatomy, physiology, and disease processes of the head and neck is a prerequisite to the appropriate practice of this medical specialty.

OTOLOGY

Anatomy

In no other area of the body are so many vital structures concentrated into so small an area as in the human temporal bone. Knowledge of the detailed anatomy of the ear and temporal bone requires years of study. The following is a presentation of basic concepts and appropri-ate management principles of disease of the ear and temporal bone.

The external, or outer, ear consists of the auricle and external auditory canal (EAC) to the level of the tympanic membrane (Fig. 1). In adults, the EAC is ~2.5 cm long and can be divided into a shorter cartilaginous portion (the external one-third) and a remaining bony portion. There is rich sensory innervation of the outer ear that includes cranial nerves V, VII, and X as well as cervical nerves C-2 and C-3.

The boundaries of the middle ear (tympanic cavity) include the tympanic membrane laterally, the floor of the hypotympanum inferiorly (within which lies the jugular bulb), the lateral wall of the inner ear (otic capsule) medially, the tegmen tympani superiorly (above which lies the brain), the mastoid air cells posteriorly, and the posterior wall of the glenoid fossa anteriorly. The carotid artery and eustachian tube course in the anterior wall of the middle ear. The eustachian tube provides drainage of the middle ear cavity to the nasopharynx and runs in an anterior/medial/inferior direction. The middle ear is also freely continuous with the mastoid air cells via the aditus ad

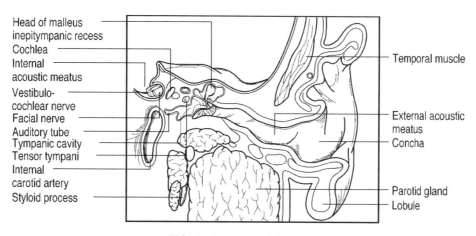

Head of malleus
inepitympanic recess
Cochlea
Internal
acoustic meatus
Vestibulo-
cochlear nerve
Facial nerve
Auditory tube
Tympanic cavity
Tensor tympani
Internal
carotid artery
Styloid process

Temporal muscle

External acoustic
meatus
Concha

Parotid gland
Lobule

FIG. 1. Anatomy of the ear.

383

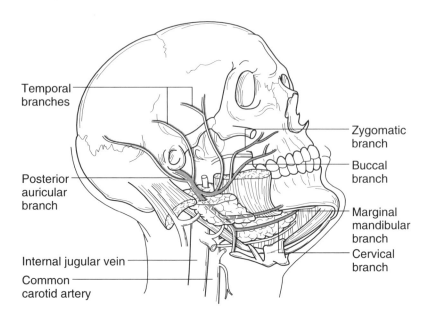

Temporal branches

Posterior auricular branch

Internal jugular vein

Common carotid artery

Zygomatic branch

Buccal branch

Marginal mandibular branch

Cervical branch

FIG. 2. The facial nerve. (Adapted from Gray JW, Skandalakis JE. *Atlas of surgical anatomy for general surgeons.* Baltimore: Williams and Wilkins, 1985.)

antrum located posterosuperiorly. The tympanic membrane is made up of an outer layer of stratified squamous epithelium, a middle fibrous layer, and an inner layer of mucosa continuous with the lining of the tympanic cavity. The middle ear contains the malleus (hammer), incus (anvil), and stapes (stirrup)—the ossicular chain (bones of hearing). The malleus handle is vertically attached to the superior half of the tympanic membrane and is often visible on otoscopy. The head of the malleus, lying in the attic or epitympanum, is attached to the incus, which is in turn attached to the stapes. The footplate of the stapes is attached to the vestibule at the oval window.

The inner ear consists of the bony labyrinth containing the membranous labyrinth. The basal turn of the cochlea forms the promontory (on the medial wall of the middle ear cavity). The cochlea contains the organ of Corti, the hearing end organ, and consists of two and a half spiral turns. It is innervated by the auditory nerve. Within the spiral turns, there are three compartments; the scala vestibuli and scala tympani contain perilymph, whereas the scala media contains endolymph. Sensory cells for signal transduction, the inner and outer hair cells lie within the scala media and rest on the basilar membrane. Posterior to the cochlea lies the vestibular system with its three semicircular canals (horizontal, superior and posterior) placed at right angles to each other as well as the utricle and the saccule. The semicircular canals are specialized for detecting acceleration directed in an angular direction; the utricle and saccule can best detect linear acceleration. These vestibular organs are innervated by the superior and inferior vestibular nerves.

Figure 2 depicts the anatomy of the facial nerve. The facial nerve (CN VII) enters the internal auditory canal (IAC) with cranial nerve VIII; the portion of the facial nerve within the IAC is known as the "labyrinthine portion." At the geniculate ganglion, the facial nerve turns posteriorly and courses within the medial wall of the middle ear; this is known as the "tympanic" or "horizontal" portion of the facial nerve. At the level of the oval window (and lateral to the horizontal semicircular canal), the facial nerve curves inferiorly and courses through the mastoid bone (the mastoid portion) to exit via the stylomastoid foramen. From this point, the facial nerve courses in the anterior parenchyma of the parotid gland to divide the gland into a superficial and deep lobes. Within the gland, the divisions of the nerve originate: temporal, zygomatic, buccal, mandibular, and cervical.

Physiology

The auditory system detects and processes sound. The shape of the auricle and the length of the EAC provide for resonance of sounds in the 2- to 5-kHz frequency range (providing a gain of 10 to 15 dB), which represents the range of frequency of human speech. The middle ear functions as an impedance matching device to convert the low impedance of the acoustic energy of air to the high impedance of fluid. This is achieved by three mechanisms. First, the most important factor is that the vibratory area of the tympanic membrane is ~20 times that of the stapes footplate; second, the handle of the malleus is longer than the long process of the incus chain by a factor of 1.3 leading to a "lever"-type amplification of gain; third and least important is the shape of the tympanic membrane. These mechanisms lead to a pressure gain of ~25 dB. Once the acoustic energy is transmitted to the fluid filled cochlea (to the perilymph of the scala vestibuli), it initiates a traveling wave on the basilar membrane. The maximum displacement of the basilar membrane occurs at a point on the membrane corresponding to the frequency of the initiating sound. High frequencies cause resonance at the basal end of the cochlea, whereas low frequencies cause apical resonance. This displacement of the basilar membrane leads to stimulation of the inner and (more important) outer hair cells via opening and closing of ion channels causing current flow and depolarization. The stimulated nerve fibers propagate the signal to the central auditory system where afferent information is processed.

The eustachian tube provides drainage and pressure equalization for the middle ear and ultimately for the mastoid air cells. It is easier for air to exit the middle ear via the eustachian tube than for air to enter the middle ear (hence the fact that airplane descents are more difficult to adjust to than ascents).

The anatomy of the facial nerve has been described in detail. Functionally, the facial nerve provides innervation to the muscles of facial expression as well as the stylohyoid, posterior belly of the digastric muscle and the stapedius muscle.

Diseases

Infections

Uncomplicated infections of the external ear canal (otitis externa or swimmer's ear) are generally treated by topical antibiotics. In an immunocompromised patient, however, care should be taken to observe for a necrotizing otitis externa, previously known as "malignant otitis externa." Immunocompromised patients, including diabetics, AIDS patients, and transplant patients, are predisposed to the condition. This disease classically causes exuberant granulation of the EAC and osteomyelitis of the bony canal. Infection can spread to adjacent areas such as the brain and vascular structures. Diagnosis is confirmed by technetium bone scan and treatment is with a long course of intravenous antibiotics directed toward the most common pathogen, *Pseudomonas aeruginosa.*

Acute infections of the middle ear are usually caused by *Streptococcus pneumoniae, Hemophilus influenzae,* and *Moraxella catarrhalis,* and can generally be treated with oral antibiotics. Recurrent acute infections usually occur in children and are related to a degree of eustachian tube dysfunction. This is attributed to the more horizontal position of the eustachian tube, its shorter length, and the presence of an enlarged adenoid pad that obstructs the eustachian tube orifice in the nasopharynx. Recurrent infections or persistent fluid in the middle ear, despite adequate antimicrobial therapy, are indications for myringotomy with tube placement.

Chronic infections of the mastoid/middle ear complex that are unresponsive to medical therapy may require mastoidectomy with exenteration of diseased mucosa and skeletonization of the sigmoid sinus, facial nerve, and adjacent dura.

Tympanic membrane perforations are caused most commonly by infection but can also accompany trauma. Treat-

ment is directed at the underlying cause (i.e., antibiotics for infection). A perforation often closes spontaneously as the tympanic membrane heals; however, persistent perforation may require surgical closure, termed "tympanoplasty." (One should recognize that tympanoplasty should not be carried out in the presence of active underlying infectious disease.) Tympanoplasty is tailored to the type and degree of perforation and can be performed through the external ear canal (transcanal approach) or via a postauricular incision (transmastoid approach). Cholesteatoma is a growth of skin in the middle ear cleft. This typically presents as layers of pearly white material. These benign tumors may be congenital or acquired and cause local destruction by migration and erosion of adjacent bony structures. They also serve as a nidus for infection. Surgical treatment involves complete removal of the cholesteatoma with preservation of adjacent structures. Early cholesteatomas can be excised via a transcanal approach, but more commonly a mastoidectomy is required. A tympanoplasty and ossiculoplasty may be performed at a later time during a "second-look" procedure in order to improve or restore hearing.

Diseases of the Ossicular Chain

Various diseases can affect the ossicular chain; these include congenital malformations, infections, trauma, and genetic diseases. Treatment that is aimed at restoring the hearing loss can be as simple as providing a hearing aid. In contrast, surgical reestablishment of an intact and mobile ossicular chain, ossiculoplasty, may be required. Infection is the most common cause of ossicular damage. The most common genetic disease affecting the ossicular chain is otosclerosis, a disease that causes absorption and then abnormal hardening of the human temporal bone. This autosomal dominant disease with incomplete penetrance affects females twice as often as males and has a peak age of incidence between 15 and 45. The most common lesion is at the anterior edge of the stapes footplate leading to fixation and therefore a conductive hearing loss. Treatment options include hearing aids or surgery. Surgical treatment involves stapedectomy or stapedotomy with placement of a prosthesis.

Hearing loss is separated into conductive deficiencies, sensorineural deficiencies, or mixed. Conductive hearing loss is caused by pathology lateral to the oval window and includes fluid or soft tissue in the middle or external ear, diseases of the tympanic membrane, and ossicular chain abnormalities. Sensorineural hearing loss is caused by pathology in the cochlea or nervous system. It can be a normal part of the aging process (presbycusis, in the high frequency ranges), or may it denote pathology in the cochlea (noise-induced damage to the fine hair cells, syphilitic infection, or trauma causing cochlear concussion) or imply central nervous system pathology (acoustic neuroma, stroke).

The treatment of sensorineural hearing loss is directed primarily at the underlying cause and then secondarily at restoring hearing by the use of assistive devices. In selected cases of anacusis (or profound hearing loss), surgical placement of a cochlear implant often improves hearing levels. A unilateral asymmetric sensorineural hearing loss should always raise suspicion of an intracranial tumor, most commonly an acoustic neuroma. The diagnosis of acoustic neuroma can be confirmed by magnetic resonance imaging. Treatment options include observation, amplification with a hearing aid, focused radiation therapy, or surgery. The surgical approach is usually coordinated with a neurosurgeon, and involves continuous intraoperative monitoring of cranial nerves VII and VIII.

Facial nerve paralysis can be caused by a multitude of diseases including trauma, infection, and tumors. Idiopathic facial nerve palsy (Bell's palsy) is common but should remain a diagnosis of exclusion after appropriate evaluation and testing rules out neoplastic or inflammatory etiologies. A viral etiology is thought to be the source of pathogenesis. Herpes zoster infection of the facial nerve, called "Ramsay Hunt syndrome," can be treated effectively with oral administration of acyclovir. If nerve dysfunction is caused by compression of the nerve within its bony canal, decompression of the nerve may be indicated; this is usually accomplished via a transmastoid approach. When there is an identifiable damaged section of nerve, the injured section may be replaced by a nerve graft; this has variable results. For patients in whom very limited or no recovery is expected, various facial slings and reanimation techniques can be offered for cosmetic improvement. It is important to remember that patients with facial nerve paralysis lose their ability to close the ipsilateral eye and are therefore at risk for corneal drying and ulceration; appropriate measures should be instituted to keep the eye moist.

NOSE AND PARANASAL SINUSES

Anatomy

The importance of the nose as an airway, humidifier, sensory organ, and central aesthetic structure of the face must be underscored. The external infrastructure of the nose includes the paired nasal bones, the upper lateral cartilages, the alar cartilages (located inferiorly), and the nasal septum. The nasal valve is the area of greatest resistance to airflow and is located at the anterior-most portion of the inferior turbinate, the lower edge of the upper lateral cartilage, and the nasal septum (you can find the nasal valve on yourself as the area that collapses when you perform forced inspiration).

There are four paired paranasal sinuses: frontal, maxillary, ethmoid, and sphenoid sinuses (Fig. 3). The frontal sinuses are in close proximity to the orbit and the frontal

lobes of the brain. Bridging veins in the posterior wall of the frontal sinus provide a route for infection into the intracranial space. The large maxillary sinuses are located below the orbits. The infraorbital nerve runs through the roof of the maxillary sinus. The ethmoid sinuses are divided into the anterior and posterior ethmoid cells, and are separated from the orbit by the lamina papyracea. The sphenoid sinuses are located posteriorly and are in close proximity to the pituitary gland, the carotid artery, the optic nerve. The lateral wall of the sphenoid sinus forms the medial wall of the cavernous sinus and its contents (cranial nerves III, IV, V1, V2, and VI).

The lateral nasal wall is composed of the medial wall of the maxilla from which the inferior, middle, and superior turbinates project; beneath each turbinate lies the corresponding meatus. The inferior meatus receives the drainage of the nasolacrimal duct. The frontal, maxillary, and anterior ethmoid sinuses drain into the middle meatus in an area known as the anterior "osteomeatal complex" (OMC). The posterior ethmoid and sphenoid sinuses drain into the posterior OMC located above the posterior edge of the middle turbinate.

The sphenopalatine ganglion provides sensory and autonomic innervation to the nasal cavity and is located postero-superior to the middle turbinate. The olfactory nerve and bulbs lie just above the cribriform plate and supply the special sense of smell.

Blood supply to the nose posteriorly comes from the sphenopalatine artery, anteroinferiorly from the greater palatine artery, and superiorly from the anterior and posterior ethmoid arteries. The sphenopalatine and greater palatine arteries are branches of the internal maxillary artery which is derived from the external carotid artery; the anterior and posterior ethmoids derive from the ophthalmic artery, a branch of the internal carotid artery. There is a rich capillary bed supplying the mucosa of the nose at the anterior-inferior portion of the nasal septum, where there is a confluence of the capillary systems of the sphenopalatine, greater palatine, and anterior ethmoid arteries. This site is the most common area of epistaxis

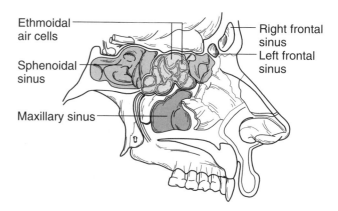

FIG. 3. The paranasal sinuses.

and has several names, among them "Little's area," "Kiesselbach's triangle," or "Woodruff's plexus."

Physiology

The right and left nasal cavities undergo alternating engorgement of the venous sinusoids within the turbinates, leading to alternating nasal obstruction every 2 to 6 hr. This is normal and is known as the "nasal cycle." The turbinates disrupt laminar airflow and create turbulence. It is thought that this helps improve humidification, warming, and filtering of inspired air. The paranasal sinuses produce ~0.5 L/day of mucus, which is actively cleared by ciliary action. The direction of ciliary movement, not gravity, determines mucus flow; for example, the ostium of the maxillary sinus is located well above the floor of the sinus, but the direction of mucociliary clearance is up, toward this ostium.

Diseases of the Paranasal Sinuses

Inflammation of the mucosa of the sinuses, sinusitis, can be caused by a variety of mechanisms, but the underlying process remains the same. Thickening of the sinus mucosa leads to blockage of the sinus ostium which leads to further mucociliary dysfunction. Allergic disease is one of the most common etiologies behind sinusitis. Infections are also common and can be viral, bacterial, or fungal. Often there is a combination of these factors with allergic or viral rhinosinusitis leading to a superimposed bacterial infection. The diagnosis of acute sinusitis is a clinical one and is defined by the classic triad of fever, sinus pain, and purulent drainage. CT scan findings during acute sinusitis include a pathognomonic air-fluid level in the affected sinus(es). The symptoms of chronic sinusitis are usually more indistinct and have been present for >3 months. Chronic sinusitis reveals mucosal thickening on CT scan.

The treatment of acute sinusitis is aimed at relieving the obstruction at the sinus ostium and treating the bacterial component; this is achieved by antibiotics and nasal decongestants. For chronic cases, any underlying pathology (e.g., allergic disorder) should be sought out and treated. The inflammatory reaction of nasal mucosa in response to nasal polyps is poorly understood and can occur in the face of allergy or infection. Nasal polyps are a poorly understood nasal inflammatory response which can occur in the face of allergy or infection. "Sampter's triad" refers to the association of nasal polyps, asthma, and aspirin sensitivity.

In a diabetic or otherwise immunocompromised patient with sinusitis, the possibility of invasive fungal sinusitis (mucormycosis) should be considered. The characteristic clinical appearance is that of a rapidly progressive disease; intranasal examination shows black or dark red areas where the fungus has invaded and caused tissue necrosis. This is a true emergency and requires immediate surgical debridement and intravenously administered antifungal antibiotics. Any delay leads to rapid involvement of the orbit or brain.

If sinusitis symptoms do not resolve upon medical management, surgery can be considered. In the past, this would include external approaches to the sinuses, such as external ethmoidectomy or maxillary sinus surgery. Today, for uncomplicated sinus disease, these procedures have been replaced by functional endoscopic sinus surgery. Various angled telescopes are used in combination with specialized instruments to enlarge the natural ostia of the various sinuses and remove diseased mucosa via an intranasal approach with no external incision. The major risks to sinus surgery include damage to nearby structures including the brain and the eyes.

Nasal obstruction is a common complaint. Again any underlying inflammatory disease should be sought and treated. Failing such treatment, the patient may be a candidate for surgical straightening of the nasal septum (septoplasty) or inferior turbinate reduction. Too aggressive removal of the nasal turbinates may cause atrophic rhinitis, a condition characterized by a chronically dry nose and the continuous production of crusts.

The otolaryngologist is often called to evaluate cases of epistaxis. Usually a thorough history and physical examination will reveal the underlying cause. Laboratory studies should include a complete blood count as well as a coagulation profile. In cases where uncontrollable bleeding occurs despite aggressive attempts to treat any underlying cause, the nose can be packed in layers with a gauze strip impregnated with antibiotics. If the patient has persistent bleeding when the packing is removed, interventional radiology aimed at selective embolization of the bleeding vessel is possible. Surgical treatment involving ligation of one or more of the arteries supplying the nasal cavity, including the internal maxillary, the anterior and posterior ethmoid arteries can be performed.

NEOPLASMS OF THE HEAD AND NECK

It is beyond the scope of this chapter to discuss the surgical anatomy and pathology of the head and neck in exquisite detail. However, certain guiding principles that are useful as a general overview are addressed.

Tumors of the Proximal Aerodigestive Tract

By far the most common malignancy of the upper aerodigestive tract (representing >75% of all malignancies) is squamous cell carcinoma (SCCA). Consistent etiologic factors in the majority of cases are excessive tobacco or ethanol abuse. When used together, a patient is at 15 times the risk of a nonsmoker and nondrinker of developing SCCA. The most common sites of origin are the oral cavity followed by the larynx. Signs and symptoms of the primary tumor include pain, dysphagia, dyspnea, voice change, bleeding, and weight loss. The natural history of SCCA is that of progressive enlargement of the primary tumor and metastasis to locoregional lymph nodes. Distant metastasis to liver, lungs, or bone is a relatively late occurrence.

Diagnosis of malignancy is ideally made by biopsy of the primary tumor. Violation of the neck to perform open biopsy of suspicious cervical nodes should generally be avoided, unless a careful search for an upper aerodigestive tract primary has been performed. Fine needle aspirate is more commonly performed. Biopsy can be done either in the office or in the operating room in the case of inaccessible lesions under general anesthesia with the use of specialized endoscopes (rigid laryngoscopes, bronchoscopes, and esophagoscopes). At that time, the remainder of the aerodigestive tract is carefully examined to exclude synchronous primaries. A relative contraindication to biopsy is the appearance of a vascular mass. Intranasal masses should not be biopsied, unless clinical examination or imaging studies rule out the possibility of intracranial communication.

Treatment of SCCA can range from attempts at cure to palliation. Small lesions of the aerodigestive tract (<2 cm) can be treated with either radiation therapy or surgical resection with adequate margins with similar cure rates. Radiation therapy, once given in maximal doses, usually can not be repeated. The effect of radiation is mainly tumor specific; there is a lesser but significant effect on the microvasculature located within the radiation field. Some exophytic tumors, or tumors known to respond well to radiation therapy (e.g., tonsillar or soft palate SCCA) may be treated primarily by radiation with surgery being reserved for salvage cases. The type of surgery is tailored to the location of the lesion. Access to tumors of the head and neck remains one of the most challenging aspects of surgical intervention. If it is known in advance that both surgery and radiation will be necessary, it is often preferable to give the radiation postoperatively in order to reduce the rate of surgical complications. Curative resection involves extirpation of the tumor with clear margins. Tumors of the oral cavity may require composite resection including portions of the tongue, mandible, floor of mouth, and lingual or hypoglossal nerves.

Tumors of the larynx may require partial or total laryngectomy. The latter involves complete dissociation of the airway from the digestive tract in which the trachea is permanently sutured to the skin of the neck, a tracheostomy. Voice rehabilitation after a total laryngectomy includes one of three options. The first option is the use of esophageal speech, wherein the patient learns to swallow air and then allows it to come up in a controlled fashion using the pharynx, tongue and lips for proper enunci-

ation. The second option is via the use of an electrically vibrating membrane that amplifies vibrations produced at the floor of mouth by enunciating the words. The third option is by the creation of an artificial one-way fistula between the posterior wall of the trachea and the anterior wall of the esophagus that allows air to enter the esophagus from the trachea; the patient then covers the stoma and forces air out through his mouth which he can then shape into the appropriate sounds. Closure of surgical defects may either be primary, with the use of skin grafts, loco-regional flaps, or distant free-flaps. Reconstruction is tailored to meet the needs of the tissue defect, the ability of the patient to tolerate the reconstruction, and the experience of the surgeon. The complex functional and aesthetic characteristics of the head and neck make complex primary reconstructions, including microvascular techniques, of paramount importance in the modern management of head and neck cancers. In particular, the treatment of advanced oral cavity tumors has been revolutionized thanks in large part to developments in primary reconstruction.

If the tumor has metastasized to locoregional lymph nodes (Fig. 4), either surgery or radiation may be used for treatment. Predictable patterns of metastases in the neck exist which depend upon the site of the primary tumor. Radiation can be effective for neck nodes up to 2 cm in size. Surgery for neck disease is classified by the structures removed as follows (Figs. 5–7):

1. Comprehensive neck dissection: removal of all five lymph node groups
   a. Radical neck dissection: sacrifice of sternocleidomastoid muscle, internal jugular vein, and spinal accessory nerve (cranial nerve XI)
   b. Modified radical neck dissection: preservation of at least one of the above three structures

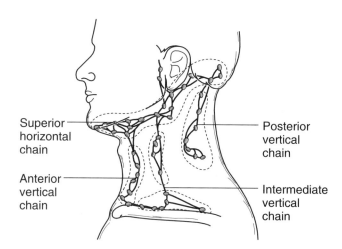

FIG. 4. The lymph node regions of the neck. (Adapted from Gray JW, Skandalakis JE. *Atlas of surgical anatomy for general surgeons.* Baltimore: Williams and Wilkins, 1985.)

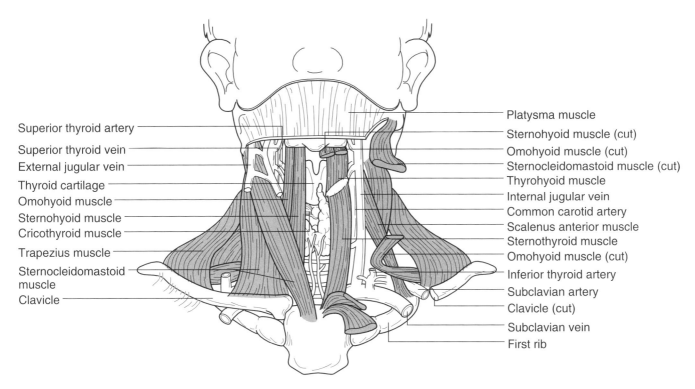

Superior thyroid artery
Superior thyroid vein
External jugular vein
Thyroid cartilage
Omohyoid muscle
Sternohyoid muscle
Cricothyroid muscle
Trapezius muscle
Sternocleidomastoid muscle
Clavicle

Platysma muscle
Sternohyoid muscle (cut)
Omohyoid muscle (cut)
Sternocleidomastoid muscle (cut)
Thyrohyoid muscle
Internal jugular vein
Common carotid artery
Scalenus anterior muscle
Sternothyroid muscle
Omohyoid muscle (cut)
Inferior thyroid artery
Subclavian artery
Clavicle (cut)
Subclavian vein
First rib

FIG. 5. Overview of anatomy of the neck. (Adapted from Gray JW, Skandalakis JE. *Atlas of surgical anatomy for general surgeons.* Baltimore: Williams and Wilkins, 1985.)

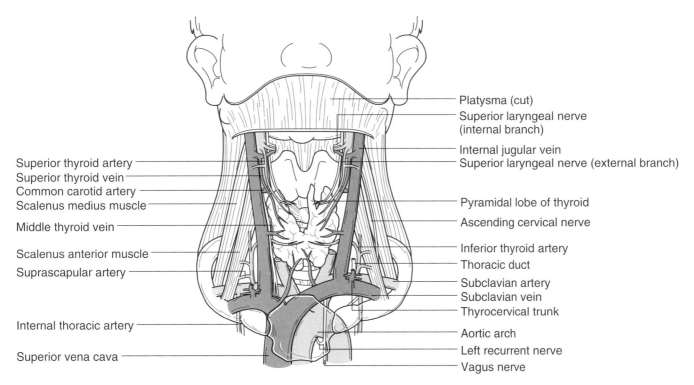

Superior thyroid artery
Superior thyroid vein
Common carotid artery
Scalenus medius muscle
Middle thyroid vein
Scalenus anterior muscle
Suprascapular artery
Internal thoracic artery
Superior vena cava

Platysma (cut)
Superior laryngeal nerve (internal branch)
Internal jugular vein
Superior laryngeal nerve (external branch)
Pyramidal lobe of thyroid
Ascending cervical nerve
Inferior thyroid artery
Thoracic duct
Subclavian artery
Subclavian vein
Thyrocervical trunk
Aortic arch
Left recurrent nerve
Vagus nerve

FIG. 6. Overview of anatomy of the neck. (Adapted from Gray JW, Skandalakis JE. *Atlas of surgical anatomy for general surgeons.* Baltimore: Williams and Wilkins, 1985.)

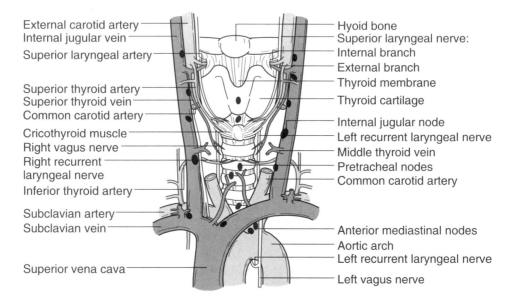

External carotid artery
Internal jugular vein
Superior laryngeal artery

Superior thyroid artery
Superior thyroid vein
Common carotid artery
Cricothyroid muscle
Right vagus nerve
Right recurrent
laryngeal nerve
Inferior thyroid artery

Subclavian artery
Subclavian vein

Superior vena cava

Hyoid bone
Superior laryngeal nerve:
Internal branch
External branch
Thyroid membrane
Thyroid cartilage

Internal jugular node
Left recurrent laryngeal nerve
Middle thyroid vein
Pretracheal nodes
Common carotid artery

Anterior mediastinal nodes
Aortic arch
Left recurrent laryngeal nerve
Left vagus nerve

FIG. 7. Deeper structures in the neck. (Adapted from Gray JW, Skandalakis JE. *Atlas of surgical anatomy for general surgeons.* Baltimore: Williams and Wilkins, 1985.)

2. Selective neck dissection: preservation of at least one of the lymph node groups. These are further subclassified based on the precise lymph node groups removed
3. Extended neck dissection: removal of additional structures (e.g., the external carotid artery, cranial nerve XII, etc.)

Removal of all five lymph node groups, the external carotid artery, internal jugular vein, and sternocleidomastoid muscle would be termed an "extended modified radical neck dissection with preservation of cranial nerve XI and sacrifice of the external carotid artery." Resection of the spinal accessory nerve, which can lead to significant shoulder dysfunction, is treated by aggressive physical therapy and pain management.

Tumors of the Salivary Glands

There are three paired major salivary glands (Fig. 8): the parotid, submandibular, and sublingual glands (in order of decreasing size). In addition, there are hundreds of minor salivary glands scattered throughout the remainder of the upper aerodigestive tract. A wide variety of tumors of salivary gland origin exist. As a general principle, the smaller the size of the gland in which a tumor is located, the higher the chance that the tumor is malignant. Parotid tumors are the most common, and the most common of these is the benign pleomorphic adenoma (mixed tumor). Because of the small chance of malignant degeneration of these tumors, surgical excision is recommended; a margin of normal gland is required in the resection because these tumors have

pseudopod extensions that account for the tendency of these tumors to recur. Papillary cystadenoma lymphomatosum (Warthin's tumor) are the second most common benign salivary tumor. These tumors may represent salivary duct tissue incorporated into lymph glands with lymphocytes. Interestingly, these lesions are isolated to the parotid glands and in 10% of cases are bilateral in distribution. Mucoepidermoid carcinoma and adenoid cystic carcinoma are the most common malignant tumors of the salivary glands. Adenoid cystic carcinoma is notable for its submucosal growth and tendency for perineural invasion.

Complications of surgical resection of the parotid gland include injury to the facial nerve (which runs between the superficial and deep lobes) as well as aberrant nerve regeneration of the parasympathetic fibers innervating the removed parotid gland. These abnormally regenerating nerve fibers innervate the sweat glands of the skin leading to gustatory sweating (Frey's syndrome). Resection of the submandibular gland may injure the marginal mandibular branch of the facial nerve, causing inability to retract the corner of the mouth inferiorly. Thyroid and parathyroid disorders are discussed elsewhere in this text, but resection of these glands may also be necessary as part of the en bloc resection of aerodigestive tract tumors.

Areas of recent progress in head and neck oncology include the availability of surgical approaches to the skull base, oral cavity, and larynx, which allow increased preservation of function. Advanced radiation techniques involving multiple treatments each day (i.e., hyperfractionation) or direct implantation of tumors with radiation catheters have expanded their use in head and neck can-

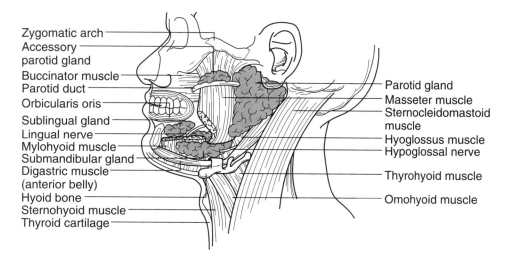

FIG. 8. Overview of glands and muscles of face. Salivary glands are shown in blue. (Adapted from Gray JW, Skandalakis JE. *Atlas of surgical anatomy for general surgeons.* Baltimore: Williams and Wilkins, 1985.)

cer treatment. Chemotherapy, in conjunction with radiation, may sometimes obviate the need for radical resection in the head and neck.

FACIAL PLASTIC AND RECONSTRUCTIVE SURGERY

Due to its emphasis on anatomic areas of obvious visible aesthetic importance, minimization of cosmetic deformity has always been a focus of many otolaryngologic procedures. Thus, the otolaryngologist needs a strong background in proper soft tissue technique and familiarity with a variety of facial cosmetic and reconstructive procedures.

Important principles to bear in mind include the following:

1. No single aesthetic procedure works for all patients. The surgery should be individualized to meet the aesthetic features of the surrounding structures, the needs of the patient, and the experience of the surgeon.
2. Proper preoperative patient education is essential. The presence of prior deformities and factors that increase complication rates, such as smoking, should be discussed with the patient.
3. Tissue trauma with instrumentation should be minimized. This includes the use of proper instruments for the delicate handling of soft tissue as well as strict aseptic technique.
4. Skin suture lines should be tension free. Any tension will lead to widening of the scar.
5. Tissue mobilization can be safely performed only if the surgeon has a clear understanding of the vascular supply of the tissues involved.

Special Complications

Rhinoplasty may lead to alar stenosis with difficulty breathing through the nose. Too aggressive resection of the nasal dorsum may lead to a "saddle-nose" deformity. If the patient has thick skin with exuberant scar tissue formation in the region above the tip of the nose (supratip region), a "pollybeak" deformity may result. Smoking has been shown to increase the chance of ischemia and death of nasal skin.

Excessive resection of eyelid skin during a blepharoplasty may lead to ectropion, or scleral "show." This usually is caused in the postoperative period by scar contracture leading to the eyelid being pulled away from the globe. Treatment is conservative initially with the use of eyelid exercises and massage but may require corrective surgery.

Proper understanding of various principles, including the position of relaxed skin tension lines and the clear understanding of aesthetic facial subunits is essential, whether the surgeon is performing a maxillectomy, open reduction of a facial fracture, or any of a myriad of other head and neck procedures.

PEDIATRIC OTOLARYNGOLOGY

Tonsillectomy and adenoidectomy remains the most commonly performed major surgical procedure in children in the United States. There are two major indications: infection and obstructive hyperplasia.

Patients with three or more infections of tonsils and/or adenoids per year despite adequate medical therapy are surgical candidates. Patients with chronic or recurrent tonsillitis associated with the streptococcal carrier refractory to appropriate antibiotics should also be advised to undergo tonsillectomy and adenoidectomy. Peritonsillar abscess unresponsive to medical therapy and drainage is another indication for tonsillectomy. A peritonsillar abscess characteristically has the findings of trismus, a "hot potato" voice, and deviation of the uvula to the opposite side (due to swelling of the soft palate); treatment of the acute abscess is with incision and drainage. Obstructive hyperplasia includes symptoms of upper airway obstruction, dysphagia, sleep disorders, alterations in orofacial growth, and any associated cardiopulmonary complications. Another indication for tonsillectomy is to rule out neoplasia in the case of asymmetric tonsils.

Recurrent acute otitis media is the most common otologic problem in the pediatric population. The pathophysiology of acute otitis media in children usually relates to eustachian tube dysfunction (either via blockage by adenoid tissue or inflammation of the mucosa during a viral infection). Gas in the middle ear is resorbed causing negative middle ear pressure which leads to a serous effusion. This then becomes superinfected by bacteria resulting in an episode of acute otitis media. When the number of acute infections per year exceeds five in a period of a year, myringotomy and tube placement may be beneficial. This prevents accumulation of serous fluid in the middle ear and subsequent superinfection. Myringotomy and tube placement should also be considered for a chronic serous otitis media that fails to respond to conservative management, as well as a chronically retracted tympanic membrane (due to negative middle ear pressure); prevention of hearing loss and speech delay are the ultimate goals of surgical intervention.

Medical progress has extended the survival of pediatric patients with previously early fatal disease but often at the expense of prolonged periods of mechanical ventilation. One of the most challenging problems facing otolaryngologists is subglottic stenosis secondary to prolonged endotracheal intubation. The diagnosis can usually be made by careful history and physical examination. Plain films of the airway are often helpful. Treatment depends on the severity of obstruction. If the child is asymptomatic, observation may suffice in the hope that the child will outgrow the stenosis. For more severe obstructions, surgery (laryngotracheoplasty and laryngotracheal reconstruction) with the use of autologous cartilage (either conchal cartilage from the ear or rib cartilage) can be of benefit. Tracheotomy is often necessary, but single-stage reconstruction with ~1 week of nasotracheal intubation is becoming standard therapy.

Children are much more apt than adults to inhale or ingest foreign objects. Foreign bodies that have entered the airway and the tracheobronchial tree are more likely to enter the right mainstem bronchus than the left due to the more direct path of the former. Plain films of the airway and of the chest as well as inspiratory and expiratory chest radiographs (in the case of a ball valve–type foreign object obstructing a bronchus) are helpful in identifying and localizing the object. Preparation of instruments in

the operating room is essential prior to beginning any procedure; having a duplicate of the inhaled object allows identification of the instrument that would best facilitate extraction. There are a variety of rigid laryngoscopes and bronchoscopes that allow visualization of the airways while still allowing ventilation of the patient under general anesthesia. Foreign bodies that are lodged in the esophagus need to be removed as soon as possible. If they have sharp ends or points or contain substances that can potentially cause more damage (i.e., batteries), emergent extraction of the foreign body is mandatory.

EMERGENCIES IN OTOLARYNGOLOGY

The otolaryngologist must be the master of all methods of airway management. In cases where the airway is obstructed and orotracheal or nasotracheal intubation is not possible, establishment of a surgical airway becomes necessary. The most rapid procedure is the cricothyroidotomy. By incising through the thin skin and tissues overlying the cricothyroid membrane, a tube may be inserted into the trachea for ventilation purposes. This method is only used at times of extreme emergency because of the proximity to the glottis and the theoretical increased risk of subglottic stenosis. If a long-term tube is necessary, this can be revised to a tracheotomy at the second tracheal ring. In skilled hands, a tracheotomy can be performed quickly. It involves incising the skin and subcutaneous tissues, the midline fascia of the strap muscles, the thyroid isthmus, and entering the trachea itself. A tube is placed within the hole thus created to maintain patency of the airway. (One should note that "tracheotomy" refers to the surgical procedure, and "tracheostomy" refers to the actual opening created in the trachea.)

Sinus and ear infections can spread by their proximity to nearby structures, including the brain and the orbits. If an abscess is identified, drainage is required to prevent systemic sepsis. As noted earlier, the diagnosis of mucormycosis in an immunocompromised patient is a surgical emergency requiring immediate debridement and antifungal therapy.

Infection may also occur and spread in any of the various fascial compartments of the head and neck. Infection and abscess formation of the enclosed submandibular space can progress and cause airway obstruction by displacement of the tongue superiorly and posteriorly (Ludwig's angina). Rapidly progressing infections of the fascial planes with liquefactive necrosis, or necrotizing fasciitis, should be treated promptly by securing the airway (by tracheotomy if necessary) and incision and drainage. CT scanning is helpful in identifying and locating fluid collections. If untreated, infection in the tissues surrounding large blood vessels may cause rupture of those structures with lethal results. After surgical drainage, treatment is aimed at resolving the infection with antibiotics and possibly hyperbaric oxygen therapy.

Hemoptysis after placement of a tracheostomy should always raise the suspicion for a tracheo-innominate fistula. Pathogenesis involves development of an abnormal connection between trachea and innominate artery secondary to high tracheal tube cuff pressure leading to tracheal necrosis and erosion into the innominate artery located anterior to the trachea. This complication from a tracheostomy and even prolonged endotracheal intubation is fortunately rare. The mortality from this complication is ~50%. There may be a small amount of bleeding initially, known as a "sentinel bleed," which should raise clinical suspicion and hopefully early diagnosis.

Intraoperative entry into the jugular vein may lead to air entering the low pressure venous system. Air emboli can lead to respiratory and hemodynamic compromise. Auscultation of the heart may reveal a "churning" sound. Treatment involves placing the patient in Trendelenburg position and in the left lateral decubitus position to trap air in the right atrium. Hyperbaric therapy may be of benefit in reducing the effects of the air embolus by directly reducing its size.

Postoperative bleeding after surgery on the neck can lead to an expanding hematoma. Only a small amount of blood within the tissue planes of the neck is sufficient to cause airway compromise. If the patient is clinically unstable, the wound should be opened emergently at the bedside and the hematoma decompressed. Endotracheal intubation may be required to maintain a patent airway. If this is impossible, cricothyroidotomy or tracheostomy may be necessary. Definitive therapy involves neck reexploration.

A catastrophic complication of neck irradiation for cancer is carotid artery rupture. Should massive pharyngeal bleeding occur, the airway should be secured as previously described. The bleeding is then tamponaded with direct external pressure with or without a throat pack. Intravascular volume resuscitation with blood products and balanced salt solutions should be performed to maintain stable vital signs. Surgical therapy is performed as soon as possible and often requires carotid artery ligation, which entails a significant risk of stroke. Bypass procedures or embolization may be possible if the problem is identified early at the time of a sentinel bleed.

SUMMARY

Otolaryngology—Head and Neck surgery requires knowledge of a wide range of surgical and nonsurgical diseases. These include, but are not limited to, otology, sinus and voice disorders, head and neck oncology, facial plastic and reconstructive surgery, and pediatric otolaryngology. Furthermore, a large percentage of chief complaints to the primary care physician is related to the ears, nose, and throat. Thus, it is important for the student of medicine to be familiar with the basics of this surgical specialty.

STUDY QUESTIONS

1. Describe the pathogenesis of tracheoinnominate fistula. What are some factors that favor the development of this clinical entity?
2. Characterize the different anatomical segments of the ear.
3. What are the typical bacteria involved in paranasal sinus infections? What is the appropriate treatment of sinusitis?
4. What are the different types of salivary gland neoplasms?
5. Describe the different types of neck dissections.

SUGGESTED READING

Bailey BJ, et al. *Head and neck surgery—otolaryngology. Vols. 1 and 2.* Philadelphia: Lippincott-Raven, 1993.

Cummings CW, et al. *Otolaryngology—head and neck surgery. Vols. 1–4.* St. Louis: Mosby–Year Book, 1993.

Glasscock ME, et al. *Surgery of the ear.* 4th ed. Philadelphia: Saunders, 1990.

Simons RL. *Coming of age—a twenty-fifth anniversary history of the American Academy of Facial Plastic and Reconstructive Surgery.* New York: Thieme Medical Publishers, 1989.

CHAPTER 30

Concepts of Anesthesia

James J. Jacque and Albert J. Varon

The development of surgical anesthesia is perhaps one of the greatest breakthroughs of modern medicine. Although Sir Christopher Wren injected wine and opium into dogs as early as the 1600s, an anesthetic suitable for surgical procedures did not exist until the 1840s, when diethyl either was introduced into clinical practice. The synthesis of ultra–short-acting barbiturates and neuromuscular blocking agents in the 1930s and 1940s allowed for more extensive surgical procedures to be performed. Since then, both pharmacologic and technical advances have formed an anesthetic armamentarium that have enabled complicated surgical procedures to be safely carried out on very sick, fragile patients.

General anesthesia is considered to have four basic components: unconsciousness/hypnosis, analgesia, amnesia, and muscle relaxation. A combination of agents may be used to produce general anesthesia. For example, unconsciousness may be produced with barbiturates, analgesia with opiates, amnesia with benzodiazepines, and muscle relaxation with neuromuscular blocking agents. A general anesthetic delivered in this manner would be considered a "balanced" anesthetic technique. Some volatile inhalational anesthetics may produce all of the above components and would be considered "complete" anesthetics.

Induction of general anesthesia may be carried out with intravenous agents such as barbiturates and benzodiazepines, or with inhalation of a volatile anesthetic agent. General anesthesia may be maintained via tight-fitting mask or endotracheal tube. Intubation of the trachea is facilitated by administration of either a depolarizing or nondepolarizing neuromuscular blocking agent. Usually, general anesthesia is maintained with a combination of inhaled nitrous oxide and a volatile anesthetic agent, and can be supplemented with the administration of a narcotic analgesic. If there is a surgical need for muscle relaxation, a nondepolarizing relaxant is administered and the lungs are mechanically ventilated.

Emergence from general anesthesia begins at the conclusion of the surgical procedure and is different for patients who are breathing spontaneously versus being mechanically ventilated. For patients breathing spontaneously, emergence begins with the cessation of administration of the volatile anesthetic and nitrous oxide. During this period, it is important to maintain the patient's airway, either by head positioning or mechanical devices such as nasal or oral airways. If the patient has been intubated, has received muscle relaxants, and has been mechanically ventilated, several criteria must be met before extubation. An adequate level of consciousness must be achieved in order to regain protective laryngeal reflexes. This is particularly important in patients who have a full stomach and are at risk for pulmonary aspiration of gastric contents. Before extubation, an adequate level of alveolar ventilation must be met since barbiturates, volatile anesthetic agents, and narcotics are all potent respiratory depressants. If muscle relaxants have been used, it is important to have an adequate level of muscle strength before extubation. Depolarizing agents are short lived, and patients quickly return to full strength spontaneously. Nondepolarizing agents may require reversal of their action by administration of an acetylcholinesterase inhibitor such as neostigmine or edrophonium. Once these criteria have been met, the patient may be extubated safely.

Regional anesthesia refers to the infiltration of a local anesthetic agent around a nerve or bundle of nerves to produce blockade of conduction of sensory and motor impulses to areas of the body subserved by those nerves. Examples of regional anesthesia include subarachnoid (spinal) or epidural blockade for procedures involving the lower abdomen or lower extremities, and peripheral nerve blockade such as femoral-sciatic nerve blocks for the lower extremity and brachial plexus blocks for upper extremity procedures. Patients undergoing regional anesthesia may or may not require supplementation with sedative/anxiolytic agents.

Some procedures may be performed with local anesthesia infiltrated into the surgical field by the surgeon.

Often, an anesthesiologist is present to sedate the patient as well as to monitor the patient for adequacy of ventilation, circulation, and level of consciousness. This type of anesthetic delivery is called "monitored anesthesia care" (MAC).

PREOPERATIVE EVALUATION OF THE SURGICAL PATIENT

The preoperative evaluation of the surgical patient enables the anesthesiologist to become familiar with the patient's past medical, surgical, and anesthetic history as well as past and current medications, allergies, and physical examination. A careful history and physical examination guide the physician to order appropriate laboratory data and other studies, all of which may have significant impact on the perioperative management of the patient.

Another important component of the preoperative evaluation is an explanation of the anesthetic plan, including the risks and benefits of that plan, an overview of the events on the day of surgery, and obtaining informed consent.

The history should center around a thorough review of systems. Careful questions regarding symptomatology of coronary artery disease and left ventricular dysfunction are important. Risk factors for occult coronary artery disease should be elucidated and the level of exercise tolerance documented. Valvulopathies and the history of a murmur may indicate the need for antibiotic prophylaxis for subacute bacterial endocarditis. A history of reactive airway disease may profoundly affect the management of an anesthetic as can tobacco use, chronic obstructive pulmonary disease, a history of recurrent pneumonia, or recent upper respiratory infection. A thorough review of other systems may suggest the presence of endocrine, renal, hepatic or central nervous system (CNS) disease. Tobacco, alcohol or drug use, current medications, and history of drug allergies must be documented.

The patient's past surgical history should demonstrate past anesthetic experiences that may reveal difficult intubations, adverse drug responses, perioperative nausea, prolonged muscle relaxation, prolonged intubation, or malignant hyperthermia. If the patient has not received a general anesthetic, then questioning should be directed to adverse anesthetic experiences of family members. The physical examination should include careful evaluation of the airway, including dentition, lungs, heart, and peripheral pulses. Any preexisting neurologic deficits should be carefully documented.

Currently, several million dollars are spent annually on unnecessary preoperative testing. For example, a cell count with differential, a complete chemistry profile, coagulation studies, chest x-ray and electrocardiogram are unnecessary tests for a healthy, nonsmoking 25-year-old patient undergoing an elective herniorrhaphy. A careful history and physical examination will serve as a guide in ordering appropriate preoperative laboratory and other studies.

The preoperative evaluation allows for allaying the anxiety of the patient. Anxiety may be further reduced by the administration of a preoperative anxiolytic agent such as a benzodiazepine. Agents such as H_2 receptor antagonists may also be administered to reduce the risk of gastric acid aspiration. In addition, the anesthesiologist may choose to continue the patient's current medications through the morning of surgery. This is particularly important in patients with a history of hypertension, coronary artery disease, pulmonary disease, and diabetes. Often problems are discovered preoperatively that may require further diagnostic tests and treatment or medical consultation. The role of the consultant is to (a) determine the presence of disease, (b) determine the extent of disease, and (c) medically optimize the disease state. Once a given disease state has been optimized, then the patient is considered to be "fit" for surgery.

AIRWAY MANAGEMENT

The evaluation of the airway and its appropriate management are the cornerstones of the delivery of any anesthetic. The evaluation of the airway involves a dental examination, evaluation of the tongue size and the ability to view pharyngeal structures, the ability to extend the atlanto-occipital joint, and the thyromental distance. The inability to view pharyngeal structures and extend the atlanto-occipital joint beyond 12 degrees, or a short thyromental distance indicate the potential for a difficult endotracheal intubation.

Patency of the airway is important to ensure adequate alveolar ventilation and oxygenation. Patency may be disrupted by supraglottic or subglottic obstruction, and its diagnosis and treatment may serve as life-saving maneuvers. Supraglottic airway obstruction may result from a large and relaxed tongue, redundant pharyngeal soft tissue, pharyngeal mass, foreign body, or laryngospasm. Subglottic obstruction can be caused by an intraluminal mass, compression of the trachea by an extratracheal mass, or aspiration of a foreign body. Signs of upper airway obstruction include stridorous or sonorous sounds with inspiration, pronounced intercostal or supraclavicular retraction upon inspiration, and paradoxical movement of the diaphragm.

Initial maneuvers for opening the airway include extension of the head (backward head tilt), with or without anterior jaw thrust and insertion of artificial airways, either oral or nasal. If the obstruction is not relieved immediately, positive pressure ventilation with 100% oxygen should be delivered with a bag-mask combination.

Indications for endotracheal intubation include the provision of a patent airway, protection from aspiration of gastric contents, difficult airway maintenance by mask, the facilitation of mechanical ventilation, and the presence of upper airway mass lesions. In addition, the operative site and operative position may indicate the need for tracheal intubation.

Endotracheal intubation may be performed either awake or asleep, either nasally or orally and may be done directly with a laryngoscope or blindly. A fiberoptic bronchoscope may be used when oropharyngeal structures prevent a direct view of the larynx.

Securing the airway in the presence of risk factors for aspiration of gastric contents requires specific management. Patients are considered to have a "full stomach" when there has been ingestion of liquids or food within 8 hrs. Other risk factors include obesity, pregnancy, hiatal hernia, bowel obstruction, acute abdomen, diabetic gastroparesis, esophageal or gastric pathology, closed head injury, and emergency surgery.

A method of securing the airway of the patient with a full stomach prior to induction of general anesthesia is an awake intubation, either directly with a rigid or fiberoptic laryngoscope or indirectly via a "blind" nasal intubation. If the airway is to be secured after the induction of general anesthesia, then a rapid sequence or "crash" induction is utilized. The patient is preoxygenated with 100% oxygen for 3 to 5 min prior to induction. Administration of an induction agent such as thiopental or etomidate is immediately followed by a rapid-acting depolarizing muscle relaxant such as succinylcholine. After the administration of the induction agent, an assistant holds posterior pressure on the cricord cartilage, functionally closing the most proximal portion of the esophagus (Sellick's maneuver). The patient is *not* ventilated with positive pressure and cricoid pressure *not* removed until the endotracheal tube cuff is inflated and its proper placement verified. Proper position is verified by the presence of bilateral breath sounds and the presence of end-tidal carbon dioxide.

Complications from tracheal intubation may occur during laryngoscopy and intubation, while the tube is in place and after extubation of the trachea. Dental and soft tissue trauma may occur. Release of catecholamines due to laryngoscopy may result in hypertension and tachycardia, cardiac dysrhythmias, and myocardial ischemia. Esophageal intubation and aspiration are also potential complications. After the tube is in place, the tube may obstruct, slip into a mainstream bronchus, or cause tracheal mucosal ischemia. After extubation, complications may be immediate or delayed. Larynogospasm and aspiration of gastric contents are life-threatening complications. Other complications include pharyngitis, laryngitis, edema of the upper airway, laryngeal granuloma formation, tracheal stenosis, vocal cord paralysis, and arytenoid cartilage dislocation.

INTRAVENOUS ANESTHETIC AGENTS

The first modern clinical use of an intravenous anesthetic occured in 1934, when Dr. John Lundy of the Mayo Clinic used sodium thiopental for surgical anesthesia. The pharmokinetic profile of the ultra–short-acting barbiturate allowed for rapid induction of general anesthesia and, after a single intravenous bolus, rapid emergence. The use of thiopental became widespread, being used not only for induction but also maintainance of general anesthesia by repeated bolus or continuous infusion. The outbreak of the Second World War accounted for even greater use of sodium thiopental, with oftentimes disastrous results. The pharmacodynamic profile of thiopental may produce further hemodynamic compromise in an already unstable patient. This is due to venous dilation, arterial vasodilation, and direct myocardial depression resulting in decreases in preload, afterload, contractility, and ultimately hypotension. Thus, thiopental is contraindicated in patients who are markedly hypovolemic, which may be due to either hemorrhage or sepsis, and in patients who have marked impairment of left ventricular function. Sodium thiopental should be used with caution in patients who have compromised coronary or cerebrovascular circulation. Although thiopental has a very short α redistribution half-time, it has a relatively long β-elimination half-time, resulting in a delayed emergence when used for maintainance by repeated boluses or infusion. These problems led pharmacochemists to search for other agents that may have more ideal pharmacodynamic and pharmacokinetic profiles. The following are agents currently in use.

Methohexital, an oxibarbiturate, is also an ultra–short-acting barbiturate. Methohexital has a much shorter β-half-time and does not produce hypotension to the same degree as thiopental. Although it has similar effects on cardiac muscle and the vasculature, it maintains the mean arterial pressure at the expense of increased heart rate, raising heart rate by ~25% after a single intravenous bolus. In addition, methohexital has been shown to produce epileptiform activity on an electroencephalogram and clinically reduces the seizure threshold. Thus, methohexital should be used with caution in patients with underlying coronary artery disease and a history of seizures.

Ketamine, a cyclohexylamine, can be used for induction and maintenance of anesthesia, and at lower doses, sedation and analgesia. It can be given intramuscularly. It produces a disassociative state of anesthesia. Patients may have their eyes open, may phonate, and may exhibit purposeless movement yet are insensate to noxious stimuli. Ketamine causes the release of catecholamines from the CNS and results in tachycardia and hypertension. This action masks the direct depressive effects on the myocardium. Ketamine has direct relaxant effects on bronchial smooth muscle and can be efficacious in patients with reactive airway disease. Unfortunately, ketamine produces a postemergence psychosis, manifesting in ~30% of patients. This psychosis occurs more frequently in younger patients and females, and its incidence is related to the total dose and the rapidity of injection. Ketamine is contraindicated in patients with intracranial hypertension and should be used with caution in patients with coronary artery disease and hypertension.

Benzodiazepines produce anxiolysis and sedation at low doses and unconsciousness at higher doses. Like barbiturates, benzodiazepines bind specifically to the γ-aminobutyric acid (GABA) receptor complex and exert inhibition of neuronal transmission. Benzodiazepines as a class are safe agents, producing little effect on hemodynamic parameters. They are not potent respiratory depressants. At doses used for conscious sedation, benzodiazepines have the ability to produce anterograde amnesia, an important component of any anesthetic. Diazepam, the prototype benzodiazepine, and midazolam are the most commonly used agents. Although diazepam can be given by mouth, midazolam has several clear-cut advantages over diazepam. Midazolam has a much shorter elimination half-time than diazepam does. This allows return of psychomotor functioning sooner and makes it more suitable for same-day surgical procedures. Midazolam is approximately three times more potent than diazepam, and when used for conscious sedation, specific responses to incremental doses are more predictable. Midazolam does not burn when given either intramuscularly or intravenously, and midazolam produces anterograde amnesia more effectively than diazepam.

Etomidate is an induction agent with short elimination and redistribution half-times and stable hemodynamic profile. Unfortunately, etomidate produces depression of plasma glucocorticord and mineralocorticoid levels, and should not be used by infusion for maintenance of general anesthesia. Etomidate is associated with burning on injection and myoclonus.

Propofol, like etomidate, has a very short β half-time, It is suitable to maintain general anesthesia when given by repeated bolus or infusion. Like thiopental, it produces vasodilation and myocardial depression. It is known to produce burning on injection. The pharmacokinetics of propofol may make it suitable for use in ambulatory surgical procedures.

The pharmacokinetics of intravenous agents are summarized in Table 1.

OPIATE ANALGESICS

Opium has been employed for centuries for the treatment of pain, diarrhea, cough, and anxiety. Morphine was first isolated in the 1800s and clinically replaced opium. The discovery of opiate receptors and the development of

TABLE 1. *Pharmacokinetic profiles of intravenous anesthetic agents*

	Redistribution half-life (min)	Elimination half-life (hr)	Clearance (ml × min^{-1})	Volume distribution
Thiopental	2–4	10–12	180–200	100–200
Methohexital	5–6	3–5	700–900	60–80
Etomidate	2–4	2–5	800–1,400	200–400
Propofol	2–4	1–3	1,400–2,800	200–500
Diazepam	10–15	20–40	15–35	60–100
Midazolam	7–15	2–4	300–550	70–130
Ketamine	11–17	2–3	1,250–1,400	200–250

synthetic opioids revolutionized the use of narcotics in the operating room, allowing more critically ill patients to be successfully operated on.

There are four populations of opiate receptors, each having specific effects: μ-receptors for analgesia, respiratory depression, euphoria, and physical dependence; κ-receptors for sedation, miosis, and spinal analgesia; σ-receptors for hallucinations, dysphoria, and cardiac stimulation; and δ-receptors for changes in affective behavior. Clinically, opioids in use today have a spectrum of effects on different receptor populations. They may be classified as agonists (morphine), antagonists (naloxone), or combined agonists-antagonists (nalbuphine).

Morphine

Morphine exerts agonism at both μ and κ receptors, resulting in analgesia, profound respiratory depression, euphoria, sedation, and miosis. The respiratory depression is dose related, preserving tidal volume but causing an overall diminution in alveolar minute ventilation. Thus, as analgesic depth is increased by agonism at μ-receptors, respiratory rate decreases proportionately. Morphine as well as other μ-receptor agonists must be used with extreme caution in patients who have respiratory failure and are not mechanically ventilated. Other CNS effects include miosis, nausea, and vomiting; which are the result of stimulation of the chemoreceptor trigger zone. Narcotic agonists are not amnestic agents, and patients receiving them may experience recall. Hemodynamic effects of morphine are related primarily to release of histamine and arteriolar and venous dilation. Histamine release may also trigger bronchoconstriction. Other effects include increases in bowel transit time and constipation, sphincter of Oddi spasm (resulting in biliary colic), and urinary retention. Morphine is metabolized by the kidney.

Meperidine

Meperidine is a synthetic opioid that has many effects like morphine. It does, however, decrease myocardial contractility and increase heart rate. Meperidine has fewer side effects on the gastrointestinal tract, less pupillary constriction, and a shorter duration of action when compared to morphine. Small doses are sometimes given intravenously to treat postoperative shivering. Like morphine, meperidine is metabolized by the kidney.

Fentanyl

Fentanyl is a synthetic agent related to meperidine. It is ~100 times more potent than morphine and has a more rapid onset and shorter duration of action than morphine. The respiratory depression caused by fentanyl may last longer than its analgesic effects. Fentanyl has no significant hemodynamic effects, but large doses may cause bradycardia. It is metabolized by the liver and excreted by the kidneys. Fentanyl may cause truncal rigidity.

Sufentanil

Sufentanil is 700 to 1,000 times more potent than morphine. Like fentanyl, it has a rapid onset and short duration of action and is rapidly eliminated by the kidneys after being metabolized in the liver. It blocks sympathetic responses to surgical stimuli better than fentanyl, is a more profound respiratory depressant, and may contribute to decreases in myocardial contractility. Its therapeutic index is higher than fentanyl.

Alfentanil

Alfentanil is less potent than fentanyl but has a more rapid onset of action and is more rapidly eliminated. These pharmacokinetic properties make it a suitable agent for ambulatory surgical procedures. Like sufentanyl, it is metabolized by the liver and small bowel and is excreted in urine and feces.

The pharmacokinetics of opiate agents are summarized in Table 2.

INHALATIONAL ANESTHETIC AGENTS

Volatile anesthetics were the first agents to be used for surgical anesthesia. Chloroform and ether combined with

TABLE 2. *Pharmacokinetic profiles of opioid analgesics*

	Elimination half-life (min)	Clearance (ml × kg^{-1} × min^{-1})	Volume of distribution (L × kg^{-1})
Morphine	114	14.7	3.2
Meperidine	180–260	15.1	3.8
Fentanyl	185–220	11.6	4.1
Sufentanil	148–164	12.7	1.7
Alfentanil	70–98	6.4	0.86

nitrous oxide were used for induction and maintenance of anesthesia until the 1930s, when intravenous agents were introduced into clinical practice. Since then, agents with more suitable pharmacokinetics and pharmacodynamics have been developed and provide smoother, safer anesthesia for patients.

Volatile inhalational anesthetics are typically vaporized in an anesthesia machine and then delivered to the patient's lungs via a breathing circuit. The gas molecules cross the alveolar capillary membrane entering the bloodstream and ultimately act on the central nervous system by crossing the blood-brain barrier. Each volatile agent has physical characteristics that affect its uptake and distribution. The pharmacokinetics of these agents are summarized in Table 3.

Alveolar uptake is governed primarily by concentration of the inspired gas, alveolar ventilation, and the functional residual capacity. The rate of rise of the alveolar partial pressure of a volatile agent is more rapid, with increased inspired concentration, increased alveolar ventilation, or decreased functional residual capacity.

The transfer of an inhaled anesthetic from the alveolus to blood is dependent on the blood/gas partition coefficient (solubility), cardiac output, and arterial-venous partial pressure difference. Induction and maintenance of an anesthetic will occur more rapidly with agents that are poorly soluble, in patients with lower cardiac outputs or when the arterial-venous partial pressure difference is greatest.

The minimum alveolar concentration (MAC) is defined as the alveolar concentration of an agent that is needed to prevent movement is 50% of patients when a standard incision is made. MAC may be considered as the ED$_{50}$. An

TABLE 3. *Pharmacokinetic properties of inhaled anesthetic agents*

	MAC (%atm; with O$_2$ only)	Vapor pressure at 20°C (mm Hg)	Partition coefficients at 37°C	
			Blood/Gas	Brain/Blood
Nitrous oxide	104	39,000	0.47	1.1
Halothane	0.74	243	2.54	1.9
Enflurane	1.68	175	1.91	1.4
Isoflurane	1.15	238	1.46	1.6
Desflurane	6.0	664	0.42	1.3
Sevoflurane	2.05	160	0.69	1.7

ED_{95} is achieved when the alveolar concentration of the agent exceeds MAC by ~30%.

Since nitrous oxide diffuses more rapidly onto the blood from the alveolus, large amounts of this gas diffusing into the blood tend to decrease the volume of the alveolar gas mixture and thus increase the relative alveolar concentration of the volatile agent. This increase in the rate of rise of the alveolar concentration of volatile agent is known as the "second gas effect."

Volatile anesthetics are predominantly eliminated via the lungs unchanged. The decrease in alveolar concentrations is influenced by many of the same factors that influence the speed of induction. Alveolar hyperventilation, low cardiac output, decreased functional residual capacity, low solubility, or a large venous-alveolar partial pressure gradient all increase the rate of elimination. A small amount of volatile agent may be metabolized by cytochrome oxidases in the liver and excreted by the kidneys.

The exact mechanism of action of volatile anesthetics is not known, but several theories have been developed. The Myerton-Overton theory states that neuronal transmission in the CNS may be disrupted because of insertion of lypophillic anesthetic molecules into neuronal cell membranes, thus changing the three-dimensional structure of these membranes and hampering transmembrane ionic flow. The receptor hypothesis suggests that volatile anesthetic agents may bind to hydophobic regions of specific membrane receptor proteins in the CNS and impair neuronal transmission. Finally, another theory proposes that volatile agents may interfere with the degradation of the inhibiting neurotransmitter GABA, thus increasing gabaminergic inhibition in the CNS.

The effects of volatile anesthetics on ventilation are similar; all produce dose-dependent decreases in alveolar ventilation. Although these agents may increase the ventilatory rate, a decrease in tidal volume results in the overall diminution of alveolar minute ventilation. Volatile anesthetic agents are bronchodilators, most likely due to decreases in vagal tone.

All volatile agents to greater or lesser degrees produce dose-dependent decreases in mean arterial pressure, cardiac index, stroke volume, and systemic vascular resistance. They also produce dose-dependent increases in heart rate.

MUSCLE RELAXANTS

Muscle relaxants are used to facilitate intubation and provide optimum exposure for surgical procedures. They do so by interrupting normal transmission of impulses at the neuromuscular junction. Muscle relaxants can be classified into two broad categories: depolarizing and nondepolarizing.

The prototype depolarizing agent is succinylcholine, a molecule structurally identical to two molecules of acetylcholine joined together. Succinylcholine mimics the action of acetylcholine, binding to nicotinic postsynaptic receptors and initially causing depolarization of the postsynaptic membrane. Because degradation of succinylcholine is slow, the postsynaptic membrane remains depolarized, preventing further depolarization by acetylcholine. The depolarization produced initially results in transient muscle contractions called "fasciculations." The onset and duration of action of succinylcholine is short, with recovery occurring in 5 to 10 min after an intubating dose. Prolonged recovery may occur in patients who have abnormal or decreased levels of plasma cholinesterase. Possible side effects include bradycardia, nodal rhythm, sinus arrest, hyperkalemia, myalgia, and increases in intragastric, intraoccular, and intracranial pressure. Myoglobinuria and trismus may also occur. Succinylcholine may also be a trigger for malignant hyperthermia. Succinylcholine is contraindicated in patients with massive crush injuries, burns, denervation injuries related to spinal cord transsection, and upper motor neuron injury.

Nondepolarizing neuromuscular blocking agents act as pure antagonists of nicotinic receptors present on postjunctional muscle membranes. They bind competitively, preventing depolarization by acetylcholine. Nondepolarizing agents are classified as short, intermediate, or long acting. Some agents, such as curare, metocurine, atracurium, and mivacurium, cause release of histamine and can cause hemodynamic compromise. Pancuronium exerts a vagolytic effect resulting in tachycardia. Metabolism and excretion of these agents occur to varying degrees in the liver and kidney depending on the agent. The degree of blockade is monitored with a peripheral nerve stimulator. The classification and pharmacology of these muscle relaxants is summarized in Table 4.

The paralysis produced by nondepolorizing neuromuscular blocking agents can be reversed by administration of an acetylcholinsterase inhibitor such as neostigmine, pyridostigmine, or edrophonium.

LOCAL ANESTHETICS

Local anesthetics block nerve conduction when infiltrated into the surgical field by the surgeon or injected in proximity of nerve bundles to produce anesthesia in regions of the body. Historically, cocaine was used clinically as the first local anesthetic in the 1880s, both as a field anesthetic and regional anesthetic. Its side effects limited its use. Procaine came into clinical use after the turn of the century; agents with more suitable pharmacokinetics and pharmacodynamics were introduced later. Their pharmacology is summarized in Table 5.

TABLE 4. *Classification and pharmacology of nondepolarizing neuromuscular blocking agents*

	ED$_{95}$ (mg × kg^{-1})	Onset to maximum twitch depression (min)	Recovery to control twitch height (min)
Intermediate action			
Atracurium	0.15–0.30	3–5	20–35
Vecuronium	0.04–0.07	3–5	20–35
Mivacurium	0.08	2–3	12–20
Long action			
D-Tubocurarine	0.51	3–5	60–90
Pancuronium	0.07	3–5	60–90
Pipercuronium	0.07	3–5	50–80
Doxacurium	0.25–0.40	4–6	60–80

Local anesthetics exist in basic and protonated forms of their hydrochloride salt. The uncharged form is lipophilic and readily diffuses through neuronal membranes. Several theories exist regarding the mechanism of action of local anesthetic agents. The membrane expansion theory suggests that local anesthetic agents insert themselves into the bilipid membrane, causing three-dimensional changes in the architecture of ion channels, thus preventing depolarization. The membrane receptor theory hypothesizes that local anesthetics displace calcium and bind to receptors within sodium channels, ultimately preventing depolarization. Finally, the surface charge theory suggests that the negatively charged membrane surface is neutralized by the protonated form of the local anesthetic. This effectively hyperpolarizes the neuron, making it more difficult for depolarization to occur.

Systemic absorption is related to the total dose, site of injection, protein binding, and whether a vasoconstrictor is used in the anesthetic solution. Ester agents are degraded by esterases in the liver and plasma, and the method of metabolism is agent specific. Amide agents are degraded completely by the liver. When plasma levels of local anesthetics reach toxic levels, their effects are seen in the CNS. Inhibitory transmission is depressed first, resulting in agitation, excitation, and potentially seizures. If plasma levels become high enough, depression of all centers occurs and coma ensues. Toxic levels of local anesthetics can cause myocardial depression and decreases in myocardial conduction, resulting in cardiovascular collapse. Allergic reactions are infrequent, with most reports being attributed to ester agents.

REGIONAL ANESTHESIA

Local anesthetics can be used to produce spinal anesthesia, epidural anesthesia, or peripheral nerve blockade. Spinal anesthesia involves injection of local anesthesia into the subarachnoid space. The procedure is performed much in the same manner as is a diagnostic lumbar puncture. After return of cerebrospinal fluid is noted to verify proper positioning of the spinal needle, a small dose of anesthetic is injected, usually lidocaine, tetracaine, or bupivicaine. The level of sensory and motor blockade is dependent on the vertebral interspace used, the position of the patient, the baricity of the solution, the total dose of the anesthetic, and the speed of injection. Achievement of very high levels of blockade can result in respiratory arrest and cardiovascular collapse, owing to paralysis of the respiratory muscles and blockade of sympathetic nerve fibers. Other complications include hypotension, postdural puncture headache, bleeding, and infections. Absolute contraindications to spinal anesthesia are coagulopathy, shock, and untreated bacteremia.

Epidural anesthesia is performed in a manner similar to spinal anesthesia except that the anesthetic is deposited in the epidural space and a larger volume of anesthetic solution is infused. A catheter may be inserted into the epidural space, and repeated doses may be given for longer procedures. In addition, this catheter may be used for administrations of a combinations of local anesthetic and opiate for postoperative analgesia. Inadvertent subarachnoid injection of the anesthetic will result in a "total spinal" with respiratory arrest and cardiovascular collapse. Like subarachnoid anesthesia, epidural techniques are contraindicated in the setting of shock, coagulopathy, and untreated bacteremia.

Upper extremities may be anesthetized by blocking the brachial plexus. Two common approaches to the brachial plexus are the interscalene and axillary approach. The interscalene technique is associated with a risk of pneumothorax, phrenic and laryngeal nerve paralysis, and vertebral artery injection. Although the axillary approach is more popular because of a lower incidence of pneumothorax, it still carries with it a risk of intravascular injection. The hand may be anesthetized

TABLE 5. *Classification and pharmacology of local anesthetic agents*

Classification	Onset of action	Duration of action (min)	Maximum adult dose (mg)
Esters			
Procaine	Slow	45–60	500
Chlorprocaine	Rapid	30–45	600
Tetracaine	Slow	60–180	100
Amides			
Lidocaine	Rapid	60–120	300
Mepivacaine	Slow	90–180	300
Bupivacaine	Slow	240–480	175

by blocking the median nerve, ulnar nerve, and the radial nerve. Lower extremity surgery can be carried out by blocking the femoral and sciatic nerves. All five nerves of the foot can be blocked at the level of the ankle. As with all regional techniques, these blocks are contraindicated when coagulopathy is present.

MONITORING

Standard monitors for any anesthetic delivered include electrocardiogram, pulse oximetry, blood pressure device, and a precordial stethoscope to ensure adequacy of ventilation. A method to measure temperature should be available. Capnography is indicated for any general anesthetic. Additional monitoring, such as invasive arterial, central venous, or pulmonary artery pressure devices may be indicated because of the patient's medical condition or the extent of the surgical procedure.

STUDY QUESTIONS

1. Characterize "appropriate" preoperative evaluation of patients to undergo elective procedures by anesthesiologists.
2. Describe basic aspects of "airway management."
3. Discuss the different types of agents (e.g., intravenous agents, inhalational agents) utilized in administering surgical anesthesia.
4. What are the advantages and disadvantages of local anesthesia?
5. What are the advantages and disadvantages of regional anesthesia?

SUGGESTED READING

Danson JK, Eckhardt WF, Perese DA. *Clinical anesthesia: procedures of the Massachusetts General Hospital.* 4th ed. Boston. Little, Brown, 1993.
Stoelting RK, Miller RD. *Basics of anesthesia.* 3rd ed. New York: Churchill-Livingstone, 1994.

CHAPTER 31

Gynecology and Gynecologic Oncology

Ricardo Estape, Marilu Madrigal, and Manuel A. Penalver

Gynecology was first created as a subspecialty of general surgery and only recently has it been combined with obstetrics. An understanding of gynecology and gynecologic oncology is essential to the study of surgery since there are many surgical diseases whose differential diagnosis includes gynecologic entities and vice versa. The pelvis is continuous with the abdominal cavity, and a good surgeon should be intimately aware of the anatomy and diseases of the pelvis to provide good patient care.

NORMAL PHYSIOLOGY

In the female reproductive cycle, ovulation is followed by menstrual bleeding in a predictable sequence if conception does not occur: beginning at puberty (11 to 13 years old) and continuing to menopause (48 to 52 years old). A regular reproductive cycle of ~28 days is usually established by age 15 and is dependent on the hypothalamic-pituitary-ovarian hormonal axis.

The hypothalamus produces hypothalamic gonadotropin-releasing hormone (GnRH) in a pulsatile fashion which induces the pituitary gland to produce follicle-stimulating hormone (FSH) and luteinizing hormone (LH). FSH stimulates the ovary to mature its follicles and produce estradiol, which prepares the endometrium for implantation. LH at midcycle stimulates ovulation of the lead follicle, which in turn becomes the corpus luteum and produces progesterone, which stabilizes the endometrium for implantation. This ongoing cycle begins at puberty and ends around 51 years of age when viable follicles have been depleted.

Increased levels of these hormones, estradiol and progesterone, are responsible for the changes of puberty. Likewise, their withdrawal is responsible for the opposite changes in the menopause. These hormones affect not only the female genital tract, but also the breasts, skin, cholesterol levels (increase HDL and decrease LDL), bones, vascular system, and psychological characteristics

in women. Each of these changes is beyond the scope of this review; however, many patients' visits are associated with cyclic changes, and the menstrual history should be a routine part of a thorough patient history.

PELVIC ANATOMY

The gynecologist and surgeon should be familiar with the Pfannenstiel, Maylard, Cherney, and midline vertical incisions. Most benign pelvic operations can be done with the transverse Pfannenstiel "bikini cut" incision. The muscle-splitting incisions such as the Maylard and Cherney are used for more difficult or extensive pelvic procedures that are limited to the pelvis and lower abdomen. The majority of pelvic cancer procedures are done through a midline incision since pelvic tumors spread cephalad via both lymphatic and intraperitoneal routes. Visualization through low transverse incisions is extraordinarily difficult.

The pelvic organs include the uterus, tubes, ovaries, bladder, and rectosigmoid colon. The support, vascular supply, and lymphatic drainage of these tissues are in the retroperitoneum, and therefore the pelvic surgeon must become intimately familiar with these structures and their exposure (Figs. 1 and 2).

The ovarian arteries arise from the aorta bilaterally and travel in the infundibulopelvic ligament to supply the ovaries and fallopian tubes. The left ovarian vein drains to the left renal vein, whereas the right ovarian vein drains into the inferior vena cava. The uterine arteries arise bilaterally from the internal iliac arteries (hypogastric arteries), and the uterine veins drain into the hypogastric veins. The hypogastric arteries can be ligated bilaterally, to decrease blood loss in the pelvis, without causing necrosis to other pelvic structures since there is a large amount of collateral circulation in the pelvis.

A large number of nerves traverse the pelvis on their way to the lower torso as well as the legs. The femoral and obturator nerves arise from the lumbar plexus and

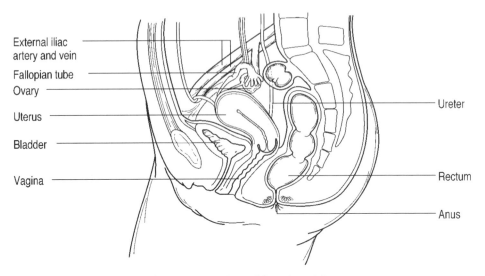

FIG. 1. Lateral view of female pelvis.

traverse the retroperitoneal area. These nerves are important landmarks in pelvic and inguinal node dissection in cancer surgery. The sciatic and internal pudendal nerves arise from the sacral plexus and must be identified to avoid injury when operating deep in the pelvis. The autonomic nerve supply of the pelvic viscera is organized in ganglia and travels through the cardinal and uterosacral ligaments to and from the spinal cord. Transection of these fibers can lead to impaired bladder and rectal function postoperatively.

The ligaments of the pelvis have several functions, which include support of the uterus as well as transport for nerve bundles, vessels, and lymphatics. The round ligament arises from the anterior/superior surface of the uterus, travels to the side wall and through the inguinal canal, and inserts on the labia majora. The broad ligament is simply the visceral peritoneum overlying the uterus and tubes. The cardinal ligaments are the main support for the uterus and travel from the lateral surface of the cervix and upper vagina to the obturator internus

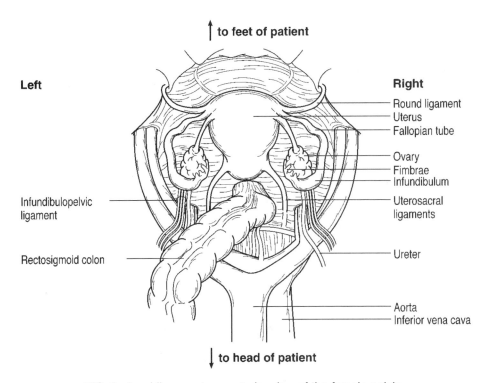

FIG. 2. An oblique, anteroposterior view of the female pelvis.

fascia. The uterosacral ligaments travel from the posterior cervix to the periosteum of the presacral space. Weakness and tears of these ligaments during childbirth and after the withdrawal of estrogen in the menopause can lead to the finding of uterine prolapse (Fig. 3) as well as cystoceles, rectoceles, and enteroceles.

With knowledge of all these structures, careful retroperitoneal dissection separates the uterus, tubes, and ovaries from the adjacent large vessels and ureters. The ureters can be traced from the pelvic brim to the pelvis and through the cardinal ligament, which they traverse before entering the bladder. The three most common areas of ureteral injury are at the level of the infundibulopelvic ligament, at the level of the cardinal ligament and at the cervico-vaginal junction, where the ureter turns towards the bladder.

The muscles of the pelvis are also important in support of the pelvic organs. The main muscle of the pelvis is the levator ani with its component pubo-, ileo-, and ischiococcygeus muscles. The levator ani arises from the arcus tendineus, which is the connective tissue sling of the obturator internus muscle. The piriformis muscle completes the inner musculature of the pelvis. The bony skeleton of the pelvis is composed of the pubis, the ilium, and the ischium anteriorly and laterally and by the sacrum posteriorly.

ABNORMAL BLEEDING

When evaluating abnormal bleeding, patient's age is of prime importance. After menopause, which is defined as cessation of menses for 12 months, vaginal bleeding is always considered abnormal, and endometrial cancer should be considered. Although the most common cause of vaginal bleeding is atrophic vaginitis in this age group, endometrial sampling or dilatation and curettage should be performed to exclude the possibility of uterine malignancy.

During the reproductive years, any abnormality of bleeding should be considered a complication of pregnancy until proven otherwise. A pregnancy test should be obtained in any females of reproductive age with complaints of irregular bleeding. A positive pregnancy test in the face of vaginal bleeding is considered a threatened or incomplete abortion, or an ectopic pregnancy, which can be life threatening. Threatened abortions are treated with bed rest; incomplete abortions are treated by uterine curettage. Ectopic pregnancies are fertilized ovum implanted in the fallopian tubes that have disastrous potential. Ruptured ectopic pregnancy is a principal diagnosis that must be considered in females of reproductive age with acute abdominal pain. Exsanguination and death can result from untreated ectopic pregnancy that has ruptured. Ectopic pregnancy has traditionally been treated with a salpingectomy; however, newer techniques allow for more conservative methods, including salpingostomy and even medical management with chemotherapy (Methotrexate) in selected patients. If pregnancy has been excluded, anatomical causes of bleeding should be considered. Fibroid uterus, cervical polyps, endometrial polyps, malignancies, and hyperplasia of the endometrium are the most commonly encountered diseases in this setting. Dilatation and curettage, in the office or operating room, as well as pelvic ultrasound are useful in the diagnosis of anatomical causes of bleeding. Although definitive treatment of a fibroid uterus is a hysterectomy, more conservative methods such as myomectomy and medical management are used in selected patients. In the absence of pregnancy and anatomical lesions, hormonal imbalance should be considered. Anovulation, the failure of ovulation, is characterized by the lack of progesterone production seen after ovulation, leads to unopposed estrogen and abnormal bleeding.

In the premenarchal age group, vaginal bleeding is abnormal and is most commonly associated with a foreign body in the vagina. Other causes of premenarchal vaginal bleeding include rape, ovarian malignancy, and hormonal ingestion. These patients should be evaluated by an examination under anesthesia to rule out a foreign body as well as other pathology. Hormonal evaluations should also be done to rule out precocious puberty.

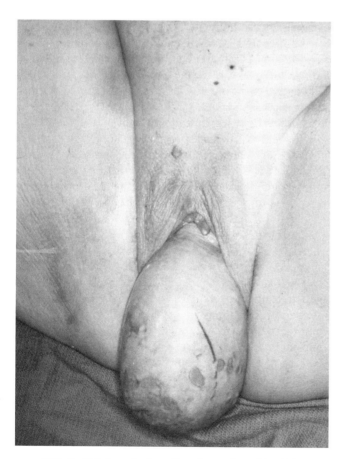

FIG. 3. Total vaginal vault prolapse (procidentia).

PELVIC INFECTIONS

Sexually transmitted diseases ranging from simple vaginitis to acquired immunodeficiency syndrome (AIDS) have become more prevalent in the past 30 years. Many of these infections are localized to the vagina, but many can ascend the vagina and enter the peritoneal cavity through the uterus and fallopian tubes. These infections can be indolent or very aggressive and cause pelvic abscesses, acute abdominal pain, and infertility as well as chronic pelvic pain long term.

The sexual habits and mode of expression that individuals choose will affect their risk for infection as well as the site of infection. For this reason, a careful sexual history can guide in the diagnosis of these pelvic infections. Risk factors include unprotected intercourse, multiple partners, low socioeconomic status, poor hygiene, history of sexually transmitted diseases, and all the same factors in the patients' partner.

Infection of the upper female genital tract, pelvic inflammatory disease (PID), is predominantly by direct ascent along the mucosal surfaces. The predominant organisms are *Chlamydia trachomatis* and *Neisseria gonorrhea*. The endocervical mucous usually prevents ascending infection, but around the time of the menses this thick mucous breaks down and may allow an ascending infection. This also explains how oral contraceptives decrease PID by creating a consistently thick mucous.

PID can range from mild symptomatology to severe infection with peritonitis from free pus in the peritoneal cavity. The relative mobility of the fallopian tube contributes to the rapid and widespread extension of the infection. In this anaerobic environment, anaerobes thrive so that the infection in the upper genital tract is usually polymicrobial with a mixture of aerobic and anaerobic bacteria. In patients with severe infections, tubo-ovarian abscesses (TOA) may form. These patients are usually acutely ill with high fevers, tachycardia, severe abdominal or pelvic pain, nausea, vomiting, and even changes in bowel habits.

On examination, patients with PID exhibit muscular guarding, rebound tenderness, purulent cervical discharge, cervical motion tenderness, and an adnexal mass. The clinical presentation mimics appendicitis, diverticulitis, ectopic pregnancy, and other less common problems. PID should always be included in the differential diagnosis of the above problems, and if there is a question as to the diagnosis, the patient can be evaluated with diagnostic laparoscopy.

Aggressive therapy for patients with PID is necessary to attempt to prevent long-term sequelae such as infertility and pelvic pain. Patients with mild symptomatology and no peritoneal irritation signs can be treated with oral doxycycline (100 mg oral for 1 week) and one intramuscular injection of ceftriaxone (250 mg) as recommended by the Centers for Disease Control. More severe symptomatology must be treated with intravenous antibiotics in a hospitalized setting. Other criteria for inpatient treatment are nulliparous patients, TOAs, paralytic ileus, previous treatment failure, immunocompromised patient, or uncertain diagnosis.

In the face of clinical uncertainty, diagnostic laparoscopy is considered the gold standard. Laparoscopy will show free pus in cul-de-sac, inflamed fallopian tubes, or possibly TOA. In contrast, the appendix as well as other intraperitoneal structures will appear normal. In more recent literature, TOA can be treated by drainage in the young nulliparous patient but should be treated with hysterectomy and bilateral salpingo-oophorectomy in the postmenopausal and in those near the menopause (>40) who have completed childbearing.

ADNEXAL MASSES AND OVARIAN CANCER

The definition of the world adnexa is "appendages to the main organ," and in the pelvis, adnexal masses refer to enlargements that are palpable and adjacent to the uterus. For the most part, these masses represent ovarian enlargements, and their evaluation is facilitated by identifying patient age. Adnexal masses found in the postmenopausal period are considered abnormal and should be evaluated for malignancy. Complex adnexal masses are malignant in up to 50% of these cases. Total abdominal hysterectomy with bilateral salpingo-oophorectomy (TAH/BSO) has minimal morbidity and is considered the standard of care. Perhaps the only situation in which postmenopausal adnexal masses can be observed is in a patient with a unilateral cystic mass that is <5 cm and a normal CA-125 (ovarian cancer tumor marker) level.

In the reproductive age group, most adnexal masses are physiologic in nature. During this time period, the ovaries fluctuate between a follicular and a luteal phase, which routinely produces fluid-filled cysts. These are physiologic cysts and should be followed conservatively with reevaluation in 2 to 3 months, with an expectation for spontaneous resolution. If, after 3 months of observation, the cyst persists, the patient should have it excised. Oral contraceptives have been shown to increase the resolution of these cysts by downregulating the FSH and LH production from the pituitary and thus removing ovarian stimulation. Situations in which adnexal masses in the reproductive age group are not considered to be physiologic include complex masses such as endometriomas, TOA, dermoid cyst, and cancer. The incidence of ovarian carcinoma in the reproductive age group is between 3% and and 5%. Ultrasound, history, and tumor markers (CA-125, β–human chorionic gonadotropin, lactic dehydrogenase, α-fetoprotein) can help distinguish benign from malignant masses.

In the premenarchal age group, adnexal masses are also considered abnormal. As in the postmenopausal period, the premenarchal girl has static ovaries and therefore should not have functional or physiologic enlargements. Enlargements are evaluated by laparoscopy with minimal morbidity. A conservative approach to ovarian cysts should be followed whenever possible. Only in extreme cases should the ovary be removed in its entirety. With improvements in reproductive technology, conservation of the uterus, tubes, and the largest amount of normal ovary can preserve fertility.

Neoplastic ovarian masses (Fig. 4) can arise from any one of three germ cell layers: the epithelial layer, the germ cell layer, or the stromal layer. Benign epithelial tumors include serous cystadenomas, mucinous cystadenomas, endometriomas, and Brenner cell tumors. Benign germ cell tumors include benign cystic teratoma (dermoid), the most common tumor of the ovary. Benign stromal masses include granulosa cell, theca cell, and Sertoli-Leydig cell tumors.

Ovarian cancer is the fifth most common cancer among females in the United States and the second most common gynecologic malignancy. It has the highest mortality rate of all gynecologic malignancies, with a 5-year survival rate of 30%. Early detection is difficult, and most patients present with advanced disease. It is most commonly found in women 50 to 60 years of age with European ethnic background and decreased fertility or delayed childbearing.

Ovarian cancer is surgically staged (Table 1) and should be treated by TAH/BSO, omentectomy, and pelvic and paraaortic lymphadenectomy if tumor is confined to pelvis and radical tumor debulking. Studies have shown that optimal debulking of the tumor, which is described as removal of all gross tumor lesions and deposits to less than 1 centimeter, provides longer disease-free survival and higher response rates to chemotherapy. All patients

beyond stage IA disease should undergo adjuvant chemotherapy with close follow-up.

Approximately 70% of patients exhibited response to chemotherapy, especially Taxol and cisplatin. Unfortunately, the 5-year survival rates have not changed in the past 30 years. The mainstay of therapy continues to be debulking for primary and resectable recurrences, followed by chemotherapy. This is true for the epithelial carcinomas, which comprise 90% of all ovarian malignancies but is not true for germ cell malignancies.

Germ cell carcinomas (i.e., dysgerminoma, immature teratoma) are treated with debulking much like the epithelial tumors, but these tumors, even in the face of advanced stage, respond well to chemotherapy. Early disease (stage I and II) have cure rates approaching 95% with current chemotherapy regimens. Aggressive therapy should therefore be undertaken in this cell type of tumor. Disease confined to the ovary can be treated with conservative surgery, e.g., oophorectomy, if future fertility is desired.

TABLE 1. *FIGO staging for ovarian carcinoma*

Stage	Criteria
I	Growth limited to the ovaries
II	Growth involving one or both ovaries with pelvic extension
III	Tumor in one or both ovaries with peritoneal implants outside the pelvis and/or positive retroperitoneal nodes or inguinal nodes, or superficial liver implants
IV	Distant metastasis, malignant pleural effusions, or parenchymal liver disease

FIGO: International Federations of Gynecologists and Obstetricians.

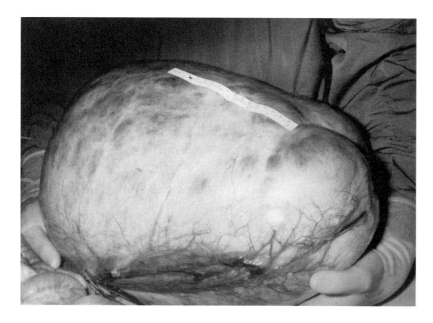

FIG. 4. An intraoperative view of an enormous mucinous cystadenoma of the ovary.

CERVICAL DYSPLASIA AND CANCER

In the early 1940s, cervical cancer was the most common gynecologic malignancy. Presently, it ranks behind endometrial and ovarian cancer in annual incidence. The death rate as well has decreased by 70%. This can all be attributed to the work of Papanicolaou and Traut, who demonstrated that cervical cancer and frequently endometrial cancer could be diagnosed by cervical smear. Although it remains a major health issue in the United States, it represents a formidable clinical problem in Third World countries. The incidence of cervical cancer in the United States is 15 per 100,000 Caucasian women and 34 per 100,000 African-American women. This is in contrast to an estimated incidence of 65 per 100,000 women in Third World countries and even higher in areas of Africa and South America. An estimated 14,900 new cases of cervical cancer will be diagnosed in the United States in 1997, with an additional 60,000 new cases of carcinoma in situ and 250,000 new cases of cervical dysplasia.

The scope of cervical neoplasia ranges from the preinvasive dysplasia to the invasive cervical cancer. This is one of a handful of cancers that have been proven to have precursor lesions that progress to invasive lesions. With this knowledge of precursor lesions, cancers can be treated in their infancy with minimally invasive procedures and cured prior to the invasive transformation.

Prior to birth, the vagina and cervix are covered with columnar epithelium, which soon becomes replaced with squamous epithelium. The junction between the squamous epithelium and the columnar epithelium originating in the endocervical canal is referred to as the squamocolumnar junction (SQJ). During adolescence as well as during the first pregnancy, the SQJ moves outward toward the external cervical os. The area between this new SQJ and the old SQJ is called the "transformation zone," and it is this area that is most susceptible to the carcinogenic effects of sexually transmitted diseases, in particular human papillomavirus (HPV) and to a lesser degree Trichomonas, *Chlamydia trachomatis,* and spermatozoal DNA.

Major risk factors for the development of dysplasia and cervical cancer are early onset of sexual intercourse (<20), multiple sexual partners (>2), smoking, and presence of HPV infection (especially subtypes 16, 18, 31, 33, 35, 39, and possibly 42). Large screening studies for HPV prevalence have demonstrated that as high as 50% to 60% of college-aged women who have been screened are positive for HPV and may or may not have cytopathologic changes suggestive of HPV infection or dysplasia.

The terminology of preinvasive disease has undergone many changes since the work of Papanicolaou. The use of class I to V, mild to severe dysplasia, and cervical intraepithelial neoplasia (CIN I to III) pap smear interpretations has fallen out of favor and has been replaced by the Bethesda system for nomenclature of pap smears.

The new Bethesda system (Table 2) has only three categories for preinvasive disease, which are as follows: (a) ASCUS, atypical squamous cells of undetermined significance that are nondysplastic cells that have some abnormal qualities; (b) SIL low grade, squamous intraepithelial lesion low grade, which accounts for minimally dysplastic cells as well as those cells that have koilocytic changes suggestive of HPV infection, a known major risk factor and possibly an etiologic agent for dysplasia; and (c) SIL high grade, which accounts for the moderate to severe dysplasia as well as the carcinoma in situ. This new system was devised to stratify those lesions that need definitive treatment from those lesions that can be evaluated and followed without invasive treatment.

TABLE 2. *1991 Bethesda system: categories of reported information*

Adequacy of the specimen
  Satisfactory for evaluation
  Satisfactory for evaluation but limited by *(specific reason)*
  Unsatisfactory for evaluation *(specific reason)*
Descriptive diagnosis
  Benign cellular changes
    Infection
      Trichomonas vaginalis
      Fungal organisms consistent morphologically with candida sp.
      Predominance of coccobacilli consistent with shift in vaginal flora
      Bacterial morphologically consistent with Actinomyces sp.
      Cellular changes associated with herpes simplex virus
    Reactive changes
      Reactive cellular changes associated with:
        Inflammation (includes typical repair)
        Atrophy with inflammation ("atrophic vaginitis")
        Radiation
        Intrauterine devices
        Other
  Epithelial cell abnormalities
    Squamous cells
      Atypical squamous cells of undetermined significance
      Low-grade squamous intraepithelial lesion (HPV, mild dysplasia/CIN I)
      High-grade squamous intraepithelial lesion (moderate-severe dysplasia, CIN II, CIN III, CIS)
      Squamous cell carcinoma
    Glandular cells
      Endometrial cells, cytologically benign, in postmenopausal woman
      Atypical glandular cells of undetermined significance
      Endocervical adenocarcinoma
      Endometrial carcinoma
        Extrauterine adenocarcinoma
        Adenocarcinoma, not otherwise specified
    Other malignant neoplasm

Pap smears are only a screening tool and as such should never be used for management decisions on patients. Any abnormal pap smear showing SIL low grade or high grade requires colposcopy and colposcopy-directed biopsies. For patients with two consecutive pap smears showing ASCUS, they too should undergo colposcopy.

Colposcopy consists of using a magnifying scope with acetic acid to identify the transformation zone and biopsy any abnormal area. Abnormal areas are seen as a continuum ranging from simple white lesions to vascular punctations to vascular mosaicism to grossly abnormal cervix and vessels. The colposcopy-directed biopsies are then used for diagnosis of the lesion. Lesions that show ASCUS or minimal dysplasia on biopsy can be followed conservatively since they have a very high regression rate (60%). Lesions that show SIL high grade require a larger biopsy—cone biopsy or loop electrosurgical excision procedure (LEEP)—which can be used to exclude a more invasive procedure. Wide excision may be definitive therapy as well. LEEP can be done in the clinic and consists of a thin wire in the shape of a loop that is used to cut and coagulate across the cervix to remove the concerning lesion. Other procedures that have been used in the past and are still used but to a lesser degree are cryotherapy of the cervix and laser ablation of the cervix. These procedures, however, do not give a tissue diagnosis and cannot rule out invasion. The clinical ease of LEEP and its ability to give tissue diagnosis have taken these other procedures out of favor except in select patients. After LEEP, patients should be monitored closely every 3 to 6 months to rule out persistence or recurrence of their dysplasia. After completion of the appropriate procedures, the diagnosis of cervical cancer can be made from the pathology report. Once the diagnosis is made, disease must be staged to decide the appropriate course of therapy.

Staging of cervical cancer, unlike ovarian and endometrial, is done using clinical and not surgical parameters. For adequate clinical staging, a thorough pelvic exam, chest radiograph, intravenous pyelogram, cystoscopy, and sigmoidoscopy are required. The criteria for cervical cancer staging (Table 3) has recently been changed by FIGO to further stratify patients by prognosis. With careful clinical staging, the majority of patients can be stratified adequately so that their prognosis correlates with their stage of disease.

Patients who have stage IA1 cervical cancer can be treated with a simple hysterectomy alone. Patients with stage IA2 or IB1 can be treated with radical hysterectomy as well as pelvic and paraaortic lymphadenectomy. Patients with stage IB2 or above may get a staging laparotomy to evaluate the extent of the disease or can be treated with radiation therapy alone if the tumor is confined to the pelvis. Chemotherapy is added if tumor is found to have metastasized outside of the pelvis and the lower abdomen.

Radical surgery and pelvic irradiation are the mainstay of cervical cancer therapy as these tumors respond very poorly to present chemotherapeutic regimens. Radical surgery was first reported by Ernst Wertheim in 1900. Radiation therapy then became standard therapy until the 1940s, when Meigs reported increased survival after radical lymphadenectomy was added to the classical Wertheim radical hysterectomy. The difference between the simple and radical hysterectomy is in the amount of parametrial and paracervical tissue that is removed. In the simple hysterectomy, the clamps are placed directly adjacent to the cervix and across the external os to remove only the uterus and cervix, and a minimal portion of the vagina. In the radical hysterectomy, the uterosacral ligaments and cardinal ligaments that support the uterus as well as carry lymphatics are transected near the pelvic side wall to allow adequate margins on the tumor. The vagina is transected ~2 cm below the external cervical os to remove the upper portion of the vagina for adequate tumor margins. The results of the Wertheim/Meig's combined procedure have been verified by several authors in large studies, and this procedure can achieve 5-year survival rates of 85% in early-stage cervical cancer. Overall 5-year survival rates correlate with stage and are shown below (Table 4).

TABLE 3. *FIGO staging of carcinoma of the cervix*

Stage	Criteria
I	Carcinoma is strictly confined to the cervix
IA	Preclinical carcinoma of the cervix (diagnosed only by microscopy)
IA1	Minimal microscopic evidence of stromal invasion (<3 mm)
IA2	Microscopic lesions that are ≥3 mm of invasion but <5 mm in depth and <7 mm in width of horizontal spread
IB	Microscopic lesions that are ≥5 mm in depth and/or 7 mm in horizontal spread but are still confined to the cervix.
IB1	IB lesions that are <4 cm in maximum diameter
IB2	IB lesions that are >4 cm in maximum diameter ("bulky IB")
IIA	Extends to the upper two-thirds of the vagina
IIB	Extends to the paracervical/parametrial tissue
IIIA	Extends to the lower one-third of the vagina
IIIB	Extends to pelvic side wall by examination, or intravenous pyelogram shows ureteral obstruction
IVA	Bladder or rectal mucosa involvement
IVB	Distant metastasis

TABLE 4. *Five-year survival for treated cervical carcinoma*

FIGO stage	Five-year survival
IA	99%
IB	85–90%
IIA	73–80%
IIB	60–68%
IIIA	40–45%
IIIB	30–38%
IVA	10–15%
IVB	1–3%

The benefits of radical surgery for early-stage cervical cancer versus radiation therapy are clear. Surgical benefits include preservation of ovarian function in young women, preservation of sexual function (which is not seen in radiation-treated patients secondary to vaginal fibrosis and stenosis), and finally prevention of long-term radiation effects. On the other hand, surgery can have some immediate complications such as hemorrhage, dysfunctional bladder and urinary fistulas. It is very important that the risks and benefits of treatment are discussed with the patient.

Patient follow-up is critical as most cervical cancers recur within the first 2 years posttreatment. Careful serial vaginal examinations and biopsies, as indicated, are necessary. CT scans have also been used to detect early recurrences and should be used routinely in the first 1 to 2 years.

Recurrent disease is associated with a very poor prognosis. Distant recurrences can be treated with isolated radiation or chemotherapy, but current protocols offer little long-term benefit. Central recurrences, in very select patients, can be treated with "pelvic exenteration," i.e., the en bloc removal of disease and all involved pelvic organs. In select patients, this procedure offers a success rate of 40% to 50%.

ENDOMETRIAL HYPERPLASIA AND CANCER

The relationship between estrogen production and endometrial growth is quite clear. Endometrial proliferation represents a normal part of the menstrual cycle and occurs during the follicular or estrogen-dependent phase. With continued estrogen stimulation, unopposed by progesterone, simple endometrial proliferation will become endometrial hyperplasia. Endometrial hyperplasia is thus defined as the abnormal proliferation of both glandular and stromal elements leading to altered histologic architecture. Unlike cervical carcinoma precursors, there is no formal agreement that these hyperplastic lesions will progress to endometrial cancer if left untreated. It is, however, clear that some types of hyperplasia have an increased tendency toward endometrial carcinoma.

Risk factors for endometrial hyperplasia include those conditions that produce unopposed estrogen stimulation of the endometrium. Exogenous estrogens without progesterone will induce hyperplasia. Other risk factors include anovulation, obesity (increased peripheral conversion of androstenedione to estrone by enzymes in fat cells), estrogen-secreting tumors, and tamoxifen. Although tamoxifen is an antiestrogen, it has weak estrogenic properties and acts as unopposed estrogen.

Endometrial hyperplasia has long been called by many names, but the International Society of Gynecologic Pathologists has recently adopted new terminology that clarifies some of the previous problems. The new terminology includes only "simple" and "complex hyperplasia" depending on the amount of glandular crowding and includes the presence or absence of nuclear atypia. Through recent studies, it has become more evident that only those hyperplasia with nuclear atypia have a propensity to undergo malignant transformation.

The diagnosis of endometrial hyperplasia can be made by taking a sample of the endometrium. The most common indication for endometrial sampling is abnormal uterine bleeding. Simple or complex hyperplasia without nuclear atypia can be easily treated with medical management. Treatment involves progestational agents for 10 to 12 days/month. Hyperplasia with nuclear atypia are more likely to become endometrial cancer and as such should be treated with simple hysterectomy.

Endometrial cancer is the most common gynecologic malignancy (Fig. 5). As with hyperplasia, it is usually a

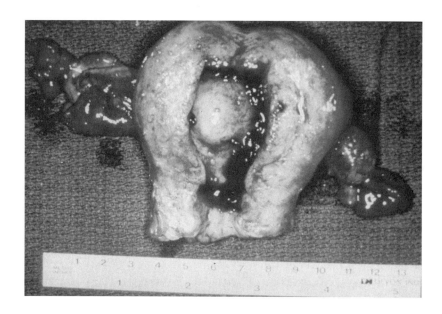

FIG. 5. Uterus (bivalved) revealing a focus of endometrial carcinoma.

TABLE 5. *FIGO staging of endometrial carcinoma*

Stage	Criteria
IA	Tumor confined to endometrium
IB	Tumor confined to inner half of myometrium
IC	Tumor extends to outer half of myometrium
IIA	Tumor extends to endocervical glands
IIB	Tumor extends to endocervical stroma
IIIA	Tumor invades serosa, adnexa, and/or positive peritoneal cytology
IIIB	Vaginal metastasis
IIIC	Positive pelvic and/or periaortic lymph nodes
IVA	Tumor invades bladder and/or bowel mucosa
IVB	Distant metastasis, including intraabdominal and/or inguinal lymph nodes

disease of postmenopausal women and the diagnosis is usually made on the basis of an endometrial sampling after abnormal uterine bleeding. Endometrial cancer staging has recently been changed to a surgical staging in order to provide a more accurate prognostic stage (Table 5). Surgical treatment includes hysterectomy with bilateral salpingo-oophorectomy as well as pelvic and periaortic lymph node sampling if the tumor invades >30% of the myometrium.

The most important prognostic factors for endometrial cancer are histologic grade and depth of myometrial invasion. There are also two aggressive types that worsen prognosis, e.g., papillary serous adenocarcinoma and clear cell adenocarcinoma. Adjuvant radiation therapy is the mainstay of therapy for patients with poor prognostic disease after surgical exploration. Chemotherapy as well as hormonal therapy can also be used to treat recurrent tumors with some success.

VULVAR CANCER

The surgical management of vulvar cancer, in particular squamous cell cancer, which accounts for 90% to 95% of vulvar cancers, has significantly changed during recent years (Fig. 6). Following the lead of the surgical oncologists with the treatment of breast cancer, a more conservative surgical approach has been adopted and has been shown to be more beneficial to patients in terms of quality-of-life issues. At the same time, there has not been a decrease in the survival advantage obtained by more radical surgery. The traditional treatment of radical vulvectomy and bilateral groin node dissection has been challenged due to the high impact on patient's self-esteem caused by the operation. The morbidity of this operation is encountered with both the radical vulvectomy and the lymph node dissection aspects of the operation. The radical vulvectomy has been associated with sexual dysfunction, and the lymphadenectomy with wound breakdown and subsequent lower extremity lymphedema. Modifica-

tions include omission of the lymph nodes in patients with invasion of ≤1 mm past the basal membrane as well as unilateral lymphadenectomy for lateralized lesions. Lateralized lesions are defined as those that are at least 1 cm away from the midline structures of the clitoris, labia minora, and the perineum. Another modification has been the omission of the pelvic lymphadenectomy. In previous years, if the inguinal lymph nodes contained metastatic disease, a pelvic lymphadenectomy was performed. Currently, due to national cooperative study results, the pelvic lymphadenectomy is omitted, and patients who have positive inguinal nodes are treated with pelvic and groin radiation therapy. Whereas in the past the operation was performed through a large incision extending from the vulva to both groins, a more conservative approach is currently used, employing separate groin incisions. An incision is made for the radical vulvectomy and then separate incisions are made for the groin lymphadenectomy. These modifications with the lymphadenectomy have shown improvement in quality of life with a decrease in morbidity. The radical vulvectomy has also been modified, and the procedure of choice is the modified radical vulvectomy, obtaining 1.5- to 2.0-cm margins of tumor resection. With a less radical vulvectomy, the patient's sexual function has been better preserved. Different centers in the United States have pub-

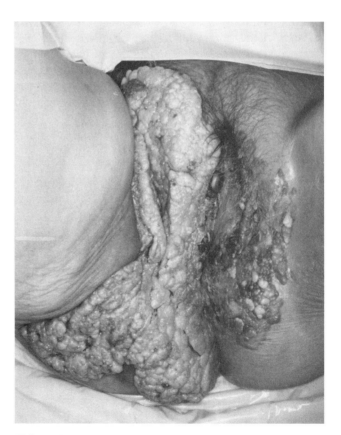

FIG. 6. Verrucous vulvar carcinoma involving a significant portion of perineum, groin, and buttock.

TABLE 6. *FIGO staging of vulvar cancer*

Stage	Criteria
I	Tumor <2 cm with negative nodes
II	Tumor >2 cm with negative nodes
III	Tumor of any size with spread to lower urethra, vagina, or rectum, or positive unilateral inguinal lymph nodes
IVA	Tumor invades upper urethra, bladder mucosa, or rectal mucosa, or bilateral positive inguinal lymph nodes
IVB	Any distant metastasis, including pelvic nodes

lished data with the more conservative approach to radical vulvectomy and have shown acceptable complication rates, with maintenance of survival rates similar to those obtained with more radical surgery.

The second most common cancer of the vulva is malignant melanoma. The most important prognostic factor of melanoma of the vulva is the depth of invasion. Classification systems such as the Clarke and Breslow staging systems have been used, and conservative therapy is used for patients who have melanoma invading <0.76 mm. In such patients, a wide local excision is sufficient and there is no need to perform a lymphadenectomy. On the other hand, patients with advanced disease and invasion of >4 mm past the basal membrane are also treated with wide local excision since these patients are considered to have systemic disease and for the most part are treated with adjuvant chemotherapy after the partial resection. For intermediate lesions, with 0.76 to 4 mm of invasion, routine lymphadenectomy is controversial. At the present time, at the University of Miami, we continue to perform lymphadenectomy for patients with intermediate depth of invasion melanomas.

Other forms of vulvar cancers include basal cell carcinoma and Paget's disease of the vulva, which can be associated with an underlying adenocarcinoma. Sarcomas of the vulva are rarely seen and tend to metastasize through lymphatics and blood vessels. Pathogenesis is similar to sarcomas in other parts of the body. Table 6 outlines the staging of vulvar cancer.

STUDY QUESTIONS

1. Adnexal masses in females especially over the age of 50 are abnormal. What is considered standard evaluation of adnexal masses?
2. The treatment of ovarian cancer has evolved in recent years. Discuss these advancements and the role of surgical resection of this malignancy.
3. Cervical cancer is the third most common gynecological malignancy. List the accepted etiologies behind this neoplasm and the common clinical symptoms. Also describe the appropriate therapy based on cancer staging.
4. After what age should pap smears be performed routinely? With abnormal or suspicious results, what diagnostic studies should be performed?
5. What is the relationship between endometrial hyperplasia and endometrial carcinoma? What are risk factors that predispose to this epithelial change?

SUGGESTED READING

Averette H, Donato D. Ovarian carcinoma: advances in diagnosis, staging and treatment. *Cancer* 1990;65:703.

Averette H, Nguyen H, Penalver M, Estape R. Radical hysterectomy: a 25-year experience at the University of Miami. *Cancer* 1993;71:1422–1437.

Burrell M, Franklin E, Campion M. The modified radical vulvectomy: an 8-year experience. *Am J Obstet Gynecol* 1988;159:715.

Koss LG. The new Bethesda system for reporting results of smears of the uterine cervix. *J Natl Cancer Inst* 1990;82:988.

Pettersson F, Coppleson M, Creasman W. Annual report on the results of treatment in gynecologic cancer. *FIGO Rep* 1994;24:1–83.

SECTION IV

Examination

CHAPTER 32

Preparation for the Oral Examination

Mark G. McKenney, Patrick C. Mangonon, and Stephen M. Cohn

Many institutions complement their surgery clerkship with an oral examination, which can unnerve even the most well-read and prepared student. Unlike the multitude of written examinations the student has successfully completed during his/her undergraduate and medical school experience, oral examinations are rarely employed. An oral examination is similar to a job or medical school admissions interview, requiring proper attitude and attire, excellent interpersonal skills, the ability to think clearly during stress, and the same superior fund of knowledge mandated to successfully complete a written examination. The oral examination is, in actuality, a realistic method of assessing the skills required to perform as a clinician.

Although there are an unlimited number of ways to administer an oral examination, most frequently two methods are employed. One format, which mimics the qualifying examination that surgeons take after completing their residency, requires the student to respond to a number of patient management problems by an examiner, frequently a surgical faculty member. The examiner can ask about any disease process that has surgical implications. There is no limit to the type and depth of questions that can be asked, and examinees must recognize that there are some questions which they cannot answer. The second format frequently employed requires the student to provide the examiner with a list of patients who the student has been involved with during clerkship. In the latter format, the examiner may only ask questions that pertain to the disease process of the patients on the list. While on first impression it seems that the second format would be dramatically easier and more limited in scope, this is not necessarily the case. For example, if a student presents a list of patients to the examiner that includes a patient with appendicitis, the examiner may discuss the disease process of appendicitis and the surgical care of patients with this disease process, but then take this as an opportunity to discuss fluid and electrolytes in a surgical

patient. Alternatively, the examiner may wish to discuss the general topics of wounds and wound healing, antibiotics, conditions that mimic the surgical abdomen, or general abdominal anatomy. A high level of preparation, therefore, is essential to enhance performance in an oral examination, irrespective of form.

If the examination is set up so that the student presents a list of patients, there are several factors to consider when preparing the list. A good analogy is that the oral examination is similar to a rodeo bull ride. To have a high score on this event, both the rider and the bull must perform well. If you answer questions well but have a very limited subject matter, then your grade will probably suffer. The best score will be obtained by having challenging patient problems and handling them well.

Understanding the philosophy of the oral examination is critical to doing well on this test. The oral examination is done in lieu of a practical examination since it is not possible for the examiner to observe you actually taking care of patients. It is an opportunity to manage patient problems and verbalize thought processes. There are a few fundamental differences between oral and written examinations. While there is a time limit on both written and oral tests, in an oral examination one must answer questions in a timely fashion and cannot return to the more difficult problems. (Generally, answering questions on four patients in 30 min is appropriate.) In order to gain experience in this testing method, it is important to practice. Several mock or practice sessions before actually taking the test will reduce your anxiety and improve your performance. Students typically perform much better after repeated mock examinations as they become noticeably more relaxed and better able to verbalize thought processes.

Guessing on the oral examination is not acceptable, as the purpose is to mimic patient care, and, clearly, conjecture in the setting of patient care can have disastrous results. When examinees have reached the limit of their

415

knowledge base and are not certain of the correct course, they should state this clearly. This would be similar to getting a consultation for a complex patient management problem. In this case, you may lose points for a deficit fund of knowledge but would not be penalized for bad judgment.

Proper attitude and dress are important for the oral examination. Taking a written test in jeans while chewing gum will not have an effect on the overall grade, but the same cannot be said of the more subjective oral test. The oral examination is more similar to a job interview, and dress and attitude can have a significant impact. A student wearing a dirty white coat, obviously needing to shave, and loudly smacking gum while slouching in his chair shows disrespect for the examiner and the process, and leads to a poor impression. Attitude is also important. An oral examination is not the appropriate time or place to get into a confrontation with the surgical attending regarding patient care. Think of the examination as a discussion of patient care with a competent colleague, and give the same respect and consideration that you would demand in return.

The oral examination is stressful, but with appropriate preparation the task can be successfully undertaken and even enjoyed. The student should investigate the format to be used well in advance. This is the starting point for reducing anxiety and allowing concentration on the test. Several practice or mock oral sessions will help immeasurably. These mock tests can be performed by individuals at almost any level. If a faculty member is not available, request a mock session with a senior resident. If you are picking the patient list, do so carefully. Pick patients who are challenging, but take the time to prepare for these patients. Take the time to dress appropriately. Think of this oral examination as a job interview. Proper attire and attitude contribute to your overall impression and are reflected in your evaluation. Following these simple suggestions can alleviate much of the stress of this test and will help make the test a superb learning experience.

CHAPTER 33

Written Examination

Patrick C. Mangonon, Mark G. McKenney, and Ara J. Feinstein

MULTIPLE CHOICE

Select the *best* answer.

1. True statements regarding the initial evaluation of a trauma patient include all of the following **except**
   A. Without exception, universal precautions must be adhered to while evaluating a trauma patient.
   B. The first concern in evaluating a trauma patient is airway patency.
   C. Application of a tourniquet is an excellent method of obtaining hemostasis.
   D. Diagnostic peritoneal lavage is a sensitive test for intraperitoneal injury.
   E. Hemodynamic instability after an isolated stab wound to the abdomen requires emergent laparotomy.

2. A 36-year-old man with a past surgical history of perforated appendicitis 10 years ago presents with abdominal distention, nausea, vomiting, colicky pain, and obstipation worsening over the past 24 hr. Which of the following is the most likely diagnosis?
   A. Crohn's ileitis
   B. Small bowel obstruction secondary to cancer
   C. Small bowel obstruction secondary to adhesions
   D. Gastroenteritis
   E. Colon cancer

3. The most common benign soft tissue tumor of mesenchymal origin is a
   A. Rhabdomyosarcoma
   B. Lipoma
   C. Rhabdomyoma
   D. Leiomyoma
   E. Ewing's sarcoma

4. Carpal tunnel syndrome is a type of compressive neuropathy involving which nerve?

A. Median nerve
B. Ulnar nerve
C. Radial nerve
D. Musculocutaneous nerve
E. Brachial nerve

5. Which of the following increases lower esophageal sphincter tone?
   A. Nicotine
   B. Caffeine
   C. Alcohol
   D. Glucagon
   E. Metoclopramide

6. Vitamin K–dependent factors include all **except**
   A. II
   B. V
   C. VII
   D. IX
   E. X

7. Benign prostatic hypertrophy (BPH) occurs in which area of the prostate?
   A. Peripheral zone
   B. Central zone
   C. Transitional zone
   D. Bulbar zone
   E. Anterior fibromuscular stroma

8. An otherwise healthy 18-year-old man presents to the emergency room with a history of vague mid-abdominal pain that now is localized to the right lower abdomen. There was some associated nausea and vomiting but without relief. His temperature is 100.2°F. Physical examination reveals exquisite rebound tenderness at McBurney's point. The next most appropriate step is
   A. Plain abdominal radiographs
   B. Abdominal ultrasound

417

C. Intravenous antibiotics and computed tomographic (CT) scanning of the abdomen
D. Intravenous fluids and antibiotics
E. Intravenous fluids and antibiotics followed by an emergent laparotomy

9. A 20-year-old thin man comes to the emergency department after being involved in an altercation in which he sustained blunt chest and abdominal trauma. On initial evaluation, he has labored breathing and appears to ventilate with paradoxical movement of the right chest wall. On further inspection, his trachea appears deviated slightly to the left and his external jugular veins are prominent. Auscultation of his lung fields reveals decreased breath sounds in the right chest. Suddenly, his blood pressure drops to 60/40 mm Hg and his breathing pattern becomes more labored. The *first* action that should be undertaken in this patient is
A. Stabilization of the "flail" chest
B. Decompression of the tension pneumothorax
C. Endotracheal intubation
D. Searching for other injuries common in this setting
E. Obtaining a chest radiograph

10. What are the two most common sites of metastatic breast cancer?
A. Liver and lung
B. Liver and bone
C. Lung and bone
D. Lung and adrenals
E. Lung and pancreas

11. Which of the following statements are correct regarding gallstones?
A. The majority of stones in the United States are pigment stones.
B. Gallstone disease is more common in men.
C. The incidence of pigment stones decreases with age.
D. A decrease in the concentration of phospholipids in bile may result in supersaturation of cholesterol.
E. Bacteria may have a role in the formation of cholesterol stones.

12. Which of the following are true regarding colonic diverticuli?
A. The vast majority are true diverticula.
B. They are more common in societies with high-residue diets.
C. False diverticula occur at the point of entry of penetrating arterial branches.
D. Nearly all cases of diverticulosis become symptomatic within a short period after diagnosis.

E. False diverticula are most commonly found in the right colon.

13. Effects of massive transfusion include all of the following **except**
A. Decreased hemoglobin affinity for oxygen
B. Citrate toxicity
C. Transmission of viral infection
D. Hypothermia
E. Pulmonary edema

14. Lidocaine and epinephrine would be used in all of the following situations **except**
A. Hemorrhoidectomy
B. Hernia repair
C. Digital nerve block
D. Suture closure of forehead laceration
E. Excision of small lipoma of back

15. A patient with known hypopharygeal cancer is receiving radiation therapy. She begins to cough up large amounts of fresh blood. The most appropriate management is the following:
A. Check her coagulation profile, and correct any underlying coagulopathy.
B. Secure the airway.
C. Administer massive blood replacement as the first step.
D. Perform carotid artery ligation.
E. Provide emergent radiation treatment.

16. Patients with sickle cell anemia are most often found to have which pair of the following bacteria associated with musculoskeletal infections?
A. Staphylococcus and Salmonella species
B. Streptococcus and Neisseria species
C. Pseudomonas and Bacteroides species
D. Proteus and coliform species
E. Staphylococcus and Streptococcus species

17. All of the following are thought to adversely affect wound healing **except**
A. Previous radiation exposure
B. Diabetes mellitus
C. Malnutrition
D. Prior surgery
E. Chronic ingestion of corticosteroids

18. The most common cause of small bowel obstruction in the Western world is
A. Malignancy
B. Adhesions
C. Midgut volvulus
D. Hernia
E. Enteritis

19. In a critically ill patient, which of the following measures would most accurately assess adequacy of protein supplementation?
    A. Oxygen consumption and carbon dioxide production
    B. 24-hr urine creatinine
    C. Midarm muscle circumference
    D. Serum prealbumin level
    E. Serum albumin level

20. Which of the following statements is true regarding burn injury depth?
    A. Third degree burns involve destruction of all epidermal and dermal elements.
    B. Blisters are characteristic of first degree burns.
    C. First degree burns involve only the most superficial layers of the dermis.
    D. Superficial second degree burn injury typically presents with an insensate burn wound.
    E. The total body surface area of burn injury is the sum of first second and third degree burn areas.

21. The ratio of fluid in the extracellular space is best described as
    A. Interstitial 90%, intravascular 10%
    B. Interstitial 75%, intravascular 25%
    C. Interstitial 25%, intravascular 75%
    D. Interstitial 50%, intravascular 50%
    E. Interstitial 40%, intravascular 60%

22. A previously healthy 18-year-old man is in an automobile accident. He loses consciousness, but regains it and appears normal to emergency rescue personnel. An hour after being brought to the emergency room, he becomes lethargic and has weakness on his right side with a dilated pupil on the left side. What is the presumptive diagnosis?
    A. Concussion
    B. Amaurosis fugax
    C. Acute epidural hematoma
    D. Transient ischemic attack
    E. Cerebellar atrophy

23. A 45-year-old previously healthy woman is found to have a small pituitary adenoma and bilateral adrenal hyperplasia. The standard treatment is
    A. Bilateral adrenalectomy
    B. Bilateral subtotal adrenalectomy
    C. Transfrontal excision of the adenoma
    D. Transcranial excision of the adenoma
    E. Transsphenoidal excision of the adenoma

24. Which of the following is the most common form of esophageal atresia?
    A. Blind proximal pouch with distal tracheoesophageal fistula (TEF)
    B. Esophageal atresia with proximal TEF
    C. Both proximal and distal pouches with separate fistulas to the trachea
    D. Atresia without fistula
    E. Midesophageal narrowing with single esophageal fistula to trachea

25. The external branch of the superior laryngeal nerve supplies
    A. Motor innervation of the "strap" muscles of the neck
    B. Sensory function to the mucous membrane above the vocal cords
    C. Motor innervation of the inferior constrictor muscles
    D. Stimulation for calcitonin release
    E. Motor innervation of the cricothyroid muscle

26. All of the following statements regarding groin hernias are true **except** which one?
    A. Femoral hernias are more common in women.
    B. The indirect inguinal hernia is the most common groin hernia in women.
    C. The direct inguinal hernia is uncommon in women.
    D. A proper repair of an inguinal hernia requires tight closure of the internal ring around the spermatic cord vessels.
    E. Direct inguinal hernia rarely enters the scrotum.

27. All of the following statements regarding hepatocellular carcinoma are true **except** which one?
    A. It is the most prevalent malignancy worldwide.
    B. Hepatomas develop in a significant percentage of patients with cirrhosis and chronic hepatitis B infection.
    C. The fibrolamellar variant has a poor survival profile.
    D. In certain cases, liver transplantation can be used to treat hepatocellular carcinoma.
    E. Elevated α-fetoprotein is a common laboratory finding.

28. In a hemodynamically stable patient with massive lower gastrointestinal (GI) bleeding, the best localization study is
    A. Barium enema
    B. Colonoscopy
    C. "Tagged" red cell scan
    D. CT scanning of the abdomen and pelvis
    E. Angiography

29. What is the **best** diagnostic test for a 4-cm mass on the lower extremity suspected to be a sarcoma?
    A. Excisional biopsy
    B. Incisional biopsy

C. Magnetic resonance imaging (MRI)
D. Needle core biopsy
E. Fine-needle aspiration (FNA) biopsy

30. Which of the following statements regarding pyloric stenosis is true?
A. It usually presents within the first 2 weeks of life.
B. It is more common in women.
C. All infants require an upper GI study or ultrasonography for diagnosis.
D. Pyloromyotomy is appropriate treatment.
E. A trial of medical therapy is warranted after diagnosis is made.

31. Clinical signs and symptoms of renal transplant rejection include all of the following **except**
A. Urinary tract infection
B. Hematuria
C. Ipsilateral leg swelling
D. Fever
E. Pain

32. A 70-year-old man with a known diagnosis of bronchogenic carcinoma is admitted to the intensive care unit in respiratory distress. Physical examination reveals tracheal deviation, jugular venous distention, and facial and upper extremity edema. A chest radiograph demonstrates a mass in the right superior mediastinum with mass effect displacing the trachea to the left. Appropriate management includes
A. Stabilizing the patient's respiratory insufficiency followed by immediate mediastinal radiotherapy
B. Immediate endotracheal intubation and broad-spectrum intravenous antibiotics
C. Immediate placement of a right thoracostomy tube
D. Immediate rigid bronchoscopy
E. Administration of 80 mg of furosemide and observation of the edema

33. Which of the following metabolic conditions predispose patients to recurrent renal stone formation?
A. Hypercalcuria
B. Short bowel syndrome
C. Hyperuricosuria
D. Primary hyperparathyroidism
E. All of the above

34. Which of the following is an **absolute** indication for surgical treatment of BPH?
A. Severe urinary frequency
B. Nocturia
C. Urinary retention
D. Urinary incontinence
E. Urinary tract infection

35. Laboratory abnormalities consistent with severe disseminate intravascular coagulopathy (DIC) include all of the following **except**
A. Elevated prothrombin time
B. Increased platelet count
C. Increased fibrin degradation product levels
D. Elevated thrombin time
E. Decreased fibrinogen levels

36. The cell responsible for wound contracture is the
A. Macrophage
B. Myofibroblast
C. Neutrophil
D. Endothelial cell
E. Sarcomere

37. A 24-year-old woman suddenly experiences excruciating and incapacitating lower abdominal pain. She is otherwise healthy. After being brought to the emergency room by emergency rescue personnel, her clinical evaluation reveals a temperature of 97.4°F, heart rate of 120 beats/min, blood pressure of 80/44 mm Hg, respiratory rate of 30 breaths/min, and a moderately distended abdomen. The most likely diagnosis is
A. Acute cholecystitis
B. Acute appendicitis
C. Pelvic inflammatory disease
D. Ruptured ectopic pregnancy
E. Ruptured ovarian cyst

38. The blood supply to the midgut originates from which of the following arteries?
A. Celiac axis
B. Superior mesenteric artery
C. Inferior mesenteric artery
D. Small intestinal artery
E. Both superior mesenteric artery and celiac axis

39. A patient with depressed left ventricular function usually has
A. Increased pulmonary capillary wedge pressure (PCWP) and decreased systemic vascular resistance
B. Decreased PCWP and decreased left ventricular stroke work index (LVSWI)
C. Increased PCWP and decreased LVSWI
D. Increased PCWP and increased ejection fraction
E. A decreased end-diastolic volume and decreased ejection fraction

40. The critical number of bacteria that is thought to promote wound infection is
A. 10^2 organisms/gram of tissue
B. 10^4 organisms/gram of tissue
C. 10^5 organisms/gram of tissue
D. 10^6 organisms/gram of tissue

E. 10^{11} organisms/gram of tissue

41. Which one of the following shifts oxyhemoglobin dissociation curve to the left?
    A. Decreased pH
    B. Increased carbon dioxide tension
    C. Increased 2,3-diphosphoglycerate
    D. Decreased body temperature
    E. Pyruvate kinase deficiency

42. A 62-year-old man with a "blue" right great toe is found to have an ipsilateral popliteal artery aneurysm measuring 3.2 cm in diameter. Which of the following is true?
    A. The popliteal artery aneurysm is not large enough to warrant repair.
    B. Aortic and contralateral popliteal artery aneurysms are common.
    C. This patient's blue toe is probably unrelated to his popliteal artery aneurysm.
    D. Simple ligation of the popliteal artery is sufficient therapy.
    E. These aneurysms are typically "false" aneurysms.

43. The best indicator of appropriate fluid replacement in burn injury is
    A. Hourly urine output
    B. Heart rate
    C. Blood pressure
    D. Serum blood urea nitrogen to creatinine ratio
    E. Measuring central venous pressure

44. A 37-year-old man is 1 day after a standard appendectomy for nonperforated appendicitis. The operation was uneventful, but he has a temperature of 101.4°F. Blood pressure is within normal limits; heart rate is 104 beats/min. The most likely diagnosis is
    A. Atelectasis
    B. Intraabdominal infection
    C. Urinary tract infection
    D. Wound infection
    E. Reaction to anesthesia

45. All of the following hormones are found in increased serum levels immediately after traumatic injury **except**
    A. Cortisol
    B. Norepinephrine
    C. Epinephrine
    D. Glucagon
    E. Insulin

46. The most common electrolyte abnormality in the patients after elective operation is
    A. Hypomagnesemia
    B. Hypocalcemia
    C. Hyponatremia
    D. Hypophosphatemia
    E. Hypochloremia

47. A 39-year-old African-American woman with hypercalcemia is being evaluated by another physician. She is referred to a thoracic surgeon because her chest radiograph demonstrates enlarged bilateral hilar lymph nodes. It is reasonable to
    A. Perform immediate incisional biopsy of the hilar lymph nodes
    B. Await completion of the hypercalcemia evaluation
    C. Start chemotherapy empirically
    D. Start radiation therapy to the mediastinum
    E. Order an human immunodeficiency virus test on this patient

48. All of the following can be part of the treatment for an air embolism during a radical neck dissection **except**
    A. Hyperventilating the patient
    B. Aspiration of air from the heart using a central venous line
    C. Hyperbaric oxygen treatment
    D. Placing the patient in Trendelenberg position
    E. Placing the patient in the left lateral decubitus position

49. A 60-year-old man with a history of recurrent left knee pain, swelling, and effusions is seen by an orthopedist. The patient states that he has not been sexually active since his wife's death 5 years ago. He also denies a recent history of fever, chills, or night sweats. Fluid drawn from the patient's left knee reveals a thin, tapered, strongly negative birefringent appearance to polarized light. The patient's white blood cell count and erythrocyte sedimentation rate are both within normal limits. The most likely diagnosis is
    A. Septic arthritis
    B. Gouty Arthritis
    C. Transient synovitis
    D. Pseudogout
    E. Ankylosing spondylitis

50. Identical HLA phenotype between siblings of the same parents occurs how often?
    A. 25%
    B. 50%
    C. 100%
    D. 75%
    E. Randomly

51. In rickets, called osteomalacia in adults, the main abnormality in this disorder usually results from a deficiency of which of the following substances?

A. Zinc
B. Vitamin A
C. Vitamin K
D. Vitamin D
E. Vitamin C

52. In patients with mitral stenosis, measurements of pulmonary artery occlusion pressure are accurate reflections of
A. Left ventricular end-diastolic pressure
B. Microvascular pulmonary pressure
C. Right atrial pressure
D. Left atrial pressure
E. Left ventricular end-diastolic volume

53. Patients with increased nasogastric tube output are prone to which of the following electrolyte and acid-base abnormalities?
A. Hyponatremic, hyperchloremic, metabolic acidosis
B. Hyponatremic, hypochloremic, metabolic alkalosis
C. Hypernatremic, hypokalemic, metabolic alkalosis
D. Isolated hypokalemia
E. Isolated metabolic alkalosis

54. A 47-year-old woman with a history of end-stage renal disease and chronic diabetes mellitus underwent an uneventful cadaveric renal transplant 3 months ago. She has developed fever and productive cough. The sputum is copious and foul-smelling. A chest radiograph demonstrates a cavitary lesion with air-fluid levels in the right lower lobe near the hilum. Appropriate management should entail
A. Immediate bronchoscopy and drainage of this lung abscess
B. Long-term oral antibiotics and reevaluation as an outpatient
C. Immediate thoracotomy and external drainage of this abscess
D. Long-term intravenous antibiotics and invasive drainage for refractory cases
E. Expectant therapy

55. The most common cyanotic congenital heart defect is
A. Tetralogy of Fallot
B. Tricuspid atresia
C. Transposition of the great vessels
D. Partial anomalous venous return
E. Total anomalous venous return

56. All of the following are indications for liver transplantation **except**
A. Biliary cirrhosis

B. Life expectancy of <1 year secondary to end-stage liver disease
C. Hemachromatosis
D. Budd-Chiari syndrome
E. Cholangiocarcinoma secondary to sclerosing cholangitis

57. Prolongation of the partial thromboplastin time occurs in all of the following **except**
A. DIC
B. Intravenous heparin administration
C. Lupus anticoagulant
D. Factor XIII deficiency
E. Liver failure

58. Which of the following is true about esophageal carcinoma?
A. Most patients present with early disease.
B. The goal of therapy is cure.
C. Adenocarcinoma is the most common type of esophageal cancer.
D. Placement of an esophageal stent is the preferred method for managing malignant TEFs.
E. Cytomegalovirus esophagitis is an associated risk factor.

59. A 32-year-old man is involved in a motor vehicle accident. He is rescued by the paramedics 2 hr after the incident. His right forearm was found to be pinned between the car and the ground. In the emergency room, the patient is noted to have an extremely tense right forearm, normal pulses, and extreme forearm pain on passive range of motion of the right hand digits. The radiographs of the right forearm do not demonstrate bony fracture. The most appropriate management for this patient's clinical presentation is the following:
A. Order the nurse to give 10 mg of intravenous morphine to the patient as soon as possible.
B. Place the patient's forearm in an cast for comfort.
C. Notify the operating room of an emergently needed operation.
D. Put ice on the right forearm and reexamine the patient in 2 hr.
E. Reassure the patient that expectant therapy is all that is needed.

60. A 68-year-old man with a chronic nonproductive cough from emphysema comes for evaluation of a productive cough and fever. He appears to have lost weight. A chest radiograph demonstrates complete collapse of the left upper lobe. The most appropriate management should include
A. Obtaining a sputum gram stain and culture and administering empiric oral antibiotics

B. Obtaining a sputum gram stain and culture, administering empiric oral antibiotics, and scheduling a CT scan of the chest
C. Immediate bronchoscopy
D. Referral to state health agency for tuberculosis quarantine protocols
E. Aggressive chest physiotherapy only

61. A thin 70-year-old man complains of vague abdominal pain and hematuria. On physical examination, a right abdominal mass is palpated. The most appropriate diagnostic study to obtain is
A. A CT scan of the abdomen
B. An intravenous urogram
C. Cystoscopy
D. Urinary cytology
E. MRI

62. A 25-year-old woman is involved in a motorcycle accident. In the emergency room, she is unconscious and does not respond to pain on the left side of the body. Her systolic blood pressure was initially 90 mm Hg but increased to 110 mm Hg after 2 L of intravenous saline and then fell again to 85 mm Hg. She has an open right femur fracture and a closed left tibia fracture. She is obese, and her abdominal girth is difficult to assess. A peritoneal lavage is performed, and 20 cc of blood is aspirated from the abdominal cavity. What should be done next?
A. CT scanning of the head
B. CT scan of the head and abdomen
C. Emergent laparotomy
D. Ventriculostomy placement in the emergency room
E. Immediate chest radiograph

63. A 40-year-old woman, whose father underwent an operation for parathyroid hyperplasia and pheochromocytoma in the remote past, is found to have primary hyperparathyroidism. Her pathology is most likely to be
A. A solitary parathyroid adenoma
B. Two parathyroid adenomas
C. Parathyroid cancer
D. Multiple endocrine neoplasia (MEN) I
E. Parathyroid hyperplasia

64. What is the average 5-year survival for women with more than four positive axillary nodes, as reported by the National Surgical Adjuvant Breast Project?
A. 10%
B. 20%
C. 30%
D. 50%
E. 70%

65. The most common cause of surgical renovascular hypertension is
A. Fibromuscular hyperplasia
B. Atherosclerosis
C. Renal artery aneurysms
D. Renal calcinosis
E. None of the above

66. All of the following statements are true regarding benign gastric ulcers **except** which one?
A. Type I is the most common.
B. Type II and type III ulcers requiring surgery should be treated with an operation appropriate for duodenal ulcers.
C. They are more common than duodenal ulcers.
D. Patients with the most common type of gastric ulcer have normal or low gastric acid secretion.
E. *Helicobacter pylori* is a causative agent in a significant percentage of cases.

67. Complications of portal hypertension may include
A. Esophageal varices
B. Ascites
C. Encephalopathy
D. Splenomegaly
E. All of the above

68. A 71-year-old woman presents to the emergency room with persistent abdominal pain and distention, voluminous vomiting, and obstipation. She has not had previous abdominal surgery. Physical examination reveals a markedly distended abdomen with hyperactive bowel sounds. The remainder of the examination is unremarkable. Abdominal radiographs demonstrate multiple dilated loops of small bowel, absence of air in the colon, but pneumobilia. The primary diagnosis is
A. Gallstone ileus
B. Mesenteric ischemia
C. Endometriosis
D. Cancer
E. Appendicitis

69. All of the following statements regarding ulcerative colitis are true **except** which one?
A. Ten years after the onset of disease, the risk of colon cancer is ~10%.
B. Painful diarrhea is a common symptom.
C. Granuloma are typically found in the transmural pathology.
D. Total proctocolectomy is completely curative.
E. The serosa is usually spared of the inflammatory process.

70. Which of the following correctly characterizes endometriosis?

A. It is unrelated to retrograde menses.
B. It may be associated with dysparunia, infertility, and dysmenorrhea.
C. Cyclical birth control pills may be effective in controlling symptoms.
D. Danazol is not effective in controlling symptoms.
E. "Moon facies" and hirsutism are commonly associated symptoms.

71. A 41-year-old man is brought to the emergency room after he "dropped to the floor" from sudden abdominal pain. His temperature is 98.6°F, his heart rate is 98 beats/min, respiratory rate 26 breaths/min, and blood pressure 124/82 mm Hg. Physical examination reveals diffuse abdominal tenderness, involuntary guarding, and obvious signs of peritonitis. An upright chest radiograph demonstrates pneumoperitoneum ("free air under the diaphragm"). The most likely diagnosis is
A. Perforated duodenal ulcer
B. Perforated gallbladder
C. Perforated sigmoid diverticulitis
D. Perforated terminal ileum from Crohn's disease
E. Perforated gastric cancer

72. All of the following are typically found in both hemorrhagic and cardiogenic shock **except**
A. Narrowed pulse pressure
B. Hypovolemia
C. Endogenous catecholamine release
D. Arteriolar constriction
E. Low cardiac output

73. Paraplegia after repair of thoracoabdominal aneurysms is
A. Caused by prolonged intraoperative hypotension
B. Usually an adverse reaction to anesthesia
C. Due to inadequate blood flow in the anterior spinal artery during operative repair
D. A result of occlusion of the native bilateral vertebral arteries
E. Less frequent than after repair of infrarenal abdominal aortic aneurysms

74. A 65-year-old man has been previously healthy despite smoking two packs of cigarettes per day for 45 years. He has recently developed a cough and episodic expectoration of blood-tinged sputum. A chest radiograph demonstrates a new 2.5-cm solitary pulmonary nodule in the periphery of the right upper lobe. There is no effusion. Which of the following are true?
A. A follow-up chest radiograph should be performed in 3 months.
B. Antituberculosis medication should be started empirically.

C. Bronchoscopy is useful in obtaining tissue for biopsy in this situation.
D. Chemotherapy should be administered to "downstage" the tumor.
E. High-resolution CT scan of the chest should be obtained.

75. A tissue biopsy was obtained from the patient in the previous question, revealing epidermoid bronchogenic carcinoma. Which should be the next appropriate management step?
A. Bone scan should be performed.
B. CT scan of the abdomen should be obtained.
C. CT scan of the brain should be obtained.
D. A baseline serum calcium and electrolytes should be obtained.
E. All of the above are true.

76. Complications from renal transplant include
A. Acute rejection
B. Lymphocele
C. Cushing's syndrome
D. Cancer
E. All of the above

77. All of the following are stages of wound healing **except**
A. Maturation
B. Inflammatory
C. Hypertrophic
D. Proliferation
E. Epithelialization

78. The most common benign esophageal tumor is
A. Lymphoma
B. Leiomyoma
C. Hemangioma
D. Polyp
E. Esophageal ring

79. A 48-year-old executive recently experienced a syncopal episode at a business meeting. Physical examination reveals a soft "crescendo-decrescendo" murmur, heard best at the right upper sternum. The murmur occurs late in systole. Echocardiogram demonstrated aortic stenosis with valve area no greater than 0.6 cm². The left ventricular ejection fraction is 45%. Which of the following is true?
A. Immediate surgical replacement of the aortic valve should be undertaken.
B. A repeat echocardiogram should be performed.
C. Medical therapy and minimally invasive therapy are equally successful in treating the vast majority of these cases.
D. A cardiac catheterization should be performed before valve replacement.

E. Because of the severely depressed left ventricular function, operative intervention cannot be performed.

80. What is appropriate therapy for a gunshot wound to the extraperitoneal rectum?
   A. Transanal repair
   B. Loop colostomy alone
   C. Diverting colostomy, distal rectal irrigation, and presacral drainage
   D. Transanal tube drainage and loop colostomy
   E. Loop colostomy and transanal repair

81. Which of the following malignancies can cause hypercalcemia **without** the presence of bony destruction?
   A. Renal cell carcinoma
   B. Stage IV breast cancer
   C. Advanced bronchogenic carcinoma
   D. Metastatic prostate cancer
   E. Multiple myeloma

82. During which week of fetal growth does the midgut return to the abdominal cavity from the umbilical cord?
   A. 3rd week
   B. 4th week
   C. 10th week
   D. 15th week
   E. 20th week

83. All of the following statements regarding gastric parietal cells are true **except** which one?
   A. They are located in the fundus and body of the stomach.
   B. They secrete hydrochloric acid.
   C. They secrete intrinsic factor.
   D. They secrete gastrin.
   E. They have a histamine (H_2) receptor at the cell membrane.

84. What is the most common *primary* liver malignancy?
   A. Cholangiocarcinoma
   B. Hepatoblastoma
   C. Neuroblastoma
   D. Hepatoma
   E. Angiosarcoma

85. Which of the following treatments should be used first in a patient with severe hypercalcemia?
   A. Furosemide
   B. Mithramycin
   C. Calcitonin
   D. Vitamin D
   E. Intravenous saline

86. The heart valvular lesion that frequently causes sudden death is
   A. Aortic stenosis
   B. Mitral stenosis
   C. Aortic regurgitation
   D. Mitral regurgitation
   E. Pulmonary stenosis

87. A 28-year-old woman is 20 weeks pregnant. She presents to the emergency room with right-sided abdominal pain. There is a history of associated nausea and vomiting. On physical examination, tenderness is localized to the right lateral abdomen at the level of the umbilicus. Fetal evaluation is normal. She is afebrile. The presumptive diagnosis is
   A. Acute cholecystitis
   B. Acute appendicitis
   C. Cecal volvulus
   D. Threatened abortion
   E. Hyperemesis gravida

88. A 74-year-old man with a history of chronic hypertension and known abdominal aortic aneurysm presents to the emergency room complaining of back pain. His measured blood pressure is 80/50 mm Hg, and a large pulsatile mass is palpable in the umbilical region. The next best step in management is
   A. Emergent laparotomy
   B. Abdominal ultrasound
   C. Diagnostic peritoneal lavage
   D. CT scan of the abdomen and pelvis
   E. Admission to an intensive care unit for aggressive intravenous fluid rehydration

89. Fractures in the pediatric (skeletally immature) patient are characterized by all of the following statements **except** which one?
   A. Greenstick and torus fractures are more likely to occur in pediatric patients than adults due to a thicker periosteum in children.
   B. Fractures in pediatric patients that involve the growth plate are at an increased risk of developing angular bony deformities.
   C. Salter-Harris type 1 and type 2 fractures usually respond to nonsurgical treatment.
   D. When compared to fractures in adults, those in pediatric patients usually take twice as long to heal.
   E. All of the above are true.

90. A 48-year-old man presents with a cough, chest pain, and hemoptysis. Chest radiograph reveals a mass in the right upper lobe. He lives in the Mississippi Valley, where he works as an earth mover. Your clinical diagnosis is
   A. Actinomycosis
   B. Blastomycosis
   C. Coccidioidomycosis

D. Histoplasmosis

E. Aspergillosis

91. A Clark's level IV melanoma penetrates into which level of the skin?
    A. Papillary dermis
    B. Reticular dermis
    C. Epidermis
    D. Subcutaneous fat
    E. Basement membrane

92. Level II axillary lymph nodes are located
    A. Superior to the axillary vein
    B. Lateral to the pectoralis minor muscle
    C. Under the pectoralis minor muscle
    D. Between the major and minor pectoralis muscles
    E. Medial to the pectoralis minor muscle

93. What is the definitive method to diagnose Hirschprung's disease?
    A. Full-thickness rectal biopsy
    B. Rectal manometry
    C. Contrast enema
    D. Stool culture
    E. CT scan of abdomen and pelvis

94. All of the following statements regarding arterial supply to the stomach are correct **except** which one?
    A. The left gastric artery is a branch of the celiac arterial trunk.
    B. The right gastroepiploic artery is a branch of the gastroduodenal artery.
    C. The gastroduodenal artery courses behind the pylorus.
    D. The left gastroepiploic artery is a branch of the superior mesenteric artery.
    E. The splenic artery gives off the vasa brevia (short gastric arteries).

95. A 43-year-old woman presents to the emergency room with complaints of postprandial abdominal pain, nausea, and vomiting. She has rebound tenderness in the right upper quadrant. After obtaining a thorough patient history and detailed physical examination, the best initial diagnostic study is
    A. CT scan of the abdomen and pelvis
    B. Barium enema
    C. Abdominal ultrasound
    D. Upper GI contrast series
    E. Endoscopic retrograde cholangiopancreatography

96. A 50-year-old man with a combined history of chronic bronchitis and emphysema has a persistent cough for many years. He presents to the emergency room with acute shortness of breath. He is hypotensive with tracheal deviation toward the right hemithorax. Breath sounds are absent in the left hemithorax. The next most appropriate step in management is
    A. Immediate chest radiograph
    B. Immediate left thoracostomy tube
    C. Immediate β_2-receptor agonist inhaler therapy with 60% FiO_2
    D. Obtain and arterial blood gas sample immediately
    E. Expectant therapy

97. Screening for prostate cancer should start at what age?
    A. At the age of 40 for African-American men or individuals with a family history of prostate cancer
    B. At age 60
    C. At age 30
    D. At age 40 for Caucasian and African-American men
    E. At age 55

98. A tumor of the salivary gland has been discovered. Which of the following describes increasing order of incidence of malignancy?
    A. Minor salivary glands, submandibular, sublingual, parotid
    B. Minor salivary glands, sublingual, submandibular, parotid
    C. Submandibular, parotid, minor salivary glands, sublingual
    D. Sublingual, submandibular, parotid, minor salivary glands
    E. Parotid, submandibular, sublingual, minor salivary glands

99. Select the correct statement regarding pancreatic trauma.
    A. Isolated pancreatic injury from penetrating trauma is common.
    B. Normal serum amylase always excludes serious pancreatic injury.
    C. Blunt transection of the pancreas typically occurs in the tail of the pancreas.
    D. Drains should not be left adjacent to parenchymal contusions.
    E. Penetrating injury to the tail of the pancreas is best treated by splenectomy and distal pancreatectomy.

100. Which of the following are current American Cancer Society recommendations for breast cancer screening?
    A. Routine yearly mammogram beginning at age 35
    B. Annual mammogram after age 50 for all women

C. Annual mammogram after age 50 only for women with a significant family history of breast cancer

D. Baseline mammogram between 25 to 30 years old

E. Annual breast examination by physician for all women older than 25 years of age

101. Risk of spontaneous bleeding becomes significant with a platelet count of less than
A. 70,000
B. 50,000
C. 20,000
D. 5,000
E. 1,000

102. A 25-year-old man presents to a family medicine clinic for routine physical examination. An incidental cardiac murmur is detected at the upper left sternal border. An echocardiogram shows an atrial septal defect (ASD) with significant pulmonary blood flow. He is otherwise healthy. What is the next most appropriate step in management?
A. Cardiac catheterization performed to evaluate coexistent coronary artery disease
B. Endovascular occlusion of the ASD with a spring coil
C. Operative closure of the ASD primarily or with a patch
D. Close observation and serial echocardiograms as an outpatient
E. Expectant therapy

103. Acute respiratory failure is best documented by
A. Bilateral interstitial infiltrates seen on chest radiograph
B. CO_2 retention
C. Cyanosis
D. Hypoxemia
E. Increased sputum production

104. A 27-year-old man has just undergone open reduction and internal fixation of a right femoral shaft fracture. Four days after the operation, his right calf region is markedly swollen. His arterial pulses are palpable throughout, and motor and sensory function of the distal extremity is normal. Which of the following is true?
A. The fact that he is young makes the possibility of deep venous thrombosis unlikely.
B. Lack of calf tenderness on manual dorsiflexion of the ankle excludes deep venous thrombosis.
C. Without hematologic abnormalities, deep venous thrombosis does not occur.
D. One must suspect right lower extremity venous injury.

E. A venous duplex of the right lower extremity should be obtained.

105. A 55-year-old man with a history of severe pancreatitis presents with abdominal bloating, weight loss, diarrhea, steatorrhea, weakness, and fatigue. The most likely diagnosis is
A. Malabsorption secondary to pancreatic exocrine insufficiency
B. Malabsorption secondary to pancreatic endocrine insufficiency
C. Pancreatic cancer
D. Peptic ulcer disease
E. Crohn's disease

106. A 4-year-old boy with a history of frequent respiratory illness is brought to the doctor's office with a complaint of progressive muscle weakness. The child on physical examination is noted to have pseudohypertrophy of the calves, a crouched gait, and a positive "Gower's sign." The most likely diagnosis of this child is
A. Legg-Calvé-Perthe's disease
B. Muscular dystrophy
C. Polio
D. Scurvy
E. Polymyositis

107. A child underwent a cardiac catheterization at 6 months of age for evaluation of severe heart failure, which revealed an isolated ventricular septal defect (VSD). She responded to digitalis and diuretics, and now, at 5 years of age, she is referred for ventricular septal closure. She is not in heart failure. Chest film reveals a normal heart size. Right and left heart catheterization is performed prior to surgery and reveals the following data:

Site	Pressure (mm Hg)	O$_2$ saturation
Superior vena cava	Mean = 5	62%
Right atrium	Mean = 5	62%
Right ventricle	100/5	64%
Pulmonary artery	110/50, mean 70	68%
Left atrium	Mean = 7	98%
Aorta	110/80, mean 90	93%

The following is most likely:
A. The VSD is closed.
B. The child has developed severe pulmonary vascular obstructive disease.
C. The defect is small and can be closed at low risk through the atrium.
D. Additional medical therapy would be beneficial.

E. The initial diagnosis was incorrect.

108. All are true statements regarding Hirschprung's disease **except** which one?
    A. It may be complicated by a fulminant enterocolitis.
    B. The diseased bowel is not dilated.
    C. The procedure of choice for a newborn with obstruction due to Hirschprung's disease is immediate "pull-through" procedure.
    D. Resection of disease and a colostomy should be performed in neonates with obstruction due to Hirschprung's disease.
    E. Multiple colonic biopsies are necessary to delineate "normal" bowel.

109. One year after antrectomy with Billroth II reconstruction performed for ulcer disease, a 45-year-old man complains of burning midepigastric pain unrelieved by antacids, aggravated by food, and associated with bilious vomiting. Endoscopy reveals diffuse superficial erythematous changes in the stomach. He likely has
    A. Alkaline reflux gastritis
    B. Afferent loop syndrome
    C. Efferent loop syndrome
    D. Recurrent anastomotic (stomal) ulcer that was missed on endoscopy
    E. Early dumping

110. A 46-year-old man in previously good health complains of a 2-month history of progressive exertional dyspnea. He denies chest pain. On physical examination, a loud diastolic rumble is heard in the apical area. The murmur disappears in the right lateral decubitus position. The most likely diagnosis is
    A. Mitral stenosis
    B. Mitral regurgitation
    C. Atrial myxoma
    D. Papillary muscle rupture
    E. VSD

111. A 39-year-old woman has just underwent an urgent cholecystectomy for acute cholecystitis. Four hours after the procedure, her temperature is 103.4°F. Her abdomen is only mildly distended, but malodorous drainage is noted from the wound. The presumptive diagnosis is
    A. Necrotizing fasciitis
    B. Simple wound infection
    C. Stitch granuloma
    D. Pylephlebitis
    E. Malignant hyperthermia

112. Dermatitis may be a manifestation of deficiency of all of the following **except**
    A. Riboflavin
    B. Folate
    C. Niacin
    D. Pyridoxine
    E. Biotin

113. Which of these hemodynamic parameters cannot be directly measured by pulmonary artery catheter?
    A. Cardiac output
    B. Pulmonary artery pressure
    C. Pulmonary vascular resistance
    D. PCWP
    E. Right atrial pressure

114. A 52-year-old woman with symptomatic biliary colic undergoes an uneventful laparoscopic cholecystectomy. Two weeks later, she presents to the emergency room with progressive shortness of breath and fever. Her temperature is 102.4°F, blood pressure is 140/88 mm Hg, and her heart rate is 104 beats/min. Physical examination reveals a patient in moderate respiratory distress. Her sclerae are anicteric. Auscultation of the lung fields shows bilateral inspiratory rales. There is a loud systolic ejection murmur heard at the left lower sternal border. Her laparoscopic incisions are unremarkable, and there is no abdominal pain on palpation. What is the most logical management choice?
    A. An ultrasound of the right upper quadrant should be performed.
    B. Intravenous antibiotics should be started, and the patient should be admitted and observed.
    C. A CT scan of the chest should be performed.
    D. The patient can be reassured that this will resolve with time.
    E. An echocardiogram should be obtained.

115. The most common acid-base abnormality seen in patients with high ileostomy output is
    A. + anion gap, metabolic acidosis
    B. + anion gap, metabolic alkalosis
    C. - anion gap, metabolic acidosis
    D. - anion gap, metabolic alkalosis
    E. None of the above

116. Factors that impact on survival from burn injury include all of the following **except**
    A. Burn injury size
    B. Age of patient
    C. Comorbid medical disease
    D. Failure to perform immediate burn wound excision
    E. Burn wound sepsis

117. An elderly woman recently underwent a transhiatal esophagectomy for esophageal cancer. The intraoperative course was unremarkable. She was advanced to an oral diet on day 8. Since then, a progressively

increasing left pleural effusion has developed. Thoracentesis was performed for moderate respiratory distress. Fluid obtained appears "milky." The next most appropriate step in managing this problem is

A. Repeated thoracentesis for symptomatic relief
B. Increasing the patient's oral triglyceride intake
C. Bilateral chest tubes for pleural drainage
D. Ceasing oral intake and administering parenteral nutrition
E. Starting a medium-chain triglyceride diet, placing a left chest tube for pleural drainage, and monitoring frequently for nutritional status and immunocompetence

118. The half-life of heparin is
A. 5 min
B. 60 min
C. 4 hr
D. 6 hr
E. 24 hr

119. All of the following are complications of parenteral nutrition **except**
A. Pneumothorax
B. Intestinal mucosal atrophy
C. *C. difficile* colitis
D. Cholestasis
E. Nonketotic hyperosmolar coma

120. Extraintestinal manifestations of Crohn's disease include all of the following **except**
A. Uveitis
B. Pyoderma gangrenosum
C. Ankylosing spondylitis
D. Vertigo
E. Erythema nodosum

121. Widely metastatic prostate cancer is best treated with
A. Bilateral orchiectomy
B. Estrogen
C. Testosterone
D. Pelvic external beam radiation
E. Retropubic radical prostatectomy

122. Which of the following are pulsion diverticuli?
A. Zenker's diverticula
B. True diverticuli
C. Meckel's diverticula
D. Midesophageal diverticuli
E. None of the above

123. Within the first 24 hr, the dominant cell in a healing wound is the
A. Endothelial cell
B. Monocyte
C. Fibroblast
D. Neutrophil
E. Lymphocyte

124. Which of the following factors most strongly influences the prognosis of patients with soft tissue sarcomas?
A. Histologic grade
B. Cell type
C. Age of patient
D. Clinical symptoms
E. Tumor size

125. A 0.70-mm-deep melanoma has approximately what risk of regional nodal metastasis?
A. 50%
B. 25%
C. 10%
D. 75%
E. <5%

126. What is the most common cause of bloody nipple discharge?
A. Trauma
B. Intraductal papillary carcinoma
C. Ductal carcinoma in situ
D. Intraductal papilloma
E. Fibrocystic mastopathy

127. All of the following are considered appropriate treatment in managing increased intracranial pressure **except**
A. Control of hypernatremia
B. Minimizing unnecessary stimulation
C. Trendelenberg position
D. Hyperventilation
E. Administration of mannitol

128. A 62-year-old woman in previously good health comes to your office for evaluation of progressively worsening right arm and shoulder pain that she has been experiencing for 3 months. She denies arthritides. She has smoked half a pack of cigarettes a day for several years. On examination, she has complete range of motion of the extremity. There is no crepitus or palpable mass in the shoulder. It is important to obtain
A. A complete forearm radiograph
B. An electrocardiogram
C. A complete chest radiograph
D. A skin biopsy of suspicious lesions
E. A rheumatology consult

129. Esophageal lesions considered to be premalignant include all of the following **except**
A. Achalasia
B. Barrett's esophagus

C. Esophageal webs associated with Plummer-Vinson syndrome

D. Epiphrenic diverticulum

E. Distal esophageal strictures secondary to lye ingestion

130. Which of the following is not considered a recognized complication of inguinal hernia repair?
    A. Hematoma
    B. Impotence
    C. Neuralgia
    D. Testicular atrophy
    E. Wound infection

131. Deficiency of what coagulation inhibitor leads to the clinical syndrome of warfarin-induced skin necrosis?
    A. Protein C
    B. VIIa
    C. Antithrombin III
    D. α_2-antiplasmin
    E. α_2-macroglobulin

132. Which of the following statements is true regarding hepatic anatomy?
    A. The falciform ligament separates the left and the right lobes.
    B. The gallbladder separates the medial and lateral segments of the right lobe.
    C. The caudate lobe is segment I.
    D. The falciform ligament contains the obliterated umbilical artery.
    E. Hepatic artery anatomy is invariably constant.

133. Pathologic analysis of adenocarcinoma of the colon reveals growth into the muscularis propria, no extension to the serosa, and one mesenteric lymph node that contains cancer cells. Using the TNM staging system, how would such a lesion be staged?
    A. I
    B. II
    C. III
    D. IV
    E. V

134. What is the average 5-year survival for the case described above?
    A. 70%
    B. 50%
    C. 35%
    D. 15%
    E. 5%

135. Which of the following is a true statement regarding Meckel's diverticuli?

A. They arise because of failure of obliteration of the umbilical vein.

B. They are the most common source of GI bleeding in the adult population.

C. They are located on the mesenteric border.

D. Approximately 50% contain ectopic pancreatic or gastric mucosa.

E. They are typically found within 2 ft of the ligament of Treitz.

136. Malnutrition should be suspected in
    A. Those patients who do not tolerate a regular diet until the third postoperative day
    B. All surgical patients
    C. Patients with minor burns
    D. Only those patients with a weight loss that approaches 30% of usual body weight
    E. All patients with major injury or critical illness

137. All of the following are thought to contribute to the development of inguinal hernia **except**
    A. Chronic cough
    B. BPH
    C. Colonic obstruction
    D. Prior abdominal surgery
    E. Strenuous activity

138. Which of the following is true regarding closed head injury?
    A. Postauricular ecchymosis (Battle's sign) is very suggestive of acute subdural hematoma.
    B. Significant blood loss can occur from simple scalp laceration.
    C. Epidural hematomas are typically the result of bony fragment laceration of the frontal artery.
    D. All subdural hematomas require emergent craniotomy.
    E. In the absence of brain injury by CT scan, decreased neurological status is always due to drug intoxication.

139. An unstable patient is admitted to the intensive care unit after a *severe* stroke. Before proceeding to obtain a CT scan of the head, you would do which of the following?
    A. Sedate the patient.
    B. Anticoagulate the patient.
    C. Intubate the patient.
    D. Cardiovert the patient.
    E. Consult Neurology.

140. The cremasteric muscle fibers are an extension of which abdominal wall layer?
    A. Internal oblique

B. External oblique
C. Transversus abdominus
D. Superficial fascia
E. Peritoneum

141. Current accepted treatment for *localized* prostate cancer is
A. Radical prostatectomy
B. High-dose chemotherapy
C. Bladder-preserving prostatectomy
D. Cryotherapy of the prostate
E. All of the above

142. Select the incorrect statement regarding soft tissue sarcomas.
A. The pseudocapsule contains tumor cells.
B. Diagnosis is best accomplished with FNA biopsy.
C. Hematogenous spread is more common than lymphatic spread.
D. Tumors frequently extend across fascial planes.
E. Simple excision is associated with 90% local recurrences.

143. A 30-year-old woman taking oral contraceptives for 9 years had a liver mass seen on ultrasound performed recently. She now presents in shock from intraabdominal bleeding. What is her liver mass most likely to be?
A. Focal nodular hyperplasia
B. Liver cell adenoma
C. Cavernous hemangioma
D. Benign congenital cyst
E. Hepatoma

144. Which of the following statements is true regarding Goodsall's rule of anal fistulas?
A. With a cutaneous opening in the left lateral posterior position, the internal opening will likely be in the posterior midline.
B. With a cutaneous opening in the left lateral posterior position, the internal opening will likely be on a radial line directly into the anus.
C. With a cutaneous opening in the right lateral anterior position, the internal opening will likely be in the anterior midline.
D. With a cutaneous opening in the right lateral anterior position, the internal opening will be in the posterior midline.
E. With a cutaneous opening in the right lateral posterior position, the internal opening will likely be on a radial line directly into the anus.

145. Which of the following is true regarding carotid artery stenosis?

A. In cases of symptomatic high-grade carotid artery stenosis, outcomes from medical and surgical therapy are equivalent.
B. Carotid endarterectomy is indicated for asymptomatic 80% stenosis of the left internal carotid artery.
C. The majority of cases are due to fibromuscular hyperplasia.
D. Amaurosis fugax depicts irreversible monocular blindness.
E. All of the above are true.

146. Which of the following statements regarding stress metabolism is true?
A. Endogenous fat stores are poorly utilized.
B. Triglyceride levels fall as turnover of free fatty acids increases.
C. There is a marked elevation in the insulin/glycogen ratio.
D. Glycerol is broken down into ketone bodies for use as peripheral fat.
E. Increased cortisol and catecholamine levels result in increased lipolysis.

147. Without exception, the first aspect of patient assessment is
A. Estimation of burn size
B. Airway patency
C. Breathing ability
D. The presence of circumferential wounds
E. The possibility of abuse as an etiology

148. A complication of cardiopulmonary bypass is
A. Pancreatitis
B. Coagulopathy
C. GI hemorrhage
D. Cerebrovascular accidents
E. All of the above

149. Symptoms of elevated intracranial pressure include all of the following **except**
A. Exophthalmos
B. Headache
C. Nausea
D. Agitation
E. Diplopia

150. The most common type of hernia in women is
A. Femoral hernias
B. Umbilical hernias
C. Indirect inguinal hernias
D. Direct inguinal hernias
E. Hiatal hernias

MATCHING

Match the numbered item with the *best* lettered choice on the right.

_____ 151. Frey's syndrome
_____ 152. Kernohan's notch phenomenon associated with soft tissue sarcomas
_____ 153. Conn's syndrome
_____ 154. Leriche syndrome
_____ 155. Zollinger-Ellison syndrome
_____ 156. Addison's disease
_____ 157. Pancoast's tumor
_____ 158. Duchenne's muscular dystrophy
_____ 159. Marjolin's ulcer
_____ 160. Charcot's triad
_____ 161. Calot's triangle
_____ 162. Li-Fraumeni syndrome
_____ 163. Reynold's pentad
_____ 164. Hesselbach's triangle
_____ 165. Beck's triad
_____ 166. Battle's sign
_____ 167. Grey-Turner sign
_____ 168. Cushing's triad

A. Gastrinoma
B. Breast cancer
C. Pseudohypertrophy of calf muscles, clumsy gait, "Gower's sign"
D. Hypertension, bradycardia, bradypnea
E. Ipsilateral hemiparesis contralateral dilated pupil
F. Cystosarcoma phylloides of the breast
G. Cystic duct, common hepatic duct, inferior border of liver
H. Aberrant regeneration of parasympathetic nerve fibers after parathyroidectomy resulting in "gustatory sweating"
I. Ecchymosis about flank
J. Right upper quadrant pain, fever, jaundice
K. Metaplastic change of distal esophageal mucosa from squamous to columnar epithelia
L. Superior sulcus tumor, ipsilateral shoulder and arm pain; Horner's syndrome
M. Hypertension, low serum potassium, low serum renin
N. Distant heart sounds, jugular venous distention hypotension
O. Hyponatremia, elevated ACTH, low serum cortisol, hyperpigmented palmar creases
P. Right upper quadrant pain, fever, jaundice, hypotension, mental obtundation
Q. Coagulopathy associated with cardiopulmonary bypass
R. Inguinal ligament, epigastric vessels, lateral border of rectus muscle sheath
S. Squamous cell carcinoma arising in chronically inflamed wound
T. Acute lower extremity ischemia secondary to thromboembolic phenomenon
U. Absence of bilateral femoral pulses, thigh and buttock claudication, impotence
V. Progressive muscular atrophy from deinnervation
W. Postauricular ecchymosis

ANSWERS

Multiple Choice

1. C	41. D	85. E
2. C	42. B	86. A
3. B	43. A	87. B
4. A	44. A	88. A
5. E	45. E	89. D
6. B	46. C	90. D
7. C	47. B	91. B
8. E	48. A	92. C
9. B	49. B	93. A
10. A	50. A	94. D
11. D	51. D	95. C
12. C	52. D	96. B
13. A	53. B	97. A
14. C	54. A	98. C
15. B	55. A	99. E
16. A	56. E	100. B
17. D	57. D	101. C
18. B	58. D	102. C
19. D	59. C	103. D
20. A	60. B	104. E
21. B	61. A	105. A
22. C	62. C	106. B
23. E	63. E	107. B
24. A	64. C	108. C
25. E	65. B	109. A
26. D	66. C	110. C
27. C	67. E	111. A
28. E	68. A	112. B
29. B	69. C	113. C
30. D	70. B	114. E
31. C	71. A	115. C
32. A	72. B	116. D
33. E	73. C	117. E
34. C	74. E	118. B
35. B	75. B	119. C
36. B	76. E	120. D
37. D	77. C	121. A
38. B	78. B	122. A
39. C	79. D	123. D
40. C	80. C	124. A
	81. A	125. E
	82. C	126. D
	83. D	127. C
	84. D	128. C

129. D	
130. B	
131. A	
132. C	
133. C	
134. C	
135. D	
136. E	
137. D	
138. B	
139. C	
140. A	
141. A	
142. D	
143. B	
144. A	
145. B	
146. E	
147. B	
148. E	
149. A	
150. C	

Matching

151. H	
152. E	
153. M	
154. U	
155. A	
156. O	
157. L	
158. C	
159. S	
160. J	
161. G	
162. B	
163. P	
164. R	
165. N	
166. W	
167. I	
168. D	

Subject Index

Page numbers followed by *t* and *f* indicate tables and figures, respectively

evaluation of, 296f–298f, 296–299
  for admission criteria, 299, 299t
  for airway patency, 296
  for social issues, 299
fluid resuscitation in, 299f, 299–300
laboratory studies in, 300
minor, 302–303
and nutrition, 301
pathogenesis of, 295
postresuscitation care in, 301–302
rehabilitation after, 302
and sepsis, 302
surgical management of, 302
wound care in, 300–301

C

CABG (coronary artery bypass grafting), 271–272
calcium
  homeostasis of, 216f
  imbalances of, 50–51, 51t
  nutritional significance of, 35
calcium pyrophosphate deposition disease (CPPD), 353
calculi, renal, 373–375
  hyperparathyroidism and, 216
capital femoral epiphysis, slipped, 350
carbohydrates
  digestion of, 133–134
  metabolism of, during stress/sepsis, 32
  oxidation of, 29, 30f
carbon dioxide consumption (VCO2), calculation of, 35
carbonic acid
  homeostasis of, 53f, 53–54, 54t
  loss of, 56
carbuncles, 64, 64f
carcinoembryonic antigen (CEA), and prognosis in colorectal cancer, 159
carcinoid syndrome, 137
carcinoid tumors, of small intestine, 136–137
carcinoma. See under specific type
cardiac. See also entries under heart
cardiac surgery, history of, 265
cardiac tamponade, 276
cardiogenic shock, 311
cardiopulmonary bypass, complications of, 272–273
cardiovascular critical care, 307–311, 308t, 309f
  adrenergic agonists in, 309
  arrhythmia management in, 310
  hemodynamic monitoring in, 308, 308t
  hypertensive emergencies in, 310
  inotropic agents in, 309
  shock in, 310
  stroke volume in, 308–309
carotid artery, rupture of, from radiation therapy, 393
carotid artery stenosis, 239–241, 341
carotid endarterectomy, 240
carpal tunnel syndrome, 353–354
cartilage, properties of, 347
catabolism, of protein, in "flow" phase of injury, 5
catgut sutures, 26

catheters, for vascular access, infections from, 314
caustic substances, esophageal injuries from, 108–109
cavernous hemangioma, hepatic, 168
cavernous malformations, 341
CEA (carcinoembryonic antigen), and prognosis in colorectal cancer, 159
central cord syndrome, 337, 356
central lines, placement of, complications of, 39
central nervous system (CNS)
  developmental anomalies of, 343, 343f
  infections of, 344–346, 345t, 346f
  neoplasms of, 338–339
cerebral abscess, 345
cerebral palsy, 349
cerebrospinal fluid (CSF)
  analysis of, in subarachnoid hemorrhage, 342
  removal of, for elevated intracranial pressure, 333
cerebrovascular accident, from carotid artery stenosis, 239–241, 341
cervical dysplasia, 408, 408t
cervical spine, fractures of, 356
Chandelier sign, 201t
Charcot's triad, 182–183, 201t
Chaussier's sign, 201t
chemical burns, pathogenesis of, 295
chemotherapy
  adjuvant
    for breast cancer, 87
    for colorectal cancer, 159
  for esophageal carcinoma, 114
  for melanoma, 72
  for ovarian cancer, 407
chest, injury to, 283–286, 287f
chest pain, in pericarditis, 276
chest tubes, placement of, 251–252, 252f
chest wall, anatomy of, 251, 251f
child abuse
  fractures from, 352
  neurologic injury from, 338
children, surgery in, 315–329. See also specific disorders
Child's classification, of liver disease, 169, 169t
chloride
  imbalance of, 48–49
  for metabolic alkalosis, 57
chlorprocaine, properties of, 401t
cholangiocarcinoma, 185–186
  with sclerosing cholangitis, 184
cholangiography
  endoscopic retrograde, 179, 179f, 183
  percutaneous transhepatic, 178f, 178–179
cholangitis, 182–183
  sclerosing, 184
cholecystectomy, 181, 181t
  for gallbladder cancer, 185
cholecystitis, 180f, 180–181
  acalculous, 181–182
cholecystography, oral, 178
cholecystostomy, percutaneous, 181
choledochoenterostomy, for biliary

strictures, 183
choledocholithiasis, 182, 182t
cholelithiasis, 179f, 179–180
cholesteatoma, 385
Christmas disease, 13
chylothorax, 253
circulation
  fetal, 265–266, 266f
  postbirth, abnormal, 266–267
circumcision, 316, 316f
cirrhosis, 169, 169t
  and hepatic malignancy, 168
Clark classification, of melanoma, 72f, 72–73, 74t
claudication, intermittent, 230–231
clean-contaminated wounds, 19
clean wounds, 19
clubfoot, 350
CNS. See central nervous system (CNS)
coagulation, 10f, 10t, 10–11
  activation of, 8
  extrinsic vs. intrinsic pathways in, 10
coagulation factors, 10f
  disorders of, 13, 13t
cobalt, nutritional significance of, 34t
coccidioidomycosis, 263
colectomy, 160f
colitis
  ischemic, 155–156
  ulcerative, 151–153, 153f
collagen
  production of, and wound healing, 22–23, 23f
  properties of, 347
Colles fracture, 355, 355f
colloid solutions, for burn patient, 301
colon
  anatomy of, 143–144, 144f
  blood supply to, 144–145, 147f–149f
  Crohn's disease in, 153–154
  digestion in, 145–146
  diverticula of, 154f, 154–155
  lymphatic drainage of, 145, 149f
  physiology of, 145–146
  trauma to, 291–292
  volvulus of, 155
colonoscopy, 150, 151f
colorectal cancer, 158–159, 159t, 160f
colorectal disease, patient evaluation in, 150–151
colorectal polyps, 156, 158, 158t
colposcopy, 409
compartment syndrome, 294, 355
complement, activation of, 6–8, 7f
compressive neuropathy, 353–354
computed tomography (CT)
  in abdominal aortic aneurysm, 235f
  in acute abdomen, 202
  in acute pancreatitis, 192–193
  in arterial disease, 229
  in blunt abdominal trauma, 289, 289f
  in central nervous system neoplasms, 339
  of gallbladder, 178
  in neurologic disease, 331
  in pancreatic carcinoma, 195
  in pulmonary nodules, 257